Comprehensive Periodontics
for the Dental Hygienist

Second Edition

Mea A. Weinberg, D.M.D., M.S.D., R.Ph.

Cheryl Westphal, R.D.H., M.S.

Stuart J. Froum, D.D.S.

Milton Palat, D.D.S., J.D.
New York University College of Dentistry

Consulting Editor
James Burke Fine, D.M.D.
School of Dental and Oral Surgery
of Columbia University
Presbyterian Hospital Dental Service
New York, New York

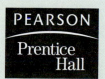
PEARSON
Prentice
Hall

Upper Saddle River, New Jersey 07458

Library of Congress Cataloging-in-Publication Data

Comprehensive periodontics for the dental hygienist / [edited by] Mea A. Weinberg ... [et al.].— 2nd ed.
  p. ; cm.
  Includes bibliographical references and index.
  ISBN 0-13-153467-X
  1. Periodontics. 2. Dental hygiene.
  [DNLM: 1. Periodontal Diseases—diagnosis. 2. Periodontal Diseases—therapy.] I. Weinberg, Mea A.

  RK361.C58 2006
  617.6'32—dc22

2004030501

Notice:
The authors and the publisher of this volume have taken care that the information and technical recommendations contained herein are based on research and expert consultation, and are accurate and compatible with the standards generally accepted at the time of publication. Nevertheless, as new information becomes available, changes in clinical and technical practices become necessary. The reader is advised to carefully consult manufacturers' instructions and information material for all supplies and equipment before use, and to consult with a health care professional as necessary. This advice is especially important when using new supplies or equipment for clinical purposes. The authors and publisher disclaim all responsibility for any liability, loss, injury, or damage incurred as a consequence, directly or indirectly, of the use and application of any of the contents of this volume.

Publisher: Julie Levin Alexander
Assistant to Publisher: Regina Bruno
Executive Editor: Mark Cohen
Associate Editor: Melissa Kerian
Editorial Assistant: Jaquay Felix
Media Editor: John J. Jordan
Director of Production and Manufacturing: Bruce Johnson
Managing Production Editor: Patrick Walsh
Production Liaison: Christina Zingone
Production Editor: Jessica Balch, Pine Tree Composition
Manufacturing Manager: Ilene Sanford

Manufacturing Buyer: Pat Brown
Design Director: Cheryl Asherman
Design Coordinator: Christopher Weigand
Cover Designer: Christopher Weigand
Director of Marketing: Karen Allman
Channel Marketing Manager: Rachele Strober
Manager of Media Production: Amy Peltier
Media Production: Tina Rudowski
Composition: Pine Tree Composition, Inc.
Printer/Binder: Courier Westford
Cover Printer: Phoenix Color Corporation

Cover image reprinted with perimission. © Dr. Michael Iott & Associates, New York, NY.

Pearson Education Ltd., *London*
Pearson Education Australia Pty. Limited, *Sydney*
Pearson Education Singapore, Pte. Ltd.
Pearson Education North Asia Ltd., *Hong Kong*
Pearson Education Canada, Ltd., *Toronto*

Pearson Educación de Mexico, S.A. de C.V.
Pearson Education—Japan, *Tokyo*
Pearson Education Malaysia, Pte. Ltd.
Pearson Education, Upper Saddle River, New Jersey

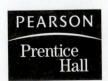

10 9 8 7 6 5
ISBN 0-13-153467-X

Contents

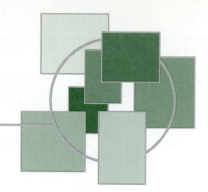

Appendices   561

Case Studies   575

Foreword

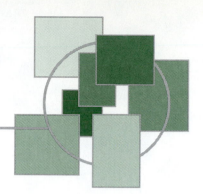

In the increasingly complicated world of periodontics, it is important that the fundamental principles of therapy and pathogenesis remain the unifying theme of any text on the subject. This text, anchored in evidence-based learning, offers these fundamental principles with concise definitions, precise objectives, and helpful lists not only of key words but also of key points. It simplifies many of the complexities of the disease process without confusing them and provides clear links back to practical aspects of therapy.

Importantly, while basic biologic principles unify the text, timely discussions of implant care, medically compromised patients, and chemotherapeutics add a high degree of relevance. Indeed, at the dawn of the new millennium, it is critical to prepare clinicians for the inevitable advances in chemotherapy and diagnostics that will be the hallmark of clinical management of periodontal diseases in the future.

The reader is urged to take full advantage of the many learning tools incorporated into this text. These tools include frequent references, definitions, key words, key points, and self-quiz questions. When more details are required than are possible in a book of this type, the reader is urged to consult the references. Hopefully, on completion of this text the reader will fully understand the evidence-based nature of periodontal diseases and their many modes of treatment. Moreover, it is the purpose of this book to be both clear and concise, and it is expected that readers will be able to use similar clear explanations of therapy and etiology when discussing periodontal problems with both patients and colleagues. This clarity of thought will inspire readers to seek further illumination of the topics through the biomedical literature, consultation with learned faculty, and a zest for lifelong learning.

Dean Michael C. Alfano, D.M.D., Ph.D.
Professor and Dean, College of Dentistry
New York University

Preface

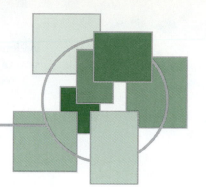

There is a significant body of knowledge about the risk factors, pathogenesis, treatment, and prevention of periodontal diseases. This knowledge is rarely applied as an evidence-based approach to the difficult problem of deciding when specific treatments or examination methods are appropriate. Classic and current references are included in each chapter, along with applicable Web sites so the reader can supplement information in the textbook with information from other sources.

This basic text has been written in an attempt to make the professions' understanding of periodontal diseases accessible to the dental hygiene student, the practicing dental hygienist, and the dentist needing to update their knowledge through a concise synopsis of clinical periodontics.

Part I deals with the anatomy of the periodontium, risk factors (e.g., dental biofilms, smoking, and diabetes mellitus) for periodontal diseases, and periodontal disease as a risk factor for systemic conditions (the periodontal/medicine relationship) such as stroke, cardiovascular disease, emphysema, and premature low-birth-weight babies. This inter-relationship between medicine and periodontology has opened new insights into the concept of oral health being an integral part of the overall general and systemic health of an individual.

Part II discusses in detail the 1999 Classification System of the Periodontal Diseases (American Academy of Periodontology).

Part III deals with the clinical assessment phase of the dental hygiene process of care. This part discusses the various assessment tools that are required to be performed on a patient for the development of a dental hygiene diagnosis.

Part IV discusses the treatment planning, implementation, and evaluation process of dental hygiene care. Nonsurgical and surgical therapy through problem-based learning (PBL) are discussed in detail. A problem-based system with basic concepts of treatment planning will be introduced to the student. A comprehensive review of halitosis is presented. In this section is an extensive review of drugs used in periodontal therapy including various controlled-release drug devices (e.g., Peri-oChip™, Atridox®, Arestin®) and enzyme suppression drugs (e.g., Periostat™). The appendices include the Health Insurance Portability and Accountability Act (HIPAA), a comprehensive listing of periodontic informatics, and how to critically assess the periodontal literature Following Chapter 31 are four problem-oriented,

ix

evidence-based case studies. Each case details the problem, followed by a discussion of the questions and answers to the problem.

We hope this book will serve as a helpful text for all dental practitioners.

Mea A. Weinberg, D.M.D., M.S.D., R.Ph.
Cheryl Westphal, R.D.H., M.S.
Stuart J. Froum, D.D.S.
Milton Palat, D.D.S., J.D.
James Burke Fine, D.M.D.

Contributors

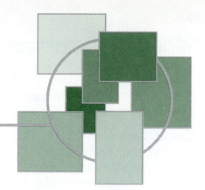

Mary Elizabeth Aichelmann-Reidy, D.D.S.
Assistant Professor
Department of Periodontics
University of Maryland
Baltimore, Maryland

Khalid Almas, B.D.S., M.Sc.
Associate Professor
Department of Periodontics
Division of Diagnostics, Infectious Diseases
  and Health Promotion
New York University College of Dentistry
New York, New York

Denise Estafan, D.D.S, M.S.
Associate Professor
Director of Clinical Esthetics
Division of Reconstructive and Comprehensive Care
New York University College of Dentistry
New York, New York

James Burke Fine, D.M.D
Associate Dean of Postgraduate Studies
Associate Professor of Clinical Dentistry
Director of Postgraduate Periodontics
Columbia University School of Dental
and Oral Surgery
New York, New York

Suzanne K. Farrar, B.S., R.D.H., H.C.M.
Clinical Instructor
Department of Periodontics
Louisiana State University School of Dentistry
New Orleans, Louisiana

Cynthia Fong, R.D.H., M.S.
Lecturer/Instructor in Periodontics
Department of Dental Hygiene
Pierce College
Tacoma, Washington

Herbert Frommer, D.D.S.
Professor
Director of Radiology
New York University College of Dentistry
New York, New York

Stuart J. Froum, D.D.S.
Clinical Professor, Director of Research
Department of Implantology
Department of Periodontics
Division of Diagnostics, Infectious Diseases
  and Health Promotion
New York University College of Dentistry
New York, New York

Diana L. Mercado Galvis, D.D.S., R.D.H., M.S.
Clinical Associate Professor
New York University College of Dentistry
New York, New York

Ann M. Goodwin, R.D.H., M.S.
Former Clinical Associate Professor
Dental Hygiene Program
New York University College of Dentistry
New York, New York

Rosemary DeRosa Hays, R.D.H., M.S.
Clinical Associate Professor
Dental Hygiene Program
New York University College of Dentistry
New York, New York

Judith Kreismann, R.D.H., B.S., M.S.
Clinical Associate Professor
Dental Hygiene Program
New York University College of Dentistry
New York, New York

Eva M. Lupovici, R.D.H., M.S.
Clinical Associate Professor
Dental Hygiene Program
New York University College of Dentistry
New York, New York

John D. Mason, B.A., D.D.S.
Assistant Professor
Department of Periodontics
Louisiana State University School of Dentistry
New Orleans, Louisiana

Trisha E. O'Hehir, R.D.H., B.S.
Editor of *Perio Reports*
Senior Consulting Editor, RHD Magazine
Vice President, Perio-Data™ Company
Assistant Visiting Professor
Northern Arizona University
Flagstaff, Arizona

Jill Rethman, R.D.H., B.A.
Visiting Clinical Instructor
School of Dental Medicine, Department of Dental
 Hygiene
University of Pittsburgh
Pittsburgh, Pennsylvania

Michael P. Rethman, D.D.S., M.S.
Past President of the American Academy
 of Periodontology
Former Chief of Periodontics
Tripler Medical Center
Honolulu, Hawaii

Robert S. Schoor, D.D.S.
Past President of the American Academy
 of Periodontology
Associate Professor
Director of Postgraduate Periodontics
Department of Periodontics
Division of Diagnostics, Infectious Diseases
 and Health Promotion
New York University College of Dentistry
New York, New York

Surendra Singh, D.D.S., M.S.
Professor
Department of Periodontics
University of Medicine and Dentistry of New Jersey
 School of Dentistry
Newark, New Jersey

Jeanne St. Germain, B.S., R.D.H.
Clinical Instructor
Department of Periodontics
Louisiana State University School of Dentistry
New Orleans, Louisiana

Mea A. Weinberg, D.M.D., M.S.D., R.Ph.
Clinical Associate Professor
Director of Second Year Periodontics
Department of Periodontics
Division of Diagnostics, Infectious Diseases
 and Health Promotion
New York University College of Dentistry
New York, New York

Cheryl Westphal, R.D.H., M.S.
Clinical Associate Professor
Assistant Dean for Allied Health Programs
Director, Dental Hygiene Program
New York University College of Dentistry
New York, New York

Raymond A. Yukna, D.M.D., M.S.
Professor, Coordinator Postgraduate Periodontics
Louisiana State University School of Dentistry
New Orleans, Louisiana

Selected Illustrations by Jesse Doscher, D.D.S.

Reviewers

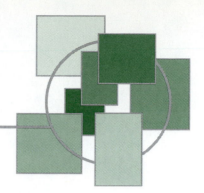

Barbara C. Bush, R.D.H., M.S.Ed.
Associate Professor
Department of Allied Health
Western Kentucky University
Bowling Green, Kentucky

Susan T. Clarke, R.D.H., B.S., M.Ed.
Assistant Professor of Dental Hygiene
Georgia Perimeter College
Dunwoody, Georgia

Alice S. Derouen, R.D.H., M.Ed.
Chair of Dental Sciences Department
Director of Dental Hygiene Program
Horry-Georgetown Technical College
Conway, South Carolina

Joan G. Ellison, R.D.H., M.S.
Instructor in Dental Hygiene
Harrisburg Area Community College
Harrisburg, Pennsylvania

Lisa Fleck, R.D.H., M.S.
Assistant Professor
Department of Dental Hygiene
Minnesota State University
Mankate, Minnesota

Nancy L. Foster, Ed.M.
Professor of Dental Health
University of Maine at Augusta
Bangor, Maine

Deborah A. Graeff, R.D.H., M.S.
Associate Professor
Erie Community College
Williamsville, New York

Leslie Hills, R.D.H., M.Ed.
Lecturer
University of Vermont
Burlington, Vermont

Mary Johnson, R.D.H., M.S.
Professor of Dental Hygiene
Clark College
Vancouver, Washington

Laura L. Justice, R.D.H., M.S.Ed.
Associate Professor of Dental Hygiene
Lexington Community College
Lexington, Kentucky

Merry LeBlond, R.D.H., M.S.
Former Chairperson
Adjunct Instructor
Middlesex County College
Edison, New Jersey

Joanne Weir, B.S.D.H., M.P.S.
Assistant Professor
Georgia Perimeter College
Dunwoody, Georgia

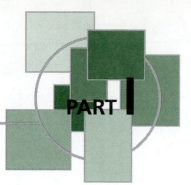

PART I

The Periodontal Diseases: Introduction and Background

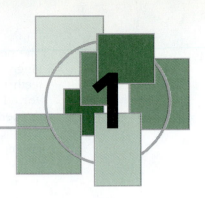

Anatomy of the Periodontal Structures: The Healthy State

Mea A. Weinberg, D.M.D., M.S.D., R.Ph.

Outline

- Clinical Anatomy of the Gingival Unit
- Microscopic Anatomy of the Gingival Unit
- Attachment Apparatus
- Physiology of the Periodontium
- Changes with Aging
- Summary
- Key Points
- Web Sites
- Self-Quiz
- References

Goal

To provide knowledge of the structures and functions of the periodontium in health.

Educational Objectives

Upon completion of this chapter, the dental hygiene student should be able to:

- Illustrate and discuss the clinical anatomy of the periodontium.
- Illustrate and describe the microscopic anatomy of the periodontium.
- List and describe the functions of the periodontium.
- Discuss the importance of the dentogingival unit.
- Describe the lymphatic, blood, and nerve supply to the gingiva and the attachment apparatus.

KEY WORDS

- periodontium
- attachment apparatus
- connective tissue attachment
- dentogingival unit
- biologic width

The periodontium, translated in Latin to mean "around the tooth," consists of the gingiva, periodontal ligament, cementum, and alveolar and supporting bone of the teeth (Fig. 1–1a■). The attachment apparatus consists of periodontal tissues involved in the attachment and support of the root in the tooth socket, specifically the periodontal ligament, cementum, and alveolar bone (Hassell, 1993). A working knowledge of the ultrastructural anatomy and biology of the periodontal tissues is an important prerequisite for practitioners to recognize and treat periodontal diseases.

In order to understand the different stages of diseases in the periodontium, it is necessary to recognize the structures and functions of the periodontium in health. This chapter describes the clinical and microscopic features of the periodontium in health and will be the foundation for ensuing discussions in this text.

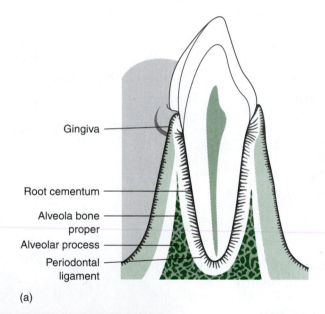

(a)

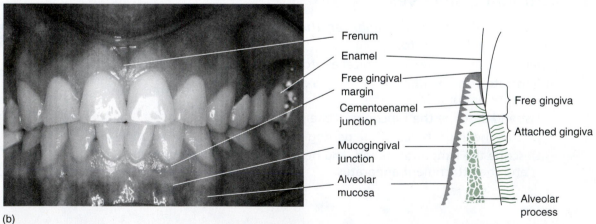

(b)

Figure 1–1   (a) Schematic drawing of a tooth with its periodontium. (b) Landmarks of the gingival unit. (*Left*) The gingiva is salmon pink, while the alveolar mucosa is thinner and redder in color. (*Right*) Schematic drawing of a cross-section of the periodontium. (Adapted from J. Lindhe and T. Karring, Anatomy of the periodontium, in *Clinical periodontology and implant dentistry,* ed. J. Lindhe. Copenhagen: Munksgaard, © 2003.)

Clinical Anatomy of the Gingival Unit

The oral mucosa is divided into three types: (1) masticatory mucosa, which includes the gingiva and hard palate; (2) lining mucosa, which consists of the alveolar mucosa, soft palate, lining of lips, cheeks, and sublingual area; and (3) specialized mucosa, which is found on the dorsum of the tongue.

Masticatory Mucosa (Gingiva)

The gingiva forms a protective covering over the other components of the periodontium and is well adapted to protect against mechanical insults (e.g., toothbrushing and chewing). The gingiva encircles the cervical portion of the teeth and covers the alveolar process. Anatomically, the gingiva is subdivided into the free gingiva, attached gingiva, and interdental gingiva or papilla (Fig. 1–1b■). The outer surface of the gingiva consists of stratified squamous epithelium. Underneath the epithelium is gingival connective tissue, which is termed the lamina propria.

Free Gingiva (Marginal Gingiva)

The free gingiva or marginal gingiva surrounds the neck of the tooth. Its boundaries are coronally, the free gingival margin; apically, the free gingival groove; and laterally, the gingival crevice and the tooth (see Fig. 1–1b). The free gingiva is approximately 1.5 mm wide and has a smooth surface. The free gingiva lies on and adapts to the enamel and can be separated from the tooth with a periodontal instrument (Schroeder & Listgarten, 1997).

The free gingival margin is the edge or the most coronal part of the free gingiva and in a fully erupted tooth is located on the enamel approximately 0.5 to 2 mm coronal to the cementoenamel junction (CEJ). In the anterior region, the free gingival margin usually has a scalloped outline following the contour of the cementoenamel junction (see Fig. 1–1b). In the posterior region the architecture becomes less scalloped. Prior to the completed eruption of permanent teeth in children, the free gingival margin usually remains located on the cervical bulge of the enamel. This is a normal situation and as the tooth erupts the free gingival margin will ultimately move apically.

Gingival Crevice   The gingival crevice is the space between the free gingiva and the tooth surface and is lined by nonkeratinized stratified squamous epithelium. In gingival health the gingival crevice is termed a sulcus; once inflamed it is termed a pocket. Healthy gingiva sulcular depth is approximately 1 to 3 mm when measured with a periodontal probe. Only in experimental conditions with germ-free animals can the sulcular depth be zero.

Gingival crevicular fluid (GCF) fills the sulcus and originates from blood vessels within the underlying connective tissue (lamina propria) and flows through the tissue into the gingival crevice. The rate of passage of this fluid is dependent upon the absence or presence of inflammation in the connective tissue of the gingiva. The flow is minimal to absent in health, but increases due to inflammation from accumulation of plaque in the gingival crevice (Alfano, 1974). Components of GCF resemble blood serum components and include elements such as calcium, sodium, potassium, and phosphorous, along with cells and bacteria. The role of GCF is both protective and destructive. While crevicular fluid flow cleanses the sulcus, it is also a source of nutrients for subgingival bacteria and supports subgingival calculus formation (Mukherjee, 1985). Certain antibiotics including tetracyclines used in the treatment of periodontal diseases have been found to concentrate in higher levels locally in the GCF (pocket area) than in the serum (Gordon, Walker, Murphy, Goodson, & Socransky, 1981).

Free Gingival Groove   The free gingival groove, a shallow depression on the outer surface of the gingiva, is about 1 to 2 mm apical from the margin of the gingiva and corresponds approximately to the level of the cementoenamel junction. This groove separates the free gingiva from the attached gingiva. The free gingival groove is present in about 30 to 40% of adults and occurs most frequently in the mandibular premolar and incisor areas. It is more pronounced on the facial than on the lingual regions. Its absence or presence is not related to the health of the gingiva.

Attached Gingiva

The attached gingiva is continuous with the free gingiva and is firmly attached to the underlying cementum and periosteum (connective tissue) covering the alveolar process. It extends apically from the free gingival groove to the mucogingival junction (MGJ). The mucogingival junction joins the attached gingiva to the alveolar mucosa (see Fig. 1–1b) except on the palate because the attached gingiva runs into the palatal mucosa. The width of the free gingiva and the attached gingiva consists of the total width of gingiva.

Attached gingiva is not movable, being bound down to the tooth and bone, making it capable of withstanding forces from toothbrushing and chewing. The width of the attached gingiva varies in different areas of the mouth and between individuals (Fig. 1–2■). On the facial aspect, the attached gingiva is widest in the incisor region and narrowest in the first premolar area. On the lingual aspect, the attached gingiva is widest in the molar region and narrowest in the incisor region.

The color of the gingiva is normally salmon pink with slight variations. The gingiva shows varying degrees of brownish-black color depending on ethnic variation (Fig. 1–3■), which is considered to be normal gingival coloring and is referred to as melanin pigmentation.

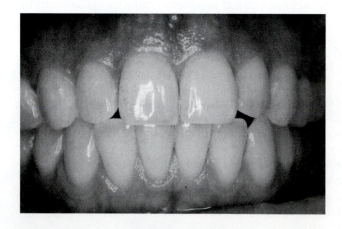

Figure 1–2 Varying amounts of attached gingiva; the narrowest width is on the mandibular premolars and the widest is on the maxillary incisors.

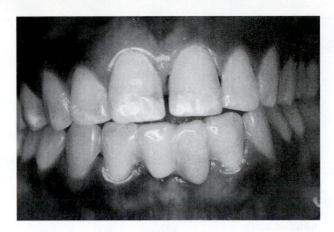

Figure 1–3
Physiological gingival pigmentation in a 30-year-old patient from India.

Stippling   Clinically, the outer surface of the attached gingiva has an appearance similar to an orange peel with shallow depressions between elevations. The free gingiva has a smooth surface and is not stippled (Fig. 1–4■). A histologic description of stippling is discussed in the following section.

Stippling may be present in health or disease. The absence of stippling does not necessarily indicate the presence of disease. On the other hand, the presence of inflammation with the loss of stippling can be considered part of the disease process, assuming stippling was present initially.

Stippling is present in only about 40% of adults and varies in different individuals, ages, and sexes. Stippling of the attached gingiva is absent in children under 5 years of age and may be more evident in men than women. It is more prominent in the anterior than the posterior region and may even be absent in the molar areas. The facial gingiva shows more prominent stippling than the lingual.

Interdental Gingiva (Interdental Papilla)

In health the interdental gingiva tightly fills the gingival embrasure, which is the space between the contact point and alveolar bone of two adjacent teeth. The margin and lateral borders of the interdental gingiva are an extension of the free gingiva, whereas the remaining parts are attached gingiva (Fig. 1–5a■).

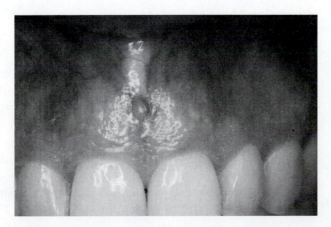

Figure 1–4   Surface stippling of the attached gingiva and the interdental gingiva. Note the dimpling or depressions on the surface. The surface of the free gingiva is not stippled.

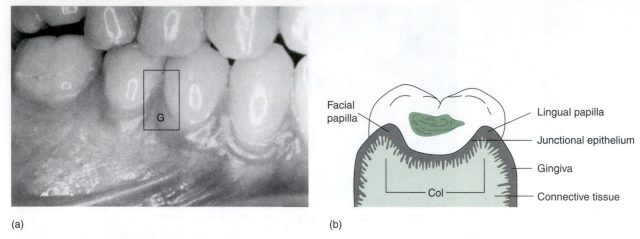

(a)   (b)

Figure 1–5   Features of the interdental gingiva. (a) In health the interdental gingiva fills the gingival embrasure (G). (b) The col is directly under the contact point of the teeth. (From P. F. Fedi, Jr., and A. R. Vernino, *The Periodontic Syllabus.* Copyright © 2000 by Lippincott Williams & Wilkins.)

The size and shape of the papillae are determined by tooth-to-tooth contact, the curvature of the cementoenamel junction, and the width (faciolingually) of the interproximal tooth surfaces. When teeth are crowded, as often seen in mandibular incisors, the papillae may be slender and narrow. Anterior papillae are pyramidal in shape while posterior papillae are rounder and slightly flatter. An anterior papilla forms a single pyramidal structure because there is only one papilla. The papillae of posterior teeth (premolars and molars) are wedge shaped, with one vestibular (facial) and one oral (lingual) papilla connected by a concave area called the col (Fig. 1–5b■). The col is directly apical to the contact point, representing the fusion of the interproximal junctional epithelia of two adjacent teeth. While an anterior papilla can form a col shape, it is more prominent in posterior papillae. When a diastema (loss of contact between two adjacent teeth) is present the interdental papilla is absent and there is no col. Since the shape of a col is concave and may not be keratinized, it may predispose the interproximal area to the accumulation of dental plaque.

Lining Mucosa

Alveolar Mucosa

Although not actually part of the periodontium, the alveolar mucosa is an important periodontal structure and deserves discussion. The alveolar mucosa extends apically from the mucogingival junction to the mucous membrane of the cheek, lip, and floor of the mouth (see Fig. 1–1b). In comparison to the attached gingiva, alveolar mucosa is thinner and redder in color, has a smooth surface, is movable, and not keratinized.

Frenum Attachments

Frenum (pleural: frena) attachments are folds of alveolar mucosa. They are not concentrations of muscle, having no more muscle fibers than alveolar mucosa. The function of a frenum is to attach lips and cheeks to the maxillary and mandibular mucosa and to limit the movement of the lips and cheeks. There are usually seven frena located in the canine/premolar area, between the central incisors and in the mandibular anterior lingual area. A frenum should originate and end in alveolar mucosa near the mucogingival junction.

Specialized Mucosa

The mucosa of the dorsum of the tongue contains numerous papillae of three types: filiform, fungiform, and circumvallate. The circumvallate papillae are located along the V-shaped groove on the back of the tongue. Each papilla is surrounded by a circular groove. The taste buds are located mainly on the sides of these papillae. The filiform papillae are slender ones and the most abundant, covering the entire top or dorsal surface of the tongue. No taste buds are associated with these papillae; they respond only to heat and mechanical stimuli. The fungiform papillae, which are broad and flat, are found chiefly at the edges of the tongue and are provided with taste buds.

Microscopic Anatomy of the Gingival Unit

Gingival Epithelium

The gingiva is covered by a layer of stratified squamous epithelium with an underlying core of connective tissue called the lamina propria (Fig. 1–6■). The gingival epithelium exists as structurally different forms specific to certain areas of the teeth. Thus, the gingival epithelium can be divided into (Fig. 1–7■):

- the oral epithelium (OE);
- the sulcular or crevicular epithelium (SE); and
- the junctional epithelium (JE).

The gingival epithelium is avascular and relies upon the underlying lamina propria for its blood supply and nutrients. The epithelium found in the oral cavity consists of several layers of cells (see Fig. 1–7):

1. stratum basale or stratum germinativum (basal cell layer); deepest layer next to the lamina propria;
2. stratum spinosum (prickle or spinous cell layer);
3. stratum granulosum (granular layer); and
4. the stratum corneum (keratinized/cornified cell layer; also called the superficial cell layer); this outermost layer serves as a barrier membrane protecting the underlying periodontal tissues from invasion by foreign substances.

Cell Renewal

Just like the epithelium of the skin, the gingival epithelium is also subject to considerable insult and thus must have a means of regular renewal. The epithelium achieves this renewal by producing a pool of cells that migrate from the basal

Figure 1–6
Photomicrograph of the gingival epithelium. (Courtesy of Dr. Harvey Wishe, New York University College of Dentistry)

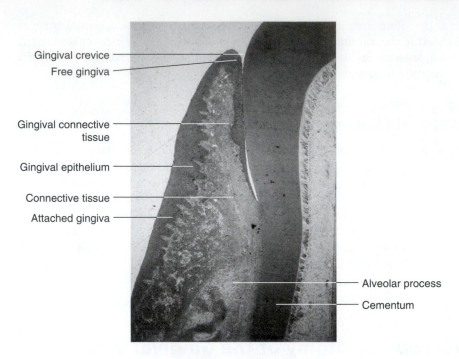

Gingival crevice
Free gingiva
Gingival connective tissue
Gingival epithelium
Connective tissue
Attached gingiva
Alveolar process
Cementum

layer to the oral environment. This process by which epithelial cells differentiate or mature is called keratinization. The type of differentiation reflects the functional demands or stimulus placed on the tissue. During keratinization, the entire thickness of the epithelium is replaced. The time it takes for this replacement or cell renewal is called the turnover time. This time differs with the various types of epithelium. Such differences become important during tissue healing after periodontal surgery or tissue damage.

The keratinization process occurs as follows (Moss-Salentijn & Hendricks-Klyvert, 1990):

- Basal cells in the basal cell layer divide and produce new cells.
- The "older" basal cells travel or move into the next layer, the spinous cell layer, on their way to the most outer epithelial cell layer.
- Once in the spinous cell layer, the basal cells becomes keratinocytes. On their way to the outer surface, the keratinocytes synthesize or produce keratin.
- Keratin is a protein that contributes to the mechanical toughness of the outer surface of the epithelium.
- When the keratinocytes reach the outer epithelial surface, they are shed from the surface into the oral cavity.

Three grades of keratinization or maturation are identified according to the completeness of the transition of the keratinocyte from the basal cell layer to the outermost, superficial cell layer. Consequently, epithelium can be keratinized, parakeratinized, or nonkeratinized. Keratinized epithelium is composed of all four layers and is primarily seen in the skin. Fully keratinized cells form keratin and lose their nuclei by the time they migrate to the outer surface. Parakeratinized

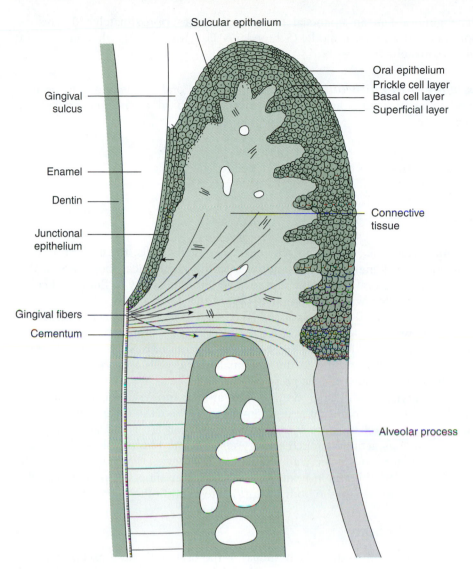

Sulcular epithelium

Oral epithelium
Prickle cell layer
Basal cell layer
Superficial layer

Gingival
sulcus

Enamel

Dentin

Junctional
epithelium

Connective
tissue

Gingival fibers
Cementum

Alveolar process

Figure 1–7   Diagram of the layers of the gingival epithelium. Underlying the epithelium is the gingival connective tissue (lamina propria).

cells, which are found in the mouth in areas such as the gingival oral epithelium, retain their nuclei but show some signs of being keratinized. The stratum granulosum is usually difficult to recognize and a surface parakeratinized outer layer is present. Epithelial cells found in the junctional epithelium and alveolar mucosas are nonkeratinized and do not undergo keratinization.

Oral Epithelium

The oral epithelium faces the oral cavity on the outer surface of the free and attached gingivae extending from the free gingival margin to the mucogingival junction. The gingiva is usually composed of parakeratinized stratified squamous epithelium.

The gingiva has an epithelial turnover time of approximately 10 days as demonstrated in an animal model (Schroeder & Listgarten 1997), while in the skin it is approximately 28 days.

Cells in the Oral Epithelium The function of the oral epithelium is to protect the underlying structures and acts as a mechanical barrier. The oral epithelium contains cells:

- keratinocytes
- nonkeratinocytes (also called clear cells)
- melanocytes
- Langerhans cells
- Merkel cells

Keratinocytes make up the majority of oral epithelial cells. Keratinocytes function to synthesize keratin, which contributes to the mechanical toughness of the outer surface of the oral epithelium and relative impermeability to fluids and cells. It is also responsible for the salmon pink color of the gingiva.

Melanocytes located in the basal cell layer secrete melanin, which is responsible for the brownish pigmentation in the gingiva. Pigmentation is more prominent in darker-skinned individuals (see Fig. 1–3). The amount of pigmentation is genetically predetermined according to the potential of the cells to produce melanin, rather than to the number of cells present.

Other cell types in the gingival epithelium are the Langerhans cells, which are located in the stratum spinosum and are involved in the early defense mechanism of the gingiva. Merkel cells are found in the basal cell layer and are associated with nerve endings acting as touch-sensory cells. White blood cells such as lymphocytes and neutrophils or polymorphonuclear leukocytes (PMNs) are transiently found in the epithelial layers in health but increase in numbers in periodontal disease, functioning to defend the body against bacteria and other invaders.

Sulcular Epithelium

The sulcular epithelum is structurally similar to the oral epithelium except that it is less keratinized. The sulcular epithelium exhibits good resistance to mechanical forces and is relatively impermeable (resistant) to the flow of fluids and cells. The sulcular epithelium has epithelial ridges as does the oral epithelium. Sulcular or crevicular epithelium lines the gingival sulcus without being attached to the tooth surface. It is generally nonkeratinized and thin but can become parakeratinized if given the appropriate stimulus. The sulcular epithelium exhibits two or three cell layers but a definitive and continuous cornified layer is absent. At the free gingival margin, the sulcular epithelium is continuous with the oral epithelium. Apically, it overlaps the coronal surface of the junctional epithelium (see Fig. 1–7).

Junctional Epithelium

The junctional epithelium is the epithelial part of the free gingiva not visible to the oral cavity. It provides the contact between the gingiva and the tooth. The junctional epithelium can be regarded as a downgrowth of the squamous epithelium of the gingiva and is continuous with the sulcular epithelium, extending from the bottom of the crevice to the cementoenamel junction. It forms a collar around the neck of the tooth on the cervical part of the enamel.

The junctional epithelium is composed of nonkeratinized stratified squamous epithelium. It is composed of only two epithelial layers, either an active basal cell layer and an inactive suprabasal cell layer or a basal cell and spinous cell layer (Hassell, 1993; Schroeder & Listgarten, 1997).

The junctional epithelium, through the epithelial attachment, contributes to the direct attachment of the gingiva to the tooth surface and thus serves a significant role in periodontal health and disease when this attachment to the tooth is lost.

At the coronal portion, the thickness of the junctional epithelium is about fifteen to thirty cells, while apically, near the cementoenamel junction, there may be only one to two cells (see Fig. 1–7). Interproximally, the junctional epithelium of adjacent teeth fuses coronally to form the lining of the col area (Schroeder & Listgarten, 1997).

Semipermeable Membrane   The junctional epithelium is more permeable than the oral or sulcular epithelium. Thus, the junctional epithelium is referred to as a semipermeable membrane allowing the movement of bacterial products, fluids, and cells of certain sizes (Kornman, Page, & Tonetti, 1997). There are fewer intercellular junctions and thus wider spaces between the cells than in the oral or sulcular epithelium, and the cells are arranged in a parallel fashion. This allows for easy passage of cells and tissue fluid from the lamina propria into the sulcus and for passage of bacteria and its by-products from the gingival sulcus into the lamina propria. It is also more permeable because the cells do not keratinize. The coronal part of the junctional epithelium that is closest to the bottom of the sulcus is the most permeable part, while the apical part is where cell division for tissue renewal occurs.

Cells in the Junctional Epithelium   In addition to keratinocytes, the junctional epithelium may contain clear cells. In health, small numbers of PMNs are transiently seen in the junctional epithelium (Tonetti, Imboden, Gerber, & Lang, 1995). They will usually pass through the junctional epithelium into the gingival sulcus, where they play a role in the defense of the host (body) against bacteria and other microorganisms.

Cellular Turnover   A unique characteristic of the junctional epithelium is its high rate of cellular turnover. As demonstrated in an animal model, the cells of the junctional epithelium undergo constant turnover every 4 to 7 days, whereby the basal cells migrate coronally out through the sulcus where the old cells are shed into the oral cavity.

Alveolar Mucosa

Alveolar mucosa is compressible and movable due to the presence of a submucosa between the thin lamina propria and the underlying tissue, usually muscle. The presence of elastic fibers, and an underlying loose connective tissue that is attached to the underlying periosteum of the alveolar process, also allows for movement.

The epithelium of the alveolar mucosa has about the same thickness as that of the gingiva, but its structure is completely different (Schroeder, 1991; Schroeder & Listgarten, 1997). A granular layer is not present and the superficial layer does not histologically stain, as does the surface of parakeratinized epithelium (Squier & Hill, 1998). The epithelium contains melanocytes, Langerhans cells, Merkel cells, and small lymphocytes.

Epithelial ridges are usually not present or if present they are indistinct because they are shorter and wider than in the gingiva, giving a smoother surface texture. The color is darker red than the gingiva because of its highly vascular underlying connective tissue. The point where there is a marked increase in elastic fibers within the underlying connective tissue demarcates the mucogingival junction.

Gingival Connective Tissue

Underlying the stratified squamous epithelium and encircling the tooth is the gingival connective tissue or lamina propria.

Connective Tissue/Epithelium Interface

The interface between the connective tissue and oral epithelium is through connecting epithelial ridges that extend into the connective tissue (Fig. 1–8■). At the intersection of epithelial ridges are pits or depressions that contain connective tissue extensions called connective tissue papillae. Clinically these depressions may be evident on the surface of the gingiva, creating a stippled appearance. Stippling is established at the areas of fusion between adjacent epithelial ridges. In periodontal health the epithelial ridges are absent from the junctional epithelium and are not well developed in the sulcular epithelium. The main purposes of stippling are to aid in the increased strength between the epithelium and connective tissue and to enable the epithelium to obtain its blood supply from the connective tissue papillae in the shortest distance possible.

Gingival Connective Tissue

The main component of the gingival connective tissue, as with all connective tissue, is collagen fibers, accounting for about 60% of the total volume. Collagen is a protein composed of amino acids. There are many different types of collagen, with Types I and III primarily found in most connective tissues. Type I collagen fibers give the gingiva its firmness and resiliency. The lamina propria provides mechanical support and nutrients for the avascular epithelium. The remainder of gingival connective tissue consists of ground substance, which is composed of proteins termed proteoglycans, in which the collagen fibers, cells, nerves, and blood vessels are embedded. Proteoglycans have a protein core with carbohydrate side chains (glycosaminoglycans) of chondroitin sulphate, heparin sulphate, and hyaluronic acid. The ground substance also allows for the transportation of water and nutrients through the tissue.

Gingival Fibers   The free and attached gingivae are attached to the tooth surface through a connective tissue attachment. Collagen fibers in the gingiva are arranged in such a way that they maintain the gingiva against the tooth and bone. The collagen fibers are organized in bundles or groups according to their origin and insertion (Schroeder & Listgarten, 1997). The collagen fibers embedded on one end in the cementum are termed Sharpey's fibers (Goldman, 1951). Collectively the gingival fiber bundles are called the gingival fibers, the supracrestal fiber apparatus (because they are located coronal to the crest of alveolar bone), or the gingival connective tissue attachment. These three terms will be used interchangeably throughout the text. Table 1–1■ reviews the primary collagen fiber groups in the gingiva (Fig. 1–9■), including the circular, dentogingival, dentoperiosteal,

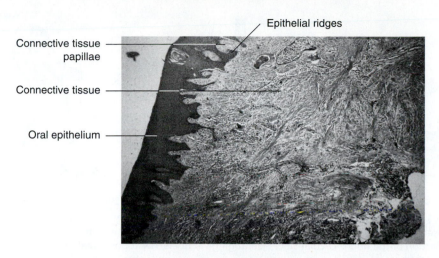

Connective tissue papillae

Connective tissue

Oral epithelium

Epithelial ridges

Figure 1–8   A photomicrograph of the gingival oral epithelium/connective tissue interface. Note prominent epithelial ridges. Intersections between the epithelial ridges under the epithelial surface correspond to depressions seen on the surface of the gingiva. Fingerlike projections termed connective tissue papillae extend into the depressions on the undersurface of the epithelium. This produces the characteristic stippled appearance of the attached gingiva. (Courtesy of Dr. Harvey Wishe, New York University College of Dentistry)

alveologingival, and transseptal fibers. Secondary gingival fiber groups include periostogingival, interpapillary, transgingival, intercrevicular, semicircular, and intergingival fibers (Ammons, Schectman, Dillinghan, & Goldman, 1951; Page, 1974). Their function is to support and give contour to the free and attached gingivae and firmly connect the attached gingiva to the underlying cementum and alveolar bone. The free gingiva is not actually free nor is it attached to the tooth, but rather it is held in close proximity to the tooth by the gingival fibers, which prevent the free gingiva from being deflected from the tooth during mastication.

Table 1–1   Classification of the Gingival Fibers

Name of Fiber	Origin and Distribution	Function
Circular	Encircles the tooth within the free gingiva	Provides support and contour to the free gingiva
Dentogingival	From the cementum at the base of the gingival sulcus, flares coronally into the free gingiva (group A), laterally into the attached gingiva (group B), and apically into the periosteum (group C); found on the facial, lingual, and interproximal surfaces	Contributes to the support of the gingiva
Dentoperiosteal	Extends from the cementum apically over the alveolar crest into the periosteum	Anchors the tooth to the bone
Alveologingival	Extends from the periosteum of the alveolar crestal bone coronally into the connective tissue	Attaches the gingiva to the alveolar bone
Transseptal	Runs from the cementum of one tooth interproximal to the cementum of the adjacent tooth	Keeps teeth in alignment and protects the interproximal bone from the inflammatory infiltrate; resistant to inflammation and will continuously reform when bone and fibers are destroyed

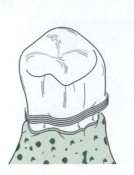
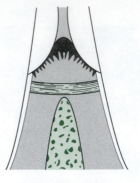
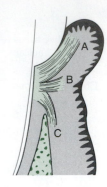

(a) Circular fibers   (b) Transseptal fibers   (c) Dentogingival fibers

Figure 1–9   The major part of the connective tissue of the free and attached gingivae are composed of collagen fibers that are arranged in groups or bundles. The name indicates the origin and insertion of the fibers: circular fibers, dentogingival fibers, dentoperiosteal fibers, and transseptal fibers.

Collagen Organization

Collagen fibers are either densely or loosely organized. Dense connective tissue that is found in the lamina propria of the gingiva consists of heavy, tightly packed fibers that function to resist tension. Loose connective tissue, as exemplified by alveolar mucosa, is composed of the collagen fibers that are thin and delicate and do not have a mechanical protective function. Collagen is constantly being synthesized and degraded as part of the normal remodeling or turnover of gingival connective tissue.

Cellular and Vascular Elements

The cellular part of the lamina propria predominately consists of

- fibroblasts;
- macrophages;
- mast cells; and
- plasma cells, lymphocytes, and neutrophils.

Fibroblasts synthesize ground substance, collagen, and collagenase. Collagenase is an enzyme responsible for the breakdown of collagen during remodeling. Thus, fibroblasts play a chief role in the maintenance and remodeling of connective tissue. Other cells in the lamina propria include red blood cells, PMNs, macrophages, lymphocytes, and mast cells, which are involved in the defense of the host against toxins.

A rich vascular complex is found in the lamina propria. Since there is no submucosa, as is found in the alveolar mucosa, the blood supply passes directly to the lamina propria.

Cell-to-Cell Tissue Junction

Epithelial Cell-to-Cell Attachment

Electron microscopy has demonstrated that epithelial cells are held together by intercellular bridges or desmosomes. A desmosome consists of two adjacent attachment plaques, which are continuous with the innermost leaflet of the cell membrane (Fig. 1–10■). A space exists between adjacent desmosomes allowing passage of material and fluid through the tissue while holding together epithelial cells. Junctional epithelium has four times fewer desmosomes than oral epithelium, so the intercellular spaces are wider.

Epithelium-Tooth Surface/ Connective Tissue Interface

The junctional epithelium adheres to the tooth surface (e.g., enamel) through the epithelial attachment. The basal cells of the junctional epithelium do not contact the enamel or the connective tissue directly. Instead, between the junctional epithelium and the tooth and connective tissue is a basal lamina and hemidesmosomes (Stern, 1965; see also Fig. 1–10). The basal lamina and the hemidesmosomes are referred to as the epithelial attachment and it provides the attachment of the junctional epithelium to the tooth surface as seen under the electron microscope. The epithelial attachment is not synonymous with junctional epithelium, which refers to the entire epithelium. The basal lamina has an outer electron lucent (lighter) zone called the lamina lucida and an inner electron dense (darker) zone called the lamina densa. The basal lamina is continuous around the base of the junctional epithelium. These structures lie in a sandwich-like arrangement, one on top of each other.

A hemidesmosome consists of one attachment plaque continuous with the cell membrane and attaches the epithelial (basal) cell to the basal lamina. This in turn

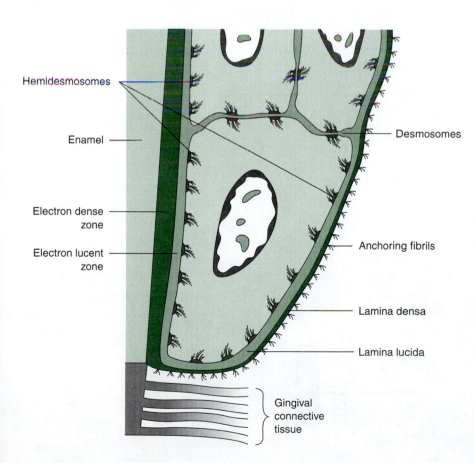

Figure 1–10 Schematic illustration showing the attachment of the junctional epithelium to the tooth surface and the underlying connective tissue and enamel. The electron-dense zone is a continuation of the lamina densa; the electron-lucent zone is a continuation of the lamina lucida; anchoring fibrils radiate out into the lamina propria. The cell membrane of the epithelial cells harbor hemidesmosomes toward the enamel and the connective tissue. Adjacent epithelial cell membranes also harbor desmosomes, which hold epithelial cells together. (Copyright © 2003 by J. Lindhe and T. Karring. Anatomy of the periodontium, in *Clinical periodontology and implant dentistry*, ed. J. Lindhe. Copenhagen: Munksgaard.)

attaches to the enamel on one side and the underlying connective tissue on the other side (see Fig. 1–10). Connective tissue fibers called anchoring fibrils attach the lamina densa to the underlying connective tissue. This same structural relationship also exists between the oral and sulcular epithelium, where a basal lamina separates the epithelium from the connective tissue.

Dentogingival Unit

The dentogingival unit collectively refers to the epithelial attachment and the gingival connective tissue attachment (gingival fibers) to the cementum, both of which are involved in the stabilization of the gingiva to the tooth. Of the two types of attachment, the gingival connective tissue (gingival fibers) forms a firmer one, supporting the epithelium and probably inhibiting movement of the epithelium apically.

The combined length of the dentogingival unit has been described in the literature as the biologic width (Fig. 1–11■). A study using human cadaver models determined that the components of the biologic width included the junctional epithelium with a mean length of 0.97 mm and gingival connective tissue attachment with a mean length of 1.07 mm (Gargiulo, Wentz, & Orban, 1961). This soft-tissue dimension is essential to maintain gingival health. Biologic width or the length (coronalapical dimension) of the soft tissue attachments becomes important during periodontal-prosthetic (restorative) treatment. The margin of a restoration should not disturb the biologic width. Thus, the margin of a restoration should not be closer than 2 mm to the alveolar bone crest.

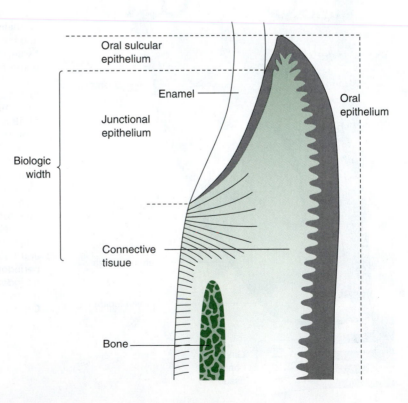

Figure 1–11
Schematic illustration of the biologic width includes the length of the junctional epithelium (0.97 mm) and the gingival connective tissue attachment (1.07 mm). (Copyright © 2003 by J. Lindhe and T. Karring. Anatomy of the periodontium, in *Clinical periodontology and implant dentistry,* ed. J. Lindhe. Copenhagen: Munksgaard.)

Formation of the Dentogingival Unit

The formation of the dentogingival unit has important clinical considerations during the periodontal evaluation and in the healing of the gingiva after periodontal treatment. After completion of the enamel, the ameloblasts produce the primary enamel cuticle as their last function before they degenerate and become part of the reduced enamel epithelium. At the time of tooth eruption, the enamel is still covered with reduced enamel epithelium, which is connected to the enamel by the primary enamel cuticle. As tooth eruption occurs, the reduced enamel epithelium fuses with the oral epithelium at the base of the sulcus forming the junctional epithelium. The reduced enamel epithelium forms the lining of the gingival sulcus. The junctional epithelium produces another cuticle between itself and the enamel called the secondary cuticle, which holds the junctional epithelium in close proximity to the tooth. While the tooth erupts into occlusion, the junctional epithelium gradually moves apically down the crown exposing it. Several stages occur during this passive eruption process. Eventually, the junctional epithelium ends at the cementoenamel junction. With gingival inflammation, the junctional epithelium also migrates onto the cementum, while the *base of the sulcus remains located on the enamel,* at the cementoenamel junction or on the root surface. In other words, the base of the epithelial attachment of the gingiva is at the cementoenamel junction in health and gingivitis. This situation changes in periodontitis, where the junctional epithelium migrates apically along the root surface. This concept of attachment level is important when performing periodontal probing and monitoring periodontal disease progression.

Attachment Apparatus

The periodontal ligament, cementum, and alveolar and supporting bone constitute the attachment apparatus (Fig. 1–12■). The function of these tissues is to support and anchor the teeth within the alveolar process (Hassell, 1993).

Periodontal Ligament

The connective tissue that extends from the cementum covering the root surface to the alveolar bone is termed the periodontal ligament. The periodontal ligament is primarily composed of collagen fibers and islands of loose connective tissue, creating interstitial spaces where blood vessels, nerves, lymphatics, and cells are embedded in a ground substance (Beertsen, McCulloch, & Sodek, 1997). The primary cell of the periodontal ligament is the fibroblast, which synthesizes collagen, collagenase, and ground substance. On one side of the periodontal ligament is the alveolar bone, where osteoblasts reside and are involved in bone formation. The other side of the periodontal ligament is the cementum, where cementoblasts reside and are involved in the formation of cementum.

Connective Tissue Attachment

The primary component of the periodontal ligament is collagen fibers. The fibers are arranged in groups or bundles that blend into one another and are collectively called the principal fibers (Fig. 1–13■). This constitutes the second type of connective tissue.

Figure 1–12
Photomicrograph of the attachment apparatus. (Courtesy of Dr. Harvey Wishe, New York University College of Dentistry)

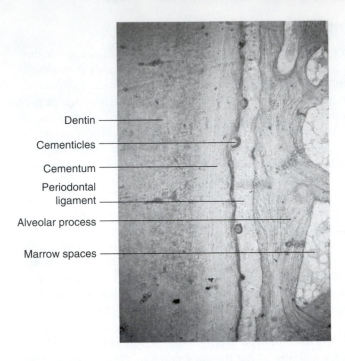

Dentin
Cementicles
Cementum
Periodontal ligament
Alveolar process
Marrow spaces

The principal fibers are a continuation of the gingival fibers or gingival connective tissue attachment (the other type of connective tissue attachment) in the gingiva and are also named according to their direction of insertion and location. Table 1–2■ reviews the principal fiber groups (Hassell, 1993). The ends of the fibers, which are embedded into alveolar bone and cementum, are termed Sharpey's fibers. The first principal fibers formed before the tooth erupts are the alveolar crest fibers. With definitive tooth-to-tooth contact, the oblique fibers mature. Eventually, with the formation of the apical fibers, the periodontal ligament is established. Since the periodontal ligament contains few elastic fibers, it is the wavy configuration of the principal fibers that permits slight movement of the tooth under function (tooth-to-tooth contact). Collagen turnover time is five times faster in the periodontal ligament than in bone or gingiva because of the greater functional demands placed upon it.

Figure 1–13
Schematic diagram showing the location of the periodontal ligament between the alveolar bone proper and the root cementum. The tooth is joined to the bone by bundles of collagen fibers, which can be divided into the following main groups: alveolar crest fibers, horizontal fibers, oblique fibers, interradicular fibers, and apical fibers.

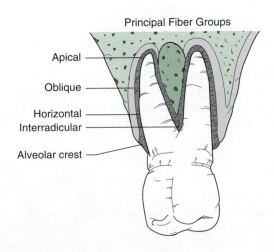

Principal Fiber Groups

Apical
Oblique
Horizontal
Interradicular
Alveolar crest

Table 1–2	Classification of the Principal Fiber Groups of the Periodontal Ligament		
Name of Fiber Bundle	**Direction**	**Function**	**Features**
Alveolar crest	Originates from the cementum and runs apically to insert into the alveolar crest	Resists lateral movement of the tooth and keeps tooth in its socket	The first fibers to be formed before tooth eruption has occurred
Horizontal	Originates from cementum and runs at right angles and inserts into bone	Opposes lateral forces	The second fibers to be formed as soon as the first tooth-to-tooth contact has occurred
Oblique	Found in the middle third of the root apical to the horizontal fibers; originates from cementum and runs coronally and diagonally into bone	Absorbs occlusal forces	The most abundant and thus the principal attachment of the tooth
Apical	Originates from cementum of the apex of the root, spreading out apically and laterally into bone	Resists tipping of the tooth	One of the last fibers to form
Interradicular	From the crest of the interradicular septum extending to the cementum in the furcation area	Resists the forces of luxation (pulling out) and tipping	Lost when bone is destroyed in the furcation area in disease

Periodontal Ligament Space

Although the width of the periodontal ligament varies from tooth to tooth and from different areas on the same tooth, the average width is approximately 0.25 mm. Seen radiographically, a tooth that has heavy occlusal loads placed upon it for long periods of time will have a thicker periodontal ligament space. A tooth that is not in function, such as a tooth without an antagonist, will have a narrower periodontal ligament space.

Functions of the Periodontal Ligament

The periodontal ligament functions include the following:

1. Suspensory: acts like a suspensory mechanism attaching the tooth to the alveolar bone.
2. Shock absorption: acts as a shock absorber transmitting occlusal forces to the alveolar bone. Axial-placed forces, which are parallel to the long axis of the tooth, are more easily absorbed than lateral or rotational forces.
3. Remodeling: serves a remodeling function by providing cells that are involved in the formation and resorption of cementum and bone and itself.
4. Formative: carries a blood supply to the rest of the periodontium for nutrition.
5. Sensory: transmits tactile pressure and pain perception via the trigeminal nerve.
6. Proprioceptive: allows the feeling of localization of pain and pressure to be transmitted through proprioceptive nerve endings (e.g., trigeminal nerve) found in the periodontal ligament. For example, when biting into a hard object, the mouth quickly opens. This quick reflex sensation is a

function of the periodontal ligament. The greatest amount of sensory receptors is found in the apical area.

Abnormalities

Histologically, besides collagen fibers, clusters of epithelial cells are found within the periodontal ligament. These clusters are called epithelial rests of Malassez. Epithelial rests of Malassez are considered to be remains of epithelium of Hertwig's epithelial root sheath, which plays an important role in the development of the cementum and the shape of the roots. Their presence and function are controversial, but they may play a role in the formation of dental cysts.

Cementicles are calcified bodies of cementum seen in the periodontal ligament of older adults (see Fig. 1–12). Either they are attached to the cementum, embedded within the cementum, or not associated with the root. It is unknown if cementicles present any clinical significance.

Cementum

The cementum is a layer of mineralized tissue covering the root of the tooth and is composed of collagen, ground substance, cells, and calcium and phosphate in the form of hydroxyapatite. The primary function of the cementum is to attach the principal fibers to the root surface.

The cementum is a product of the periodontal ligament and forms in layers or increments. As a layer of uncalcified cementoid forms, adjacent cementoblasts found in the periodontal ligament stop producing. When the layer of cementoid becomes 80 to 90% calcified, more cementoid is laid down. Therefore, the cementum is never fully calcified. Cementoid serves a protective function, resisting resorption. Sharpey's fibers are embedded into cementoid allowing for repositioning of the tooth in response to biting forces.

The surface of the cementum is soft and relatively permeable, allowing bacterial by-products and toxins to easily penetrate the cemental surface. However, it is now recognized that the toxins are actually not as deeply penetrated into the root surface as was once thought (Nakib, Bissada, Simmelink, & Goldstine, 1982). The cementum is avascular and does not contain lymph vessels or nerves.

Relationship of Cementum and Enamel

The relationship of the cementum to the enamel margin varies (Fig. 1–14■). In 60 to 65% of the population, the cementum overlaps the enamel. In 30% of the population, the cementum meets exactly with the enamel in an edge-to-edge relationship, and in 5 to 10% of the population, the cementum and enamel do not meet and the dentin is exposed, leaving an area of possible sensitivity.

Types of Cementum

Two kinds of cementum are identified under the light microscope. Acellular cementum, which is formed before tooth eruption, is found on the coronal two-thirds of the root and is approximately 0.1 mm in thickness, with the cementoenamel junction being the thinnest area. Since acellular cementum does not contain cementocytes, it is not involved in the laying down of new cementum.

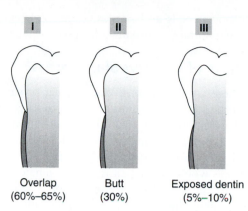

Figure 1–14   Schematic illustration of the relationships of the cementum to the enamel at the cementoenamel junction. (Adapted from P. F. Fedi, Jr., and A. R. Vernino, *The Periodontic Syllabus.* Copyright © 2000 by Lippincott Williams & Wilkins.)

Cellular cementum, which covers the apical third of the root and furcations, has a thickness of about 0.5 mm and is formed much faster than acellular cementum. Cellular cementum can be laid down on top of acellular cementum or it can comprise the entire thickness of the cementum.

Physiologic Features

As teeth wear down (attrition) on either the occlusal surface or incisal edge, there is a compensatory deposition of cellular cementum in the apical area in addition to deposition of bone at the alveolar crest and in the socket. This acts to maintain the vertical dimension of the face and maintain the length of the root. Instead of remodeling (resorption and deposition) like bone, cementum is deposited continuously. Cementum thickens with increasing age, but the production of cementum slows.

Cementum does not resorb as readily as bone due to its avascularity and protective layer of cementoid. This property makes orthodontic movement possible without normally resorbing the roots. However, cementum can be resorbed under certain circumstances such as inappropriate orthodontic movement, cysts, tumors, trauma, replanted teeth, periapical disease, and periodontal disease or for no known reason. Therefore, instead of resorption followed by deposition, a new layer of cementum is formed on the most superficial or oldest layer.

Abnormalities

Hypercementosis is a condition characterized by an atypical thickening of the cementum. It may be localized to one tooth due to factors such as excessive and rapid orthodontic movement or may result from excessive occlusal force placed on a tooth. It can also involve numerous teeth such as in a systemic hereditary disease like Paget's disease. Usually, the thickening occurs on the apical part or the entire root surface of the cementum.

Alveolar Process

The alveolar process constitutes that part of the maxilla and mandible that forms and supports the sockets or alveoli of the teeth. Periosteum is connective tissue that covers the outer surface of the alveolar process and is well supplied with blood vessels and nerves, some of which enter the bone. Endosteum covers the inner surface of the alveolar process facing the tooth surface.

Parts of the Alveolar Process

There are two parts to the alveolar process: the alveolar bone proper and the supporting bone. It is important to distinguish between the alveolar process and the alveolar bone proper. The alveolar bone proper or cribriform plate is hard compact bone that lines the tooth socket, which is contained within the alveolar process (Fig. 1–15■). Radiographically, it is referred to as the lamina dura. The bone where Sharpey's fibers terminate is called bundle bone and is found at the inner surface of the tooth socket. The cribriform plate is perforated by numerous openings that carry blood, nerves, and lymphatics from the bone to the periodontal ligament.

The supporting bone is composed of two parts: compact bone and cancellous bone (also called spongy or trabecular bone). Compact bone, which covers the alveolar process, consists of buccal (outer) and lingual (inner) cortical plates that are continuous with the cribriform plate (Fig. 1–16a■). The buccal and lingual cortical plates vary in thickness. Generally, the cortical plate is thicker in the mandible than in the maxilla. In the maxilla, the compact bone is thicker on the palatal than on the buccal surfaces. In the mandible, the bone is thicker in the buccal area of the premolar and molar areas and thinnest in the incisor area.

Cancellous bone fills the area between the buccal and lingual cortical plates and between the alveolar bone proper of adjacent teeth. There may be little or no cancellous bone when there is close root proximity of adjacent teeth. In these cases, the interdental septum is thin and the alveolar bone proper is fused with the cortical plate of bone.

Figure 1–15   A section through the mandible after removal of all teeth. The thin bone lining the tooth socket (cribriform plate or alveolar bone proper) is clearly seen. (Reprinted with permission from A. Schroeder, F. Sutter, D. Buser, and G. Krekeler, *Oral implantology.* Copyright © 1996 by Thieme Medical Publishers, Inc., New York.)

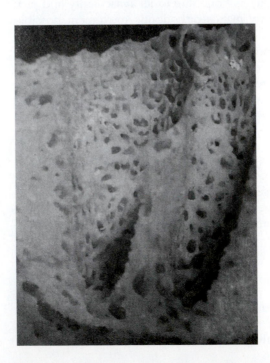

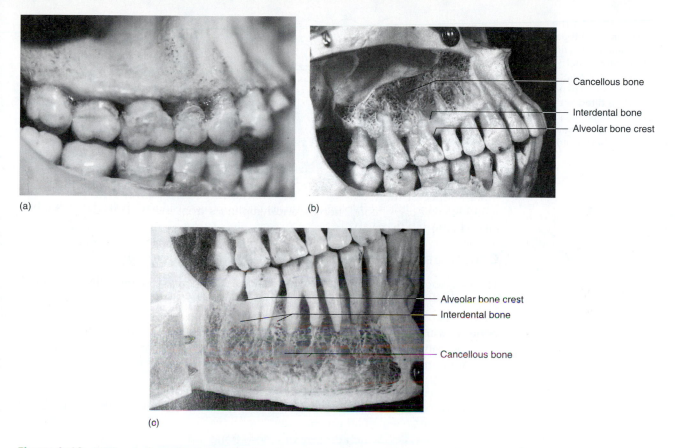

(a)   (b)

(c)

Figure 1–16   (a) Dry skull specimen showing the outer cortical plates of bone covering the roots of the teeth. (b) Dry skull of the maxilla. The cortical plates of bone are removed. (c) Dry skull of the mandible. The cortical plates of bone are removed. (Figure 1–16b and c reprinted with permission from A. Schroeder, F. Sutter, D. Buser, and G. Krekeler, *Oral implantology.* Copyright © 1996 by Thieme Medical Publishers, Inc., New York.)

Morphology

The cortical plate of bone covering the roots of the teeth is called radicular bone. Interradicular bone is found between roots of the same teeth (e.g., bi- and trifurcation areas of multirooted teeth). The interdental septum or interproximal bone consists of the cribriform plate of two adjacent teeth and some cancellous bone (Fig. 1–16b,c■). The alveolar bone crest is the most coronal part of the alveolar bone. It is where the outer cortical plate is continuous with and fuses with the cribriform plate. At this area cancellous bone is absent.

Alveolar Bone Crest   The shape of the alveolar bone crest is influenced by the width of the interdental space, stage of eruption, position of the teeth in the arch, and shape of the cementoenamel junction. By following the contour of the cemento-enamel junction, the alveolar bone crest is relatively flat in the posterior and more convex and pointed in the anterior. In health, the shape of bone takes on a form where the alveolar bone crest is more coronal than the radicular bone. The slope of the alveolar bone crest follows an imaginary parallel line connecting the cementoenamel junction of adjacent teeth (Ritchey & Orban, 1953) and is approximately

Figure 1–17 The alveolar crest is parallel to a line connecting the cementoenamel junctions of adjacent teeth, even when a tooth is tilted and the cementoenamel junction on one tooth may be lower than the adjacent tooth.

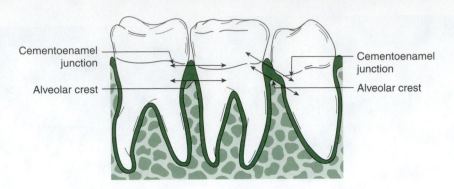

2 mm apical to it if the biologic width is taken into consideration (Fig. 1–17■), but this relationship may vary.

Composition of Bone

The alveolar process is primarily composed of collagen fibers and cells embedded in a ground substance (proteoglycans), which make up the organic component. The inorganic salts of bone are principally calcium and phosphate. The salts allow bone to withstand compression. The combination of fibers and salts makes bone exceptionally strong without being brittle. The cells present in the alveolar and supporting bone are

1. osteoblasts, which synthesize and secrete bone;
2. osteocytes, which are osteoblasts that are embedded within lacunae as bone is being laid down; and
3. osteoclasts, which destroy or resorb bone.

Metabolism

Despite its rigid physical characteristic, bone is a vascular tissue and the least stable of all the periodontal tissues. There is a constant remodeling with formation and resorption of bone due to the functional demand placed upon it. This occurs more rapidly in cancellous than compact bone. The normal remodeling of bone occurs by resorption by osteoclasts followed by deposition by osteoblasts. During orthodontic movement, bone is resorbed on the pressure side and laid down on the tension side.

Variations in Anatomy

Roots of teeth are usually contained entirely within the alveolar bony plates. Frequently, the bone may not completely encircle prominent roots of teeth that are rotated, in facioversion, in lingoversion, tipped, or crowded. The resulting defects take the form of windows (fenestrations) where the radicular cortical bone is lost except for the most coronal edge or clefts (dehiscences) where the cortical bone, including the marginal bone (most coronal edge of bone), is lost over the root (Fig. 1–18■). The etiology of these defects is not definitive. These defects occur more frequently on facial bone than on lingual bone.

Buttressing bone occurs at the margin of bone where it thickens in response to increased functional demands. This is a response to the repair process, with bone resorption and deposition occurring.

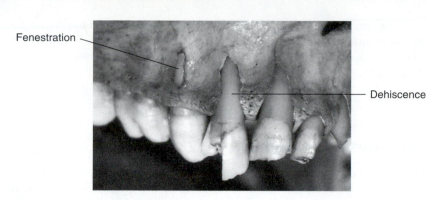

Fenestration

Dehiscence

Figure 1–18 Dry skull specimen of a dehiscence showing loss of radicular cortical bone involving the marginal bone and a fenestration with loss of radicular bone but not involving the marginal bone.

Physiology of the Periodontium

The blood to the gingiva is primarily supplied by the vessels of the periosteum, periodontal ligament, and alveolar bone (Fig. 1–19■). The supraperiosteal vessels run along the facial and lingual surfaces of the alveolar bone and give off many little branches as they make their way toward the gingiva. These finally join with blood vessels of the alveolar bone and periodontal ligament to form a gingival plexus located just under the oral epithelium.

The inferior and superior alveolar arteries supplying the periodontal ligament originate from the apical foramen, the alveolar bone, and the gingiva.

The blood supply to the cortical bone is via branches of the supraperiosteal blood vessels. The vessels that enter the interdental septum in addition to the vessels that supply the remainder of the alveolar bone supply blood to the cancellous bone.

Lymphatic drainage from the gingiva starts in the papillae of the connective tissue and drains into the regional lymph nodes, primarily the submandibular nodes. The lymphatic vessels follow the course of the blood vessels.

The nerves supplying the periodontium branch off from the trigeminal nerve (fifth cranial nerve). The nerves follow the course of the blood vessels that supply blood to the periodontium. Gingival branches of the anterior superior alveolar nerve innervate the gingiva overlying the maxillary incisors and canines. The gingival branches of the middle superior alveolar nerve supply the gingiva around the maxillary premolars. The posterior superior alveolar nerve supplies the gingiva around the maxillary molars.

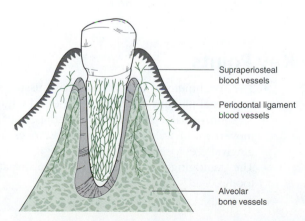

Supraperiosteal blood vessels

Periodontal ligament blood vessels

Alveolar bone vessels

Figure 1–19 The blood supply to the periodontium comes from three sources: (1) supraperiosteal blood vessels, (2) blood vessels from the periodontal ligament, and (3) blood vessels of the alveolar process.

The gingival branches of the inferior alveolar nerve supply the facial gingiva of the mandibular incisors, canines, premolars, and molars. The mental nerve supplies the mandibular facial gingiva of the incisors, canines, and premolars. The gingival branches of the buccal nerve supply the facial gingiva of the mandibular molars. The lingual nerve supplies the mandibular lingual gingiva.

Changes with Aging

With increasing age certain changes in the hard-and soft-tissue components of the periodontium occur, as well as a thinning of the gingiva with reduced keratinization. The amount of stippling is either reduced or unchanged. Within the lamina propria, there is a decrease in the number of cells and the gingival fibers become less dense.

Cementum increases in thickness throughout life, with a greater deposition in the apical area in response to the continuing tooth eruption that compensates for tooth attrition.

Cells within the periodontal ligament decrease in number, while the number of elastic fibers increases. The width of the periodontal ligament can be either increased or decreased.

Changes in the alveolar bone occur with aging just as in any other bone in the body. There may be a decrease in vascularity and healing.

A physiologic tendency with increasing age is for the proximal surface contacts of teeth to wear down (attrition), causing the teeth to migrate in a mesial direction (mesial drifting) while retaining tooth-to-tooth contact. Accordingly, bone is laid down on the distal surface, which is the tension side, and bone is resorbed on the mesial surface, which is the pressure side.

Summary

This chapter reviewed the structure and functions of the periodontal soft and hard tissues including the gingiva, periodontal ligament, cementum, and supporting and alveolar bone. The periodontium is a dynamic, highly specialized structure that is constantly changing with the demands placed upon it. Knowing the macro and microstructure of the periodontium in health will help to understand the process that leads to pathological destruction.

Key Points

- The attachment of the soft and hard tissues to the tooth surface contributes to the stability and health of the periodontium.
- The junctional epithelium is a semipermeable membrane involved in the movement of fluids, cells, and substances from the lamina propria into the gingival crevice and vice versa.
- The dentogingival unit is involved in the attachment of the gingiva to the tooth.

Web Sites

www.temple.edu/dentistry/perio/periohistology (histology of the periodontium)

www.usc.edu/hsc/dental/ohistol

www.dentalarticles.com

Self-Quiz

1. Which one of the following structures comprises the attachment apparatus? (p. 19)
   a. gingiva, cementum, alveolar and supporting bone, periodontal ligament
   b. gingiva, cementum, periodontal ligament
   c. cementum, alveolar and supporting bone, periodontal ligament
   d. cementum, alveolar and supporting bone

2. Which one of the following areas is the width of attached gingiva greatest? (p. 6)
   a. mandibular second premolars
   b. mandibular canines
   c. maxillary lateral incisors
   d. maxillary first premolars
   e. maxillary second molars

3. Which one of the following substances is the primary component of the connective tissue of the periodontium? (p. 14)
   a. gingival crevicular fluid
   b. calcium
   c. collagen
   d. proteoglycans

4. Which one of the following structures directly attaches the junctional epithelium to the enamel? (pp. 16–17)
   a. desmosomes
   b. hemidesmosomes
   c. basal lamina
   d. gingival fibers

5. Which one of the following structures is involved in the attachment of the gingiva to the tooth surface? (p. 17)
   a. alveolar mucosa
   b. dentogingival unit
   c. mucogingival junction
   d. desmosomes

6. Which one of the following structures comprises the biological width? (p. 18)
   a. gingival sulcus, junctional epithelium, gingival connective tissue attachment
   b. gingival sulcus, sulcular epithelium, gingival connective tissue attachment
   c. junctional epithelium, gingival connective tissue attachment
   d. sulcular epithelium, gingival connective tissue attachment
   e. sulcular epithelium, junctional epithelium, principal fibers

7. Which one of the following types of bone lines the tooth socket? (p. 24)
   a. alveolar
   b. interradicular
   c. interdental
   d. trabecular

8. Which one of the following structures is referred to as a semipermeable membrane? (p. 13)
   a. junctional epithelium
   b. oral epithelium
   c. sulcular epithelium
   d. lamina propria
   e. cementum

9. All of the following structures are avascular except one. Which one is the exception? (p. 22)
   a. enamel
   b. cementum
   c. junctional epithelium
   d. lamina propria

10. Arteries that supply blood and lymphatics to the free gingiva originate from all of the following parts of the periodontium except one. Which one is the exception? (pp. 27–28)

    a. supraperiosteal

    b. periodontal ligament

    c. alveolar bone

    d. cementum

References

Alfano, M. 1974. The origin of gingival fluid. *J. Theor. Biol.* 47:127–136.

Beertsen, W., C. A. G. McCulloch, and J. Sodek. 1997. The periodontal ligament: A unique, multifunctional connective tissue. *Periodontology 2000* 13:20–40.

Gargiulo, A., F. Wentz, and B. Orban. 1961. Dimensions and relations of the dento-gingival junction in humans, *J. Periodontol.* 32:261–267.

Goldman, H. M. 1951. The topography and role of the gingival fibers. *J. Dent. Res.* 30:331–336.

Gordon, J. M., C. B. Walker, J. C. Murphy, J. M. Goodson, and S. S. Socransky. 1981. Tetracycline: Levels achievable in gingival crevice fluid and in vitro effect on subgingival organisms. Part 1. Concentrations in crevicular fluid after repeated doses. *J. Periodontol.* 52:609–612.

Hassell, T. M. 1993. Tissues and cells of the periodontium. *Periodontology 2000* 3:9–38.

Kornman, K., R. Page, and M. Tonetti. 1997. The host response to the microbial challenge in periodontitis: Assembling the players. *Periodontology 2000* 14:33–53.

Moss-Salentijn, L., and M. Hendricks-Klyvert. 1990. Oral mucosa-epithelium. In *Dental and oral tissues,* eds. L. Moss-Salentijn and M. Hendricks-Klyvert, 27–44. Philadelphia: Lea & Febiger.

Mukherjee, S. 1985. The significance of crevicular fluid. *Compendium Cont. Educ. Dent.* 6:611–616.

Nakib, N., N. M. Bissada, J. W. Simmelink, and S. N. Goldstine. 1982. Endotoxin penetration into root cementum of periodontally healthy and diseased human teeth. *J. Periodontol.* 53:368–378.

Page, R. C., W. F. Ammons, L. R. Schectman, and L. A. Dillingham. 1974. Collagen fibre bundles of the normal marginal gingiva in the marmoset. *Arch. Oral. Biol.* 19:1039–1043.

Ritchey, B., and B. Orban 1953. The crests of the interdental alveolar septa. *J. Periodontol.* 24:75–87.

Schroeder, H. E. 1991. Oral mucosa. In *Oral structural biology,* ed. H. E. Schroeder, 350–391. Stuttgart and New York: Georg Thieme Verlag.

Schroeder, H. E., and M. A. Listgarten. 1997. The gingival tissues: The architecture of periodontal protection. *Periodontology 2000* 13:91–120.

Squier, C. A., and M. W. Hill. 1998. Oral mucosa. In ed. A. R. Ten Cate, *Oral histology.* St. Louis, MO: Mosby.

Stern, I. B. 1965. Electron microscopic observations of oral epithelium I. Basal cells and the basement membrane. *Periodontics* 3:224–238.

Tonetti, M. S., M. Imboden, I. L. Gerber, and N. P. Lang. 1995. Compartmentalization of inflammatory cell phenotypes in normal gingiva and peri-implant keratinized mucosa. *J. Clin. Periodontol.* 22:735–742.

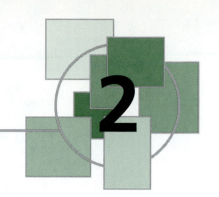

Classification of the Periodontal Diseases

Surendra Singh, D.D.S., M.S.

Outline

Classification System
Summary
Key Points

Web Sites
Self-Quiz
References

Goal

To provide knowledge of the most current classification system of the periodontal diseases.

Educational Objectives

Upon completion of this chapter, the dental hygiene student should be able to:

Describe the current 1999 classification of periodontal diseases.
Discuss the changes in the classification system for periodontal diseases.
List and describe the different periodontal diseases.

<table>
<tr><td>KEY WORDS</td></tr>
<tr><td>

• classification system
• periodontal diseases
• gingivitis
• periodontitis
</td></tr>
</table>

Inflammatory periodontal diseases are a major cause of tooth loss. Periodontal diseases are not a single disease entity, but a group of lesions affecting the tissues that form the attachment apparatus of teeth. These diseases are microbial infections caused by the host's immune response to bacterial plaque and its by-products. When classifying periodontal diseases, it is important to include not only diseases that have primary manifestation and etiology in the periodontium but also periodontal manifestations of systemic diseases. In this chapter a comprehensive classification of chronic inflammatory periodontal diseases or conditions affecting periodontal tissues is presented. This chapter is intended to *briefly introduce* the dental clinician to the classification of the periodontal diseases. Further discussion related to each type of disease is discussed in Part II.

Classification System

Over the years a number of classification systems have been developed to organize and name various disease entities or conditions affecting the periodontium. In 1989, the American Academy of Periodontology (AAP) recommended a classification based on the data from periodontal research that was used by the dental community to describe different forms of periodontal diseases (Table 2–1■). This was modified in 1992 (American Academy of Periodontology) in a position paper published by the Academy to include gingival diseases. In 1999 at the International Workshop for a Classification of Periodontal Diseases and Conditions the American Academy of Periodontology proposed a new classification system (Armitage, 1999) (Table 2–2■). *This new classification system is not based on the age of the patient at*

Table 2–1	1989 Classification of Inflammatory Periodontal Diseases

  I. Adult Periodontitis
 II. Early-Onset Periodontitis
    A. Prepubertal Periodontitis
      1. Generalized
      2. Localized
    B. Juvenile Periodontitis
      1. Generalized
      2. Localized
    C. Rapidly Progressive Periodontitis
III. Periodontitis Associated with Systemic Disease
IV. Necrotizing Ulcerative Periodontitis
 V. Refractory Periodontitis

Gingival Diseases (Added in the 1992 AAP Classification)

Gingivitis
- Plaque-Associated Gingivitis
- Chronic or Long-Standing Gingivitis
- Acute Necrotizing Gingivitis
- Steroid Hormone-Influenced Gingivitis
- Medication-Influenced Gingival Overgrowth
- Desquamative Gingivitis

Source: American Academy of Periodontology 1989, 1992.

Table 2–2	1999 Classification of Periodontal Diseases and Conditions

I. Gingival diseases
   A. Dental plaque–induced gingival diseases*
      1. Gingivitis associated with dental plaque only
         a. Without other local contributing factors
         b. With local contributing factors (see VIIIA)
      2. Gingival diseases modified by systemic factors
         a. Associated with the endocrine system
            (1) Puberty-associated gingivitis
            (2) Menstrual cycle–associated gingivitis
            (3) Pregnancy-associated
               (a) Gingivitis
               (b) Pyogenic granuloma
            (4) Diabetes mellitus–associated gingivitis
         b. Associated with blood dyscrasias
            (1) Leukemia-associated gingivitis
            (2) Other
      3. Gingival diseases modified by medications
         a. Drug-influenced gingival diseases
            (1) Drug-influenced gingival enlargements
            (2) Drug-influenced gingivitis
               (a) Oral contraceptive–associated gingivitis
               (b) Other
      4. Gingival diseases modified by malnutrition
         a. Ascorbic acid–deficiency gingivitis
         b. Other
   B. Non-plaque-induced gingival lesions
      1. Gingival diseases of specific bacterial origin
         a. *Neisseria gonorrhea*–associated lesions
         b. *Treponema pallidum*–associated lesions
         c. *Streptococcal* species–associated lesions
         d. Other
      2. Gingival diseases of viral origin
         a. Herpes virus infections
            (1) Primary herpetic gingivostomatitis
            (2) Recurrent oral herpes
            (3) Varicella-zoster infections
         b. Other
      3. Gingival diseases of fungal origin
         a. Candida species infections
            (1) Generalized gingival candidiasis
         b. Linear gingival erythema
         c. Histoplasmosis
         d. Other
      4. Gingival lesions of genetic origin
         a. Hereditary gingival fibromatosis
         b. Other
      5. Gingival manifestations of systemic conditions
         a. Mucocutaneous disorders
            (1) Lichen planus
            (2) Pemphigoid
            (3) Pemphigus vulgaris
            (4) Erythema multiforme   *(cont.)*

Table 2–2	1999 Classification of Periodontal Diseases and Conditions (*cont.*)

   (5) Lupus erythematosus
   (6) Drug-induced
   (7) Other
  b. Allergic reactions
   (1) Dental restorative materials
    (a) Mercury
    (b) Nickel
    (c) Acrylic
    (d) Other
   (2) Reactions attributable to
    (a) Toothpastes/dentifrices
    (b) Mouthrinses/mouthwashes
    (c) Chewing gum additives
    (d) Foods and additives
   (3) Other
  6. Traumatic lesions (factitious, iatrogenic, accidental)
   a. Chemical injury
   b. Physical injury
   c. Thermal injury
  7. Foreign-body reactions
  8. Not otherwise specified
 II. Chronic periodontitis[†]
  A. Localized
  B. Generalized
 III. Aggressive periodontitis[†]
  A. Localized
  B. Generalized
 IV. Periodontitis as a manifestation of systemic diseases
  A. Associated with hematologic disorders
   1. Acquired neutropenia
   2. Leukemias
   3. Other
  B. Associated with genetic disorders
   1. Familial and cyclic neutropenia
   2. Down syndrome
   3. Leukocyte adhesion deficiency syndromes
   4. Papillon-Lefèvre syndrome
   5. Chediak-Higashi syndromes
   6. Histiocytosis syndromes
   7. Glycogen storage disease
   8. Infantile genetic agranulocytosis
   9. Cohen syndrome
   10. Ehlers-Danlos syndrome (Types IV and VIIIAD)
   11. Hypophosphatasia
   12. Other
  C. Not otherwise specified (NOS)
 V. Necrotizing periodontal diseases
  A. Necrotizing ulcerative gingivitis (NUG)
  B. Necrotizing ulcerative periodontitis (NUP)
 VI. Abscesses of the periodontium
  A. Gingival abscess
  B. Periodontal abscess
  C. Pericoronal abscess

| Table 2–2 | 1999 Classification of Periodontal Diseases and Conditions (*cont.*) |

VII. Periodontitis associated with endodontic lesions
    A. Combined periodontal–endodontic lesions
VIII. Developmental or acquired deformities and conditions
    A. Localized tooth-related factors that modify or predispose to plaque-induced gingival diseases/periodontitis
        1. Tooth anatomic factors
        2. Dental restorations/appliances
        3. Root fractures
        4. Cervical root resorption and cemental tears
    B. Mucogingival deformities and conditions around teeth
        1. Gingival/soft tissue recession
            a. Facial or lingual surfaces
            b. Interproximal (papillary)
        2. Lack of keratinized gingiva
        3. Decreased vestibular depth
        4. Aberrant frenum/muscle position
        5. Gingival excess
            a. Pseudopocket
            b. Inconsistent gingival margin
            c. Excessive gingival display
            d. Gingival enlargement (see IA3 and IB4)
        6. Abnormal color
    C. Mucogingival deformities and conditions on edentulous ridges
        1. Vertical and/or horizontal ridge deficiency
        2. Lack of gingiva/keratinized tissue
        3. Gingival/soft tissue enlargement
        4. Aberrant frenum/muscle position
        5. Decreased vestibular depth
        6. Abnormal color
    D. Occlusal trauma
        1. Primary occlusal trauma
        2. Secondary occlusal trauma

*Can occur on a periodontium with no attachment loss or on a periodontium with attachment loss that is not progressing.

†Can be further classified on the basis of extent and severity. As a general guide, extent can be characterized as localized ≤ 30% of sites involved and generalized ≥ 30% of sites involved. Severity can be characterized on the basis of the amount of clinical attachment loss (CAL) as follows: slight = 1–2 mm CAL; moderate = 3–4 mm CAL; and severe = ≥ 5 mm CAL.

Source: Armitage, G.C. 1999. Development of a classification system for periodontal diseases and conditions. *Ann Periodontal* 4:1–6.

the time of presentation but rather describes distinct forms of periodontal diseases based on clinical, radiographic, and historical data. Table 2–2 reviews the current classification system (Armitage, 1999).

A section on gingival diseases (1A) was added to the current 1999 system. This includes plaque-induced gingivitis and non-plaque-induced diseases (1B). Also included in this classification system are gingival diseases that can be modified by systemic factors such as medications or diabetes mellitus.

Periodontitis is an inflammatory lesion mediated by host/microorganism interactions, and results in clinical attachment loss and alveolar and supporting bone loss. Adolescents as well as adults can develop periodontitis. One of the changes that were made in the periodontitis classification was replacing the term "Adult Periodontitis" with "Chronic Periodontitis." Chronic Periodontitis is subdivided as localized (≤ 30% of the sites affected) and generalized (> 30% of the sites affected). Disease severity is divided into three groups, which are based on the amount of clinical attachment loss (CAL): slight = 1–2 mm CAL; moderate = 3–4 mm CAL; and severe = ≥ 5 mm CAL. The Academy decided that adults, as well as adolescents could develop periodontitis and "adult" was too restrictive. *Thus, the age factor is eliminating from the criteria for periodontal diseases.*

The term "Early-Onset Periodontitis" was replaced with "Aggressive Periodontitis." Again, the age-dependent nature of the patient was a factor in changing the terms. The older term "early-onset periodontitis" included prepubertal periodontitis, juvenile periodontitis (localized or LJP and generalized), and rapidly progressive periodontitis. Localized juvenile periodontitis is now termed localized aggressive periodontitis and generalized juvenile periodontitis is now referred to as generalized aggressive periodontitis. Prepubertal periodontitis with complicating systemic involvement is now included under the heading of periodontitis as a manifestation of systemic diseases (IV). If there are no modifying systemic conditions it is referred to as chronic periodontitis or aggressive periodontitis.

Refractory periodontitis will no longer have a separate disease classification because any periodontal case can be considered refractory (e.g., localized aggressive periodontitis can be a refractory periodontitis case) or unresponsive to periodontal treatment (e.g., refractory chronic periodontitis).

Necrotizing ulcerative diseases include necrotizing ulcerative gingivitis (NUG) and necrotizing ulcerative periodontitis (NUP). The term acute necrotizing ulcerative gingivitis (ANUG) was changed to necrotizing ulcerative gingivitis (NUG). The Academy decided that the term "acute" was a clinical descriptive term and should not be used as a diagnostic classification and since there is no chronic form of NUG.

New classifications that were added include periodontal abscesses (VI), periodontitis associated with endodontic lesions (VII), developmental or acquired deformities and conditions (VIIIA), mucogingival deformities and conditions (VIIIB, C), and occlusal trauma (VIIID).

The "Abscesses of the Periodontium" includes gingival, periodontal, and pericoronal abscesses. These were added to the new classification system because these lesions involve special diagnostic and treatment challenges.

Table 2–1 describes the previous 1989 classification of the periodontal diseases, which is no longer used in current clinical or research aspects of periodontics; however, since older literature used these terms it is important for the clinician to realize the former names of these diseases. Discussion of the different types of the periodontal diseases will be discussed in length in subsequent chapters.

Summary

The most current classification of the periodontal diseases was a collaboration of the 1999 International Workshop for a Classification of Periodontal Diseases and Conditions. This new classification system for periodontal diseases and conditions replaced the 1989/1992 system. This classification, rather than using the age of the patient, describes different forms of periodontal diseases based on clinical presentation. This chapter is intended to introduce the clinician to periodontal disease classification terminology that will be used throughout the textbook and in periodontal literature. Each specific disease is discussed further in depth in subsequent chapters.

Key Points

- New 1999 classification of the periodontal diseases
- Periodontal diseases are broadly classified into gingivitis and periodontitis.
- Classification is based on clinical and radiographic findings rather than age of onset of disease.
- Gingival diseases are classified into plaque-induced and non-plaque-induced.
- Periodontitis is classified as chronic and aggressive.
- Necrotizing periodontal diseases includes necrotizing ulcerative gingivitis/periodontitis.
- Addition of a category on abscesses of the periodontium.
- Addition of a category on periodontitis associated with endodontic lesions.
- Addition of a category on developmental or acquired deformities and conditions.
- Addition of a category on occlusal trauma.

Web Sites

www.perio.org

www.guideline.gov/summary

http://nnd40.med.navy.mil/ndsbethesda/01August.html

www.dentalarticles.com

Self-Quiz

1. The most current classification of periodontal diseases is based on all of the following factors except one. Which one is the exception? (pp. 32, 35)
   a. age of patient
   b. clinical presentation
   c. radiographic survey
   d. historical data

2. Which one of the following terms replaces adult periodontitis? (p. 36)
   a. aggressive periodontitis
   b. necrotizing ulcerative periodontitis
   c. chronic periodontitis
   d. refractory periodontitis
   e. recurrent periodontitis

3. Which of the following conditions was included in the 1999 classification system but not in the 1989 classification system? (pp. 32, 35)

   a. drug-induced gingivitis

   b. periodontitis associated with diabetes mellitus

   c. necrotizing ulcerative conditions

   d. periodontitis associated with AIDS

4. Which of the following terms replaces the older term "localized juvenile periodontitis"? (p. 36)

   a. dental plaque-induced gingivitis

   b. chronic periodontitis

   c. localized aggressive periodontitis

   d. generalized refractory periodontitis

   e. necrotizing ulcerative periodontitis

5. Which of the following conditions is listed as a mucogingival deformity? (pp. 33–35)

   a. secondary occlusal trauma

   b. periodontal abscess

   c. lack of keratinized gingiva

   d. allergy to toothpaste

   e. recurrent oral herpes

References

American Academy of Periodontology. 1989. *Proceedings of the World Workshop in Clinical Periodontics,* I-2–I-4. Chicago: Author.

American Academy of Periodontology. 1992. *The Etiology and Pathogenesis of Periodontal Diseases* (Position paper), 1–9. Chicago: Author.

Armitage, G. C. 1999. Development of a classification system for periodontal diseases and conditions. *Ann. Periodontol.* 4:1–6.

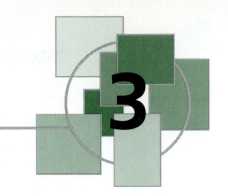

Epidemiology of the Periodontal Diseases

Mary Elizabeth Aichelmann-Reidy, D.D.S.

Outline

Introduction and
 Definitions

Indices

Accuracy of
 Methodology

Prevalence of
 Periodontal Diseases

Incidence and Disease
 Progression

Epidemiologic
 Variables

Treatment Needs

Future Trends

Key Points

Web Sites

Self-Quiz

References

Goal

To provide an understanding of the prevalence, extent, and severity of periodontal diseases in the population.

Educational Objectives

Upon completion of this chapter, the dental hygiene student should be able to:

Describe epidemiology and its descriptive terms: prevalence, incidence, extent, and severity.

Explain the significance of epidemiologic data to future treatment.

Describe the role of indices in private practice and population surveys.

Describe the prevalence and incidence of periodontal diseases.

Identify risk factors and risk indicators for periodontal diseases.

Discuss future periodontal treatment needs and future trends that may have an impact on dental hygiene practice.

KEY WORDS
• epidemiology
• risk factors
• periodontal diseases
• population surveys
• prevalence
• incidence
• severity
• extent
• indices
• risk indicators
• risk factors

Introduction and Definitions

Epidemiology is the study of health and disease in the human population. The rationale for the study of epidemiology is to identify events and risk factors in populations that lead to disease so that future health problems can be anticipated, prevented, and controlled. A risk factor is an event or characteristic associated with a given disease. It is important to identify risk factors so that health care measures can target people at risk for a particular disease, perhaps altering the future course of the disease.

Epidemiologic studies focus on populations rather than individuals. Much of what we know about periodontal diseases comes from national or population surveys. Population surveys evaluate representative samples of individuals within a study population to assess the true risk for disease and quantify how many individuals are or will be affected by disease. This quantification of disease is referred to as disease prevalence and incidence. Prevalence is the proportion or number of individuals in a population having the disease (old and new cases) at a given time. Incidence is defined as the rate of new cases occurring within a certain period of time. Disease prevalence and incidence can only be understood by looking at a large number of individuals within a population. Population surveys also provide insight into the severity and extent of a particular disease, say, periodontal disease, in populations. Severity is defined as the degree or amount of periodontal disease involvement and quantifies the amount of attachment loss, bone loss, or probing depth (Oliver, Brown, & Löe, 1998). The extent of periodontal disease refers to the number or percentage of diseased teeth or sites per individual.

Epidemiologic research is used to detect the underlying patterns of a disease and its associated factors to help find the cause of the disease. Trends are detectable when data collected from large numbers of individuals from within a study population are combined. For a survey to be useful, the clinical assessments must be standardized so that population means (averages) can be determined.

Epidemiologic data are collected through the use of a specific methodology that differs from patient evaluations in private practice. Complete, full-mouth periodontal examinations, which are necessary to establish an individual's diagnosis and to determine treatment needs, are too time-consuming for use on a large scale in an epidemiologic survey. The survey methods used to evaluate periodontal diseases in a population usually involve screening tools designed to quantify and simplify the disease assessment. These tools are referred to as indices (singular: index). An index is a numerical expression of values, with upper and lower limits, that is used to describe a specific condition. Indices are used in both clinical practice and research as the system of measurement for collecting data. They provide the private practitioner with information for patient treatment planning and the researcher with information about the prevalence and incidence of disease.

Indices

Significance of Indices

Epidemiology is used to identify disease patterns, and indices are the measurement systems used for collecting the necessary data. For the study of periodontal diseases, assessments of plaque, calculus, gingival inflammation, periodontal attachment level, bleeding, and mobility are necessary to determine individual disease status. An index is a tool for standardized data collection and can measure the presence, absence, or severity of a disease condition on a specific tooth, area, or whole mouth and then can be extrapolated to the population. Unlike subjective clinician assessments of parameters of disease, an index is a numerical expression given to conditions that can then be quantified, tabulated, and used in comparisons to predict disease patterns, progression, and trends in study populations.

If a dental hygienist examines a patient and subjectively describes the condition of oral cleanliness in the mouth as "a fair amount of plaque and calculus on the teeth," this description could be interpreted differently by another clinician and might be interpreted as light or moderate plaque levels. Terms such as fair, light, moderate, and heavy have different meaning for different practitioners and therefore need to be standardized. The use of indices can help to standardize and reproduce findings for the purpose of assessment and monitoring patients' progression in private practice.

Dentists and dental hygienists formulate treatment plans based on full-mouth data collection. Becoming aware of the periodontal problem, assessing its severity, and presenting the findings to the patient require the practitioner to record and chart data in formats that can be compared over time. Periodontal charting forms and indices tabulate the measurements to be interpreted for treatment plans.

Indices measure disease outcomes and so measure past disease. When a dental hygienist supplements a patient's clinical examination with index scores to monitor patient conditions over time, these data, along with information gleaned from population surveys, can help the clinician predict future disease progression and establish a prognosis for the individual patient.

Criteria for Indices

There are many types of indices a practitioner can select from depending on the specific method of data collection and the meaning to be given to the data collected. When selecting an index or set of indices, the following properties should be considered:

1. Simplicity or ease of use is critical to provide a fast and reproducible method to collect the data. Reproducibility creates a reliable instrument that can be used by different examiners or the same examiner over time to produce the same results.
2. The index should be quick to perform and practical. Whether in the field for research purposes or in a dental practice, the method of data collection must not be time-consuming, costly, or involve many instruments.

3. Sensitivity requires the index to detect small changes. Sensitivity determines if the disease is really present and can be seen. A true-positive result would indicate that the disease or condition exists.
4. Validity provides the correlation of the disease with the measure employed. If bleeding on probing is to be measured, then the index can be confounded by other variables such as probing pressure, spontaneous bleeding, or instrumentation differences. A valid index must measure what it intended to measure.
5. Reliability
6. Acceptable to subjects involved
7. Amenable to statistical analysis
8. Clinically significant and meaningful to researchers

There is no perfect index or one that assesses all categories of inquiry. There are numerous indices, and the practitioner must select the best ones to represent the disease under examination or the health of the patient. There are over 40 types of indices in periodontics. They fall into four general categories: oral hygiene indices (plaque and calculus), gingival indices, periodontal (destruction) indices, and treatment needs indices. An overview of historically important and commonly used indices is presented in Table 3–1■ and is reviewed briefly below.

Plaque and Debris Indices

Oral cleanliness is quantified by indices that measure plaque and debris and indices that measure calculus. Since plaque is considered the primary cause or risk factor of periodontal diseases, methods of measuring plaque (debris) are important epidemiologically and are useful to practitioners treating the disease. Many plaque indices are used today. Some are meant simply as screening tools in clinical practice to assess home-care practices, whereas others are designed to quantify and locate plaque as needed for the evaluation of plaque-control devices or products before and after use.

One of the simplest methods of monitoring patient plaque levels is the use of the O'Leary Plaque Index (O'Leary, Drake, & Naylor, 1972), also called the plaque control record. A visual record of plaque control is made using a disclosing agent. A diagram is made of plaque-covered surfaces that can be shared with patients to visually help them identify problem areas and focus their efforts at home. O'Leary and colleagues (1972) recommended reduction of plaque levels to 10% of the available tooth surfaces as the patient's goal for home-care mastery.

Other common plaque indices are the Plaque Index (PlI) (Silness & Löe, 1964), the Debris Index (DI-S) of the Simplified Oral Hygiene Index (Greene, 1967), and the modified Quigley-Hein Plaque Index (Turesky, Gilmore, & Glickman, 1970). These plaque indices provide subjective numerical values that quantify the amount of plaque present, unlike the O'Leary Index, which merely indicates the presence or absence of plaque and is most suited for patient education and motivation in private practice rather than epidemiologic surveys.

The Plaque Index (PlI) (Silness & Löe, 1964) scores the plaque thickness along the gingival margin of the tooth, whereas the Debris Index (DS-I) measures plaque surface area. The Debris Index is a component of the Simplified Oral Hygiene Index (OHI-S) developed by Greene and Vermillion (1964). The other component

(text continues on p. 49)

Table 3–1   Indices Used for Periodontal Disease Assessments

Index	Type of Measure	Teeth Measured	Method of Measurement	Scale of Measurement	Purpose	Advantages	Disadvantages	Uses
O'Leary (O'Leary, Drake, and Naylor, 1972)	Plaque	All teeth are scored at the cervical third of the tooth. Four surfaces of each tooth (M, B, D, L,) are measured.	A plaque record is made by marking a tooth diagram with the surface location of plaque. Mark each tooth surface with plaque as positive (disclosing agent used).	Calculation: Surfaces with plaque divided by the total number of surfaces. Multiply by 100 to get the percent of surfaces with plaque. Patient goal of 10% or less of plaque is ideal.	Visual record of plaque distribution; shows patients where they are insufficient in plaque removal; patient motivation.	Complete assessment of all tooth surfaces to determine areas of cleaning deficiency.	Will not pick up changes in plaque quantity at each tooth surface; time-consuming.	Private practice.
Plaque Index (PlI) (Silness and Löe, 1964)	Plaque	All teeth (distal, facial, mesial, lingual) or selected teeth.	Sweep a probe along the tooth surface at the gingival margin. (No disclosing agent is used.) The score (0, 1, 2, or 3) per tooth is obtained by summing the four different surface scores and dividing by four. Adding each tooth score and dividing by the number of teeth evaluated generates a patient score. Excellent: 0 Poor: 2.0–3.0	0 No plaque 1 A thinly adherent layer of plaque visible only when a probe is run across the tooth 2 A visible layer of plaque which is thin to moderately thick 3 Heavy plaque accumulation in the crevice and the gingival margin	Measures the thickness or amount of plaque along the gingival margin.	Good for research purposes because qualitative changes can be measured; not as time-consuming if selected teeth are used.	Somewhat subjective; limited to the cervical portion of the tooth, not for patient motivation.	Clinical studies, epidemiologic surveys.
Simplified Debris Index (DI-S) of the Simplified Oral Hygiene Index (OHI-S) (Greene and Vermillion 1964)	Soft debris	Six tooth surfaces per mouth are scored: facial surfaces of teeth nos. 3,8,14,24, and lingual surfaces of teeth nos. 19,30. If the first molars are missing, choose the first fully erupted tooth distal to the second premolar.	Each tooth is divided into gingival, middle, and incisal thirds. Scoring is done by moving a no. 23 explorer from the incisal third toward the gingival third of the tooth. No disclosing agent is used.	0 No stain or debris 1 Soft deposit covering ≤ 1/3 of the surface or the presence of extrinsic stain 2 Soft deposit covering more than 1/3 but less than 2/3 of the tooth surface 3 Soft deposit covering > 2/3 of the tooth surface.	Measures plaque surface area.	Measures the quantity of debris rather than the presence or absence; not as time-consuming.	Somewhat subjective.	Epidemiologic and research projects.

(continued)

Table 3–1 Indices Used for Periodontal Disease Assessments (cont.)

Index	Type of Measure	Teeth Measured	Method of Measurement	Scale of Measurement	Purpose	Advantages	Disadvantages	Uses
			Score as 0, 1, 2, 3. Calculation: total of surface scores divided by the number of surfaces scored Good score: 0.0–0.6 Poor score: 1.9–3.0					
Turesky Modification of the Quigley-Hein Index (Turesky, Gilmore, and Glickman 1970)	Plaque	Facial and lingual surfaces of all teeth excluding the third molars.	Score as 0, 1, 2, 3, 4, 5. Disclosing agent is used. Calculation: Total of all scores divided by the number of surfaces examined	0 No plaque 1 Flecks of plaque at the cervical margin 2 Thin, continuous band of plaque (≤ 1 mm) at the cervical margin 3 Band of plaque wider than a 1 mm but covering less than 1/3 of crown. 4 Plaque covering at least 1/3 but less than 2/3 of the crown 5 Plaque covering more than 2/3 of the crown	Measures surface area of plaque.	The additional scoring categories allow the researcher to quantify improvement or change in plaque levels after the use of a plaque-control device or topical antimicrobial.	Somewhat subjective; time-consuming.	Index of choice in clinical trials.
Simplified Calculus Index (CI-S); part of the OHI-S (Greene 1967)	Calculus	Six tooth surfaces per mouth are scored: facial surfaces of teeth nos. 3, 8, 14, 24, and lingual surfaces of teeth nos. 19, 30. If the first molars are missing, choose the first fully erupted tooth distal to the second premolar.	Score as 0, 1, 2, 3. Calculation: total calculus scores divided by the number of surfaces scored. To tabulate the total OHI-S, add the DI-S + CI-S. Combined OHI-S: Good: 0.0–1.2 Poor: 3.1–6.0	0 No calculus present 1 Supragingival calculus covering ≤ 1/3 of the exposed tooth 2 Supragingival calculus covering more than 1/3 but 2/3 or less of exposed tooth or separate flecks of subgingival calculus in the cervical region 3 Supragingival calculus covering more than 2/3 of exposed tooth or a continuous heavy band of sub gingival calculus	Quantifies calculus.	Well-defined criteria, allows for interexaminer reproducibility.	Combines location and quantity.	Epidemiologic and longitudinal studies.

Index		Area	Method	Scoring	Measures	Advantage	Disadvantage	Uses
Volpe Manhold Calculus Assessment (Volpe, Manhold, and Hazen 1965)	Calculus	Mandibular incisors and cuspids (lingual surfaces).	With a probe, the coronal extension of supragingival calculus is measured in millimeters. Three readings are made bisecting the dimension of calculus at the direct lingual and mesial and distal line angles. These readings are averaged to generate a tooth score, and the individual tooth scores are averaged to provide the total patient score.	Readings are scored in millimeter markings from the probe.	Measures the height or dimension of calculus.	Ability to measure the rate of calculus formation.	Difficult to master.	Clinical studies and epidemiologic studies.
Calculus Index of the National Institute of Dental Research (Miller et al. 1987)	Calculus	Mesiobuccal and midbuccal surfaces of all fully erupted permanent teeth present in two randomly selected quadrants (one mandibular and the other maxillary).	Detected by explorer or probe.	0 No calculus 1 Supragingival calculus only (calculus on the crown and root not extending more than 1 mm below the gingival margin) 2 Subgingival calculus is detected with or without supragingival calculus	Presence or absence and location supra- or subgingival.	Simple.	Unable to quantify amount of calculus.	Used in the National Health and Nutrition and Examination Survey (NHANES III).
Gingival Index (GI) (Löe 1967)	Gingival inflammation	Four gingival areas (buccal, mesial, distal, and lingual) for all teeth or select teeth.	Probe is inserted into the gingival crevice and moved with a sweeping along the pocket wall. Probe is also pressed lightly against the gingiva to determine its firmness. Calculation: Each of the four gingival areas per tooth is given a GI score of 0 to 3. Total the scores for each	0 Normal gingiva 1 Mild inflammation with slight changes in color and edema (swelling); no bleeding on probing 2 Moderate inflammation with redness, edema, and glazing; bleeding on probing 3 Severe inflammation with marked redness and edema; tendency to spontaneously bleed	Measures severity of gingivitis.	Can detect change in degree of inflammation.	Somewhat subjective, time-consuming.	Epidemiologic and clinical studies.

(continued)

45

Table 3-1 Indices Used for Periodontal Disease Assessments (cont.)

Index	Type of Measure	Teeth Measured	Method of Measurement	Scale of Measurement	Purpose	Advantages	Disadvantages	Uses
			area and divide by the number of teeth scored. Good: 0.0–1.0 Fair: 1.1–2.0 Poor: 2.1–3.0					
Sulcus Bleeding Index (Mühlemann and Son 1971)	Gingival inflammation	Three gingival areas (facial and lingual marginal gingival and mesial and distal interdental papillae) for all teeth.	Insert probe in the sulcus and withdraw it. Wait 30 seconds to score the area. Calculation: Total the scores for each tooth, and divide by the number of teeth.	0 Healthy appearance with no bleeding on probing 1 Healthy but with bleeding on probing 2 Bleeding on probing and color change but no swelling 3 Bleeding on probing, color change, and slight edema 4 Bleeding on probing and obvious swelling with or without color change 5 Bleeding on probing and spontaneous bleeding and color change, marked swelling with or without ulceration	Presence or absence and severity of gingival inflammation.	Less subjective, more gradations of severe inflammation.	Criticized for scores beyond clinical gingivitis.	Clinical and epidemiologic studies.
Periodontal Index (PI) (Russell 1967)	Inflammation, pocket depth, tooth mobility (visual assessment, without periodontal probing)	All teeth.	Each tooth is given a score from 0 (no disease) to 8 (severe disease) Calculation: Add up the scores for all teeth, and divide by the number of teeth scored.	0 Tooth with healthy periodontium 1 Mild gingivitis, localized and does not involve the entire tooth 2 Gingivitis encircling the entire tooth 6 Gingivitis with pocket formation	Measures the severity of the periodontal condition.	Objective measures.	Visual assessment that often underestimates disease; evaluates both gingivitis and periodontitis in the same index.	National epidemiologic surveys including the National Health and Nutrition Examination Survey (1971–1974).

					Simple.	

				with no loss of function or mobility 8 Advanced destruction with tooth mobility		Only selective teeth are measured, which may underestimate the disease.	Epidemiologic surveys (specifically designed by the WHO to compare population surveys internationally).
			0.0–0.2: normal periodontal condition 0.3–0.9: simple gingivitis 0.–1.9: early destructive periodontitis 1.6–5.0: established periodontitis 3.8–8.0: terminal disease				
Community Periodontal Index of Treatment Needs (Ainamo et al. 1982)	Periodontal pockets, calculus, gingival bleeding	Ten teeth: 2, 3, 8, 14, 15, 18, 19, 24, 30, 31	A 0.5-mm ball-tip probe with demarcations for shallow (3.5-mm) and deep (5.5-mm) pockets (CIPTN probe) is used to detect and record the presence of bleeding, calculus, and periodontal pockets. The individual is scored by sextant assigning the worst tooth score per sextant as the overall sextant score. Treatment needs are assigned based on the highest code received by each sextant. 0 No further therapy needed. 1 Patient only requires oral home-care instruction 2 Patient requires oral hygiene improvement and professional scaling 3 Patient requires oral hygiene improvement and professional scaling 4 Patient requires complex treatment (scaling and root	Code 0: No pocketing or inflammation Code 1: Bleeding on probing Code 2: Calculus present Code 3: Pocketing extending in to the black area of the probe (4–5 mm) Code 4: Pocketing extending beyond the black area of the probe (≤ 6 mm)	Measures severity of the periodontal condition and treatment needs.		

47

Table 3–1 Indices Used for Periodontal Disease Assessments (*cont.*)

Index	Type of Measure	Teeth Measured	Method of Measurement	Scale of Measurement	Purpose	Advantages	Disadvantages	Uses
Periodontal Screening and Recording (PSR) (AAP 1992)	Periodontal pockets, calculus, bleeding, and defective restorations	Mouth is divided into sextants. All teeth are measured.	Each tooth in the sextant is probed, and the tooth with the worst score determines the sextant score. The highest-scoring sextant determines the individual's overall management. If two or more sextants have a score of 3 or any one sextant has a score of 4, then a complete periodontal charting is advised. Scores of 0 or 1 require preventive measures inclusive of home-care instructions. Scores of 2 or greater require the patient to have additional professional cleaning and correction of defective restorations.	Code 0–No calculus, defective margins, or bleeding, and the black band of the probe is completely visible (probing depth less than 3.5 mm) Code 1–No calculus or defective margins, but there is bleeding, and the black band of the probe is completely visible Code 2–Supragingival or subgingival calculus or defective markings are present, but the black band is still visible Code 3–Calculus, defective restorations, and bleeding may or may not be present, and the black band is partly visible (probing depth more than 3.5 mm but less than 5.5 mm) Code 4–The black band of the probe is not visible (probing depth more than 5.5 mm) An asterisk (*) is added if any additional pathology is present, such as furcations.	Screening of periodontal disease in private practice.	Simplifies the charting of an individual's periodontal condition when extensive treatment is not required.	Cannot be substituted for a complete periodontal charting necessary for the treatment of periodontitis	Private practice.

planing with dental anesthesia and may require periodontal surgery)

of the OHI-S is a Calculus Index (CI-S). The OHI-S is used primarily for epidemiologic and longitudinal dental studies.

Another plaque index used more specifically for clinical trials is the Turesky Modification of the Quigley-Hein Index (Turesky, et al., 1970). Plaque is assessed on all facial and lingual tooth surfaces (excluding third molars) after a disclosing agent is applied. The additional scoring categories of this index allow researchers to quantify improvement or change in plaque levels after the use of a plaque-control device or topical antimicrobial. Both the modified Quigley-Hein Index and the Plaque Index (PlI) are suitable for the evaluation of topical antimicrobials and plaque-removal devices (Fischman, 1986).

In summary, a number of plaque indices are used today. Four plaque indices were presented, and each serves different purposes. The plaque control record (O'Leary et al., 1972) is used most commonly in periodontal practice, whereas the others are used more frequently in clinical trials and population surveys.

Calculus Indices

In clinical practice, calculus is not monitored by a numeric index, but is in epidemiologic surveys. Numerous methods have been devised to quantify this deposit, and three commonly used calculus indices will be presented here (see Table 3–1).

The simplified Calculus Index (CS-1), which is part of the OHI-S mentioned previously (Greene, 1967), is valuable for epidemiologic surveys and longitudinal studies and quantifies calculus by location and surface area. Another common calculus evaluation is the Volpe Manhold Calculus Assessment (Volpe, Kupczak, & King, 1967; Volpe, Manhold, & Hazen, 1965), which measures the height and dimension of the calculus present. It was designed originally for use on the lingual surfaces of the mandibular incisors but can be used throughout the mouth.

National epidemiologic studies, conducted through the National Institute of Dental Research (NIDR), have developed and used their own calculus index (Miller, Brunelle, Carlos, Brown, & Löe, 1987). The NIDR Index merely indicates the presence or absence of calculus supragingivally or subgingivally. This index was used for the third National Health and Nutrition Examination Survey (NHANES III), conducted by the National Center for the Health Statistics in collaboration with the National Institute for Dental Research from 1988 to 1991.

Gingival Indices

The epidemiologic tool used to quickly assess gingival inflammation is the gingival index. A gingival index is designed to measure the degree of visible inflammation of the gingival tissues. Visible signs of gingival inflammation are bleeding, redness, and swelling. These are accepted clinical signs of inflammation and also have been incorporated into indices for evaluation of the periodontal status of individuals and populations.

The Gingival Index (GI) of Löe and Silness (Löe, 1967) is based on the subjective assessment of the visual indicators of gingival inflammation. The degree of inflammation is subdivided into three categories, with moderate inflammation determined by the presence of bleeding and severe inflammation determined by spontaneous bleeding. The GI historically has been used for epidemiologic studies. Lobene, Weatherford, Ross, Lam, and Menaker (1986) modified this index for use in clinical trials evaluating plaque-control products. The Modified Gingival Index (Lobene et al., 1986) assesses gingival health by looking only at qualitative changes in the gingiva. Unlike the GI, which uses bleeding as an indicator of increasing severity of gingival inflammation, this index does not use bleeding on probing and has more gradations. The Modified Gingival Index is scored to pick up subtle changes earlier with four different scores for gingival inflammation.

Other gingival indices based primarily on bleeding include the Sulcus Bleeding Index (Mühlemann & Son, 1971) and the Eastman Interdental Bleeding Index (Caton & Polson, 1985). Gingival bleeding as a measure of gingival inflammation is considered a more objective measure, whereas gingival color and consistency are more subjective. For this index, gingival bleeding is determined by gently inserting a probe in the sulcus and withdrawing it. Mühlemann and Son (1971) based the Sulcus Bleeding Index on bleeding being the earliest symptom of gingivitis, but it has been criticized because distinctions are not made beyond the clinical point of gingivitis.

A novel approach to determining bleeding is the use of a triangular toothpick (e.g., Stimudent) rather than a periodontal probe. The Interdental Bleeding Index (Caton & Polson, 1985) uses interdental cleaners to evaluate bleeding in the mid-proximal gingival tissues where periodontal changes are most likely to be found. The interdental cleaner is inserted between teeth and removed, depressing the interdental papilla 1 to 2 mm. Fifteen seconds after insertion and removal, bleeding is recorded.

In an attempt to achieve a more objective measure, gingival bleeding is being used increasingly for the determination of gingival changes in epidemiologic studies. The presence or absence of bleeding has been used in current demographic studies, in the NIDR Adult Survey (1985–1986) (Brown, Oliver, & Löe, 1989), and in NHANES III (1988–1991) (Brown, Brunelle, & Kingman, 1996). Gingival bleeding also has been used to monitor patient home oral hygiene practices. The percentage of bleeding sites is considered a more accurate representation of the patient's true level of daily home care. Bleeding and gingival indices also have been monitored along with individual attachment levels and pocket bacteria to find markers or predictors of disease activity.

Indices of Periodontal Destruction

Another essential measure employed in epidemiologic studies is evaluation of periodontal destruction. Indices of periodontal destruction are designed to measure disease severity and extent by observing the outcomes of periodontal destruction. This is done by measuring clinical attachment loss and probing depth and recording bone loss and loss of function. Current national studies use direct measures of these disease outcomes. These measures are taken at the midbuccal and mesiobuccal levels of all fully erupted teeth (Brown et al., 1996). Even though current national surveys do not employ periodontal indices or directly measure the outcome of destruction, much of the historical data pertinent to periodontal diseases in the United States have been compiled using periodontal indices.

The Periodontal Index (PI) (Russell, 1967) has been a standard measure for the large national surveys that are responsible for early views of periodontal disease prevalence and incidence in the United States. The PI is a visual index and does not use a periodontal probe. The presence of inflammation, pocket formation, and loss of function is assessed visually as criteria for numeric scoring of teeth.

Two additional indices of epidemiologic importance evaluate periodontal destruction and designate treatment needs. The Community Periodontal Index of Treatment Needs (CPITN; Ainamo, Barmes, Beargie, Cutress, & Martin, 1982) was developed by an initiative of the World Health Organization (WHO) expressly for population studies. Its primary focus is to assess treatment needs.

The CPITN was modified to the Periodontal Screening and Recording (PSR) system for general-practice use. The PSR system was developed to evaluate individual treatment needs and to be used as a quick screening tool to document new patient periodontal findings in lieu of a complete periodontal charting. It has been endorsed by the American Academy of Periodontology and the American Dental Association as a quick and easy method to record the periodontal status of a patient in the private-practice setting. This screening tool reduces the number of patients that need a complete periodontal charting simply by identifying those with periodontal treatment needs and therefore the need for a complete periodontal charting.

The CPITN probe is used in the PSR system, and the same parameters employed by the CPITN are evaluated—bleeding, calculus, and probing depth. The CPITN probe has a ball tip to aid in calculus detection and a black band that demarcates probing depth from 3.5 to 5.5 mm. It was developed to increase the recognition and treatment of periodontal disease in the general dental practice. Generation of the PSR score is the responsibility of the dental hygienist, especially for recall visits.

Accuracy of Methodology

Thus far the tools used for assessing the periodontal condition in epidemiologic studies have been described. These tools define or identify individuals within a population with periodontal disease. The sampling methodology for population studies differs from that used in clinical periodontics and can influence the accuracy of the data obtained. Epidemiologic data-collection tools do not measure all the periodontal findings a clinician might use to establish a diagnosis and prognosis, such as furcation involvement or tooth mobility. Population studies, because of their large sample sizes, use indices as assessment tools, unlike diagnostic evaluations in clinical practice, and thus only score a portion of the mouth. To streamline the examination process, partial mouth scores are incorporated into indices. Partial mouth observations improve study efficiency but reduce the accuracy of overall reporting of periodontal disease prevalence and incidence.

For example, the CPITN measures only ten teeth in the mouth. Baelum, Manji, Fejerskov, and Wanzala (1993) found that the prevalence of teeth with moderate to deep pockets was underreported in the partial mouth scores of the CPITN. This was especially true for severe periodontal conditions. In another report, Baelum, Manji, Wanzala, and Fejerskov (1995) concluded that the CPITN scores tend to underestimate prevalence and severity in younger age groups and overestimate the same in the elderly. The methodology employed by the NIDR for the most recent survey, NHANES III, also involves a partial mouth evaluation. As described earlier, periodontal probing is performed in half the mouth. When half-mouth and full-mouth scores were compared (Hunt & Fann, 1991), the results were similar. Half-mouth examination was considered accurate in estimating the prevalence of periodontal disease but still underestimated the percentage of the population with more advanced disease (periodontal attachment loss). A review by Papapanou (1996) concluded that the current NIDR methodology is inadequate because it is a combination of partial scores (e.g., only two sites per tooth are measured in only one-half of the mouth). Papapanou contended that the location of the pocket and the number of probing measures could have a profound influence on the outcome of the study. Partly because previous studies comparing half-mouth scores with full-mouth scores had used partial scores for their comparison, not all probing sites encircling a tooth were measured. When combining partial mouth scores with measures at only the midbuccal and mesiobuccal sites, current methodology actually could produce a mean percentage underestimation of deep pockets of 40% and an underestimation of the prevalence of these deep pockets of 58%.

The validity of an index in describing a population also can be affected by tooth loss. Missing teeth may have been the ones most severely affected by periodontitis. Since they are no longer present to be measured, there is a built-in selection bias for the healthier teeth still present, potentially underestimating both severity and prevalence of the disease (periodontitis). Thus the overall reliability of an index is affected by the method of data collection. It is difficult to have one tool that will be representative, accurate, and efficient at the same time for all periodontal measures. Historical and modern data are based on methodologies that have been criticized, but some researchers contend that they still render an adequate estimation of disease.

Prevalence of Periodontal Diseases

National surveys have helped build our knowledge of the prevalence, severity, and extent of periodontal diseases in the United States. Based on the results of these surveys, the commonly accepted model for periodontal diseases has changed and evolved. Historically, periodontal disease was considered inevitable, and all individuals were susceptible to advanced periodontal disease, gingivitis being its precursor. In essence, periodontal disease was considered universal, and the susceptibility to periodontitis increased with age (Waerhaug, 1966).

Information gathered from more recent national surveys, however, suggests otherwise. More severe disease (advanced periodontitis) was found in only 5 to 20% of adults (U.S. Public Health Service, 1987), and moderate disease (periodontitis) was found in the majority of adults (U.S. Public Health Service, 1987). Thus only a few individuals will be susceptible to advanced disease. Today, periodontitis is not considered part of the aging process but occurs because of the interaction of bacteria and the immune response of the individual.

Prevalence of Gingivitis

Gingivitis is the most common form of periodontal disease found in individuals of all ages; it can even occur in early childhood (Ayers, Abrama, & Lausten, 1979). In the U.S. Health and Resources and Service Administration (HRSA) study of 1981 (Brown, Oliver, & Löe, 1989), 54% of adults over age 18 were affected with gingivitis involving at least six or more teeth. Another national study of employed adults between the ages of 18 and 64, the NIDR Adult Survey (1985–1986), reported less gingivitis, finding that 44% of the sample had gingivitis (defined by gingival bleeding) (Miller et al., 1987). The average involvement was 2.7 sites per person, and the extent of gingivitis increased with age. In the more recent NHANES III study (Brown et al., 1996), gingival bleeding was present in 63% of those examined, and 12% of all sites examined bled on probing. Gingivitis was slightly more prevalent in teenagers (13–17 years). The extent was similar among all age groups, ranging from 10 to 15% of the sites examined. Plaque and calculus deposits correlated with the prevalence of gingivitis, and subgingival calculus were found in 67% of the population and at 22% of the sites evaluated.

When compared with earlier national surveys, gingivitis has declined in the United States most likely due to the current focus on oral hygiene as part of a daily personal hygiene routine (Burt, 1996). In the early 1960s, visual assessments revealed that 85% of men and 79% of women had gingivitis. Current surveys report that 63% of the population has gingival bleeding and that gingivitis is found in 44 to 54% of the population. This differs considerably from reports from Third World countries, where gingivitis in the presence of extensive plaque and calculus is considered normal among adults (Löe, Anerud, Boysen, & Smith, 1978).

Prevalence of Periodontitis

Chronic periodontitis, a more severe form of periodontal disease, is not commonly found among young individuals and is more prevalent with age. The NHANES III study (Brown et al., 1996) (n = 7,447 surveyed) found that over 90% of individuals over age 13 had some attachment loss, with only 15% of the population having advanced disease (defined as 5 mm or more of attachment loss). If the definition of attachment loss were limited to 3 mm or more, the prevalence was 40%. One-quarter of the individuals surveyed showed moderate attachment loss (3–4 mm). With increasing age, the prevalence of moderate and severe attachment loss increased, but the prevalence of pockets 4 mm or greater and 6 mm or greater in size remained the same. Since the extent and prevalence of attachment loss were found to increase with age and the prevalence of 4-mm or greater pocket depths did not, increased gingival recession was deemed responsible for the increased attachment loss experienced with age (Oliver et al., 1998).

In the HRSA survey (Brown et al., 1989), periodontitis (at least one tooth with a pocket 4 mm or deeper) was found in 36% of the 7,078 individuals examined. The prevalence of the disease increased with age. Twenty-nine percent of individuals in the 19- to 44-year-old age group were affected, whereas almost 50% of individuals 45 years of age or older were affected. The percentage of elderly individuals (age 65 and older) with pockets was similar to that of the 45- to 64-year-old age group, although the number of teeth present decreased. Periodontitis, when present, usually involved only a few teeth, and advanced periodontitis was relatively rare.

In the NIDR study of employed adults between the ages of 18 and 64 (Brown et al., 1990), almost all had some attachment loss, with 44% experiencing attachment loss of 3 mm or more. Moderate pocket depths (4–6 mm) were present in only 13.4% of those examined, generally affecting only one to two sites. More advanced disease again was considered rare and was found in only 0.6% of the study population. Males experienced more disease than females, and blacks were more affected than whites.

In the NHANES III study (Brown et al., 1996), racial and gender differences were reported as well. Females overall were in better periodontal health than their male counterparts, and non-Hispanic whites had less periodontal disease than non-Hispanic blacks or Mexican Americans. Overall, the United States has a relatively low prevalence and severity of periodontal disease compared with the rest of the world, and the severity and extent of disease have declined in the past 30 years (Oliver et al., 1998).

Prevalence of Aggressive Periodontitis

The prevalence of aggressive periodontitis (replaces the older term "early-onset periodontitis"), has been estimated to be less than 1% of the general population (Papapanou, 1996). It is considered a rare form of periodontal disease. A review of national population studies indicates that approximately 3.6% of individuals between the ages of 18 and 34 (NIDR Adult Survey, 1985–1986; Oliver et al., 1998) have moderate periodontal disease. Among 14- to 17-year-olds (Löe & Brown, 1991), the prevalence of all forms of aggressive periodontitis was 2.27%, 0.53% were affected by localized aggressive periodontitis (older term is localized juvenile periodontitis) and 0.13% were estimated to be affected by generalized aggressive periodontitis (replaces the older term "generalized juvenile periodontitis").

Racial differences also have been reported. Blacks were affected more often than whites by all forms of aggressive periodontitis. Ironically, racial and gender prevalences reported by recent national surveys do not match diagnostic criteria used to define and distinguish forms of aggressive periodontitis from chronic periodontitis. In a national (NIDR) study of over 11,000 adolescents between the ages of 14 and 17, gender differences existed and were influenced by race. For example, black males were 2.9 times more likely to have localized aggressive periodontitis than black females, and white females were more frequently affected by localized aggressive periodontitis than white males by the same amount. Males, in general, were 4.3 times more likely to have generalized juvenile (aggressive) periodontitis than females. When these results were extrapolated to the racial mix of the U.S. population in general, about 87,000 cases of localized and generalized aggressive periodontitis were estimated among 13 million 14- to 17-year-olds (Oliver et al., 1998).

Traditionally, black females have been reported to be two to three times more likely to have aggressive periodontitis than white females. It has been suggested that clinical trials and case reports used to establish this racial and gender predilection may have been skewed by ascertainment bias because more females will seek dental treatment and participate in clinical trials than males (Oliver et al., 1998). Thus a national survey that does not start out with this selection bias may more accurately reflect the national population prevalence.

In summary, the national status of periodontal disease has been gleaned by three recent national surveys: the NIDR, NHANES III, and HRSA surveys. About 50% of all American adults have gingivitis involving three to four teeth. Periodontitis is experienced in over 90% of the population over 13 years of age, but only 15% have severe disease. There is a specific small subset of the population that has more advanced disease. Aggressive periodontitis is considered a rare disease in the United States and affects only 0.53 to 3.6% of individuals under age 35. Overall, the national prevalence of gingivitis has declined over the past 30 years, but the prevalence of periodontitis has remained the same, but the severity of disease has decreased (Capilouto & Douglass, 1988).

Incidence and Disease Progression

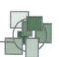

National surveys used to estimate disease prevalence are cross-sectional, which means that the study population is evaluated at only one point in time. To determine the natural progression of periodontal diseases, longitudinal studies are necessary, where individuals are examined at multiple intervals. Few longitudinal studies are available because of the difficulty of conducting them. In a 15-year longitudinal study by Löe and colleagues (1986), 480 Sri Lankan tea workers with untreated disease were evaluated. About 8% had rapid progression of their periodontitis, and most had a moderate rate of disease progression. A small portion of this population (11%) showed no progression beyond gingivitis despite the presence of heavy plaque and calculus.

A parallel study run in Norway (Löe et al., 1978) showed a different rate of disease progression. No cases of aggressive (juvenile) periodontitis were found, unlike the Sri Lankan study. The mean annual rate of attachment loss was 0.08 mm for interproximal and 0.1 mm for buccal surfaces as individuals approached 40 years of age. In patients with moderate periodontitis, progression occurred slowly at any given site. The rate of periodontal destruction did not increase with age, and therefore, the progression of periodontitis (extent and severity) appeared to be slow and continuous in this population.

In a report by Beck, Koch, and Offenbacher (1994) detailing a longitudinal study of adults identified with extensive attachment loss between the ages of 65 and 80 in North Carolina, additional evidence of slow disease progression also can be found. Only 12% of this population experienced 3 mm or more of attachment loss on one or more teeth during the 3-year study period. Again, it appears that subjects with a past history of periodontitis can be quite resistant to future disease (breakdown). Future attachment loss was associated with greater baseline probing depths, but the vast majority of sites that lost attachment had probing depths of 3 mm or less at baseline. Individuals who experienced attachment loss in the first 18 months of the study were more likely to experience attachment loss in the subsequent 18-month period.

Racial differences also were detected. Blacks tended to experience more attachment loss during both 18-month periods of the study. Only 45% of blacks had no attachment loss during the 3-year period, whereas 63% of whites were free of attachment loss. Despite having advanced attachment loss at the outset of the study, both blacks and whites had a high frequency of no further disease progression. Similarly, adult subjects with gingivitis monitored over a 3-year period had no detectable increase in probing depth (Listgarten, Schifter, & Laster, 1985). In a review by Stamm (1986), the incidence of gingivitis was greatest at puberty, declined through age 17, and then remained steady.

These studies imply that only select individuals or a small portion of the population will have new disease or disease progression. In another U.S. study by Löe and Brown (1991), only a small portion of the study population had the highest rate of disease progression, as noted by attachment loss; this subset of the population was identified with aggressive periodontitis. In the Beck and colleagues (1994) study of elderly adults, disease progression was more likely when extensive bone loss and tooth loss were experienced at a young age, again alluding to a specific subset of the population with a higher incidence of disease. In sum, only a small portion of the population will experience incidence and progression of severe attachment loss. This attachment loss will not progress at the same rate but may be episodic. The progression of periodontal disease appears to be influenced by education level, socioeconomic factors, gender, and race. These variables will be discussed in the next section of this chapter.

Epidemiologic Variables

Risk Indicators

Risk indicators are demographic, behavioral, and socioeconomic characteristics that are associated with disease but not considered causal for the disease. Aging is considered a risk indicator for periodontal disease, but does not cause periodontal disease. With increasing age, the prevalence of periodontal disease increases, but the aging process is not responsible for the disease. It is believed that there is more disease with age because there is more exposure to plaque-induced inflammation over time. Other characteristics associated with an increased frequency of disease are the level of education, gender, and race. Females have less periodontal disease than males (Sheiham & Striffler, 1970). Caucasians were found to have less periodontal disease than Hispanics, Mexicans, Indians, and African Americans. It is hypothesized that these differences are due to the availability and use of dental services, oral home care, and preventive practices. For example, the higher levels of periodontal disease reported in males versus females are attributed to higher levels of plaque and less use of dental services. More education, higher income, and dental insurance reduce the risk of oral disease. Where extensive plaque, calculus, and gingival inflammation are considered normal among adults in Third World countries, an association is found with less education and low income, and generally, there is more attachment loss than in industrial nations of the Western world.

Risk Factors

Risk factors are characteristics that have been shown to directly cause periodontal disease. Causal links are established by longitudinal and cross-sectional studies. It is important to identify causal relationships so that oral disease can be prevented if a risk factor is modifiable. For example, it is accepted that dental plaque causes gingivitis, and thus plaque is considered a risk factor for gingivitis. Poor oral hygiene has been correlated strongly with periodontal disease. The NHANES I data showed an inverse relationship between tooth loss and good oral hygiene. The periodontal index (PI) and oral hygiene (OHI-S) index scores were significantly better in individuals with the least tooth loss (Burt, Ismail, & Eklund, 1985). However, the causal relationship is not clear-cut with periodontitis. Supragingival plaque and supragingival calculus are not as strongly correlated with periodontitis as with gingivitis (Bakdash, 1994; Löe et al., 1978). In a recent appraisal by Oliver and colleagues (1998), the presence of subgingival calculus appeared to be a better predictor of periodontitis but was not considered causal because there was an inconsistent relationship among the epidemiologic data regarding oral hygiene, plaque and calculus, and periodontitis. Sites with dental calculus frequently do not bleed or display attachment loss. In the NHANES III survey (Brown et al., 1996), no bleeding was found 88% of the time when subgingival calculus was present. Additionally, gingivitis does not always progress to periodontitis, which means that periodontitis will not always occur in the presence of plaque and calculus. One could infer from this inconsistency that poor oral hygiene is an important risk factor in individuals who are more susceptible based on their immune response to bacterial plaque.

Other risk factors for periodontitis are diabetes and tobacco use. The prevalence and extent of periodontal pockets are greater in diabetics than in nondiabetics. This is especially true for poorly controlled diabetics, who experience more attachment and bone loss than well-controlled diabetics with similar plaque levels (Seppälä, Seppälä, & Ainamo, 1993). Oliver and Tervonen (1994) outlined diabetes as a risk factor for extensive, severe periodontitis when the individual's diabetes is poorly controlled and the individual has extensive subgingival calculus from poor home care and lack of professional cleanings. In a recent report (Taylor et al., 1998), subjects with non-insulin-dependent diabetes mellitus (NIDDM) had more severe alveolar bone loss progression over a 2-year period than those without NIDDM.

Smoking has been well documented as a risk factor for periodontitis. An early National Health and Nutrition Survey (NHANES I) in 1971–1974 first demonstrated the relationship between smoking and periodontitis (Ismail et al., 1983) in the United States. More recent longitudinal studies confirm this relationship. One longitudinal study showed that smokers lost proximal bone twice as fast as nonsmokers (Bolin, Eklund, Frithiof, & Lavstedt, 1993). Even when plaque accumulation is minimal, smokers have more teeth with deeper pockets and alveolar bone loss than nonsmokers (Bergström & Eliasson, 1987; Bergström & Floderus-Myrhed, 1983). In a 3-year study conducted by Beck, Koch, and Offenbacher (1995), disease was more likely to progress if the subject was a cigarette smoker, had the presence of gram-negative anaerobes in his or her subgingival microbiota (especially *Porphyromonas gingivalis*), or had financial stress. All led to an increased risk for disease progression. Thus it is apparent that microbiota and stress could be considered risk factors for periodontitis.

Another longitudinal study running from 1959 to 1985 in Tecumseh, Michigan (Ismail, Morrison, Burt, Cafesse, & Kavanaugh, 1990), reported age, smoking, and the presence of tooth mobility as risk markers for future attachment loss (2 mm or more). It has been hypothesized (Papapanou, 1996) that periodontitis actually may have different factors associated with its initiation than those involved in its progression. Multiple factors may play a role in the induction and progression of periodontal disease. The commonly accepted risk factors are lack of oral cleanliness, smoking, and systemic disease (diabetes). Specific subgingival bacteria and socioeconomic stress also have been linked causally to periodontal disease through epidemiologic studies, but further evaluation is ongoing. Gender, race, and age may play a role in disease expression but are not causally linked to periodontal disease.

Treatment Needs

Information provided by epidemiologic surveys regarding gingival bleeding (gingival inflammation), subgingival calculus, and probing depths of 4 mm or greater is of great importance to the dental hygienist. These data represent clinical parameters used to decide when treatment of periodontal disease is necessary. Most individuals will need periodontal preventive care (Oliver et al., 1998), which is provided by the hygienist. Over 90% of people surveyed (NHANES III) have attachment loss, and only 15% of the population has advanced disease, suggesting that much of the treatment needs of the United States can be fulfilled by hygienists. More extensive, severe disease is found among minorities and those with less income and education. However, these are the same individuals who are less likely to seek or perceive the need for dental services. Tooth loss due to periodontal disease remains high in the United States (Brown et al., 1989). This suggests that public awareness and education about the preventive services of dental hygienists are paramount if those individuals who are most affected are to be treated before tooth loss due to periodontitis occurs.

Future Trends

The hygienist in the general dentist's office plays an important role in the treatment of periodontal patients. The general dentist office handles the management of early and some moderate cases of periodontitis, with delegation of preventive care to the hygienist. Prevention and education are important responsibilities of the dental hygienist. As epidemiologic studies elaborate and refine the interrelationship between periodontal infections and the systemic health of the patient, hygienists will need to include this information in patient education sessions. The impact of periodontal disease on the overall health of a patient has been the subject of recent news media attention. Periodontal infections as risk factors for other diseases such as coronary heart disease and preterm low-birth-weight babies and its interrelationship with diabetes will most likely trigger increased demand for dental hygiene services. As patient awareness of periodontal disease and its systemic implications increases, more individuals will specifically seek the preventive and periodontal scaling services of the dental hygienist.

Key Points

- Epidemiologic measurements used to assess periodontal diseases include plaque, calculus, gingival, and periodontal indices.
- Indices measure past disease activity rather than current disease activity or future periodontal breakdown.

- Gingivitis is the most common form of periodontal disease.
- Aggressive periodontitis is not common in the general population.
- Chronic periodontitis is prevalent in the general population.
- Numerous contributory risk factors influence the development and prevalence of periodontal diseases.

Web Sites

www.dentalarticles.com

www.perio.org

www.ada.org

Self-Quiz

1. Which one of the following modalities would best determine disease prevalence? (p. 40)
   a. comprehensive periodontal charting
   b. epidemiologic population surveys
   c. patient questionnaires
   d. national dental hygiene expenditures

2. Which one of the following terms describes the rate of new cases of periodontal disease occurring in a given time period? (p. 40)
   a. prevalence
   b. incidence
   c. severity
   d. extent
   e. index

3. An individual has been identified with advanced attachment loss at one point in time. Is it highly unlikely (infrequent) that this individual will again experience rapid attachment loss (>3 mm) within the next three years? (pp. 53–54)
   a. The first statement is true, and the second statement is false.
   b. The first statement is false, and the second statement is true.
   c. Both statements are true.
   d. Both statements are false.

4. Which one of the following indices is best used to monitor a patient's plaque control in private dental practice? (pp. 42, 49, 50, Table 3–1)
   a. Quigley-Hein Plaque Index
   b. Plaque Record (O'Leary)
   c. Periodontal Screening and Recording (PSR) system
   d. Sulcus Bleeding Index

5. Which one of the following best measures the severity of periodontal disease in a population? (pp. 40–42)
   a. radiographs
   b. intraoral cameras
   c. indices
   d. surgical costs

6. All of the following are risk factors for periodontal disease except one. Which one is the exception? (pp. 56–57)
   a. age
   b. smoking
   c. diabetes
   d. oral cleanliness

7. A risk indicator differs from a risk factor in that there is no causal relationship of the associated characteristic with the disease. Low income and less education are risk indicators for periodontal disease. (pp. 56–57)
   a. The first statement is true, and the second statement is false.
   b. The first statement is false, and the second statement is true.
   c. Both statements are true.
   d. Both statements are false.

8. According to recent surveys, which of the following percentages of the U.S. adult population has severe periodontal disease (advanced periodontitis)? (pp. 53–54)

   a. 5–20

   b. 40–50

   c. 70–80

   d. 90–100

9. Which one of the following describes how has the prevalence of gingivitis changed over the past 30 years? (p. 53)

   a. increased

   b. decreased

   c. remained the same

   d. increased in the first 10 years and then decreased

10. Which one of the following describes the prevalence of aggressive periodontitis in the general population? (p. 54)

    a. rare

    b. frequent

    c. universal

    d. nonexistent

References

Ainamo, J., D. Barmes, G. Beargie, T. Cutress, and J. Martin. 1982. Development of the World Health Organization (WHO) Community Periodontal Index of Treatment Needs (CPITN). *Int. Dent. J.* 32:281–291.

American Academy of Periodontology. 1992.

Ayers, C., A. Abrama, and L. Lausten. 1979. Oral health assessment of inner city preschoolers. *Dent. Hygiene* 53:465–468.

Baelum, V., F. Manji, O. Fejerskov, and P. Wanzala. 1993. Validity of CPITN's assumptions of hierarchical occurrence of periodontal conditions in a Kenyan population aged 15–65 years. *Commun. Dent. Oral Epidemiol.* 21:347–353.

Baelum, V., F. Manji, P. Wanzala, and O. Fejerskov. 1995. Relationship between CPITN and periodontal attachment loss findings in an adult population. *J. Clin. Periodontol.* 22:146–152.

Bakdash, B. 1994. Oral hygiene and compliance as risk factors in periodontitis. *J. Periodontol.* 65:539–544.

Beck, J., G. Koch, and S. Offenbacher. 1994. Attachment loss trend over 3 years in community-dwelling older adults. *J. Periodontol.* 65:737–743.

Beck, J., G. Koch, and S. Offenbacher. 1995. Incidence of attachment loss over 3 years in older adults: New and progressing lesions. *Commun. Dent. Oral Epidemiol.* 23:291–296.

Bergström, J., and S. Eliasson. 1987. Cigarette smoking and alveolar bone height in subjects with high standard oral hygiene. *J. Clin. Periodontol.* 14:466–469.

Bergström, J., and B. Floderus-Myrhed. 1983. Co-twin study of the relationship between smoking and some periodontal disease factors. *Commun. Dent. Oral Epidemiol.* 11:113–116.

Bolin, A., G. Eklund, L. Frithiof, and S. Lavstedt. 1993. The effect of changed smoking habits on marginal alveolar bone loss: A longitudinal study. *Swed. Dent. J.* 17:211–216.

Brown, L., J. Brunelle, and A. Kingman. 1996. Periodontal status in the United States, 1988–91: Prevalence, extent, and demographic variation. *J. Dent. Res.* 75 (spec issue): 672–683.

Brown, L., R. Oliver, and H. Löe. 1989. Periodontal diseases in the U.S. in 1981: Prevalence, severity, extent and role in tooth mortality. *J. Periodontol.* 60:363–371.

Brown, L., R. Oliver, and H. Löe. 1990. Evaluating periodontal status of U.S. employed adults. *J. Am. Dent. Assoc.* 121:226–232.

Burt, B. 1996. Epidemiology of periodontal diseases. *J. Periodontol.* 67:935–945.

Burt, B., A. Ismail, and S. Eklund. 1985. Periodontal disease, tooth loss and oral hygiene among older Americans. *Commun. Dent. Oral Epidemiol.* 13(2):93–96.

Capilouto, M., and C. Douglass. 1988. Trends in the prevalence and severity of periodontal disease in the U.S.: A public health problem? *J. Public Health Dent.* 48:245–251.

Caton, J., and A. Polson. 1985. The Interdental Bleeding Index: A simplified procedure for monitoring gingival health. *Comp. Cont. Educ. Dent.* 6:88–92.

Fischman, S. 1986. Current status of indices of plaque. *J. Clin. Periodontol.* 13:371–374.

Greene, J. 1967. The Oral Hygiene Index. Development and uses. *J. Periodontol.* 38:625–637.

Greene, J., and J. Vermillion. 1964. The Simplified Oral Hygiene Index. *J. Am. Dent. Assoc.* 68:7–13.

Hunt, R., and S. Fann. 1991. Effect of examining half the teeth in a partial periodontal recording of older adults. *J. Dent. Res.* 70:1380–1385.

Ismail, A., B. Burt, and S. Eklund. 1983. Epidemiologic patterns of smoking and periodontal disease in the United States. *J. Am. Dent. Assoc.* 106:617–621.

Ismail, A., E. Morrison, B. Burt, R. Cafesse, and M. Kavanaugh. 1990. Natural history of periodontal disease in adults: Findings from the Tecumseh Periodontal Disease Study, 1959–1987. *J. Dent. Res.* 69(2):430–435.

Listgarten, M., C. Schifter, and L. Laster. 1985. Three-year longitudinal study of the periodontal status of an adult population with gingivitis. *J. Clin. Periodontol.* 12:225–238.

Lobene, R., T. Weatherford, N. Ross, R. Lam, and L. Menaker. 1986. A modified gingival index for use in clinical trials. *Clin. Prev. Dent.* 8(1):3–6.

Löe, H. 1967. The gingival index, the plaque index, and the retention index. Systems (Part II). *J. Periodontol.* 38:610–616.

Löe, H., A. Anerud, H. Boysen, and E. Morrison. 1986. Natural history of periodontal disease in man: Rapid, moderate and no loss of attachment in Sri Lankan laborers 14–46 years of age. *J. Clin. Periodontol.* 13:431–446.

Löe, H., A. Anerud, H. Boysen, and M. Smith. 1978. The natural history of periodontal disease in man: The rate of periodontal destruction before 40 years of age. *J. Periodontol.* 49(12):607–620.

Löe, H., and L. Brown. 1991. Early-onset periodontitis in the United States of America. *J. Periodontol.* 62:608–616.

Miller, A., J. Brunelle, J. Carlos, L. J. Brown, and H. Löe. 1987. *Oral health of the United States Adults. National findings 1985–1986.* Bethesda, MD: U.S. Public Health Service, U.S. Dept. of Health and Human Services.

Mühlemann, H. R., and S. Son. 1971. Gingival sulcus bleeding: A leading symptom in initial gingivitis. *Helv. Odont. Acta* 15:107–113.

O'Leary, T. J., R. Drake, and J. Naylor. 1972. The Plaque Control Record. *J. Periodontol.* 43(1):38.

Oliver, R., L. Brown, and H. Löe. 1998. Periodontal disease in the United States population. *J. Periodontol.* 69:269–278.

Oliver, R., and T. Tervonen. 1994. Diabetes: A risk factor for periodontitis in adults. *J. Periodontol.* 65:530–538.

Papapanou, P. 1996. *Annals of Periodontology, Section 1A: Periodontal diseases: Epidemiology.* 1996 World Workshop in Periodontics, Lansdowne, VA.

Russell, A. L. 1967. The Periodontal Index. *J. Periodontol.* 38:585–591.

Seppälä, B., M. Seppälä, and J. Ainamo. 1993. A longitudinal study on insulin-dependent diabetes mellitus and periodontal disease. *J. Clin. Periodontol.* 20:161–165.

Sheiham, A., and D. Striffler. 1970. A comparison of four epidemiological methods of assessing periodontal disease: I. Population findings. *J. Periodont. Res.* 5:148–154.

Silness, J., and H. Löe. 1964. Periodontal disease in pregnancy: II. Correlation between oral hygiene and periodontal condition. *Acta Odontol. Scand.* 22:121–135.

Stamm, J. 1986. Epidemiology of gingivitis. *J. Clin. Periodontol.* 13:360–366.

Taylor, G. W., B. A. Burt, M. P. Becker, R. J. Genco, M. Schlossman, et al. 1998. Non-insulin-dependent diabetes and the progression of bone loss over a two-year period. *J. Periodontol.* 68:76–83.

Turesky, S., N. Gilmore, and I. Glickman. 1970. Reduced plaque formation by the chloromethyl analogue of victamine C. *J. Periodontol.* 41:41–43.

U.S. Public Health Service, NIDR. 1987. *Oral health in United States adults: National findings* (NIH Publication No. 87-2868), pp. 1–168. Bethesda, MD: National Institute of Health, NIDR.

Volpe, A., L. Kupczak, and W. King. 1967. In vivo calculus assessment: III. Scoring techniques, rate of calculus formation, partial mouth exams versus full mouth exams, and intra-examiner reproducibility. *Periodontics* 5:184–193.

Volpe, A., J. H. Manhold, and S. P. Hazen. 1965. In vivo calculus assessment: I. A method and its examiner reproducibility. *J. Periodontol.* 36:292–298.

Waerhaug, J. 1966. Epidemiology of periodontal disease: A review of literature. In *world workshop in periodontics,* pp. 179–212. Ann Arbor: University of Michigan.

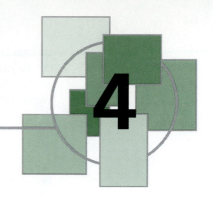

4

Dental Biofilms: Microbiology of the Periodontal Diseases

Raymond A. Yukna, D.M.D., M.S.
John D. Mason, B.A., D.D.S.

Outline

Goal

To introduce the concept of dental biofilms as one of the primary risk factors for periodontal diseases.

Educational Objectives

Upon completion of this chapter, the dental hygiene student should be able to:

Describe dental plaque formation as well as its composition in the supra- and subgingival environment.

Describe the features of subgingival biofilms.

Describe the bacteria associated with the periodontal diseases.

Describe the relationship between the mechanisms of bacterial action and host responses in the initiation and progression of periodontal diseases.

> ### KEY WORDS
> - periodontal diseases
> - risk factors
> - evidence-based approach
> - dental plaque
> - microorganisms
> - biofilm
> - etiology

The authors are indebted to Connie Holland Gandy and Marianne Gabb for assistance with the preparation of this chapter.

Inflammatory periodontal diseases are not a single entity and are not caused by a single causative factor. Risk factors are characteristics that have been shown to directly cause periodontal diseases. Causal links are established by longitudinal and cross-sectional studies. Causal relationships are important to identify so that oral disease can be prevented if the risk factor is modifiable. For example, it is accepted that dental biofilms cause gingivitis and so is considered a risk factor for gingivitis. A major triad of etiologic and risk factors exists in affecting periodontal health (Table 4–1■) (Page, Offenbacher, Schroeder, Seymour, & Kornman, 1997): (1) local factors—environmental forces that predispose to inflammatory periodontal diseases; (2) systemic factors—those medical conditions that predispose to inflammatory periodontal diseases; and (3) host factors—the influences of one's own body (e.g., individual susceptibility to disease).

Primary Etiology—Bacteria and Their Products

Inflammatory periodontal diseases are initiated and progress as the result of the accumulation of dental plaque in the area of the gingival sulcus (Fig. 4–1■). Dental plaque is defined as a dense, nonmineralized, complex mass of bacterial colonies living in a gel-like intermicrobial matrix. Microorganisms besides bacteria can live in this mass, including yeasts and viruses. Other constituents of dental biofilms include cells of various types.

The degree of tissue damage is dependent on the interaction between plaque bacteria and host defense mechanisms. Local contributing factors (e.g., calculus) may encourage the accumulation of dental biofilms, and systemic and local modifying factors may alter the host response to the bacterial challenge. However, if dental plaque is regularly removed and not allowed to accumulate, then gingival health can be maintained, in spite of other factors.

Bacterial Factors

Dental plaque (biofilm) is the major etiologic or risk factor in the initiation and progression of inflammatory periodontal diseases. Löe, Theilade, and Jensen (1965) provided the first direct scientific evidence of the causal relationship between plaque and gingival inflammation. In this classic "experimental gingivitis model" study, when subjects with excellent gingival health and little plaque did not perform oral hygiene procedures for 21 days, plaque accumulation increased and gingivitis developed. Resuming good oral hygiene eliminated dental plaque, resolved gingival inflammation, and restored gingival health. Many other studies have since

Table 4–1	Risk Factors for Periodontal Diseases
• Poor oral hygiene	• Male gender
• Tobacco smoking	• Compromised host defense
• Genetics/heredity	• Advancing age
• Stress	• Race, ethnicity
• Past history of periodontitis	• Regularity of dental care
• Systemic diseases	• Interleukin-1 production

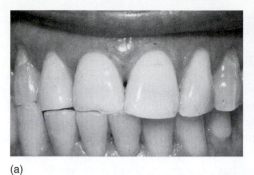
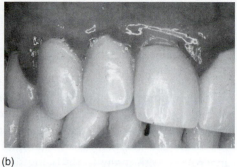

(a)   (b)

Figure 4–1   Clinical cases of healthy gingiva and inflamed gingiva: (a) healthy gingiva with good color, contour, and texture; (b) inflamed gingiva with bluish red color, puffiness, and altered contour due to dental plaque accumulation.

demonstrated a similar strong positive association between plaque accumulation and the presence of gingivitis.

Dental Biofilms

Dental plaque has all of the characteristics of a biofilm. Dental biofilms are defined as matrix-enclosed bacterial populations adherent to each other and/or to surfaces or interfaces (Costerton et al., 1994). Microorganisms in biofilms are not evenly distributed and are arranged in microcolonies surrounded by an intermicrobial matrix, which serves as a protective barrier to protect the bacteria in the biofilm from systemically and locally applied antimicrobials. Currently, the only way to remove dental biofilms is mechanically with tooth brushing, or scaling/root planing; however, once it is removed it quickly reforms. Bacteria in the film communicate with one another, build intricate intertwined structures, and even have a primitive circulatory system. Biofilms contain multiple microenvironments that vary greatly in pH, oxygen tension, and availability of specific nutrients. Subgingival dental biofilms have some loosely attached and unattached bacteria on its surface that contact the adjacent epithelium of the pockets. Microorganisms in biofilms are resistant to antibiotics and antimicrobials unless the biofilms are mechanically disrupted.

Morphology/Types

Over 500 kinds of bacteria present in biofilms normally inhabit the oral cavity, and only about twenty species (< 10%) are considered to be pathogenic for periodontal diseases (Fine, 1995; Moore & Moore, 1994; see Table 4–2a,b■). The rest constitute normal oral biota. The mere presence of one or more pathogenic species is not necessarily associated with progressing disease. Both protective host factors and interactions among the components of the dental plaque limit their pathogenicity. For individual species or groups of bacteria to be considered important in the etiology of periodontal diseases, the following criteria are considered important:

1. They are found in high numbers in advancing lesions or sites, and in relatively low numbers at healthy or nonprogressing sites.

2. Clinical healing occurs with elimination of the pathogen.
3. They are present prior to clinical changes becoming evident.
4. They create a tissue reaction.
5. They can be shown to produce disease in experimental animal or human studies.

Bacteria present in the oral cavity come in a wide variety of shapes from round coccoid forms to simple, short rods to complicated corkscrew shapes. Both Gram-positive (cell wall intact) and Gram-negative (permeable cell wall) forms are present. Some are oxygen using (aerobic) and some cannot tolerate any oxygen (anaerobic), with many forms being somewhat in between (facultative aerobic, microaerophilic, or facultative anaerobic). Within each category are both motile and nonmotile forms. Some bacteria utilize carbohydrates as food (saccharolytic), while others prefer proteins obtained in part from the tissue destruction they cause as a substrate (asaccharolytic). Some bacteria, such as spirochetes, do not readily fit any of these categories. In general terms, health-associated bacteria are Gram-positive, aerobic, saccharolytic, and nonmotile, while disease-associated bacteria tend to be Gram-negative, anaerobic, asaccharolytic, and motile (Table 4–3■).

The right combination of bacteria must be present in sufficient numbers to produce periodontal diseases. The presence of beneficial or good bacteria may modify the effects of known pathogens, thereby reducing the likelihood of disease progression. The presence of a single pathogen does not indicate active disease.

In health, the primary bacteria that live in the oral cavity are *Streptococcus sanguis, Streptococcus mitis, Veillonella* sp. *Actinomyces naeslundii,* and *Actinomyces viscosus*. In gingivitis there are increased numbers of all of the bacteria seen in health, especially *Prevotella intermedia* and spirochetes. Table 4–2b lists specific bacteria associated with various forms of periodontal diseases.

Table 4–2a	Nomenclature of Common Periodontal Microorganisms
Gram-Positive Bacteria	**Gram-Negative Bacteria**
Gram-positive facultative cocci	Gram-negative facultative rods
Streptococcus sanguis, mitis, and *salivarius*	*Eikenella corrodens*
Gram-positive anaerobic cocci	*Capnocytophaga ochracea*
Peptostreptococcus micros	*Actinobacillus actinomycetemcomitans*
Gram-positive facultative rods	Gram-negative obligate anaerobic rods
Actinomyces viscosus, israelii, and *naeslundii*	*Porphyromonas gingivalis*
Corynebacterium matruchotii	*Prevotella intermedia*
Gram-positive obligate anaerobic rod	*Bacteroides forsythus**
Eubacterium lentum	*Fusobacterium nucleatum*
	Gram-negative obligate anaerobic cocci
	Veillonella alcalescens
	Gram-negative anaerobic spirochetes
	Treponema denticola

Yeasts

Candida albicans

*In 2002 Sakamoto, Suzuki, Umeda, Ishikawa, and Benno proposed a new genus for *Bacteroides forsythus*. This new genus is *Tannerella* and the species is *Tannerella forsythensis*.

Table 4–2b	Specific Bacteria Associated with Periodontal Diseases
Strong Evidence for Etiology	**Primary Association**
Actinobacillus actinomycetemcomitans	Aggressive periodontitis
Porphyromonas gingivalis	Chronic periodontitis
Bacteroides forsythus (Tannerella forsythensis)	Chronic periodontitis
Moderate Evidence for Etiology	
Campylobacter rectus	
Eubacterium nodatum	
Fusobacterium nucleatum	
Prevotella intermedia	Pregnancy gingivitis, necrotizing ulcerative periodontal diseases
Peptostreptococcus micros	
Streptococcus intermedius-complex	
Treponema denticola	Chronic periodontitis, necrotizing ulcerative periodontal diseases
Capnocytophaga species	Aggressive, localized periodontitis

Microorganisms of Dental Biofilms

The types of microorganisms found in dental biofilms vary among individuals and sites within the mouth. Based upon the surface of the tooth in relationship to the gingival margin, dental biofilms can be identified as supragingival or subgingival.

Supragingival Plaque

The sequence of events involved in the formation of deposits on teeth starts with the deposition of a pellicle, also called salivary or acquired pellicle. When the tooth erupts, it has the organic coating of the enamel cuticle. This is lost early due to abrasion or digestion from bacteria. Within seconds after the saliva contacts the natural tooth, a coating of salivary glycoproteins forms on the tooth as an amorphous, tenacious membrane. The pellicle is thought to be acellular in that bacteria are not needed for its formation. The pellicle allows and encourages the colonization of bacteria on the tooth surface, and therefore it participates in plaque formation. Adsorption of bacteria to the pellicle is important since the pellicle is formed from glycoproteins that bind selectively to the tooth, and not all of the bacteria available in the saliva can attach to the pellicle. The pellicle can form on the surface of the tooth as surface pellicle, or it can adhere in fingerlike projections to the

Table 4–3	Health and Disease Associated Bacterial Characteristics
Health	**Disease**
Gram-positive	Gram-negative
Aerobic	Anaerobic
Nonmotile	Motile
Saccharolytic	Assaccharolytic

millions of imperfections of the enamel or areas of demineralization. This pellicle is called subsurface pellicle. Subsurface pellicle is significant because it connects the protein of the pellicle with the protein of the component of the enamel. The pellicle can be removed during prophylaxis but begins to reform within minutes. The formation is complete in 2 hours.

Bacteria adhere to the tooth surface via molecules called adhesins located on the bacterial cell surface. Adhesins that are proteins and those that recognize carbohydrate structures are called lectins. These adhesins, or lectins, recognize and then link to specific carbohydrate structures in the glycoproteins of the pellicle.

Dental Biofilm Formation Dental biofilm formation begins as the bacteria adhere to the pellicle and begin to colonize. The pellicle serves as a nutrient source for the bacteria. As the salivary proteins are metabolized, they release peptides and amino acids.

The general pattern of bacterial succession in supragingival plaque is coccoid forms followed by short rods followed by larger rods and then motile forms including spirochetes. The majority of these bacteria are Gram-positive and aerobic (living entirely in an oxygen environment); however, most aerobic bacteria do not survive on total oxygen but rather are considered facultative, living with or without oxygen. Then a shift toward increased numbers of Gram-negative microorganisms and more motile forms occurs. Supragingival plaque is usually detected by visual inspection of the teeth, with or without disclosing solution (Fig. 4–2■).

When a tooth begins to erupt, it is exposed to saliva, which contains all the acquired bacteria. At this point, the formation of dental plaque begins (Newman & Listgarten, 1999). The initial plaque formation is characterized by the numbers and kinds of bacteria that colonize the pellicle. Phase I, or initiation, begins in 1 to 2 days of plaque accumulation with no removal techniques. The microorganisms form as individual clones that extend both laterally and perpendicularly from the tooth surface to form parallel, palisading layers of bacteria (Fine, 1995; Fig. 4–3■). The first colonies of bacteria are Gram-positive cocci and short rods, including *Streptococcus mutans* and *Streptococcus sanguis*.

Phase II begins in 2 to 4 days after abstaining from daily toothbrushing or leaving individual areas undisturbed. The early plaque masses provide the base for the next phase of colonies to infiltrate. The next bacteria to form are Gram-positive rods and Gram-negative cocci. The space between the layers of the first plaque provides an anaerobic environment for the arrival of anaerobic and facultative anaerobic (liv-

Figure 4–2 Clinical picture of supragingival plaque on teeth made more evident with disclosant.

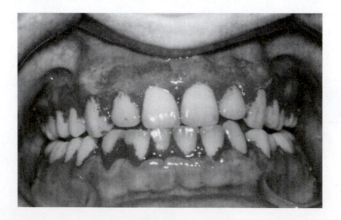

ing with or without oxygen) bacteria. The cocci still dominate the plaque; however, filamentous forms and slender rods compete for the space (Fine, 1995; see Fig. 4–3).

The matrix begins to form around the bacterial colonies derived mainly from salivary material, exudates (e.g., gingival crevicular fluid), and intermicrobial sub-

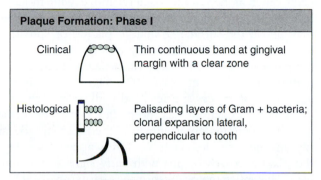

Plaque Formation: Phase I

Clinical — Thin continuous band at gingival margin with a clear zone

Histological — Palisading layers of Gram + bacteria; clonal expansion lateral, perpendicular to tooth

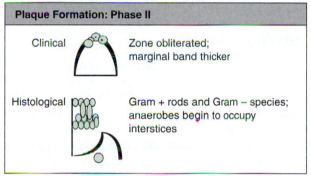

Plaque Formation: Phase II

Clinical — Zone obliterated; marginal band thicker

Histological — Gram + rods and Gram – species; anaerobes begin to occupy interstices

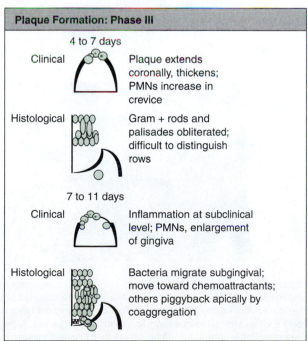

Plaque Formation: Phase III

4 to 7 days

Clinical — Plaque extends coronally, thickens; PMNs increase in crevice

Histological — Gram + rods and palisades obliterated; difficult to distinguish rows

7 to 11 days

Clinical — Inflammation at subclinical level; PMNs, enlargement of gingiva

Histological — Bacteria migrate subgingival; move toward chemoattractants; others piggyback apically by coaggregation

Figure 4–3 Illustration of different phases of plaque formation. (From D. Fine, *Periodontology*, 8:89 [1995]. Copyright © 1995 by Munksgaard International Publishers Ltd., Copenhagen. Reprinted by permission.)

stances. Bacteria can form extracellular polysaccharides (carbohydrates) from sucrose. These glucan, levans, and fructans are significant to the adhesion process and their insolubility increases the plaque resistance to removal. The levans and soluble glucans are an energy source for bacteria.

Days 4 to 7 mark Phase III of plaque formation with an increase in the filamentous bacteria. The rods, filaments, and fusobacteria comingle and interact with each other as nonmotile bacteria move with motile bacteria around the gingival margins. As the plaque matures, vibrios and spirochetes can colonize. New plaque may lie on the surface of mature plaque or spread coronally at the margin. This new plaque is characterized by cocci as before. The filaments at the edge of the plaque serve as binding sites for these cocci and a corncob formation appears (Listgarten, Mayo, & Tremblay, 1975; Fig. 4–4■). Gram-positive facultative filaments such as *Actinomyces* species bind with cocci such as *Streptococcus sanguis*.

Phase III continues as the plaque continues to mature over days 7 to 11. Due to a change in the environment at the tooth surface, spirochetes continue to multiply and new species such as vibrios appear (see Fig. 4–3). The host response to the plaque masses begins with early signs of inflammation observable in the gingiva. This inflammatory response is easily reversed by plaque removal.

Subgingival Biofilms

Bacteria living without oxygen are considered strict or obligate anaerobes. Anaerobic microbes thrive in the depths of subgingival biofilms. As the days progress from 14 to 21, the vibrios and spirochetes remain prevalent in the depths of the mass. The growth, accumulation, and pathogenicity of subgingival plaque are strongly influenced by the presence of supragingival plaque. Inflammation of the gingiva caused by supragingival plaque changes the relationship between the gingival margin and the tooth. In addition, swelling (edema) causes gingival enlargement, which alters the anatomic relationship between the tooth surface and the gingival margin and allows bacteria to invade the subgingival space and to form

Enamel ——

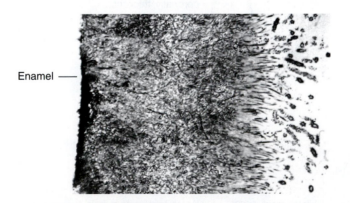

Figure 4–4 Electron micrograph of 3-week-old supragingival plaque. The central filament is attached to the enamel surface. The filaments are usually composed of *Actinomyces* sp. or *Fusobacterium nucleatum.* Corncob formations extend from the enamel surface and are usually cocci such as *Streptococcus sanguis.* (From M. Listgarten, *J. Periodontol.* 51:1–18 [1976]. Copyright 1976 by the American Academy of Periodontology. Reprinted by permission.)

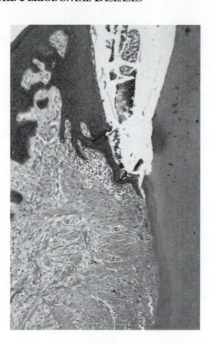

Figure 4–5   Histology of shallow pocket with plaque present.

subgingival dental plaque on the root surface or adjacent to the epithelial tissue in the sulcus (Fig. 4–5■). This newly created subgingival space, which is protected from physiologic and mechanical oral cleansing mechanisms, facilitates further bacterial multiplication. The microbiota of subgingival plaque is generally more anaerobic, more Gram-negative, more motile, and more asaccharolytic. There are also many motile organisms that are completely unattached to the plaque matrix. These microbes produce toxins, enzymes, and metabolic products that cause direct injury to the periodontium. More importantly, they act as antigens, and as the host responds to the irritant present, some destruction of the periodontal tissues occurs. Thus, elimination of subgingival plaque is critical to the prevention of periodontal diseases.

Types of Subgingival Plaque   Subgingival plaque can be separated into three types based on location: (1) tooth associated (attached), (2) tissue associated, and (3) unattached subgingival plaques. They have been identified with varying characteristics (Table 4–4■; Fig. 4–6■). *Unattached Gram-negative anaerobic microorganisms are in close proximity to the epithelium and appear to play an important role in the initiation and progression of periodontitis.* Filaments surrounded by rods can occur, creating a test-tube or bristle-brush effect on the surface plaque (Fig. 4–7■).

Nutrients

Nutrients from the crevicular fluid in the pocket are readily available, so bacteria that use proteins as energy sources are favored over those that require carbohydrates. For example, hemin-containing compounds found in crevicular fluid enhance the growth of *Porphyromonas* and *Prevotella* species; *Prevotella intermedia* use menadione, a by-product of estrogen metabolism. Thus, the final proportions of various bacteria found in the subgingival area are the sum of a large variety of intertwining processes.

Table 4–4	Types of Subgingival Plaque

Tooth Associated

Densely packed strongly adherent to tooth surface (biofilm)
Gram-positive rods, cocci, and filamentous bacteria
Facultative aerobic or facultative anaerobes
Removed by scaling and root planing
Less virulent (limited ability to cause disease)

Tissue Associated

Loosely packed, loosely adherent to soft tissue wall
Gram-negative, motile, anaerobic
Spirochetes, "bottle-brush" types
More virulent (able to cause disease)
Cannot be removed by scaling and root planing; needs to be surgically removed

Unattached

Free swimming in pocket (not a biofilm)
Gram-negative, motile, anaerobic
Spirochetes and others
More virulent (able to cause disease)
Removed by flushing

Tissue Invasion

Several studies have shown that plaque bacteria such as *Actinobacillus actinomycetemcomitans, Porphyromonas gingivalis,* and spirochetes can be found within the tissues, including the epithelium, gingival connective tissues, and the alveolar bone (Renvert, Wikström, Dahlen, Slots, & Egelberg, 1990; Saglie, Carranza, New-

Figure 4–6 Schematic of the three types of subgingival plaque plus the depiction of "invading" microorganisms.

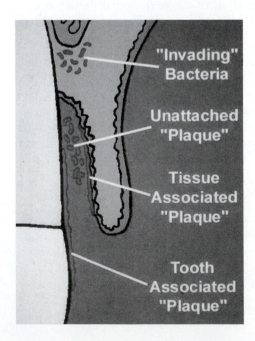

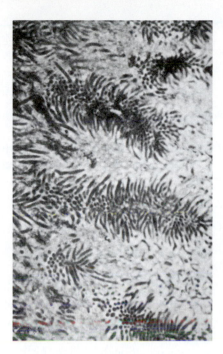

Figure 4–7   Electron micrograph of subgingival plaque. Subgingival bacteria gather to form a test-tube or bristle-brush configuration composed of Gram-negative rods (bristles) attaching to filamentous bacteria such as *Actinomyces* sp. (From M. Listgarten, *J. Periodontol.* 51:1–18 [1976]. Copyright by the Academy of Periodontology. Reprinted with permission.)

man, Cheng, & Lewin, 1982). Although the bacteria seem to be present in these tissues, they have shown no evidence of local activity or multiplication, so they may be inactive in those locations. In addition, the severity of the periodontal disease and associated tooth mobility, as well as the trauma associated with tooth extraction, suggest that the bacteria may actually be pushed into the tissues, rather than invading. However, invasion of the deeper periodontal tissues by bacteria may be important to the pathogenesis of certain periodontal diseases.

Microorganisms of Dental Implants

Clinical studies have demonstrated that the microbiota of healthy, stable dental implants are similar to that of healthy teeth, while implants that are unstable and failing have bacteria similar to natural teeth with periodontitis (Rams & Link, 1983). Dental plaque must be removed around implants just as for natural teeth, but using special dental implant instruments (i.e., plastic) that will not scratch the implant.

Other Components of Plaque

Cells

Although bacteria are the primary constituents of plaque, several types of cells are also present. Epithelial cells are found almost universally in samples of plaque in a variety of anatomic forms ranging from cells recently shed from the surface with discrete nuclei and clearly defined cell walls to what may be described as empty "ghosts" of cells filled with bacteria. White blood cells, particularly polymorphonuclear neutrophils (PMNs), are often also found in plaque. Red blood cells are commonly seen in samples taken from tooth surfaces adjacent to pockets with bleeding on probing, indicating a break in the pocket epithelial lining.

Other Tooth-Accumulated Materials

Several other tooth-accumulated materials (TAMs) besides dental plaque and pellicle are found in the region of the gingival sulcus. Food debris is the most commonly found TAM. Materia alba is also a bacterial aggregation with food debris, but it differs from plaque in that it is not strongly adherent to the tooth. There is no definite architecture as with dental plaque, and it is minimally implicated in periodontal diseases. While these tooth-accumulated materials may stain with disclosant and be visible on the tooth surface, they are readily dislodged by rinsing or a water spray, unlike pellicle or dental plaque.

Mechanisms of Bacterial Action

Different combinations of indigenous (living-in-the-mouth) bacteria, rather than just a single species, produce the pathogenic potential necessary to cause progression from gingivitis to destructive periodontitis.

Once pathogenic microbiotas are established, the microorganisms appear to incite destruction of the supporting structures by both direct toxic effects on adjacent tissues and by the indirect activation of host immune and inflammatory cells.

Direct Effect

Cytotoxic Agents The subgingival unattached plaque has endotoxins, which are lipopolysaccharides (LPS) (now called lipooligosaccharide [LOS]). Lipooligosaccharides, which are found in the cell wall of Gram-negative bacteria, can initiate inflammation, cause soft-tissue destruction, and stimulate bone resorption. Endotoxins are released from the cell wall upon death of Gram-negative bacteria. LOS is found in the cementum of untreated periodontally involved root surfaces.

Enzymes Many of the bacteria present in the various plaque environments of the sulcus/pocket produce a variety of enzymes, which can adversely affect the gingival and periodontal tissues. These enzymes accumulate in the sulcus and can penetrate through intact epithelium into the deeper tissues. Enyzmes function to destroy the connective tissue by breaking down collagen and ground substance. Some of the enzymes that have been identified as important products of plaque bacteria are shown in Table 4–5■.

Host-Derived Enzymes New information regarding *host-mediated* degradation (breakdown) of connective tissues has focused on the matrix metalloproteinases (MMPs) (Birkedal-Hansen, 1993). This group of structurally similar enzymes is produced by stimulated host cells and includes the collagenases, gelatinases, and stromelysins. These enzymes are responsible for cleaving the collagen molecule (the major component of connective tissue), degrading proteoglycans (part of the ground substance) and other proteins making up the connective tissues, and causing osteoclastic bone resorption.

Table 4–5	Common Enzymes that Break Down Periodontal Tissues

Collagenase—this degrades collagen fibers, the major-formed elements in the gingiva and periodontal ligament. Produced by both bacteria and the host cells in the body (e.g., PMNs and fibroblasts). Included in the family of enzymes called matrix metalloproteinases (MMPs).

Hyaluronidase—this breaks down hyaluronic acid, an important polysaccharide (carbohydrate) that helps hold tissue and cells together. Can act as a "spreading" factor to increase tissue permeability. This enzyme is also produced both by bacteria and by the host.

Chondroitin sulfatase—this breaks apart chondroitin sulfate, another cell- and tissue-cementing polysaccharide (carbohydrate).

Proteases—a large group of enzymes that contribute to the breakdown of noncollagenous proteins (proteins in the connective tissue other than collagen) and increase capillary permeability.

Elastases—this affects the elastin (elastic) fibers of the mucosa and blood vessels, thereby reducing tissue integrity.

Indirect Effect

Immunopathologic Mechanisms Several bacterial antigens induce inflammation in the periodontal tissues by stimulating the immune response. Both the humoral (antibody-based) and the cell-mediated (lymphocyte-based) types of immune responses have been observed in patients with periodontitis. The role of the immunologic response in periodontal disease is not completely understood; however, the potential to cause tissue destruction, as well as to be protective, is apparent. Rather than always being protective, the host immune response may contribute to the tissue destruction.

Combined Mechanisms

While not truly contagious, transmission of pathogenic bacteria has been shown to occur between individuals. *Actinobacillus actinomycetemcomitans* can be transmitted from parent to child and from dogs to humans (Asikainen, Chen, Alaluusua, & Slots, 1997). There is some evidence that *Porphyromonas gingivalis* is transmitted among individuals in a household including spouses (Asikainen et al., 1997). The most common route of transmission is via saliva. It is probable that more than one mechanism is involved in the initiation and progression of gingivitis and periodontitis. It is possible that bacterial enzymes and/or cytotoxic substances exert a direct effect on the sulcular and subsulcular tissue, and at the same time initiate an indirect immune response. Therefore, there are multiple mechanisms of action of dental plaque.

Periodontal Diseases: The Future

The scenario following the accumulation of oral biofilms on tooth surfaces will continue unless treatment is started. Without treatment the supporting structures may be destroyed. Thus, current periodontal disease is a local contributing factor for further and future periodontal disease.

Summary

Periodontal diseases have multiple risk factors. Therefore, it should not be expected that one risk factor will consistently be associated with the development of this kind of disease, and it should not be expected that control of one risk factor will completely eliminate the risk of developing the disease.

Dental plaque is the primary etiologic factor in periodontal diseases. However, other local and systemic factors play an important role. By taking a thorough health and social history, and correlating known local and systemic risk factors with periodontal clinical findings, clinicians can make patients who are at increased risk aware of the impact of these factors and the influence the factors have on their periodontal condition. Especially when treatment is unsuccessful, reevaluation of primary and secondary risk factors might improve future treatment results.

The *Parameters of Care* published by the American Academy of Periodontology (2000) suggest that the initial therapy for patients with periodontal inflammation should include the elimination, alteration, or control of risk factors that may contribute to chronic periodontitis. This represents significant progress since it is clear that periodontal diseases are infections initiated by bacteria and may have several associated risk factors. Management of these risk factors is likely to be the most successful approach to preventing periodontitis in the future.

Also, since the presence of periodontitis is recognized as a risk factor for future and more severe periodontal disease (past attachment loss is a risk factor for future attachment loss), proper diagnosis and therapy of an existing condition is very important in helping prevent future occurrences.

Key Points

- Dental plaque is a biofilm.
- Currently, evidence-based dentistry supports the use of risk assessment techniques to guide clinical decisions in the treatment of periodontal diseases.
- Important risk factors for periodontal diseases include certain periodontal bacteria (plaque biofilm).
- Formation of dental plaque begins with tooth eruption.
- Inflammatory periodontal diseases are infections caused by bacteria.
- Attempts to manage risk factors are important in the prevention and treatment of periodontal diseases.

Web Sites

www.dentalcare.com

www.perio.org

www.personal.psu.edu

www.eastman.uc/ac.uk

www.dimensionsofdentalhygiene.com

www.ncbi.nlm.nih.gov

Self-Quiz

1. All of the following are harmful products produced by bacteria that affect the periodontal tissues except one. Which one is the exception? (pp. 74–75)

   a. enzymes

   b. lipooligosaccharides

   c. waste products

   d. crevicular fluid

2. Which one of the following types of bacteria found in subgingival plaque is considered pathogenic for periodontitis? (pp. 66–67)

   a. *Porphyromonas gingivalis*

   b. *Actinomyces viscosis*

   c. *Streptococcus sanguis*

   d. *Corynebacterium matruchotii*

3. Which one of the following is the primary risk factor for periodontal diseases? (p. 64)

   a. dental calculus

   b. dental biofilms

   c. diabetes mellitus

   d. HIV/AIDS infection

   e. systemic drugs

4. Which one of the following criteria makes bacteria an important risk factor for periodontal diseases? (p. 64)

   a. found in high numbers in advancing sites

   b. irritates the epithelial lining of the pocket

   c. breakdowns in the epithelial cells in the gingiva

   d. causes tissue erosion

5. Which of the following deposits is laid down first during biofilm development? (pp. 66–67)

   a. dental calculus

   b. dental plaque

   c. acquired pellicle

   d. materia alba

6. Löe and coworkers proved that there is a direct relationship between dental plaque and periodontal diseases because the removal of dental plaque improves gingival health. (p. 64)

   a. Both the statement and reason are correct and related.

   b. Both the statement and reason are correct but not related.

   c. The statement is correct, but the reason is not.

   d. The statement is not correct, but the reason is correct.

   e. Neither the statement nor reason is correct.

7. From which of the following sources do subgingival bacteria receive nutrition? (p. 71)

   a. saliva

   b. dental calculus

   c. cervicular fluid

   d. by-products of bacterial metabolism

   e. endotoxins from supragingival plaque

8. Which of the following types of subgingival plaque is found closely associated with the epithelium and thus play a role in the initiation of periodontitis? (p. 72)

   a. tooth associated

   b. tissue associated

   c. unattached

   d. attached

   e. invading

9. In which of the following phases of plaque formation does supragingival bacteria migrate subgingivally? (pp. 68–70)

   a. Phase I

   b. Phase II

   c. Phase III/4 to 7 days

   d. Phase III/7 to 11 days

10. All of the following bacteria are strongly associated with invading epithelium and gingival connective tissue except one. Which one is the exception? (pp. 70–72)

    a. spirochetes

    b. *Actinobacillus actinomycetemomitans*

    c. *Prevotella intermedia*

    d. *Porphyromonas gingivalis*

References

American Academy of Periodontology. 2000. Parameters of Care. *J. Periodontal* 71(5):847–883.

Asikainen, S., C. Chen, S. Alaluusua, and J. Slots. 1997. Can one acquire periodontal bacteria and periodontitis from a family member? *J. Am. Dent. Assoc.* 128:1263–1271.

Birkedal-Hansen, H. 1993. Role of matrix metalloproteinases in human periodontal diseases. *J. Periodontol.* 64:474–484.

Costerton, J. W., Z. Lewandowski, D. DeBeer, D. Caldwell, D. Korber, and G. James. 1994. Biofilms, the customized microniche. *J. Bacteriol.* 176:2137–2142.

Fine, D. 1995. Chemical agents to prevent and regulate plaque development. *Periodontology* 8:87–107.

Listgarten, M. A., H. E. Mayo, and R. Tremblay. 1975. Development of dental plaque on epoxy resin crowns in man. A light and electron microscopic study. *J. Periodontol.* 46:10–26.

Löe, H., E. Theilade, and S. Jensen. 1965. Experimental gingivitis in man. *J. Periodontol.* 49:117–187.

Moore, W. E. C., and L. V. H. Moore. 1994. The bacteria of periodontal diseases. *Periodontology 2000* 5:66–77.

Newman, M. G. 1996. Improved clinical decision making using the evidence-based approach. *Ann. Periodontol.* 1:i–ix.

Newman, H. N., and M. A. Listgarten. 1999. The development of dental plaque: From preeruptive primary cuticle to acquired pellicle to dental plaque to calculus formation. In eds. N. O. Harris and F. Garcia-Godoy, *Primary preventive dentistry,* 5th ed., 21–39. Stamford, CT: Appleton and Lange.

Page, R. C., W. Offenbacher, H. E. Schroeder, G. J. Seymour, and K. S. Kornman. 1997. Advances in the pathogenesis of periodontitis: Summary of developments, clinical implications and future directions. *Periodontology 2000* 14:216–248.

Rams, T. E., and C. C. Link, Jr. 1983. Microbiology of failing dental implants in humans: Electron microscopic observations. *J. Oral Implantol.* 11:93–100.

Renvert, S., M. Wikström, G. Dahlen, J. Slots, and J. Egelberg. 1990. On the inability of root debridement and periodontal surgery to eliminate *Actinobacillus actinomycetemcomitans* from periodontal pockets. *J. Clin. Periodontol.* 17:351–355.

Saglie, R. F., F. A. Carranza, Jr., M. G. Newman, L. Cheng, and K. J. Lewin. 1982. Identification of tissue-invading bacteria in human periodontal disease. *J. Periodontol. Res.* 17:452–455.

Sakamoto, M., M. Suzuki, M. Umeda, L. Ishikawa, and Y. Benno 2002 Reclassification of *Bacteroides forsythus* as *Tannerella forsythensis corrig., gen. nov., comb. nov. Int J Syst Evol Microbiol.* 52(Pt 3):841–849.

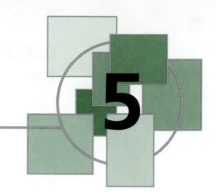

Local Contributory Risk Factors for the Periodontal Diseases

Raymond A. Yukna, D.M.D., M.S.
John D. Mason, B.A., D.D.S.

Outline

Goal

To introduce the role of local contributory risk factors for the periodontal diseases.

Educational Objectives

Upon completion of this chapter, the dental hygiene student should be able to:

List and explain contributing local risk factors.

Describe the clinical significance of dental calculus.

Discuss the specific role of dental calculus as a contributory risk factor for the periodontal diseases.

KEY WORDS
• contributory risk factors
• dental calculus
• anatomic factors
• iatrogenic factors
• traumatic factors

The authors are indebted to Connie Holland Gandy and Marianne Gabb for assistance with the preparation of this chapter.

Local Contributory Risk Factors for the Periodontal Diseases

Many local factors can increase plaque deposition and retention, inhibit plaque control, and contribute to the development of gingivitis and periodontitis. These factors are termed contributory because they do not by themselves initiate gingival inflammation, but foster increased or long-standing plaque accumulation and make plaque removal more difficult. Awareness of these local risk factors can help the dental hygienist to design more specific plaque-control activities, encourage patients to seek further corrective dental treatment, and contribute to the comprehensive care of periodontal patients.

Perhaps the most significant dentally related local factor strongly associated with an increased probability of developing periodontal diseases, but not directly involved in causing the disease, is the presence of established periodontal disease. Sites already or previously affected by periodontitis are at the greatest risk for future episodes (Douglass, 1998). More frequent professional care has been shown to reduce the risk.

Dental Calculus

Calculus is considered the most important local contributing factor. Calculus is essentially calcified dental plaque, but may form even in the absence of bacteria. Mineralization within plaque initially occurs supragingivally, but the rate of formation varies between individuals. Subgingival calculus forms more slowly in a thinner layer and, being firmly attached to the root, is usually more difficult to remove. Calculus is always covered by plaque and retains toxic bacterial products (Fig. 5–1■).

Subgingival calculus is commonly deposited in rings or ledges on root surfaces, but may also appear in a veneer form, and is associated with progressive periodontal disease (Fig. 5–2■). It is porous and can provide a reservoir of bacteria and endotoxin. Long-term studies of periodontal patients support calculus removal to promote healing and prevent further loss of attachment (Pihlstrom, McHugh, Oliphant, & Ortiz-Campos, 1983).

"Tartar" is the common "laymen" term for dental calculus, and is often used by patients when referring to calculus. Tartar is used to describe the sediment or crust on the side of a wine cask. The term was coined by a Swiss-German physician who identified all stony accretions in humans as tartars because they were similar in composition of the potassium bitartrate deposits on wine casks (Mandel, 1990). The term "calculus" is a Latin-rooted word meaning "pebble" or "stone." Needless to say, the population has become more aware of the word tartar because of the advertising of "tartar-control" toothpaste and rinses, which reinforces the use of the common name.

Radiographic evaluation of calculus is not an effective diagnostic method. Only about 45% of surfaces with clinically visible calculus are detected radiographically, but tooth surfaces visibly free of calculus show no calculus radiographically (Fig. 5–3■).

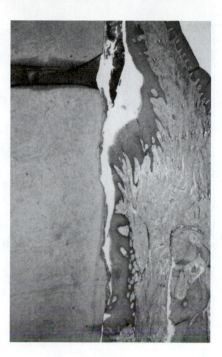

Figure 5–1 Histology of calculus with a plaque coating in a deep periodontal pocket.

Clinical Significance of Calculus

The population is more aware of supragingival plaque and calculus and its relationship to gingivitis than it is of subgingival plaque and calculus and its relationship to periodontitis. Awareness is still lacking in the need to remove plaque to prevent periodontal disease and how to remove supragingival and subgingival plaque. The situation becomes increasingly confusing when descriptions are added of mineralized plaque becoming calculus or of loosely adherent plaque residing on top of mineralized calculus. Because calculus that forms above the gingival margin is both hard and visible, it has become the focus of consumers for removal based for aesthetic reasons. Rather than being a mechanical irritant, as was once thought (Carranza, 1996), calculus contributes to the accumulation of plaque by having a porous surface. It is unknown if calculus covered with bacterial plaque is more damaging to tissues than plaque alone (Mandel, 1995).

Dental calculus can be defined as mineralized plaque, although calculus has been shown to result in germ-free animals. As with plaque, described according to its location in relationship to the gingival margin, calculus is also described as supragingival and subgingival. The mineralization process occurs separately for supragingival and subgingival plaque, and because of this, varying amounts of calculus can be found in the supragingival and subgingival areas.

Supragingival calculus can occur on any clinical crown, exposed root surface, prosthesis, or restoration. It is associated most frequently with sites that are adjacent to a salivary source, such as the parotid gland (maxillary molar area) or floor of the mouth and salivary caruncle (lingual surfaces of mandibular anterior teeth; Fig. 5–4■). Any retention site, such as a maligned tooth, a missed area of plaque

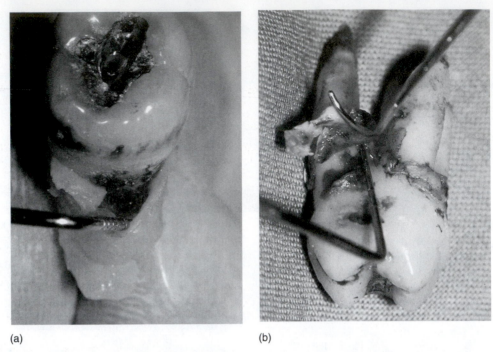

(a)   (b)

Figure 5–2   Clinical photographs of nodular calculus vs. veneer-type calculus. (a) Nodular calculus is evident more coronally while (b) veneer-type calculus is often found more apically.

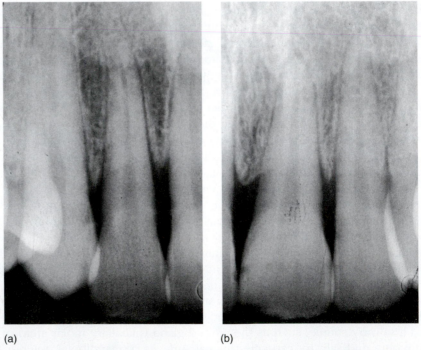

(a)   (b)

Figure 5–3   Radiographs of teeth in the same patient (a) with and (b) without calculus evident. Absence of calculus on radiographs does not mean that it is not present clinically (radiographs produce many false negatives).

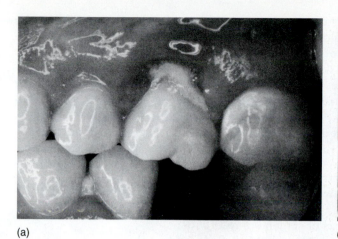
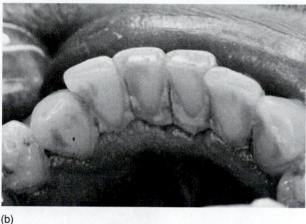

(a)   (b)

Figure 5–4   (a) Supragingival calculus on the maxillary first molar opposite Stensen's duct. (b) Supragingival calculus on the lingual surface of the mandibular anteriors in relation to the opening or orifice of the submandibular and sublingual salivary glands.

removal, or an area where mastication does not remove all debris, is a primary site for supragingival calculus formation. The mineral components of calculus are derived from saliva.

The formation of supragingival calculus occurs in layers beginning closest to the tooth. The minerals are deposited within 24 to 72 hours of plaque formation. Minerals from the saliva are deposited in the plaque matrix and around the filamentous bacteria. The process can take approximately 12 days or less for rapid formers. The actual mineralization process can occur in as few as 24 to 48 hours. Formation time varies according to the individual, the contents of the saliva, and the ability to remove plaque on all surfaces or various retention sites.

Subgingival calculus is derived from gingival crevicular fluid and any inflammatory exudates. There are more minerals available as the inflammatory process continues, and the calculus contains more calcium, magnesium, and fluoride than supragingival calculus (Mandel, 1990). It most often forms in rings around the roots of the tooth or in ledges.

The mineralization process continues as crystals of hydroxyapatite, brushite, and whitlockite form. These crystals have different proportions of calcium and phosphate in combination with other ions, such as magnesium, zinc, fluoride, and other carbonates (Ellwood, Melling, & Rutter, 1979). The crystals form in the matrix and then on the surface of the bacteria; finally, they calcify the bacteria.

Other differences in subgingival calculus and supragingival calculus are the hardness of the calculus and the difficulty in removing it. Supragingival calculus is 30% mineralized, whereas subgingival calculus is 60% mineralized. Subgingival calculus is more difficult to remove because of this hardness. The color of the two calculus types varies from yellow-white for supragingival calculus to gray or black for subgingival calculus. Unless the subgingival calculus is minutely visible at the gingival margin, this coloration adds little to its removal. The gray or black color derives from the bacterial and blood pigments.

The structure of calculus was described as layers in supragingival calculus. These layers build into incremental lines on the surfaces of a tooth. The surface of the calculus is irregular and rough. Plaque accumulates on the surface of the calculus. It can lodge in the pits and valleys of the calculus surface. In the subgingival calculus the outer surface may be less calcified. Again, subgingival plaque can accumulate. In either case, the plaque on the surface of the calculus contains living bacteria and is detrimental to the tissue. In this sense, calculus is a contributing risk factor for periodontal diseases. The calculus acts as an irritant to the gingival margin or the sulcular tissue. The overlying bacterial plaque continues to be the etiologic factor in periodontal disease.

Because of the complex attachment of calculus to root surfaces, removal is difficult. A classic article recognizes four modes of attachment of subgingival calculus to root surfaces (Zander, 1953):

1. attachment by means of mechanical locking into irregularities in the cementum;
2. attachment into areas of cementum resorption;
3. attachment by means of an organic pellicle; and
4. attachment by penetration into bacteria (not accepted by all researchers).

Anatomic Factors

Dental anatomic factors of importance to the accumulation of dental plaque include root morphology (size and shape) and position of teeth in the arch.

Root Morphology

Knowledge of dental morphology, supplemented by radiographs and the patient's dental history, is needed to identify dental anomalies. An anomaly is defined as a deviation from normal tooth development or function. Examples of dental anomalies include cervical enamel projections (CEPs), enamel pearls, and palatogingival grooves.

Several deviations in the shape or form of the tooth root can occur, and often contribute to increased plaque accumulation and more severe periodontal disease. Palatal grooves (also called palatogingival grooves or lingual grooves) are present on about 5 to 8% of maxillary incisors, tend to accumulate plaque, and can become the focus of a narrow, deep pocket (Hou & Tsai, 1993; see also Fig. 5–5■). Likewise, plaque may accumulate undisturbed in the deep mesial groove of the upper first premolars.

Enamel in the furcation area of the root surface may manifest as cervical enamel projections (CEPs) (Fig. 5–6a■) or enamel pearls (Fig. 5–6b■). These ridges of enamel may allow increased plaque accumulation. Essentially, a CEP is an extension of enamel from the cementoenamel junction apically to the entrance of the furcation, which may predispose periodontal destruction within the furcation. It may be difficult to detect a CEP clinically because the area is covered by gingiva. The highest incidence of CEPs is on the buccal aspect of the mandibular second molars. An enamel pearl is similar to a CEP except that it consists of a clump of enamel most commonly located in the bifurcation of molar roots just apical to the cementoenamel junction. It is often mistaken for calculus.

Furcation involvements create a complication because they form a cul-de-sac that creates a plaque trap. Difficult access in this protected area fosters increased

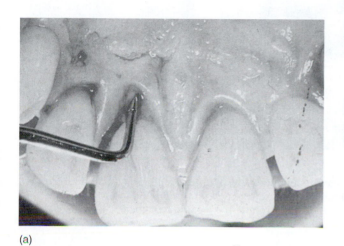

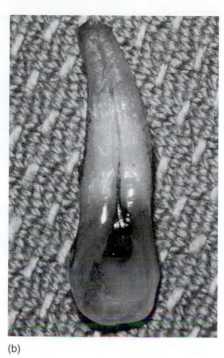

(a)

(b)

Figure 5–5 Clinical photographs of (a) a palatogingival groove with a deep pocket associated with it, and (b) an extracted lateral incisor exhibiting a deep palatal groove.

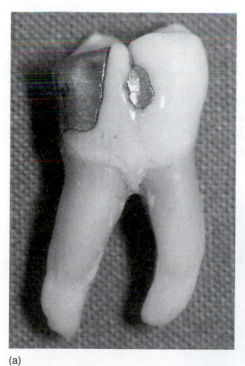

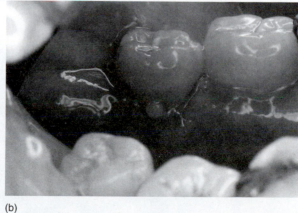

(a)

(b)

Figure 5–6 (a) Clinical photograph of a cervical enamel projection (CEP) at the furcation entrance. (b) Enamel pearl located at the lingual bifurcation on the mandibular first molar resembles a pearl. It is a potential plaque trap.

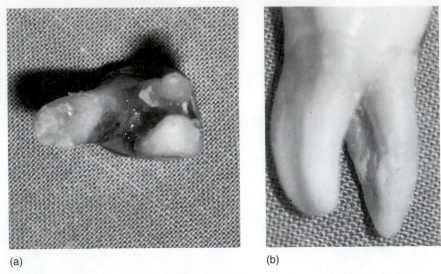

(a)   (b)

Figure 5–7   Clinical photographs of calculus within furcations: (a) dark calculus evident on all internal surfaces of maxillary molar furcations; (b) more veneerlike calculus in internal groove of mesial root of the mandibular molar.

bacterial deposits and often leads to more severe periodontal disease. Proximal furcations on maxillary molars present particular problems because of even more limited access (Fig. 5–7■).

Tooth Position

Tooth position may influence plaque accumulation and access for oral hygiene and therapy. Most studies that have evaluated the influence of crowding, tilting, rotations, and so on, have found that such tooth position anomalies lead to increased plaque accumulation (and more tissue inflammation), especially in patients who do not have excellent oral hygiene practices (Fig. 5–8■). Open contacts allow for food impaction, which may contribute to plaque-induced inflammation.

Figure 5–8   Crowded teeth with inflammation of the gingiva.

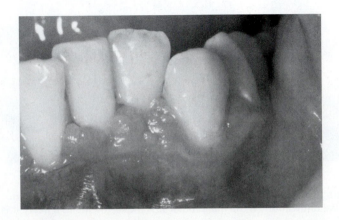

Iatrogenic Factors

There are a number of procedures, techniques, and materials used in dentistry that indirectly, and on occasion directly, contribute to the initiation and/or progress of periodontal disease.

Restorative Dentistry

Rough-surfaced and overcontoured amalgams, composites, crowns, bridges, and other types of restorations have been associated with increased gingival inflammation and periodontal disease. Plaque accumulation is enhanced by subgingival placement of restorations because of problems with greater surface roughness of the materials, fit of the margin to the remaining tooth structure, and contour of the restoration. Subgingival restorations, especially those with defective or overhanging margins, may have a profound effect on periodontal health by retaining plaque within a gingival pocket (Fig. 5–9■).

Injuries to the gingiva can occur during restorative dentistry procedures. For example, a large portion of the interdental papilla can be destroyed by the careless use of a wedge during matrix stabilization. Also, retraction cord, impression material, and temporary restorations may result in irreversible damage to the periodontium.

Fixed partial dentures must be designed such that the patient can clean all surfaces of the restoration, including the pontic area. If removable partial dentures are designed so that they impinge on the soft tissue or they exert torque on the teeth, traumatic injury to the periodontium can occur. In the presence of dental plaque, these insults can result in more rapid, more severe destruction of periodontal structures.

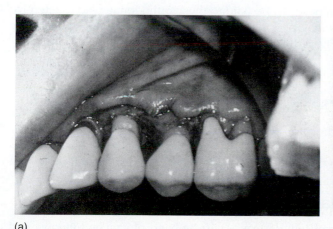

(a)

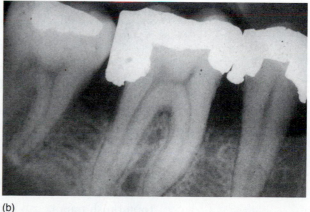

(b)

Figure 5–9   Overhanging restorations contributing to more advanced periodontitis: (a) clinical photograph of deficient crown margins exposed at surgery; (b) radiograph of large overhang on mandibular molar resulting in more advanced bone loss on that tooth surface.

Figure 5–10 Clinical photograph of orthodontic bands and brackets with increased plaque and inflammation.

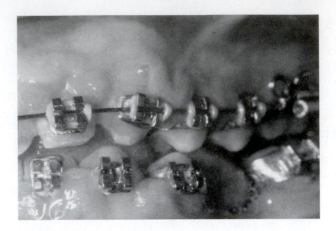

Exodontics

Extractions can adversely affect adjacent teeth if their attachment apparatus is damaged. The soft tissue and bone supporting an adjacent tooth can be irreversibly destroyed. Failure to remove calculus from adjacent tooth surfaces during the extraction may negate the chance for proper healing on the adjacent teeth. An environment may be set up that actually fosters plaque accumulation. Frequently, patients stop eating on the side where teeth have been extracted. In addition to the decrease in masticatory (chewing) stimulation to the periodontium, plaque begins to form on those teeth, and patients avoid brushing the area.

Orthodontics

Orthodontic appliances have long been associated with increased plaque accumulation, gingivitis, and caries. Fixed appliances (bands, brackets, and wires) present excellent retentive areas for bacterial growth and can contribute significantly to inflammation. Special attention needs to be paid to these orthodontic plaque-retentive areas. More frequent recalls may be indicated for patients undergoing orthodontic therapy, especially adults (Fig. 5–10■).

Traumatic Factors

Trauma to the periodontium from several sources can result in the loss of the attachment apparatus, changes in the local anatomy, and increased plaque accumulation and can contribute to the initiation and progression of periodontal diseases.

Toothbrush Trauma

Toothbrush trauma can completely destroy a narrow band of attached gingiva and result in extensive recession. In fact, toothbrush abrasion is one of the two most common factors associated with recession, the other being permanent tooth position. Such abrasion also results in extensive grooving of the root surfaces, creating plaque traps and causing cleaning problems for the patient (Fig. 5–11■).

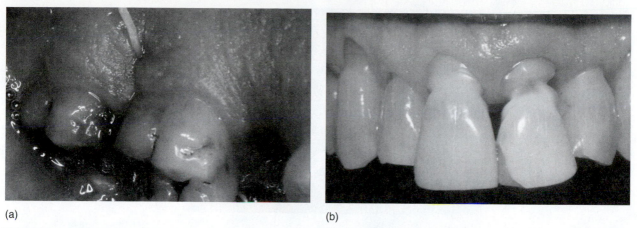

(a)   (b)

Figure 5–11   Examples of trauma to tissues from home-care procedures due to overzealous use of devices: (a) dental floss lesions between maxillary molars; (b) toothbrush abrasion in cervical area of teeth.

Factitious Disease

Occasionally, patients may persistently gouge or "scratch" their gingiva with their fingernails or other devices (factitious disease). This action usually results in extensive exposure of the root surface and localized inflammation. Although relatively rare, whenever isolated areas of recession are noted and a thorough evaluation fails to identify the etiology of the condition, factitious disease should be considered. The change in the local gingival anatomy often leads to greater plaque accumulation and inflammation (Fig. 5–12■).

Food Impaction

Food impaction is one of the more common local factors that may contribute to the initiation and progression of inflammatory periodontal disease. Open contacts, uneven marginal ridges, irregular positions of teeth, and nonphysiologic contours of teeth and restorations can result in the impaction of food on the gingiva and into

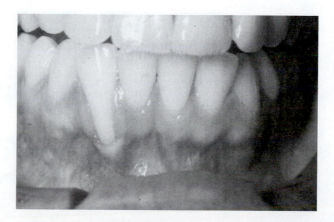

Figure 5–12   Clinical photograph of a factitious habit; recession area on the mandibular right canine.

Figure 5–13 Example of uneven marginal ridges that can cause food impaction. Lower panel shows condition after reshaping of marginal ridges.

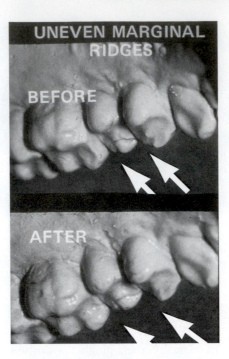

the gingival sulcus (Fig. 5–13■). The cause of the initial breakdown in an area of food impaction or food retention is not clear. Forceful wedging of food beneath the gingival tissues may produce inflammation from physical trauma, and/or food retention leads to food degradation and chemical irritation that affords an excellent breeding ground for bacteria that can initiate and perpetuate the disease process.

Chemical Injury

Indiscriminate use of topically applied aspirin tablets, strong mouthwashes, and various other topical drugs (including cocaine) may result in ulceration of the gingival tissue. Injuries of this nature are usually transient, but may temporarily interfere with plaque control and contribute to periodontal inflammation (Fig. 5–14■).

Figure 5–14 Clinical photograph of local cocaine application mimicking an aspirin burn.

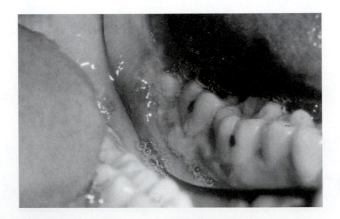

Occlusion

In the past, occlusal trauma was considered to be a major factor in the initiation of periodontal diseases. It has been conclusively proven that occlusal trauma does not initiate gingival or periodontal inflammation or pocket formation. Heavy occlusal forces can, however, cause clinical tooth mobility and the radiographic appearance of bone loss. However, these changes involve the periodontal ligament and bone, and not the marginal gingival surface tissues.

Occlusal trauma may increase the rate of progression of periodontitis if plaque-induced inflammation is also present. In this regard, trauma from occlusion acts as a contributing local risk factor in the presence of inflammation, but is not a primary etiologic factor by itself.

Key Points

- Inflammatory periodontal diseases are infections caused by bacteria.
- Certain secondary local and systemic corisk factors influence the initiation and progression of the disease.
- Dental calculus is not a primary risk factor for the periodontal diseases, but a secondary risk factor.

Web Sites

www.perio.org

www.dent.ucla.edu

www.dentalarticles.com

Self-Quiz

1. Which one of the following sources accounts for the mineralization of subgingival calculus? (p. 83)

   a. salivary proteins

   b. crevicular fluid

   c. dental plaque

   d. acquired pellicle

2. Which one of the following reasons explains the finding of supragingival calculus on the lingual surfaces of the mandibular incisors? (p. 83)

   a. difficulty in cleaning the area with a toothbrush

   b. inability of efficient salivary flow to that area

   c. presence of the parotid duct

   d. presence of Warton's duct

3. Which one of the following reasons makes calculus an important local risk factor for periodontal diseases? (p. 81)

   a. it is porous and can provide a reservoir for bacteria

   b. it directly irritates the epithelial lining of the pocket

   c. minerals cause a breakdown in the epithelial attachment

   d. the presence of lipooligosaccharides causes the tissues to erode

4. All of the following anatomic factors may predispose a site to periodontal disease except one. Which one is the exception? (pp. 84–86)

    a. tooth position

    b. furcation area

    c. crown surface

    d. root surface

5. On which of the following teeth do palatogingival grooves usually appear? (p. 84)

    a. lingual surface of mandibular lateral incisor

    b. lingual surface of mandibular central incisor

    c. palatal surface of maxillary lateral incisor

    d. palatal surface of maxillary central incisor

    e. palatal surface of maxillary canine

References

Carranza, F. A., Jr. 1996. Dental calculus. In eds., F. A. Carranza, Jr., and M. G. Newman, *Clinical periodontology,* 9th ed., 150–160. Philadelphia: W. B. Saunders.

Douglass, C. 1998. Risk assessment for periodontal disease in adults. *Oral Care Report* 8:1–11.

Ellwood, D., J. Melling, and P. Rutter. 1979. The accumulation of organisms on the teeth. In ed., Society for General Microbiology, *Adhesion of micro-organisms to surfaces,* 137–164. New York: Academic Press.

Hou, G.L., and C.C. Tsai. 1993. Relationship between palato-radicular grooves and localized periodontitis. *J. Clin. Periodontol.* 20:668–682.

Mandel, I. D. 1990. Dental calculus (calcified dental plaque). In eds., R. J. Genco, H. M. Goldman, and D. W. Cohen, *Contemporary periodontics,* 135–146. St. Louis, MO: Mosby.

Mandel, I. D. 1995. Calculus update: Prevalence, pathogenicity and prevention. *J. Am. Dent. Assoc.* 126: 573–580.

Pihlstrom, B. L., R. B. McHugh, T. H. Oliphant, and C. Ortiz-Campos 1983. Comparison of surgical and nonsurgical treatment of periodontal disease. A review of current studies and additional results after 6½ years. *J. Clin. Periodontol.* 10:524–541.

Zander, H. 1953. The attachment of calculus to root surfaces. *J. Periodontol.* 24:16–19.

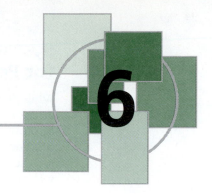

Periodontal Medicine

Raymond A. Yukna, D.M.D., M.S.
John D. Mason, B.A., D.D.S.

Outline

Systemic Risk Factors
for Periodontal
Diseases
Periodontal Diseases as
Risk Factors for
Systemic Conditions
Periodontal Diseases:
The Future

Summary
Key Points
Web Sites
Self-Quiz
References

Goal

To introduce the concept of risk factors for periodontal diseases and the relationship of periodontal diseases as a risk factor for other medical diseases.

Educational Objectives

Upon completion of this chapter, the dental hygiene student should be able to:

List and discuss possible systemic risk factors for periodontal diseases.

Discuss periodontal diseases as a risk factor for specific disease entities such as diabetes mellitus, cardiovascular disease, and preterm low-birth-weight babies.

Describe the role of diabetes mellitus as a primary risk factor for periodontal diseases.

Discuss the importance of smoking as a risk factor for periodontal diseases.

Discuss the association of hormones and periodontal diseases.

KEY WORDS
• periodontal diseases
• risk factors
• systemic diseases
• genetics
• social factors

The authors are indebted to Connie Holland Gandy and Marianne Gabb for assistance with the preparation of this chapter.

Systemic Risk Factors
for Periodontal Diseases

While it must be assumed that general health affects a patient's resistance to the development of periodontal diseases, no specific systemic disease has been shown to produce periodontal diseases in the absence of local irritating factors. In fact, the presence of certain systemic conditions may actually enhance or intensify the response to the oral biofilms beyond what would occur if the systemic condition were not present.

While it is not possible to include every systemic disorder that has an impact on periodontal disease progression, numerous conditions potentially modify biofilm accumulation and disease progression.

Periodontal diseases are no longer regarded as infections to which everyone is equally susceptible. Research is trying to determine why some patients are more "at risk" than others for destructive periodontal diseases. Although bacteria are essential for the development of periodontitis, they are insufficient by themselves. A susceptible host is also necessary, so host factors play a substantial role. Advances in the understanding of the pathogenesis of many chronic systemic diseases have increased awareness of the significant interactions and association that can occur between oral diseases such as periodontal diseases, and systemic diseases (Barnett, 2003). A rather large number of genetic and environmental or acquired factors place individuals at risk for periodontitis (Table 6–1■).

Genetics

It is now known that host susceptibility factors play an important role in high-risk periodontal patients. Evidence for genetic control of risk factors for some forms of periodontal disease includes:

1. a consistent association of periodontitis with certain genetically transmitted traits;
2. studies of separated twins with chronic onset forms of periodontitis; and
3. genetic studies of aggressive forms of periodontitis.

Periodontal diseases can no longer be thought of as a prevalent condition for which all people are at equal risk if they fail to practice good oral hygiene. It appears that microbial and host factors are both important to disease susceptibility, but neither, independently, accounts for all degrees of periodontal disease. Because periodontal diseases are more than likely diverse in etiology, any thought of a universal host risk factor is probably also inappropriate. An association has been found between the susceptibility and severity to periodontitis and the presence of a substance called *interleukin-1* (IL-1). IL-1 is a cytokine that is released from inflammatory cells in the body for the purpose of altering either its own function or those

Table 6–1	Social Factors

- Tobacco
- Stress
- Alcohol
- Drugs

of adjacent cells. An IL-1 gene-positive patient is about seven times more likely to develop or have advanced periodontal disease than a gene-negative patient, and this genotype occurs in approximately 30% of the population (Newman, 1998).

As with many other diseases, susceptibility to periodontal diseases may, to some extent, be genetically determined. Several congenital diseases with periodontal manifestations have been identified, such as hereditary gingival fibromatosis, cyclic neutropenia, Down syndrome, Papillon-Lefévre syndrome, Chediak-Higashi disease, and hypophosphatasia, among others.

It is now clear that genetic factors that act on and modify host responses to the microbial challenge are major determinants of susceptibility to periodontitis, as well as determinants of the rates and extent of disease progression and disease severity. Roughly 50% of the enhanced risk for severe periodontitis can be accounted for by heredity alone. Studies of families with aggressive periodontitis and groups of individuals with chronic periodontitis have shown that certain chromosomes and, in some cases, specific gene loci are linked to enhanced susceptibility for periodontitis (Newman, 1998).

Periodontal findings in twins who were reared together or apart have shown a significant genetic component for probing depth, attachment loss, and plaque that could not be explained by differences in family environment such as oral hygiene practices and frequency of dental visits (Michalowicz et al., 1991).

Age, Gender, and Race

Epidemiologic studies have shown that the incidence (rate of occurrence) of periodontal diseases increases with age (Abdellatif & Burt, 1987). This is likely the result of the cumulative effects of bacterial irritation of the tissues over many years, rather than a reduction in host resistance as a function of the aging process. Evidence strongly suggests that periodontal health can be maintained throughout life if local etiologic factors are controlled.

The National Institute of Dental and Craniofacial Research Survey of Oral Health of Adults in the United States shows that males have a greater incidence and severity of periodontal diseases.

No firm evidence documents that race is a significant risk factor in destructive forms of periodontitis other than as it may be related genetically within particular families.

Stress

Being under long-term physical and psychological stress seems to increase susceptibility to periodontal infection. Stress (along with depression, financial problems, social isolation, and other psychosocial factors) is another systemic risk factor for periodontitis because it may depress the immune response to periodontal pathogens, thereby increasing the severity of periodontal disease (Genco, Ho, et al., 1998). Stressful life events such as divorce, joblessness, and lifestyle factors have been correlated with increased severity of periodontal disease. Stress works in two ways. People under stress change their behavior and may pay less attention to oral hygiene. Also, their bodies increase the production of glucocorticosteroids (hormones made in the body that have anti-inflammatory actions and protect against stress) and cortisone, a type of glucocorticosteroid, which results in immunosuppression and a reduced resistance to infection. Stress variables also seem to have an effect on healing.

Endocrine

Diabetes

Diabetes mellitus is a group of diseases that results in hypgerglycemia (high blood sugar or glucose). Diabetes mellitus is classified into type 1 diabetes and type 2 diabetes. Type 1 is caused by a severe insulin deficiency resulting from a destruction of beta-cells of the pancreas, which produce and secret the hormone called insulin. Insulin is needed to control blood glucose levels since it helps bring blood glucose from the diet and that produced in the liver into the cells. The cells utilize glucose for energy. These patients are treated with insulin injections.

In type 2 diabetes, which is more common than type 1, insulin is being secreted from the pancreas, but not in sufficient amounts. Most probably, the insulin receptors on the cells surface of the tissues are not sensitive enough for the insulin to bind to the cell and allow for glucose uptake into the cell. This is referred to as insulin resistance.

Diabetes is associated with a reduced ability to cope with infections and with impaired wound healing. The balance of evidence suggests that both type 1 diabetes and type 2 diabetes carry an increased risk of severe gingivitis and periodontitis (Page & Beck, 1997). The relationship between diabetes and periodontal diseases is more likely to be observed in poorly controlled individuals (Nishimura, Takahashi, Kurihara, Takashiba, & Murayama, 1998; Taylor et al., 1996). Patients with chronic, poorly controlled diabetes appear to have more attachment loss and bone loss than diabetics with good metabolic control (Safkan-Seppälä & Ainamo, 1992).

Epidemiologic studies on type 1 and type 2 diabetic patients indicate that although persons on optimal control are at equal risk for developing periodontal disease, too few diabetics are optimally controlled, and maintaining strict control is difficult in the long term.

Elevated blood sugar levels (hyperglycemia) may suppress the host's immune response and lead to poor wound healing and recurrent infections such as multiple or recurrent periodontal abscesses. Impaired polymorphonuclear leukocyte chemotaxis (McMullen, Van Dyke, Horoszewicz, & Genco, 1981; Manouchehr-Pour, Spagnuolo, Rodman, & Bissada, 1981) and phagocytosis (Cutler, Eke, Arnold, & Van Dyke, 1991) have been implicated as a factor in the predisposition of patients to severe periodontal destruction. Women with a family history of type 2 diabetes or diagnosed as prediabetic may be at higher risk for gestational diabetes. Close periodontal supervision would seem prudent and early intervention vital. Recent evidence indicates that *meticulous control* of the diabetic state is associated with periodontal health (Grossi & Genco, 1998).

A recent article concluded that poor metabolic control of type 1 diabetes together with smoking is extremely detrimental for clinical attachment loss (Syrjala, Ylostalo, Niskanen, & Knuuttila, 2003).

Hormones

Gingivitis and periodontitis have been noticed clinically to be more severe in some patients during periods of change or imbalance in estrogen/progestin levels (Amar & Chung, 1994). In pregnant, pubertal, and postmenopausal patients, an exaggerated inflammatory response to local irritation may be evident. Hormonal status in general does have an influence on the inflammatory response.

Pregnancy   While evidence suggests that pregnancy itself may not be associated with an increased risk of periodontitis, pregnant patients often exhibit exaggerated gingival inflammatory changes in the second and third trimesters, sometimes called pregnancy gingivitis (Fig. 6–1■). Teeth often become more mobile during pregnancy due to changes in the periodontal ligament, but return to normal after delivery.

Oral Contraceptives   Oral contraceptives act by elevating hormonal levels simulating pregnancy to prevent ovulation. Thus, it is expected that the same gingival changes seen during pregnancy will also be seen in women taking oral contraceptives. Gingival changes may include inflammation and enlargement with increased amount of fluid flow into the tissue. As with pregnancy-associated gingivitis, gingival inflammation in women on oral contraceptives occurs in the presence of very little plaque. The most profound gingival changes are seen in the first few months of initially taking the contraceptive. If the condition worsens, a different formulation may be tried. Maintenance of meticulous oral hygiene is important. Once the woman discontinues the contraceptive, the gingival condition usually reverses.

Since the inception of oral contraceptives, the newer formulations contain less concentration of hormones. Unfortunately, most of the clinical studies investigating oral contraceptive usage were done in the 1960s. One report suggests that because of the lower concentrations in the current oral contraceptive formulations, the inflammatory response of the gingiva to dental plaque was not affected so no gingival changes were found (Preshaw, Knutson, & Mariotti, 2001). Perhaps more research is needed to evaluate these current formulations.

Puberty   Hormonal imbalance is also felt to contribute to the increased severity of gingivitis seen at puberty, when there is an exaggerated response to plaque. The mechanisms are probably similar to those present in pregnancy. Gingival inflammation and enlargement can occur in both males and females, but it is more prevalent in females. Changes in hormonal levels (estrogen and progesterone) and gingival inflammatory changes are transitory and will revert to normal levels post circumpubertal period.

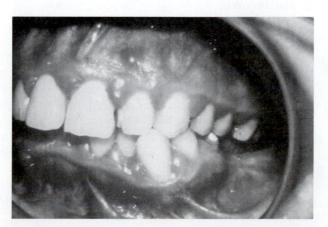

Figure 6–1   Example of pregnancy gingivitis exhibiting proximal puffiness and easy bleeding on probing, reflecting an exaggerated response to local irritants due to hormonal factors.

Menopause/Osteoporosis   Osteoporosis as a result of estrogen depletion causes bone to become more porous, with less trabeculation and decreased thickness of the cortical plate (Jeffcoat, 1998). Under sufficient dental plaque stimulus, this can lead to more severe periodontal disease, including tooth loss. A correlation has been found between osteoporosis and both periodontal disease and tooth loss in postmenopausal women (Bando, Nitta, Matsubara, & Ishikawa, 1998; Jeffcoat, 1998), but it is not considered a definitive risk factor.

Certain risk factors associated with osteoporosis include age, calcium intake (e.g., through the consumption of milk, yogurt, cheese, fish, and calcium supplements), physical activity (e.g., walking, tennis), body build, and smoking status. In a recent study, Bando and Colleagues (1998) found that normal masticatory function in periodontally healthy postmenopausal women might inhibit or delay the progress of osteoporotic changes in skeletal bone.

A study by Jeffcoat (1998) related systemic osteoporosis to oral bone loss, and Kribbs (1990) and Nitta and coworkers (1997) discussed the impact of periodontal health on osteoporosis in postmenopausal women. In the latter study, 12 edentulous postmenopausal women were compared with 14 periodontally healthy postmenopausal women: "The edentulous patients had less bone mineral density of the lumbar spine and less occlusal force." Preliminary evidence suggests that supplementation with biphosphonates, such as alendrolate (Fosamax®, Merck & Co., West Point, PA), may be helpful in stabilizing dental supporting bone because it helps improve total bone mineralization. Calibrating dental radiographs (i.e., subtraction radiography) as a diagnostic tool for systemic osteoporosis may help in early detection of both oral and systemic bone loss (Jeffcoat, 1998).

Hematologic

Several blood dyscrasias have been associated with uncommon, unusual, extreme forms of periodontal diseases. Agranulocytosis and neutropenia (including cyclic neutropenia) are associated with an increased severity of gingivitis and periodontitis as well as necrotic ulcerations. Acute leukemia is characterized by purple-colored gingival enlargement, ulceration, inflammation, and spontaneous severe bleeding. These changes are attributable to infiltration of malignant cells, neutropenia, impaired phagocytosis, platelet deficiency, and decreased effectiveness of associated immune mechanisms. Patients with these medical problems require special attention.

HIV/AIDS

Human immunodeficiency virus (HIV) seropositive individuals appear to be vulnerable to aggressive necrotizing periodontal diseases including linear gingival erythema (LGE), necrotizing ulcerative gingivitis (NUG), and an aggressive necrotizing ulcerative periodontitis (NUP) (Murray, 1994). The development of severe forms of gingivitis and periodontitis is focused on an impairment of the host response (i.e., functional defects in the host's neutrophils) to combat infections. It appears that the degree of immunodeficiency influences the prevalence and severity of these periodontal diseases in the HIV-infected population, and may also influence treatment expectations and prognosis (Fig. 6–2■). This subject is discussed in detail in Chapter 11.

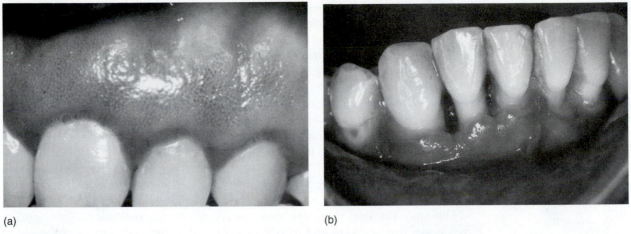

(a)   (b)

Figure 6–2   Periodontal lesions associated with HIV infection: (a) inflammation of the gingiva with characteristic lesions; (b) more advanced lesions that resemble necrotizing ulcerative periodontitis (NUP) and that are nonresponsive to typical therapy.

Nutritional

Nutritional Status

Nutritional deficiencies have not been shown to cause periodontal diseases. Nutrition studies are commonly done by inducing a deprivation state of a single nutrient or a group of related nutrients in laboratory animals that result in decreased formation of the periodontal ligament, bone, and cementum. Very few patients have a diet that is totally lacking in a single nutrient or group of related nutrients; therefore, the information gained from these experimental laboratory studies in animals may not apply to the human clinical situation.

Vitamin deficiencies are probably given more significance in the etiology of periodontal diseases from a clinical standpoint than other nutritional substances. The vitamin most often studied is ascorbic acid (vitamin C), which plays an important role in the normal functions of fibroblasts, osteoblasts, and odontoblasts. When vitamin C levels are greatly reduced (i.e., scurvy), wound healing is impaired.

Some other considerations concerning the diet may be important in the overall dental problems of some patients. Tough or coarse foods do not provide functional stimulation to the gingiva, nor do they help to remove plaque below the contact points or cervical bulge on the teeth.

Patients who regularly eat between meals present a problem in that they constantly provide a food source for the bacteria and may have difficulty in maintaining good oral hygiene.

Drug Induced

Tobacco Products

Cigarette smoking is a major (and may be the most significant) risk factor for severe periodontal diseases. Smokers are about 2.5 times more likely to have periodontal destruction than nonsmokers, yet exhibit less gingival bleeding on probing (Krall, Hayes, Garvey, & Garcia, 1997; Tonetti, 1998). A study by Krall and colleagues (1997) found that current male cigarette smokers had significantly fewer teeth than those men who reported never smoking. The number of missing teeth was positively related to pack/years of cigarette use, age, and coffee consumption and inversely related to level of education. It is more accurate to use the term "pack/years" rather than "pack/day" because it describes the exposure to toxins in a cumulative way. The study also found that current smokers had higher levels of tooth mobility, calculus deposition, and probing depth than men who had never smoked. Former cigarette smokers and men who smoked pipes or cigars were similar to men who never smoked in regard to tooth loss.

Generally, the periodontal status of former smokers has been found to be intermediate between that of never smokers and current smokers (Haber & Kent, 1992; Haber et al., 1993). It has been suggested that the past effects of smoking on the periodontium cannot be reversed, but that smoking cessation is beneficial to periodontal health (American Academy of Periodontology, 1999).

Although smoking does not dramatically affect the oral microbiota, studies have shown that smoking and tobacco products directly modulate the subgingival microflora by favoring colonization with periodontal pathogens (Grossi et al., 1996). Thus, smoking increases the risk for periodontal diseases and interferes with the ability of the gingiva and bone to respond to treatment (Gunsolley et al., 1998; Tonetti, 1998). This mechanism is probably through an altered host response. Effects of smoking seem to be related not only to the local effects in the oral cavity (heat, dryness, and increased plaque and calculus deposits), but also to a suppression of the immune system altering the host response to periodontal pathogens. To adequately deal with bacterial infections, functioning neutrophils are necessary. It has been well documented that cigarette smoke can have harmful effects on various neutrophil functions (Kenny, Kraal, Saxe, & Jones, 1977). For example, tobacco smoke can impair the chemotaxis and phagocytosis of neutrophils (Lannan et al., 1992). Thus, the PMNs do not function properly in eliminating invasive, pathogenic bacteria. Individuals with alterations in their host defense system would then be more susceptible to periodontal infections by preexisting pathogenic bacteria.

Another problem associated with smoking is that products of cigarette smoke remain on the root surfaces and in the gingival crevicular fluid, thereby providing a reservoir of irritants for the soft tissue and preventing tissue attachment.

Research has found that the presence of a specific gene (interleukin-1 beta) has been associated with risk for periodontal disease severity. It has also been reported that in heavy cigarette smokers, carriage of interleukin-1 gene complex was associated with an increased risk for peri-implant (around the implant) bone loss (Feloutzis et al., 2003).

Smokeless tobacco for some may be an alternative to cigarette smoking. However, research has shown that smokeless tobacco may also contribute to periodontal diseases and may eventually lead to cancerous changes in the soft tissues (Fig. 6–3■). A common finding is gingival recession adjacent to the site of tobacco placement. More research is needed to determine whether smokeless tobacco use is associated with an increased level of plaque-associated gingivitis. New studies have found that cigar and pipe smoking may be as harmful to periodontal tissues as cigarette smoking (Krall, Garvey, & Garcia, 1999).

Alcohol

Alcohol abuse may also contribute to periodontal diseases. Chronic alcohol intake presents an increased risk for periodontitis because of increased bleeding tendencies, poor oral hygiene due to overall neglect, and a tendency to malnutrition.

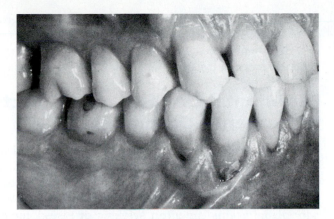

Figure 6–3 Clinical example of smokeless tobacco lesions damaging the periodontium.

Alcohol consumption is related to increased incidence (Drake, Hunt, & Koch, 1995) and prevalence of tooth loss, especially in men (Krall et al., 1997; Kranzler, Babor, Goldstein, & Gold, 1990).

Xerostomia Due to Drugs

Several medications, such as diuretics (antihypertensive drugs) and psychotropic drugs (i.e., anti-anxiety drugs such as Valium; antidepressants such as Elavil; and antipsychotic drugs such as Clozaril and Risperdal) can cause xerostomia or dry mouth, which can be uncomfortable for the patient, interfere with plaque control, and thereby increase periodontal inflammation. The reduced salivary flow has also been associated with increased caries.

Gingival Overgrowth Due to Drugs

Gingival enlargement or overgrowth in response to plaque accumulation can be exaggerated by medications such as phenytoin (used for seizures), calcium channel blocker such as nifedipine (for cardiovascular problems and hypertension), cyclosporine (in transplant patients), and several others. The alveolar bone and attachment apparatus are not affected by these drugs (Ciancio, 1996; Fig. 6–4■).

The areas of enlargement generally begin interproximally, and slowly grow to form triangular tissue masses that eventually unite in a continuous curtain of firm gingival tissue across facial and lingual surfaces. The enlarged tissue interferes with

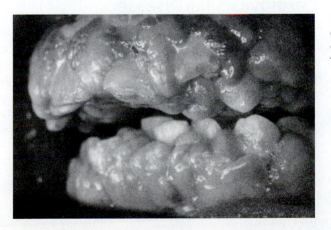

Figure 6–4 Example of drug-induced gingival overgrowth related to the use of cyclosporine.

oral hygiene and is often inflamed. Gingival overgrowth has been reported to occur in about 50% of patients receiving phenytoin (Ciancio, Yaffe, & Catz, 1972), 15% of patients receiving nifedipine (Barak, Engelberg, & Hiss, 1987), and 25% of patients receiving cyclosporine (Daley, Wysocki, & May, 1986).

Periodontal Diseases as Risk Factors for Systemic Conditions

Although inflammatory periodontal diseases are local infections of the gingiva and bone, it has been shown that the presence of periodontitis may *itself* be a risk factor for other infections in the body, systemic diseases, and pregnancy-related problems (American Academy of Periodontology, 1998). This means that oral (periodontal) infections can affect systemic diseases. However, more definitive clinical trials need to be done to confirm the role of periodontitis as a risk factor for systemic diseases.

Diabetes

A conference on oral health and systemic health that was held in Switzerland in December 2002 (Barnett, 2003) concluded that evidence showed that untreated periodontitis can complicate metabolic control of patients with diabetes. Of all the systemic diseases, diabetes and periodontal diseases have been the most extensively studied. It has been shown that periodontal diseases are responsible for higher levels of blood glucose in diabetics (Grossi & Genco, 1998). A recent study that evaluated periodontitis in diabetics with different interleukin (IL-1) genotypes concluded that the prevalence of severe attachment loss increased with decreasing diabetic control (Guzman, Karima, Wang, & Van Dyke, 2003) When these infections are controlled or eliminated in diabetic patients, their insulin requirements can often be reduced. Effective treatment of periodontal diseases can result in a reduced need to gear up tissue metabolism to fight the infection and lower blood sugar levels, thereby reducing insulin requirements and helping in diabetic control with an additional benefit of reducing other complications (e.g., blindness, renal failure, neuropathy, and coronary artery disease) of diabetes. Therefore, control of infections, including periodontal diseases, may be essential to the establishment of good metabolic control in diabetics (American Academy of Periodontology, 1998).

Cardiovascular Disease

In the late 1990s, researchers found a link between periodontal diseases and coronary heart disease (CHD) with an increased risk for atherosclerosis and thromboembolisms, independent of other risk factors for these cardiovascular diseases (Genco, Glurich, Haraszthy, Zambon, & DeNardin, 1998). This link may have been explained by the systemic inflammatory burden caused by inflammatory periodontal diseases (Nakib et al., 2004). Men with periodontitis, especially those under age 50, are 25% more likely to develop coronary heart disease (CHD) (American Academy of Periodontology, 1998; Beck, 1996). Two different surveys have shown that heart disease is the most common condition shared by periodontitis patients (Umino & Nagao, 1993).

In the late 1990s, the connection between heart attacks and periodontal disease was felt to be so convincing that proper plaque control might actually be an exercise that saves a patient's life. Although it may seem unlikely that an infection in the mouth may result in heart disease, there are several possible links that might explain this association. For example, it is well known that if a person has periodontal disease, oral bacteria will enter the blood stream even after chewing or tooth brushing. When bacteria from the inflamed gingival tissue enter the blood stream they trigger platelets to gather around them in a clump, and possibly infect and obstruct the blood vessels in the heart and the brain. Forty percent of those bacteria, especially *Streptococcus sanguis* and *Porphyromonas gingivalis,* have been traced to the mouth (Genco, Glurich, et al. 1998). Patients have a 50% increased risk for heart disease (DeStefano, Andda, Kahn, Williamson, & Russell, 1993) and 30% increased risk for stroke if they also have periodontitis.

Periodontitis and cardiovascular diseases are both associated with a systemic inflammatory response. C-reactive protein (CRP) is an inflammatory serum marker for cardiovascular disease. A study by D'Aiuto, Ready, and Tonetti in 2004 found that periodontitis may result in an increased cardiovascular risk based on serum CRP levels and that successful periodontal therapy could decrease these serum inflammatory markers.

In 2004 Nakib and colleagues reported on a study that was performed between 1996 and 1998 on 6,931 subjects. Results found that compared to subjects with no or mild periodontitis, subjects with moderate or severe periodontitis were more likely to have coronary artery calcification (CAC), but the difference was not statistically significant. Thus, these researchers suggested that periodontitis may not be strongly associated with CAC (Nakib et al., 2004). Future studies need to be conducted on this subject.

Low-Birth-Weight Babies

Women with periodontal disease may be seven to eight times more predisposed to deliver premature (< 37 weeks) infants with low birth weight (< 5.5 lb) (Davenport et al., 1998). Periodontal disease in the mother may be responsible for many of the low-birth-weight, premature births (PLBW). Current data suggest a relationship between elevated prostaglandin E_2 levels in the gingival crevicular fluid (GCF) as a marker of current periodontal disease activity and decreasing birth weight (Offenbacher et al., 1998). The increased production of PGE_2 by the mother is due to a response to the anaerobic periodontal infection. This twofold elevation in PGE_2, which is seen in the GCF and amniotic sac, was observed in PLBW compared with normal-birth-weight mothers (Hill, 1998). One-hundred and twenty-four pregnant or postpartum mothers were examined for periodontitis at the University of North Carolina (Offenbacher et al., 1996). Mothers with a defined preterm low-birth-weight delivery demonstrated that periodontal disease was a "statistically significant risk factor for PLBW." PLBW status is defined as a birth weight of less than 2500 g and/or a gestational age of less than 37 weeks at delivery or premature rupture of membranes. "PLBW cases had significantly worse periodontal disease than respective normal birth weight (NBW) controls." PLBW is a major health problem because it occurs in 1 in 10 deliveries and results in infant mortality, long-term morbidity, and 5 million neonatal intensive care unit hospital stays per year. The emotional, social, and financial burdens on families are extraordinary (Dasanayake, 1998).

A clinical pilot study published in 2003 was conducted to determine whether treatment of periodontitis reduces the risk of spontaneous preterm birth. This study concluded that although this pilot study found that performing scaling and root planing in pregnant women with periodontitis might reduce spontaneous preterm birth, larger trials need to be done (Jeffcoat et al., 2003) to confirm that periodontal therapy decreases the frequency of preterm delivery and neonatal complications.

Confirmatory research will mandate early periodontal diagnosis and dental treatment before and during pregnancy. This information will require obstetrical awareness and collaboration with dental professionals.

Respiratory Diseases

Patients with periodontal disease may be at risk for respiratory diseases (Hayes, Sparrow, Cohen, Vokonas, & Garcia, 1998). Periodontal disease is added to the list of other risk factors for this problem, including the elderly, people who smoke, and individuals confined to nursing homes or hospitals. Examples of respiratory diseases include pneumonia, bronchitis, and emphysema. Bacteria (oral biofilms) found in the oral cavity can be taken up into the lung to cause respiratory diseases. In hospital and nursing home environments, there may be less attention paid to oral hygiene. Pneumonia may be the result of infection by anaerobic bacteria, which is a component of dental plaque (American Academy of Periodontology, 1998; Scannapieco & Mylotte, 1996)

Summary

It is well known that certain medical conditions such as diabetes mellitus may cause periodontal disease in certain individuals. Additionally, periodontal diseases have been documented to cause certain medical conditions including coronary heart disease, diabetes mellitus, low-birth-weight babies, and respiratory diseases. It then becomes apparent that periodontal clinicians are treating the "whole" patient and attempting to control both periodontal diseases and medical conditions.

Key Points

- Currently, evidence-based dentistry supports the use of risk assessment techniques to guide clinical decisions in the treatment of periodontal diseases.
- Important risk factors for periodontal diseases include certain periodontal bacteria, diabetes mellitus, and smoking.
- Other risk factors not strongly related but still associated with increased probability of periodontal diseases include aging, gender, genetic predisposition, stress, nutrition, and systemic diseases including immunosuppression.
- Not only do certain medical conditions predispose individuals to periodontal diseases, but also periodontal diseases predispose people to certain medical conditions.
- Attempts to manage risk factors are important in the prevention and treatment of periodontal diseases.

Web Sites

www.perio.org
www.nidr.nih.gov/health

www.ada.org
www.grc.uri.edu
www.pharmaceutical-business-review.com
www.dentalarticles.com

Self-Quiz

1. Which one of the following is the primary risk factor for periodontal diseases? (p. 94)
   a. dental calculus
   b. dental biofilms
   c. diabetes mellitus
   d. HIV/AIDS infection
   e. respiratory diseases

2. Which one of the following evidence exists to support the concept of a genetic predisposition to periodontal diseases? (pp. 94–95)
   a. presence of a specific type of bacteria
   b. increased levels of bacterial enzymes in the blood
   c. association of periodontitis with certain transmitted traits
   d. transmission of bacteria through saliva from mother to child

3. Which one of the following mechanisms explains how increased stress adversely affects the periodontium? (p. 95)
   a. increases in subgingival pathogenic bacteria
   b. increases in estrogen levels results in gingivitis
   c. less compliance with home care of teeth and gums
   d. shifts in the concentration of available endotoxins

4. The hormonal changes associated with pregnancy cause an increased incidence of gingival disease because these changes are associated with an increase in sex hormone levels. (pp. 96–97)
   a. Both the statement and the reason are correct and related.
   b. Both the statement and the reason are correct but not related.
   c. The statement is correct, but the reason is not.
   d. The statement is not correct, but the reason is correct.
   e. Neither the statement nor the reason is correct.

5. Smoking affects the periodontium by which one of the following mechanisms? (pp. 99–100)
   a. decreasing the number of melanocytes
   b. suppressing of the immune system
   c. altering the metabolism of fibroblasts
   d. increasing the amount of fibrotic tissue
   e. decreasing the number of periodontal pathogens

6. Periodontal diseases are thought to be an important risk factor for all of the following medical conditions except one. Which one is the exception? (pp. 94–104)
   a. stroke
   b. hypertension
   c. diabetes mellitus
   d. low-birth-weight babies
   e. kidney failure

7. Which of the following statements is true about smoking and periodontal diseases? (pp. 99–100)

   a. Smoking dramatically effects the oral microflora.

   b. Smoking cessation is beneficial to periodontal health.

   c. Past effects of smoking on the periodontium is usually reversible.

   d. Current smokers have a low level of tooth mobility.

   e. Smokeless tobacco does not increase the incidence of periodontal disease.

8. Which of the following substances may be related to periodontal disease activity and low birth weight babies? (p. 103)

   a. blood

   b. suppuration

   c. gingival crevicular fluid

   d. protaglandin E_2

   e. saliva

9. Which of the following bacterium in the mouth has been found to possibly infect and obstruct blood vessels in the heart and the brain? (pp. 102–103)

   a. *Prevotella intermedia*

   b. *Fuscobacterium nucleatum*

   c. *Porphyromonas gingivalis*

   d. *Campylobacter rectus*

   e. *Bacteroides forsythus* (new name: *Tannerella forsythensis*)

10. Which of the following explains why patients with periodontal disease may be at risk for respiratory diseases especially in hospitals and nursing homes? (p. 104)

   a. neglected oral hygiene

   b. decayed teeth

   c. collapsed circulatory system

   d. increased risk for heart failure

   e. increased risk for other systemic diseases

References

Abdellatif, H. M., and B. A. Burt. 1987. An epidemiological investigation into the relative importance of age and oral hygiene status as determinants of periodontitis. *J. Periodontol.* 66:16–33.

Amar, S., and K. M. Chung. 1994. Influence of hormonal variation on the periodontium in women. *Periodontology* 6:79–87.

American Academy of Periodontology. 1998. Periodontal disease as a potential risk factor for systemic disease (Position Paper). *J. Periodontol.* 69:841–850.

American Academy of Periodontology. 1999. Tobacco use and the periodontal patient (position paper). *J. Periodontol.* 70:1419–1427.

Bando, K., H. Nitta, M. Matsubara, and I. Ishikawa. 1998. Bone mineral density in periodontally healthy and edentulous postmenopausal women. *Ann. Periodontol.* 3:322–326.

Barak, S., I. S. Engelberg, and J. Hiss. 1987. Gingival hyperplasia caused by nifedipine—histopathologic findings. *J. Periodontol.* 58:639–642.

Barnett, M. L. 2003. Coordination Meeting on Oral Health and Systemic Health Periodontal Medicine: Health Policy Implications. Geneva, Switzerland. *J. Periodontol.* 74:1081–1086.

Beck, J. D. 1996. Periodontal implications: Older adults. *Ann. Periodontol.* 1:322–457.

Ciancio, S. G. 1996. Medications as risk factors for periodontal disease. *J. Periodontol.* 67:1055–1059.

Ciancio, S. G., S. J. Yaffe, and C. C. Catz. 1972. Gingival hyperplasia and diphenylhydantoin. *J. Periodontol.* 43:411–414.

Cutler, C. W., P. Eke, R. R. Arnold, and T. E. Van Dyke. 1991. Defective neutrophil function in an insulin-dependent diabetic patient. A case report. *J. Periodontol.* 62:394–401.

D'Aiuto F., D. Ready, and M.S. Tonetti. Periodontal disease and C-reactive protein-associated cardiovascular risk. 2004. *J. Periodontol. Res.* 39:236–241.

Daley, T. D., G. P. Wysocki, and C. May. 1986. Clinical and pharmacological correlations in cyclosporin-induced gingival hyperplasia. *Oral Surg. Oral Med. Oral Patho.* 62:417–421.

Dasanayake, A. P. 1998. Periodontal disease as a risk factor in pregnancy. *Ann. Periodontol.* 3:206–212.

Davenport, E. S., C. E. C. S. Williams, J. A. C. Sterne, V. Sivapathasundram, J. M. Fearne, and M. A. Curtis. 1998. The East London study of maternal chronic periodontal disease and preterm low birth weight infants: Study design and prevalence data. *Ann Periodontol.* 3:213–221.

DeStefano, F., R. F. Andda, H. S. Kahn D. F. Williamson, and C. M. Russell. 1993. Dental disease and risk of coronary heart disease and mortality. *Br. Med. J.* 306:688–691.

Drake, C. W., R. J. Hunt, and G. G. Koch. 1995. Three-year tooth loss among black and white older adults in North Carolina. *J. Dent. Res.* 74:675–680.

Feloutzis A., N. P. Lang, M. S. Tonetti, W. Burgin, U. Bragger, et al. 2003. Il-1 gene polymorphism and smoking as risk factors for peri-implant bone loss in a well-maintained population. *Clin. Oral Implants Res.* 14:10–17.

Genco, R. J., I. Glurich, V. Haraszthy, J. Zambon, and E. DeNardin. 1998. Overview of risk factors for periodontal disease and implications for diabetes and cardiovascular disease. *Compendium* (special issue) 19:40–45.

Genco, R. J., A. W. Ho, J. Kopman, S. G. Grossi, R. G. Dunford, and L. A. Tedesco. 1998. Models to evaluate the role of stress in periodontal diseases. *Ann. Periodontol.* 3:288–302.

Grossi, S. G., and R. J. Genco. 1998. Periodontal disease and diabetes mellitus: A two-way relationship. *Ann. Periodontol.* 3:51–61.

Grossi, S. G., F. B. Skrepcinski, T. DeCaro, J. J. Zambon, D. Cummins, and R. J. Genco. 1996. Responses to periodontal therapy in diabetics and smokers. *J. Periodontol.* 67(Suppl.):1094–1102.

Gunsolley, J. C., S. M. Quinn, J. Tew, C. M. Gooss, C. N. Brooks, and H. A. Schenkein. 1998. The effect of smoking on individuals with minimal periodontal destruction. *J. Periodontol.* 69:165–170.

Guzman S., M. Karima, H. Y. Wang, and T. E. Van Dyke. 2003. Association between interleukin-1 genotype and periodontal disease in a diabetic population. *J. Periodontol.* 74:1183–1190.

Haber, J., and R. L. Kent. 1992. Cigarette smoking in periodontal practice. *J. Periodontol.* 63:100–106.

Haber, J., J. Wattles, M. Crowley, R. Mandell, K. Joshipura, and R. L. Kent. 1993. Evidence for cigarette smoking as a major risk factor for periodontitis. *J. Periodontol.* 64:16–23.

Hayes, C., D. Sparrow, M. Cohen, P. S. Vokonas, and R. I. Garcia. 1998. The association between alveolar bone loss and pulmonary function: The VA dental longitudinal study. *Ann. Periodontol.* 3:257–261.

Hill, G. B. 1998. Preterm birth: Associations with genital and oral microflora. *Ann. Periodontol.* 3:222–232.

Jeffcoat, M. K. 1998. Osteoporosis: A possible modifying factor in oral bone loss. *Ann. Periodontol.* 3:312–321.

Jeffcoat, M.K., J.C. Hauth, N.C., Geurs, M. S. Reddy, S. P. Cliver, et al. 2003. Periodontal disease and preterm birth: results of a pilot intervention study. *J. Periodontol.* 74:1214–1218.

Kenny, E. G., J. H. Kraal, S. R. Saxe, and J. Jones. 1977. The effect of cigarette smoke on human oral polymorphonuclear leukocytes. *J. Periodont. Res.* 12:227–234.

Krall, E., A. Garvey, and R. Garcia. 1999. Alveolar bone loss and tooth loss in male cigar and pipe smokers. *J. American Dent. Assoc.* 130:57–64.

Krall, E., C. Hayes, A. J. Garvey, and R. I. Garcia. 1997. Study finds a correlation between smoking and tooth loss. *J. Mass. Dent. Soc.* 46:20–23.

Kranzler, H. R., T. F. Babor, L. Goldstein, and J. Gold. 1990. Dental pathology and alcohol-related indicators in an outpatient clinic sample. *Community Dent. Oral Epidemiol.* 18:204–207.

Lannan, S., A. McLean, E. Drost, M. Gillooly, K. Donaldson, et al. 1992. Changes in neutrophil morphology and morphometry following exposure to cigarette smoke. *Int. J. Exp. Pathol.* 73:183–191.

Manouchehr-Pour, M., P. J. Spagnuolo, H. M. Rodman, and N. F. Bissada. 1981. Comparison of neutrophil chemotactic response in diabetic patients with mild and severe periodontal disease. *J. Periodontol.* 52:410–414.

McMullen, J. A., T. E. Van Dyke, H. U. Horoszewicz, and R. J. Genco. 1981. Neutrophil chemotaxis in individuals with advanced periodontal disease and a genetic predisposition to diabetes mellitus. *J. Periodontol.* 52:167–173.

Michalowicz, B. S., D. P. Aeppli, R. K. Kuba, J. E. Bereuter, J. P. Conry, et al. 1991. A twin study of genetic variation in proportional radiographic alveolar bone height. *J. Dent. Res.* 70:1431–1435.

Murray, P. 1994. Periodontal diseases in patients infected by human immunodeficiency virus. *Periodontology 2000* 6:50–67.

Nakib, S.A., J.S., Pankow, J.D. Beck, S. Offenbacher, G. W. Evans, et al. 2004. Periodontitis and coronary artery calcification: the Atherosclerosis Risk in Communities (ARIC) study. *J. Periodontol.* 75(4):505–510.

Newman, M. 1998. Genetic, environmental, and behavioral influences on periodontal infections. *Compendium* (special issue) 19:25–31.

Nishimura, F., K. Takahashi, M. Kurihara, S. Takashiba, and Y. Murayama. 1998. Periodontal disease as a complication of diabetes mellitus. *Ann. Periodontol.* 3:20–29.

Nitta, H., K. Bando, M. Matsubara, and I. Ishikawa. 1997. *Impact of periodontal health on osteoporosis in post-*

menopausal women. Periodontal Diseases and Human Health: New directions in Periodontal Medicine. Sunstar–Chapel Hill, Chapel Hill, NC, March 24–25.

Offenbacher, S., H. L. Jared, P. G. O'Reilly, S. R. Wells, G. E. Salvi, et al. 1998. Potential pathogenic mechanisms of periodontitis-associated pregnancy complication. *Ann. Periodontol.* 3(1): 233–250.

Offenbacher, S., B. Katz, G. Fertik, J. Collins, D. Boyd, et al. 1996. Periodontal infection as a possible risk factor for preterm low birth weight. *J. Periodontol.* 67: 1103–1113.

Page, R. C., and J. D. Beck. 1997. Risk assessment for periodontal diseases. *Int. Dent. J.* 47:61–87.

Preshaw P.M., M.A. Knutsen, and A. Mariotti. Experimental gingivitis in women using oral contraceptives. *J Dent Res* 80:2011–2015.

Safkan-Seppälä, B., and J. Ainamo. 1992. Periodontal conditions in insulin-dependent diabetes mellitus. *J. Clin. Periodontol.* 19:24–29.

Scannapieco, R. A., and J. M. Mylotte. 1996. Relationships between periodontal disease and bacterial pneumonia. *J. Periodontol.* 67:1114–1122.

Syrjala. A.M., P. Ylostalo, M.C. Niskanen, and M.L. Knuuttila. 2003. Role of smoking and HbA1c level in periodontitis among insulin-dependent diabetic patients. *J. Clin. Periodontol.* 30:871–875.

Taylor, G. W., B. A. Burt, M. P. Becker, R. J. Genco, M. Shlossman, et al. 1996. Severe periodontitis and risk for poor glycemic control in patients with noninsulin-dependent diabetes mellitus. *J. Periodontol.* 67: 1085–1093.

Tonetti, M. S. 1998. Cigarette smoking and periodontal diseases: Etiology and management of the disease. *Ann. Periodontol.* 3:88–101.

Umino, M., and M. Nagao. 1993. Systemic disease in elderly dental patients. *Int. Dent. J.* 43:213–218.

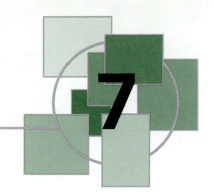

Bacteria–Host Response: Inflammatory and Immunology Fundamentals

Mea A. Weinberg, D.M.D, M.S.D., R.Ph.

Outline

Periodontal Disease
   Activity
The Bacteria–Host
   Challenge
Oral Defense
   Mechanisms
The Inflammatory
   Response and the
   Immune Response

Host Response to the
   Periodontal Diseases
Summary
Key Points
Web Sites
Self-Quiz
References

Goal

To provide an understanding of host response to the bacteria present in dental biofilms (plaque).

Educational Objectives

Upon completion of this chapter, the dental hygiene student should be able to:

List three theories of periodontal disease activity.

Describe the progression of gingivitis into periodontitis.

Discuss bacterial components that stimulate the initiation of the inflammatory and immune systems.

Describe the different levels of oral defense mechanisms.

Describe the inflammatory/immune host responses to plaque-induced periodontal diseases.

Describe the process of phagocytosis.

Compare and contrast humoral immunity and cellular immunity.

KEY WORDS

- periodontitis
- clinical connective tissue attachment loss
- gingivitis
- inflammatory process
- immune response
- periodontal disease activity
- host response
- antigens

Gingivitis is defined as inflammation confined to the gingiva without clinical connective tissue attachment loss and bone loss. Gingivitis is a direct response of the host (body) to the accumulation of supragingival dental biofilms at the gingival margin. Periodontitis is defined as the loss of clinical connective tissue attachment (also referred to as clinical attachment loss) and alveolar bone loss with the formation of a periodontal pocket. Clinical connective tissue attachment loss refers to the pathological detachment of collagen fibers from the cemental surfaces with the concomitant apical migration of the apical part of the junctional epithelium onto the root surface (Armitage, 1995). The events leading to clinical connective tissue attachment loss also result in the destruction of alveolar and supporting bone. The *inflammatory process* involved in the development of gingivitis and periodontitis is influenced by the *immune response* of the individual.

 ## Periodontal Disease Activity

The development of chronic inflammatory periodontal diseases involves a series of host responses or reactions of the body to bacteria present in the dental biofilm, which is considered the invader or irritant. Host cells or cells normally found in the body are needed to fight this infection. Examples of host cells include blood cells present in the body, such as macrophages, lymphocytes, and polymorphonuclear leukocytes (PMNs) or, as they are sometimes called, neutrophils. PMNs are a type of white blood cell involved in the host defense system. The host defense is constantly being called upon to ward off attacks of the microorganisms that are colonizing the oral cavity at any given time. This balance of host defense mechanisms against the microbial attack is kept in check until the microorganisms overtake the defense system, at which time infection and tissue damage develop. It is assumed that host cells mediate the destruction of soft and hard connective tissue because of the reaction to bacteria in the plaque.

Periodontal disease activity (PDA) is defined as the *ongoing* loss of clinical connective tissue attachment and alveolar and supporting bone (Greenstein & Caton, 1990) at a certain point in time (e.g., at the clinical examination appointment). Detection of areas in the mouth that are in the active stage of destruction may be important in the implementation of treatment. However, it is extremely difficult to determine at a given time if a site is actively breaking down or will break down in the future.

Models of Disease Activity

Currently, three theories of periodontal disease activity have been described:

- the continuous model theory;
- the random burst theory; and
- the asynchronous multiple burst theory.

The continuous model theory is based on the concept that periodontal destruction is slow and constant until tooth loss and the severity of the disease increase with age (Löe, Anerud, Boysen, & Morrison, 1986). However, epidemiologic studies have not demonstrated whether destruction is continuous or new diseased sites actually develop (Greenstein & Caton, 1990).

The next theory is the random burst theory (Socransky, Haffajee, Goodson, & Lindhe, 1984). This theory states that periodontal diseases progress in short bursts of exacerbation (actively losing attachment) followed by a period of remission or quiescence where there is no progressive attachment loss (Goodson, 1992; Socransky et al. 1984). Another proposed name for this theory is the episodic burst theory, which reflects the fact that periodontal diseases are site specific and not all sites in the mouth are equally susceptible (Zimmerman, 1986).

The third concept, the asynchronous multiple burst hypothesis, states that periodontal disease activity occurs during a limited time period (e.g., acne during childhood may resolve during adulthood) followed by remission (Greenstein & Caton, 1990; Socransky et al., 1984).

In reality, all of the above theories may be interacting to explain periodontal disease progression. No one theory alone can explain the disease progression. It cannot be assumed that all sites will continuously get worse. Also, treatment should not wait until a burst of bone destruction has occurred. Periodontal destruction is cumulative over time. Since it is difficult to actually determine if a site is disease active, it is prudent to treat all inflamed sites (Greenstein & Caton, 1990).

Progression of Gingivitis into Periodontitis

Gingivitis must precede periodontitis. That is, periodontitis does not develop unless gingivitis existed previously. However, gingivitis may, but does not always, progress to periodontitis.

Why does periodontitis develop in some individuals while in others gingivitis does not progress into periodontitis? Currently, the *exact* cause for the progression of gingivitis into periodontitis is relatively unclear. Approximately 80% of the population is susceptible to periodontal diseases (Brown & Löe, 1993). Susceptibility to periodontal diseases involves changes in bacteria–host equilibrium. A failure of this equilibrium results in the initiation of periodontal disease. However, although bacteria are essential to this process, their presence alone is not enough to cause destructive periodontal disease. There must be a decrease in the number of beneficial (good) bacteria such as *Streptococcus* sp., a critical mass of pathogenic (disease-producing) bacteria, a conducive or favorable environment to cause disease, and a susceptible host that reacts to the pathogen. Gingivitis may progress into periodontitis if the host resistance decreases and if bacteria overwhelm the defense system and penetrate soft tissue. Some reasons for a decrease in host resistance include stress, chemotherapy, local tissue trauma, uncontrolled diabetes, leukemia, steroids, and fully developed acquired immunodeficiency syndrome (AIDS).

The host response is in nature a defense mechanism. It is a natural response of the body to protect and defend the individual after the person's body has been challenged by an injurious agent such as a bacterium or virus. This same host response that provides protection to host tissues frequently also causes host tissue destruction (Fig. 7–1■). When the repair of tissue is greater than its destruction, the tissue starts healing. Fortunately, host tissue destruction usually is not permanent since tissues have a great capacity for healing.

Poor oral hygiene with/without contributing
environmental systemic and acquired factors (a susceptible host)

↓

Accumulation of dental biofilms and other antigens
at the gingival margin and in the gingival crevice; bacteria release antigenic
substances through the crevice into the connective tissue

↓

Host's inflammatory and immune systems activated

↙   ↘

Protective
PMN and macrophage phagocytosis;
plasma cell production of antibodies

Destructive
Prostaglandin E_2, cytokines, collagenases
(matrix metalloproteinases (MMPs)) and
lysosomal enzymes cause connective tissue
destruction including bone destruction

Figure 7–1 Pathway of the pathogenesis showing the sequence of events leading to periodontal destruction.

The Bacteria–Host Challenge

Microbiology

Bacteria that colonize early on the tooth surface at the gingival margin are predominately supragingival Gram-positive facultative (i.e., can live with or without oxygen) *Streptococci* and *Actinomyces* species. If plaque is not disrupted by toothbrushing and flossing, a more established and varied microbial colony develops. With increasing time and poor plaque control, periodontitis-associated microbiota populate the subgingival pocket area, including Gram-negative anaerobes (oxygen intolerant) such as *Fusobacterium nucleatum, Porphyromonas gingivalis, Eikenella corrodens, Actinobacillus actinomycetemcomitans,* and *Prevotella intermedia* (Listgarten, 1994). In addition to the subgingival anaerobic bacteria found in the deeper subgingival plaque, the bacteria found in a layer of unattached plaque in direct contact with the junctional epithelium may be or has the potential to become pathogenic and cause disease. Anaerobic bacteria become established as the bacteria multiply and become thicker with less oxygen available to the bacteria. The rate of subgingival plaque recolonization may depend upon supragingival plaque accumulation.

Bacteria, their metabolic wastes or by-products, and toxins they synthesize and release into the subgingival environment are foreign to the body and are termed antigens. Long-standing, chronic bacterial accumulation causes an excessive and persistent antigenic stimulus to the host response mechanisms. Thus, while bacteria initiate the disease process, it is enzymes and by-products produced by the host that are actually responsible for most of the breakdown of periodontal tissues. As a side effect, the reactions activated by the host response result in tissue inflammation in which surrounding cells, connective tissue, and bone are destroyed. Thus, host responses are basically protective by destroying antigens, but if the body is overwhelmed then the host responses are destructive, causing soft- and hard-tissue destruction.

Bacterial Components

Bacteria release metabolic substances proven to be toxic to cells and tissues. These stimulate the initiation of the inflammatory and immune systems. The following substances are released from bacteria that affect the host:

1. Endotoxin, a lipopolysaccharide (also termed lipooligosaccharide), is part of the outer membrane of all Gram-negative bacteria. Endotoxins, which are released when the bacteria die and lysis (break apart), stimulate biologic activities that cause tissue damage and bone destruction.
2. Leukotoxin, an exotoxin produced by *Actinobacillus actinomycetemcomitans,* can kill PMNs.
3. Bacteria synthesize and release various waste products (by-products) such as ammonia, which is toxic to many host cells, and hydrogen sulfide, which increases the permeability of the epithelium so that antigenic substances can more easily enter the lamina propria.
4. Bacteria synthesize and secrete enzymes, which can break down tissue. Hyaluronidase, an enzyme found in periodontal pockets, may break down or degrade the "cementing substance" between epithelial cells causing widening of the intercellular spaces and increased permeability. Collagenase may break down collagen and proteases degrade the connective tissue ground substance. Host cells such as PMNs and fibroblasts also secrete collagenase. Thus, these enzymes that bacteria and host cells synthesize and release prepare the tissues for absorption of toxic and otherwise harmful bacterial products.

Oral Defense Mechanisms

The host interacts with microorganisms at three different areas in the periodontium:

- the supragingival environment;
- the gingival crevice; and
- the gingival connective tissue.

The first attempt at self-protection comes from the supragingival environment and involves nonspecific defenses. These responses are important in the prevention of the extension of supragingival plaque into the subgingival area (the gingival crevice). Defense mechanisms include:

1. Saliva, which contains numerous defensive substances such as antibacterial factors (lysozyme, lactoferrin, lactoperoxidase, myeloperoxidase) and antibodies (secretory immunoglobulin A [sIgA]). Antibodies called immunoglobulins are proteins present in the blood serum and mucosal secretions (e.g., saliva, tears, sweat, nasal fluids) produced following interaction with an antigen.
2. Gingival crevicular fluid (GCF) functions as an outward flow cleansing the sulcus. The increased volume of GCF produced during the inflammatory process also serves to deliver more antimicrobial products from the deeper tissue toward the main site of supragingival bacterial colonization (e.g.,

tooth surface). These are the first substances to interact with the antigenic challenge (bacteria) to try to neutralize, isolate, or kill it.

3. Oral epithelium also serves to prevent bacteria and their by-products from entering the underlying tissues. This is attained by the surface keratin and the close attachment of the epithelial cells.

4. Shedding of epithelial cells from the oral mucosa into the oral cavity.

The Inflammatory Response and the Immune Response

If the body is unsuccessful in eliminating the pathogenic bacteria at the supragingival level, the inflammatory/immune response, working together, is further stimulated to eliminate the irritant and prevent the spread of infection. This system is activated when antigens (e.g., endotoxins, bacterial enzymes, and by-products) present in the plaque mass in the gingival crevice pass through the protective wall of PMNs (leukocyte wall) interposed between the plaque mass and the lining of the gingival crevice and junctional epithelium. After the antigens cross the junctional epithelial barrier, the deeper tissues are penetrated (Miyasaki, 1991; see Fig. 7–2■). Only a few bacteria themselves actually enter the connective tissue. Usually, it is the products from the bacteria that enter the tissues while the bacteria remain in the crevice. However, it has been demonstrated that *Actinobacillus actinomycetemcomitans, Porphyromonas* gingivalis, and spirochetes invade connective tissue (Winström, Dahlén, Slots, & Egelberg, de Graaf, van Winkelhoff, & Goené, 1989; Renvert, 1990; Saglie, Carranza, Newman, Cheng, & Lewin, 1982). Activation of the inflammatory/immune system results in the following: (1) elimination or retardation of the invader (bacteria); (2) the limiting of further tissue destruction; and (3) the beginning of healing.

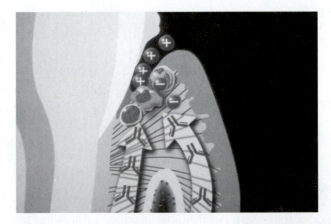

Figure 7–2   As the protective wall of neutrophils between the plaque mass and the gingival crevice and junctional epithelium becomes compromised, the inflammatory response becomes magnified by the immune system. Once the antigens in the pocket pass through the wall of white blood cells and touch or penetrate the gingival connective tissue, a burst of immunological response results in gingival tissue, periodontal ligament damage, and alveolar and supporting bone destruction. (Courtesy of Procter & Gamble, Cincinnati, OH.)

The Inflammatory Response

The inflammatory response to a bacterial challenge is a nonspecific reaction intended to prevent the spread of invading bacteria and, if possible, destroys the damaging agent. This is accomplished through the process of inflammation.

When bacteria cause irritation to the gingival or periodontal tissues, a series of responses mediated by host defense cells is initiated. First, an acute inflammatory response occurs. Table 7–1■ lists the cells involved in the inflammatory response. If this is ineffective and the stimulus is not removed and healing does not occur, inflammation becomes chronic and additional defense cells from the immune system become involved. After the events in the periodontal areas subside, the tissues are cleansed, repaired, and rebuilt. Unfortunately, sometimes the damage to some of these tissues is permanent and is present even after the infection is eliminated.

Elements of the Inflammatory System

Clinically healthy gingiva that is relatively plaque-free is characterized by a salmon pink color, firm consistency, no bleeding from the gingival crevice, and shallow sulci. In healthy gingiva the junctional epithelium does not have long epithelial ridges and overlies the highly oriented collagen fiber bundles. Although clinically there may appear to be no inflammation, at a microscopic level there may be a mild inflammatory reaction. Thus, in the junctional epithelium of clinically healthy gingiva there are always inflammatory cells, primarily PMNs, which form a protective wall between the epithelium and the bacteria. PMNs constantly migrate from the junctional epithelium into the gingival crevice where the older cells are shed into the oral cavity. With severe inflammation, a greater number of these cells are present.

The Inflammatory Process

Table 7–2■ describes three phases of the inflammatory process. If dental plaque is allowed to accumulate at the gingival margin and is not disrupted, inflammation or gingivitis results. Plaque removal every 48 hours can prevent gingivitis, but if allowed to accumulate for 72 hours, gingivitis will develop (Van Dyke, Offenbacher, Pihstrom, Putt, & Trummel, 1999). The gingiva reacts to the bacteria and its products by the first 3 days of plaque accumulation at the gingival margin with signs of acute inflammation. The first inflammatory response to injury is vascular changes in the gingival connective tissue; the epithelium is avascular. Vasodilation of the blood vessels in the connective tissue results in the outflow of blood, fluids, proteins, and cells (PMNs) into the connective tissue (Fig. 7–3■). The primary substance responsible for the vasodilation and increased permeability of the blood vessel wall is histamine, which is released from mast cells found in the connective

Table 7–1	Key Elements in the Inflammatory Response

- Polymorphonuclear leukocytes (PMNs) or neutrophils
- Macrophages
- Mast cells
- Cytokines
- Serum complement
- Gingival crevicular fluid

Table 7–2	Phases of the Inflammatory Process
Phase	**Features**
Acute transient phase	Local vasodilation and increased capillary permeability
Delayed subacute phase	Migration of PMNs and other phagocytic cells into the tissue
Chronic phase	Tissue destruction

tissue. Another substance that is involved in the vasodilation is prostaglandin. Prostaglandins are fatty acids found in most cell membranes, are synthesized in large amounts during gingivitis and periodontitis, and may be responsible for the pain and bone loss seen in periodontal diseases (Offenbacher, Heasman, & Collins, 1993). Vasodilation clinically shows as gingival edema. Thus, tissue edema or swelling is due to the increase of permeability of blood vessels, which causes the migration and accumulation of cells and fluid from the vessels to surrounding tissue. With the initiation of inflammation, the flow of gingival crevicular fluid increases from the connective tissue out through the junctional epithelium into the gingival crevice. Migration of PMNs through the junctional epithelium into the

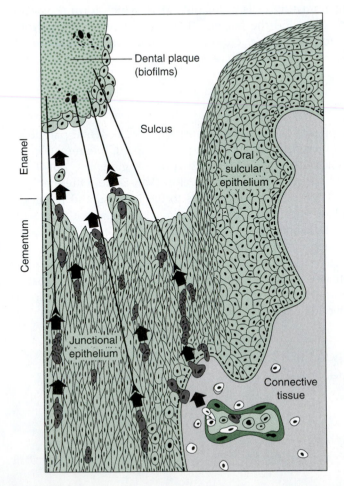

Figure 7–3 Schematic drawing of the relationship of the gingival sulcus to the epithelium and connective tissue in health. Note the dental plaque on the tooth surface at the entrance to the gingival sulcus. Neutrophils are leaving blood vessels in the connective tissue and moving chemotactically through the semipermeable junctional epithelium but not through the oral sulcular epithelium of the lateral wall of the sulcus. (Copyright © 1997 by Munksgaard, Copenhagen. Reprinted with permission of *Periodontology 2000.*)

gingival sulcus and crevicular fluid flow both peak 6 to 12 days after the onset of clinically detectable gingivitis (Kowashi, Jaccard, & Cimasoni, 1980; Zappa, 1995).

Gingival bleeding at the gingival crevice is an early and important sign of gingival inflammation. When the crevice is probed or stroked, it may bleed immediately because the sulcular epithelium (epithelium lining the sulcus) becomes ulcerated with tears in the epithelial lining. The bleeding on probing comes from the underlying vascular gingival connective tissue (lamina propria), which is engorged with blood because of the disease process (Rizzo, 1970).

The Neutrophil: The Phagocytic Cell   The neutrophil has been referred to as a "first line of defense" and the "hallmark of acute inflammation," meaning that it is one of the first defensive cells to be recruited to a site of inflammation. PMNs are the first cells to migrate from inside the blood vessels into the surrounding connective tissue and enter the gingival crevice and junctional epithelium in response to chemotactic substances such as toxins released by the bacteria and complement, which are proteins found in the serum (Miyasaki, 1991). Chemotaxis is the movement of cells in the direction of a chemical attractant. The PMNs create a wall between swimming, unattached bacteria and the junctional and sulcular epithelium. Once in the tissue, the neutrophil is ready to kill the foreign invader. Once the PMN comes in contact with the bacteria, phagocytosis occurs. The PMN is the major phagocytic cell, whose fast arrival from the blood vessels in the connective tissue into the junctional epithelium and crevice plays an important part in removing bacteria and other foreign substances. Neutrophils live a very short time. They come out of the bone marrow programmed to die in an average of about 5 days. Once at the site of injury, phagocytosis occurs where PMNs recognize the foreign material (bacteria, toxins, and by-products) and "eat and digest" it. Once inside the PMN, the bacteria are degraded by enzymes called lysosomes. As the bacteria are engulfed, lysosomal enzymes "leak" out of the cell into the surrounding tissue causing destruction of host tissue. Examples of lysosomal enzymes include collagenase, beta-glucuronidase, and alkaline phosphatase. High levels of these enzymes can be detected in the GCF during periodontitis.

Genetically, impaired PMN function is seen in patients with certain medical conditions. A depressed PMN chemotaxis and depressed phagocytic ability is seen in localized juvenile periodontitis and insulin-dependent diabetes mellitus. A depressed PMN chemotaxis is seen in Chediak-Higashi syndrome and Papillon-Lefévre syndrome. A decreased number of circulating PMNs are seen in drug-induced agranulocytosis, cyclic neutropenia, and leukemia (Genco & Slots, 1984).

The Macrophage: The Other Phagocytic Cell   The other important phagocytic cell is the macrophage. Monocytes (a type of white blood cell) in the blood differentiate or change into macrophages and migrate from the blood vessel into the inflamed connective tissues by chemotaxis and a few continue into the gingival crevice. Similar to PMNs, macrophages kill bacteria by phagocytosis. Although neutrophils and macrophages arrive at the same time at the site of inflammation, neutrophils predominate initially because of their higher concentration in the circulation. The majority of macrophages remain in the inflamed connective tissue for months, where they function to clean up the body's damaged tissue and secrete prostaglandins and cytokines. *Cytokines* are proteins that are involved in regulating the activity of the cells that release them, as well as other cells (Kjeldsen, Holmstrup, & Bendtzen, 1993). The major cytokine released by macrophages as a result of phagocytosis is interleukin (IL-1) and tumor necrosis factor (TNF).

IL-1 worsens inflammation by stimulating mast cells to release histamine and attracts more PMNs and macrophages into the tissues (Offenbacher, 1996). As with PMNs, macrophages can also damage host tissue most likely a result of cytokines. IL-1 can increase the number of osteoclasts, which stimulate bone resorption seen in periodontitis (Ishikawa et al., 1997; Tatakis, 1993;), and stimulates other cells to secrete prostaglandins, which are also involved in bone resorption. TNF is a less potent stimulator of bone resorption (Stashenko, Dewhirst, Peros, Kent, & Apo, 1987).

Phagocytosis: Opsonization   The process of phagocytosis is more effective if opsonins are present. Opsonins are antibodies or complement that bind to the surface of the bacteria, coating the bacteria so they are easier to be identified by PMNs and to be "swallowed."

The Complement System: A Group of Proteins   Besides blood cells (e.g., PMNs) and fluids migrating from the blood vessels into the gingival tissues and crevicular area during inflammation, there is also a series of about twenty to thirty different plasma proteins called the complement system. The complement system works together with the rest of the immune system to destroy invaders and to signal to other immune system cells that the attack is occurring. The complement system plays an important role in the inflammatory and immune response by generating chemotactic factors, which attract PMNs, macrophages, and other leukocytes to the inflamed area. Also, it directly kills and lysis (breaks apart) bacteria.

As with everything else in the immune system, the complement system must be activated before it can function. One way it is activated is when antibodies (proteins produced by plasma cells during the immune response) bind to the surface of bacteria (the antigen). This is called the "classical" pathway. The second way is called the "alternative" pathway, whereby endotoxins (lipooligosaccarides) activate the system. A third pathway involves the binding of specific proteins to proteins or carbohydrates on bacteria (Dennison & Van Dyke, 1997).

The Immune Response

If for any reason inflammation does not subside within several days, it will become a chronic reaction. Usually gingival inflammation progresses quickly into a chronic condition. When the PMNs and macrophages are not strong enough to destroy the invaders, the immune system is further activated, although the inflammatory cells remain in the area.

Activation of the "specific host response" or adaptive immune system is the next line of defense, with the purpose of the host developing immunity or resistance to specific antigens (e.g., bacteria and toxins). The objective of the immune response is to recognize the antigen and communicate with other defense cells to destroy or suppress the antigen. There is an interrelationship between the inflammatory and immune reactions. The same reactions and cells seen in the inflammatory level are also seen in the chronic state (e.g., PMNs and macrophages also belong to the immune system), but more cells are involved. There are two parts to the immune reaction: humoral immunity and cellular immunity.

Immune System: Cells

The major cells in the immune system are white blood cells called lymphocytes (Table 7–3■). The role of the immune system is to "patrol" the body, identifying foreign pathogens such as bacteria and viruses, cancer cells, or damaged tissue and

Table 7–3	Key Elements in the Immune Response

- B lymphocytes
- Antibodies
- Macrophages
- Cytokines

eliminating them. There are two kinds of lymphocytes that originate in the bone marrow and travel to other areas of the body. In fact, all cells in the inflammatory and immune systems including blood cells are made in the bone marrow from a stem cell. A stem cell is a cell from which all blood cells "stem" or originate. Lymphocytes predominate in the gingival connective tissue (Page & Schroeder, 1976). T lymphocytes, also referred to as *T cells,* are the mediators of cellular immunity. B lymphocytes, or *B cells,* are the mediators of humoral immunity.

Humoral Immunity

Humoral immune mechanisms are most effective against bacteria such as those found in periodontitis. Although both the humoral and cellular immunity reactions occur almost at the same time, one or the other cells may predominate during a particular stage of periodontal diseases.

B lymphocytes or B cells are so named because much of the early research was done on chickens, in which the bursa (hence "B") of Fabricius is a center of B cell activation; there is no direct equivalent of this bursa in human beings. B cells originate and mature in the bone marrow and then migrate and deposit in the blood and various lymphatic tissues (e.g., lymph nodes).

Humoral Immunity and Periodontal Disease   The following are events depicting the humoral response to plaque accumulated at the gingival margin:

1. In periodontal diseases, bacteria and their products, such as toxins and enzymes, accumulate in the gingival crevice. Then they penetrate through the protective wall of neutrophils and through the junctional epithelium, entering the lamina propria. Once this happens an inflammatory/immune response is set off. As previously stated, if the inflammatory reaction cannot eliminate the antigens effectively, the immune response comes into play.
2. From the tissues, these antigenic substances are carried to the local lymph nodes, probably by macrophages.
3. In the lymph nodes, the macrophages either present the antigens to B cells or the B cells by themselves recognize the antigens. The B cells then transform into plasma cells and memory cells.
4. Plasma cells make antibodies in the lymph nodes with the assistance from T_H cells. They also circulate in the blood to seek out and destroy the antigens.
5. The memory B cells remain inactivated, ready to respond should the same antigens appear again.
6. The plasma cells remain in the lymph nodes and secrete antibodies into the bloodstream. A local antibody response is also seen in the gingival tissues.

7. The primary antibody produced by the plasma cells is IgG (Note: "Ig" stands for immunoglobulin) with lesser amounts of IgM.
   - There are five classes of immunoglobulins found in the serum, secretions, and tissues. IgG and IgM are primarily found in the periodontal tissues and SIgA ("S" stands for secretory) is found in the saliva. IgE is found on mast cells and is responsible for the release of histamine causing vasodilation and allergy. Additionally, there is IgD.
   - Antibodies (e.g., IgG) are proteins that directly bind to and neutralize bacterial toxins (foreign antigens) forming an immune complex. This immune complex may activate the complement system or be phagocytosed by PMNs or macrophages for elimination.
8. Once the antigens and the surrounding tissue are destroyed, the tissue macrophages phagocytize and digest the debris and stimulate repair.
9. After the antigens have been eliminated, the short-lived plasma cells disappear into the gingival crevicular fluid and out through the gingival crevice, but the long-lived memory cells remain in circulation and are capable of maturing very rapidly into plasma cells if the antigens are encountered again.

Antibodies to various periodontal pathogens have been found in both serum and gingival crevicular fluids of patients with periodontal diseases (Ebersole & Taubman, 1994; Genco & Slots, 1984). Immune complex and complement will cause the release of prostaglandins from cell membranes of macrophages and PMNs. Prostaglandins of the E series (PGE_2) are potent stimulators of osteoclast activity responsible for bone resorption. B lymphocytes also release cytokines such as IL-1. Humoral immunity is activated in severe gingivitis and periodontitis. Thus, the proportion of B cells in connective tissue at sites with periodontitis can be as high as 90%.

Cellular Immunity

T cells undergo further maturation in the thymus gland located in the chest cavity. From the thymus gland, the T cells migrate into the bloodstream and lymph nodes. From the bloodstream, T cells enter the gingival tissues where they "watch" the tissues.

There are two major types of T cell: helper T cells (T_H) and cytotoxic T cells. Both T cells have protein receptors on the surface of their plasma membranes. The helper T cells have a CD4 receptor and the cytotoxic T cells have a CD8 receptor. There is a reduction in CD4 T_H cells in AIDS patients. Once the helper T cells are stimulated, they secrete cytokines that activate phagocytic cells to destroy target antigens. They also activate other immune cells such as B cells. Cytotoxic T cells are sometimes called killer T cells, and they can directly kill virus-infected cells, cancer cells, parasites, and certain bacteria by making holes in them. Thus, cellular immunity is most effective against fungi, viruses, cancer, and foreign tissue such as transplanted organs and does not play an important role in periodontal diseases.

Cellular Immunity: Process   When a macrophage presents a foreign antigen to a T cell, it is stimulated to produce more T cells and cytokines. T cells are the target of the human immunodeficiency virus (HIV). AIDS is a manifestation of what happens when T cells are destroyed, showing the importance of T cells for a properly functioning body. This type of response is responsible for organ or tissue rejection in a transplant case. Few lymphocytes within the gingival connective tissue are seen in healthy gingiva, with T lymphocytes mostly seen in gingivitis. The T cells actually kill other cells on contact when the latter are recognized as foreign or have antigens attached. Unfortunately, T cells also have the capacity to contribute to permanent tissue damage by the production of cytokines, which activate macrophages.

Summary

The pathway of destruction of inflammatory periodontal diseases is complicated, involving the host inflammatory and immune cells. Ideally, the overall outcome of these reactions is to eliminate harmful pathogens and prevent the spread of infection, while protecting the host tissues.

Key Points

- Overall, the host defenses are extremely successful in preventing infection around the teeth and in preventing destructive inflammatory periodontal diseases.
- There are two separate functions that lead to the damage seen in periodontal diseases: (1) direct effects of bacteria (e.g., enzymes, endotoxins) and (2) indirect effects of the body's own immune response.
- The host immune defense and inflammatory reactions are a double-edged sword; while being protective, they can also cause the host to suffer tissue damage.
- Bacterial products can enter the connective tissue and cause direct damage, but their effects are limited by the effectiveness of the host response.
- Weakened host defenses (e.g., because of a systemic disease) will not allow the host to ward off infection; the host will then develop signs and symptoms of destructive periodontal diseases.
- Neutrophils and macrophages are considered capable and efficient agents of phagocytosis.
- Clinical signs of gingival inflammation are first evident in the early lesion of gingivitis.
- B cells/plasma cells predominate in the body's response to periodontitis.
- Elevated serum antibodies are seen in periodontitis.

Web Sites

www.perio.org

www.vcu.edu/micro/immunology.htm

www.grants.nih.gov/grants/guide

www.dent.ucla.edu/pic/members/immunology

Self-Quiz

1. Which one of the following types of cells is primarily recruited in high numbers to the site of acute inflammation? (pp. 115–117)

   a. mast

   b. macrophage

   c. neutrophil

   d. lymphocyte

2. Which one of the following cells is phagocytic? (pp. 117–118)

   a. mast

   b. lymphocyte

   c. macrophage

   d. melanocyte

3. Which one of the following cells is mainly involved in the body's immune response to invading bacteria? (pp. 118–121)

   a. lymphocytes

   b. mast

   c. macrophages

   d. neutrophils

4. Periodontal diseases are considered a group of infections characterized by destruction of the periodontium. The direct effects of the bacteria and indirect effects by the body's own immune response are primarily responsible for the destruction. (p. 112)

   a. Both statements are true.

   b. Both statements are false.

   c. The first statement is true, the second is false.

   d. The first statement is false, the second is true.

5. The first attempt at self-protection from bacterial invasion comes from which one of the following areas in the oral cavity? (p. 113)

   a. supragingival environment

   b. subgingival environment

   c. gingival connective tissue

   d. tonsillar area

References

Armitage, G. C. 1995. Clinical evaluation of periodontal diseases. *Periodontology 2000* 7:39–53.

Brown, L. J., and H. Löe. 1993. Prevalence, extent, severity and progression of periodontal disease. *Periodontology 2000* 2:57–71.

de Graaf, J., A. J. van Winkelhoff, and R. J. Goené. 1989. The role of *Actinobacillus actinomycetemcomitans* in periodontal disease. *Infection* 17:269–271.

Dennison, D. K., and T. E. Van Dyke. 1997. The acute inflammatory response and the role of phagocytic cells in periodontal health and disease. *Periodontology 2000* 14:54–78.

Ebersole, J. L., and M. A. Taubman. 1994. The protective nature of host responses in periodontal diseases. *Periodontology 2000* 5:112–141.

Genco, R. J., and J. Slots. 1984. Host response in periodontal diseases. *J. Dental Res.* 63:441–451.

Goodson, J.M. 1992. Diagnosis of periodontitis by physical measurement: Interpretation from episodic disease hypothesis. *J. Periodontol.* 63:373–382.

Greenstein, G., and J. Caton. 1990. Periodontal disease activity: A critical assessment. *J. Periodontol.* 61:543–552.

Ishikawa, I., K. Nakashima, T. Koseki, T. Nagasawa, H. Watanabe, et al. 1997. Induction of the immune response to periodontopathic bacteria and its role in the pathogenesis of periodontitis. *Periodontology 2000* 14:79–111.

Kjeldsen, M., P. Holmstrup, and K. Bendtzen. 1993. Marginal periodontitis and cytokines: A review of the literature. *J. Periodontol.* 64:1013–1022.

Kowashi, Y., F. Jaccard, and G. Cimasoni. 1980. Sulcular polymorphonuclear leukocytes and gingival exudate during experimental gingivitis in man. *J. Periodontol. Res.* 15:151–158.

Listgarten, M. A. 1994. The structure of dental plaque. *Periodontology 2000* 5:52–65.

Löe, H., A. Anerud, H. Boysen, and E. Morrison. 1986. Natural history of periodontal disease in man. Rapid, moderate and no loss of attachment in Sri Lankan laborers 14 to 46 years of age. *J. Clin. Periodontol.* 13:431–440.

Miyasaki, K. T. 1991. The neutrophil: Mechanisms of controlling periodontal bacteria. *J. Periodontol.* 62:761–774.

Offenbacher, S. 1996. Periodontal diseases: Pathogenesis. *Ann. Periodontol.* 1:821–878.

Offenbacher, S., P. A. Heasman, and J. G. Collins. 1993. Modulation of host PGE_2 secretion as a determinant of periodontal disease expression. *J. Periodontol.* 64:432–444.

Page, R. C., and H. E. Schroeder. 1976. Pathogenesis of inflammatory periodontal disease. A summary of current work. *Lab Investigations* 33:235–249.

Renvert, S., M. Wikström, M. Dahlén, G. Slots, and J. Egelberg. 1990. On the inability of root debridement and periodontal surgery to eliminate *Actinobacillus actinomycetemcomitans* from periodontal pockets. *J. Clin. Periodontol.* 17:351–355.

Rizzo, A. 1970. Histologic and immunologic evaluation of antigen penetration into oral tissues after topical application. *J. Periodontol.* 41:210–213.

Saglie, F. R., F. A. Carranza, Jr., M. G. Newman, L. Cheng, and K. J. Lewin. 1982. Identification of tissue-invading bacteria in human periodontal disease. *J. Periodontol. Res.* 17:452–455.

Socransky, S. S., A. D. Haffajee, J. M. Goodson, and J. Lindhe. 1984. New concepts of destructive periodontal diseases. *J. Clin. Periodontol.* 11:21–32.

Stashenko, P., F. E. Dewhirst, W. J. Peros, R. L. Kent, and J. Apo. 1987. Synergistic interactions between interleukin-1, tumor necrosis factor and lymphotoxin in bone resorption. *J. Immunol.* 138:1484–1468.

Tatakis, D. N. 1993. Interleukin-1 and bone metabolism: A review *J. Periodontol.* 64:416–431.

Van Dyke, T., S. Offenbacher, B. Pihstrom, M. Putt, and C. Trummel. 1999. What is gingivitis? Current understanding of prevention, treatment, measurement, pathogenesis and relation to periodontitis. *J. International Acad. of Periodontol.* 1:3–10.

Zappa, U. 1995. Histology of the periodontal lesion: implications for diagnosis. *Periodontology 2000* 7:22–38.

Zimmerman, S. O. 1986. Discussion: Attachment level changes in destructive periodontal diseases. *J. Clin. Periodontol.* 13:473–475.

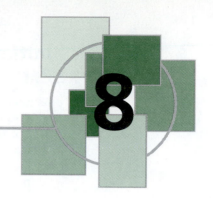

8

Histopathogenesis of the Periodontal Diseases

Mea A. Weinberg, D.M.D, M.S.D., R.Ph.

Outline

Initiation of
   Inflammatory
   Periodontal Diseases
Histopathogenesis of
   Inflammatory
   Periodontal Diseases

Summary
Key Points
Web Sites
Self-Quiz
References

Goal

*To provide an understanding of the histologic develop-
ment and progression of the periodontal diseases.*

Educational Objectives

*Upon completion of this chapter, the reader should be
able to:*

Describe the histopathogenesis of periodontal diseases.

List and describe the different stages in the histopathogenesis of
   periodontal diseases.

Discuss the clinical and histological relationship of the
   inflammatory and immune host responses to inflammatory
   periodontal diseases.

Describe the course of the progression of periodontal diseases.

KEY WORDS
• histopathogenesis
• Page and Schroeder's Lesions
• gingivitis
• periodontitis

Initiation of Inflammatory Periodontal Diseases

As discussed in previous chapters, the reaction of the host to the presence of dental plaque (biofilm) is inflammatory in nature, initially developing into inflammation of the gingival unit. Inflammation confined to the gingivia (epithelium and lamina propria) results in gingivitis. If the gingivitis is not resolved the inflammatory reaction spreads into the gingival connective tissue attachment, alveolar and supporting bone, and the principal fibers. At this stage, the disease is periodontitis.

The histopathogenesis or the events that occur in the *periodontal tissues* that lead to the development of gingivitis and periodontitis is best explained by reviewing the different stages occurring in the initiation and progression of the periodontal disease as it relates to clinical signs. In the previous chapter, the role of the host immune system in the inflammatory process and periodontal disease progression was reviewed. In this section, the *microscopic tissue changes* seen as a result of periodontal diseases are discussed. It is important to remember that all of these inflammatory and immunological events that occur during the time frame in the development of periodontal lesions are intermingled and must not be considered as separate entities. This chapter deals primarily with the tissue changes that occur during the initiation and development of gingivitis and periodontitis. When these tissue changes occur within the periodontal tissues, the inflammatory and immune responses are also triggered. Thus, the features that are reviewed in this chapter occur as part of the entire inflammatory and immunological events.

These histological lesions presented in this chapter were initially classified and published in 1976 by Page and Schroeder. Page and Schroeder classified gingivitis and periodontitis according to histopathology from animal and some human adolescent specimens. This classification is still used in periodontic literature; however, it is not a realistic, up-to-date classification. The initial early and established lesions reflected the histopathology of clinically early and chronic gingivitis. The advanced lesion reflected the histopathology of the progression of gingivitis into periodontitis.

Histopathogenesis of Inflammatory Periodontal Diseases

Stages in the Histopathogenesis

Page and Schroeder (1976) described the development of periodontal diseases as a progression of inflammation through four different stages: *initial lesion, early lesion, established lesion,* and *advanced lesion* (Table 8–1■; Fig. 8–1■). The initial and early lesions are representative of acute inflammation, while the established lesion is considered to be chronic gingivitis and the advanced lesion is periodontitis (Page & Schroeder, 1976). The information from the research by Page and Schroeder was obtained from animal specimens and a few human juvenile tissue samples. Also, since there are many factors involved in the initiation and progression of periodontal diseases, it is difficult to exactly pinpoint a clear delineation between the different stages, especially in humans. Also, it is unclear when and if an established lesion develops into an advanced lesion. Thus, even though this classic

Table 8–1	Page and Schroeder's Stages of Pathogenesis of Periodontal Disease		
Stage	**Onset Time after Plaque Accumulation**	**Histopathological Signs**	**Features**
Initial	2 to 4 days	Acute inflammation; PMNs, machrophages; vasculitis	Subclinical; no signs of gingivitis; increased flow of GCF
Early	4 to 7 days	T cell lesion	Clinical signs of gingivitis first seen (redness, bleeding, edema)
Established	2 to 3 weeks	B cell lesion; plasma cells	Chronic gingivitis
Advanced	Undetermined	Alveolar bone loss, periodontal pocket formation; B cell lesion	Periodontitis

work by Page and Schroeder is primarily with nonhuman tissues, it is still the foundation from which the histopathogenesis of inflammatory periodontal diseases can be studied. The inflammatory and immune changes discussed above are involved in the histopathogenesis of periodontal diseases.

The following are Page and Schroeder's Stages of the Histopathogenesis of Periodontal Diseases.

Initial Lesion (PMN Dominated)

The initial lesion develops after 2 to 4 days of plaque accumulation (Löe, Theilade, & Jensen, 1965; Page & Schroeder, 1976). Dental plaque accumulates on the tooth surface at the free gingival margin level (Fig. 8–1b). The protective wall of PMNs (leukocyte wall) between the plaque mass and the junctional and sulculur epithelium becomes compromised (Miyasaki, 1991). Bacterial antigens cross the permeable junctional epithelium and enter the gingival connective tissue. The response of the tissue to the antigens is acute inflammation, developing within minutes of the insult. It is characterized by a dilation of blood vessels within the connective tissue subjacent to the junctional epithelium (Page & Schroeder, 1976). There is an increased flow of GCF into the crevice, and migration of PMNs from the connective tissue into the junctional epithelium (Payne, Page, Ogilvie, & Hall, 1975) and gingival crevice in response to chemotactic factors released by bacteria and inflammatory cells. There is some loss of collagen in the lamina propria because of the action of collagenase that is replaced with inflammatory cells such as PMNs. This lesion is not clinically seen and is reversible with appropriate oral hygiene (Löe et al., 1965).

Early Lesion (T Cell Dominated)

The early lesion evolves from the initial lesion after approximately 7 days of plaque accumulation and can continue for up to 14 days. Clinically this lesion is observable as gingivitis (Seymour, Powell, & Davies, 1979). The presence and accentuation of the features in the initial lesion characterize the early lesion (see Fig. 8–1b). PMNs continually migrate from the blood vessels through the junctional epithelium

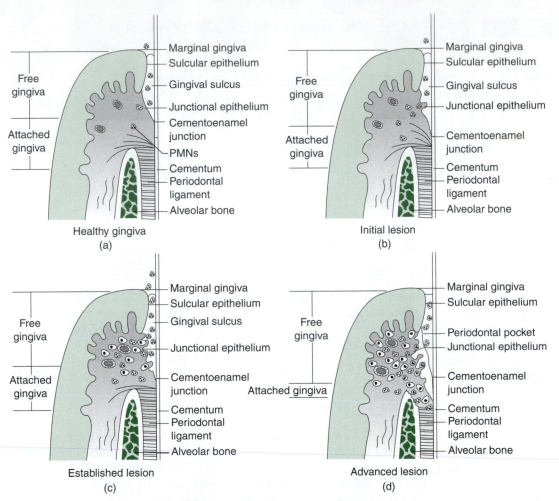

Figure 8–1 Page and Schroeder's histopathologic periodontal lesions. (a) Healthy gingiva: Little supragingival plaque accumulation; a few defense cells, primarily PMNs, migrate through the junctional epithelium into the gingival crevice and out into the oral cavity. (b) Initial lesion: This develops 2 to 4 days after plaque accumulation at the gingival margin. Vasodilation results in an increased emigration of PMNs from the blood vessels into the connective tissue and entering the gingival crevice. This is gingivitis but the lesion is not clinically visible. Early lesion: This lesion appears at the site of the initial lesion within 4 to 7 days following plaque accumulation. The same features seen in the initial lesion appear in the early lesion but they are accentuated with an increased number of PMNs and macrophages. T lymphocytes begin to migrate into the tissue and gingival crevice. A greater area of gingival connective tissue is affected. About 60 to 70% of collagen is destroyed. Acute inflammation features continue in the early lesion. This is still gingivitis. (c) Established lesion: This is characterized by the presence of PMNs, macrophages, and antibody-producing plasma cells (B lymphocytes), which comprise 10 to 30% of the infiltrate. More collagen has been destroyed. The bulk of plaque bacteria and cells in the gingival crevice cause the junctional epithelium to detach from the tooth. The pocket epithelium is mostly derived from junctional epithelium with the formation of epithelial ridges and microulcerations. This is chronic gingivitis and is still reversible if oral hygiene is reinstated. (d) Advanced lesion: This is periodontitis. Plasma cells (>50%) are the primary cells involved in periodontitis. There is clinical attachment loss with loss of clinical connective tissue attachment to the tooth and apical migration of the junctional (pocket) epithelium, resulting in a periodontal pocket. In addition, the alveolar and supporting bone has been destroyed.

into the gingival crevice, and there is increased gingival crevicular flow. T lymphocytes accumulate immediately subjacent to the junctional epithelium. There is no apparent dividing line between the initial and early lesions. Approximately 60 to 70% of collagen is lost in the connective tissue. Changes start to occur in the junctional epithelium. As a result of the downgrowth of accumulating plaque, the gingival sulcus begins to deepen. This is still an acute gingivitis without clinical connective tissue attachment loss and no bone loss as yet. This lesion is reversible with adequate oral hygiene, healing without adverse consequences.

Established Lesion (Few B Cells/Plasma Cells)

As adverse clinical conditions progress, the early lesion develops into the chronic or established gingivitis lesion (Page & Schroeder, 1976). The gingiva responds to massive accumulations of plaque, which affects a greater area of tissue (see Fig. 8–1c). The time period for the initiation of the established lesion has not actually been determined, but it can start within 2 to 3 weeks after plaque accumulation (Page & Schroeder, 1976). The manifestations of acute inflammation still persist. Established lesions may persist for months or years without progressing into periodontitis (Page, 1986; Zappa, 1995). As gingivitis becomes clinically more severe, the proportion of T cells decreases, and B cells and plasma cells increase within the lamina propria (Zappa, 1995). More collagen is lost and replaced by an inflammatory cell infiltrate. The gingival fibers are still attached to the root surface; there is no clinical connective tissue attachment loss at this stage. Because of the massive amounts of subgingival plaque that advance in an apical direction, the junctional epithelium detaches laterally from the tooth surface to become pocket epithelium with elongation of epithelial ridges deeper into the connective tissue in an attempt to maintain epithelial integrity (Kinane & Lindhe, 1998); this leads to the formation of microulcerations, which may increase its permeability to bacteria and their by-products.

The gingival margin becomes swollen and enlarged, and the gingival margin can be separated easily from the tooth surface, forming a gingival pocket. No alveolar bone loss occurs at this stage. Clinical signs are present and more severe than in the early lesion. Most of the changes that occur in the established lesion are still reversible.

Advanced Lesion (Plasma Cell/ Antibody Dominated)

The advanced lesion is characteristic of periodontitis. The inflammatory infiltrate extends into the alveolar and supporting bone and periodontal ligament (see Fig. 8–1d). Periodontal pocket formation occurs with the clinical connective tissue attachment loss to the root surface and the apical migration of the apical aspect of the junctional epithelium along the root surface that was previously occupied by connective tissue; attachment loss occurs. Subsequently there is alveolar and supporting bone loss. The apical and lateral migration of the junctional or pocket epithelium permits extension of subgingival plaque on the root surface. The lymphocytic infiltrate in the subjacent connective tissues is primarily B cells (Seymour & Greenspan, 1979). The advanced lesion may become stable or progress continuously (Goodson, 1992).

Summary

The evidence and concepts presented in Chapters 7 and 8 on the inflammatory/immune response and histopathogenesis of periodontal diseases suggests that the periodontal diseases are complex, multifactorial diseases caused by bacterial pathogens. All of the events presented in the last two chapters are going on simultaneously. These concepts were separated into different chapters because of ease of understanding.

Essentially, since the periodontal diseases are inflammatory diseases it is obvious that inflammation/immune reactions to the invading bacterial pathogens will occur. A clinical/immune/pathological concept indicates that gingivitis and periodontitis are two pathological entities, one being the extension of the other.

Thus, the histopathologic changes (Page and Schroeder's lesions) and the inflammatory/immune reactions take place within the periodontal tissues simultaneously. That is to say, the tissue changes that occur during the initiation and progression of the inflammatory periodontal diseases also involve inflammatory and immune responses of the host.

Thus, all of these events are occurring together to cause periodontal destruction and should be reviewed together. More research needs to be done to gain a better understanding of the multifactorial nature of the periodontal diseases.

Key Points

- Page and Schroder's Stages of Histopathogenesis describes the pathologic (tissue) changes associated with the inflammatory periodontal diseases.
- The tissue changes that occur during the initiation and progression of the inflammatory periodontal diseases also involve inflammatory and immune responses of the host.
- Clinical signs of gingival inflammation are first evident in the early lesion of gingivitis.
- B cells/plasma cells predominate in the body's response to periodontitis.
- T4 helper cells play a role in the defense of the disease (periodontitis).
- Periodontal pocket formation occurs when there is clinical connective tissue attachment loss to the tooth surface with apical migration of the junctional epithelium. The inflammatory events leading to attachment loss also result in alveolar and supporting bone loss.

Web Sites

www.perio.org
http://nnd40med.navy.mil/ndsbethesda/01August.htm
www.dentalarticles.com

Self-Quiz

1. Which one of the following features differentiates periodontitis from gingivitis? (p. 126)
   a. engorged lamina propria
   b. redness of the gingiva
   c. loss of connective tissue attachment
   d. number of bacteria present in the gingival crevice

2. Which periodontal lesion, according to the classification of Page and Schroeder (1976), is characterized by chronic gingival inflammation and the presence of plasma cells? (pp. 127–128)
   a. initial
   b. early
   c. established
   d. advanced

3. Which periodontal lesion, according to the classification of Page and Schroeder (1976), is characterized by attachment loss and bone resorption? (pp. 127–129)
   a. initial
   b. early
   c. established
   d. advanced

4. During the disease process, the junctional epithelium transforms into: (p. 128)
   a. alveolar bone
   b. periodontal ligament
   c. pocket epithelium
   d. sulcular epithelium
   e. oral epithelium

5. Which of the following lesions features a predominance of plasma cells? (pp. 127–129)
   a. initial
   b. early
   c. established
   d. advanced

References

Goodson, J.M. 1992. Diagnosis of periodontitis by physical measurement: Interpretation from episodic disease hypothesis. *J. Periodontol.* 63:373–382.

Kinane, D.F., and J. Lindhe. 1998. Pathogenesis of periodontitis. In eds. J. Lindhe, T. Karring, and N. P. Lang, *Clinical periodontology and implant dentistry,* 189–225. Copenhagen: Munksgaard.

Löe, H. J., E. Theilade, and S. B. Jensen. 1965. Experimental gingivitis in man. *J. Periodontol.* 36:177–187.

Miyasaki, K. T. 1991. The neutrophil: Mechanisms of controlling periodontal bacteria. *J Periodontol.* 62:761–774.

Page, R. C. 1986. Gingivitis. *J. Clin. Periodontol.* 13:345–355.

Page, R. C., and H. E. Schroeder. 1976. Pathogenesis of inflammatory periodontal disease. A summary of current work. *Lab Investigations* 33:235–249.

Payne, W. A., R. C. Page, A. L. Ogilvie, and W. B. Hall. 1975. Histopathologic features of the initial and early stages of experimental gingivitis in man. *J. Periodont. Res.* 10:51–64.

Seymour, G. J., and J. S. Greenspan. 1979. The phenotypic characterization of lymphocyte subpopulations in established human periodontal disease. *J. Periodont. Res.* 14:39–46.

Seymour, G. J., R. N. Powell, and W. I. R. Davies. 1979. Conversion of a stable T cell lesion to a progressive B cell lesion in the pathogenesis of chronic inflammatory periodontal disease: An hypothesis. *J. Clin. Periodontol.* 6:267–277.

Zappa, U. 1995. Histology of the periodontal lesion: implications for diagnosis. *Periodontology 2000* 7:22–38.

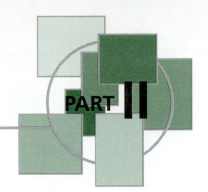

PART II

The Periodontal Diseases: Classification

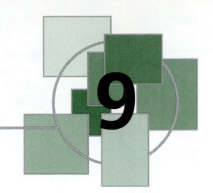

The Gingival Lesion

Surendra Singh, D.D.S., M.S.

Outline

Gingival Diseases

Pathogenesis of
   Gingivitis

Summary

Key Points

Web Sites

Self-Quiz

References

Goal

To provide an understanding of the clinical features and histopathogenesis of gingival diseases.

Educational Objectives

Upon completion of this chapter, the dental hygiene student should be able to:

List and compare the plaque-induced gingival diseases and non-plaque-induced gingival diseases.

Explain the host response to the presence of microorganisms within dental plaque.

Explain the relationship of hormones and medications with periodontal diseases.

Describe the clinical and histologic features of gingival inflammation.

> **KEY WORDS**
> - plaque-induced gingival diseases
> - non-plaque-induced gingival diseases
> - gingival pocket

The periodontal diseases are a major cause of tooth loss. Periodontal diseases are not a single disease entity, but a group of lesions affecting the tissues that form the attachment apparatus of a tooth or teeth. These diseases are microbial infections wherein the microorganisms act in concert with a host's reduced capacity to resist disease. To successfully treat periodontal diseases, it is essential that one is able to recognize different types of the diseases. When classifying inflammatory periodontal diseases, it is important to include not only diseases that have primary manifestation and etiology in the periodontium but also periodontal manifestations of systemic diseases. In this chapter a comprehensive classification of the gingival diseases or conditions affecting gingival tissues is presented.

 # Introduction

Gingivitis is defined as an inflammatory lesion, mediated by host/microorganism interactions, which remains limited to the gingival tissues and does not involve the underlying periodontal ligament, cementum, or alveolar and supporting bone (American Academy of Periodontology, 2003). In this broad condition the apical extent of the junctional epithelium and the coronal gingival connective tissue attachment remains at the cementoenamel junction; hence there is no attachment loss. Gingivitis can affect children, adolescents, and adults.

Gingivitis has been further defined based on clinical manifestations, duration of the disease, and association with either dental plaque or systemic factors such as medical conditions or medications (Page, 1986). Some professionals question whether gingivitis should be considered a periodontal disease, since it does not cause loss of significant amounts of periodontal support or tooth mortality (loss). However, most researchers have concluded otherwise (Page, 1986; Ranney, 1993, 1986).

Periodontitis is an inflammatory lesion mediated by host/microorganism interactions, and results in clinical attachment loss and alveolar and supporting bone loss. Periodontitis primarily affects adults, but children and adolescents can be afflicted. Periodontitis will be discussed in Chapter 10.

 # Gingival Diseases (Table 9–1■)

Dental Plaque-Induced Gingival Diseases

Gingivitis Associated with Dental Plaque

Gingivitis is a reaction of the host (body) to the bacteria present in the dental biofilm (plaque). Gingivitis, which exemplifies itself as inflammation of the gingiva, is the most common of the periodontal diseases (Page, 1985). Dental biofilms is the etiology or cause of gingivitis has been confirmed in Löe's classic "Experimental Gingivitis in Man" study (Löe, Theilade, & Jensen, 1965). Plaque-associated gingivitis begins at the gingival margin and can spread throughout the remaining gingival unit. Plaque-induced gingivitis will not develop unless there are bacteria present (American Academy of Periodontology, 1992); however, the composition of the

(text continues on p. 139)

Table 9–1   Common Features of the Periodontal Diseases (Using 1989 Classification System)

Disease	Patient Population	Clinical Features	Causes of the Disease	Microbiologic Features	
Dental plaque induced gingivitis (Figure 9–1■)	Adolescents, adults	Gingival redness, bleeding, and enlargement Absence of clinical attachment loss and bone loss	Inadequate oral hygiene	No specific bacteria are demonstrated although high levels of *Streptococcus sanguis*, *S. mitis*, *Fusobacterium nucleatum*, *Actinomyces viscosus*, and *Veillonella parvula* have been detected	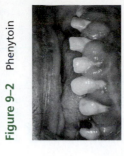 **Figure 9–1** Plaque-induced
Drug influenced gingivitis (Figures 9–2 to 9–4■)	Patients taking phenytoin, calcium channel blockers, cyclosporine	Gingival enlargement or overgrowth Absence of clinical attachment loss and bone loss	Medications and dental plaque	No specific bacteria demonstrated	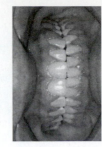 **Figure 9–2** Phenytoin **Figure 9–3** Nifedipine **Figure 9–4** Cyclosporine

Continued

137

Table 9–1　Common Features of the Periodontal Diseases (Using 1989 Classification System) (cont.)

Disease	Patient Population	Clinical Features	Causes of the Disease	Microbiologic Features
Gingival diseases associated with the endocrine system (Figure 9–5■)	Pregnant patients, adolescents, diabetics	Intense gingival inflammation Absence of clinical attachment loss and bone loss	Changes in sex hormone level; exaggerated response to plaque	*Prevotella intermedia*
Gingival manifestations of systemic conditions, mucocutaneous disorders (Figure 9–6■)	These includes skin disease including pemphigus, lichen planus, benign mucous membrane pemphigoid (BMMP), and others	Gingiva may appear blotchy red, have blisters or vesicles, or slough (peel) off from the underlying connective tissue	Abnormality in the immune system	None

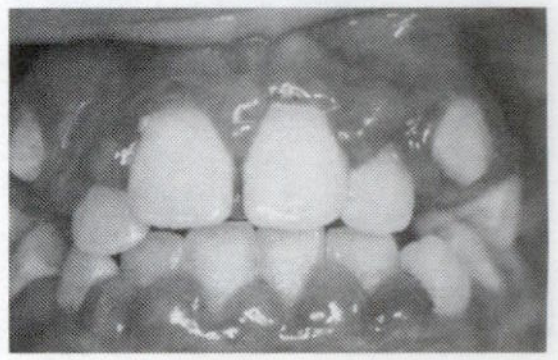

Figure 9–5　Puberty

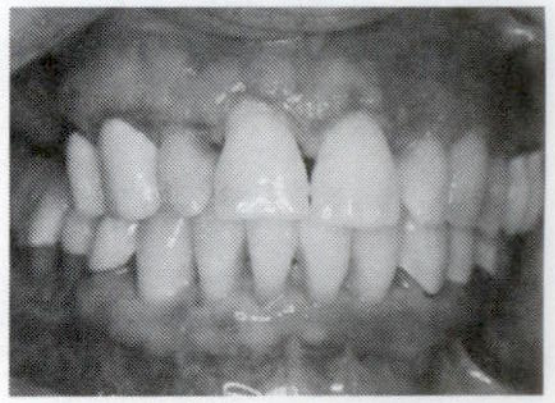

Figure 9–6　Lichen planus

required oral microbiota is not specific (Moore, Moore, & Cato 1987). Gingivitis is reversible following the removal of dental biofilms and maintenance of good oral hygiene self-care. However, if oral hygiene procedures are discontinued and the level of oral hygiene is not adequate, allowing the accumulation of biofilms, clinical signs of acute gingivitis develop within 1 to 3 weeks. This classic model of gingivitis induction is used in clinical trials to test antigingivitis oral rinses.

Since the bacteria associated with chronic, long-standing, plaque-induced gingivitis are not very specific, recognition of gingivitis is primarily made clinically. However, the earliest changes may not be seen clinically and only histologically under the microscope. With the development of gingivitis, the healthy gingiva changes in color, contour, consistency, and surface texture. Plaque-associated gingivitis starts within the interdental papilla and is clinically characterized by gingival redness, gingival bleeding, swelling, and gingival sensitivity and tenderness (Löe et al., 1965; Suzuki, 1988). The features of dental plaque-induced gingivitis can be summarized in Table 9–2■ (Mariotti, 1999).

Treatment of gingivitis includes maintenance of adequate oral hygiene self-care and regular professional mechanical debridement.

Gingival Diseases Modified by Systemic Factors

Gingivitis Associated with the Endocrine System   Altered hormonal balances elicit an apparent exaggerated response to dental plaque. Hormonal-influenced gingivitis manifests as puberty-associated gingivitis, menstrual cycle-associated gingivitis, and pregnancy-associated gingivitis. Additionally, poorly controlled plasma glucose levels resulting in a diabetes-associated gingivitis may aggravate the inflammatory response of the gingiva to plaque.

Puberty Gingivitis   During puberty, the dramatic elevation in steroid hormones often can cause a gingival response that is similar to what has been described for pregnancy gingivitis. In addition to a rise in hormones (estrogen and progesterone), the incidence and severity of gingivitis in adolescents are influenced by a number of factors, including plaque levels, dental caries, mouth breathing, tooth crowding, and tooth eruption (Stamm, 1986). The distinguishing feature between plaque-induced gingivitis and puberty gingivitis is the development of gingival inflammation in the presence of a small amount of dental plaque. Meticulous oral hygiene is the recommended treatment.

Table 9–2	Features of Gingival Diseases

- Caused by nonspecific bacteria (although certain types of bacteria are associated with gingivitis, the condition is currently still considered of nonspecific bacterial origin)
- Dental plaque present at the marginal gingiva
- Clinical signs of inflammation are limited to the gingiva
- No clinical attachment loss
- It is reversible to health following the removal of the dental plaque causing it
- Even though bacteria are the primary risk factors, secondary factors apparently modify the clinical characteristics of the disease. This has resulted in many subclassifications.

Menstrual-Cycle Gingivitis   During the menstrual cycle there are increased levels of estrogen and progesterone. These changes in hormone levels cause gingival inflammation characterized as enlarged, red interdental papilla. Connective tissue attachment loss and alveolar and supporting bone loss are not evident. All gingival changes are reversible after ovulation. It is important to note that gingival changes primarily are seen when plaque is present. Also, not every female patient will have this inflammatory response during menstruation.

Pregnancy Gingivitis   Pregnancy gingivitis is inflammation of the gingiva associated with pregnancy. The incidence of gingivitis during pregnancy ranges between 30 and 100%. The effects of pregnancy on preexisting gingivitis are seen by the second month of gestation and are most severe in the eighth month at the time of peak hormone levels (American Academy of Periodontology, 1992; Silness & Löe, 1963). Pregnant patients with healthy gingiva usually do not develop gingivitis but, if gingivitis or periodontitis is present, the course of the disease is aggravated by pregnancy.

The degree of gingival inflammation is related to the state of oral hygiene of the patient. Accumulation of dental plaque parallels the gingival changes. The severity of the gingivitis is greater in pregnant than in nonpregnant women (Löe, 1965) but is not associated with more destructive periodontitis (Cohen, Shapiro, Friedman, Kyle, & Franklin, 1971). The condition regresses postpartum (Silness & Löe, 1963). However, gingivitis during pregnancy can be prevented or be resolved by adequate plaque control starting early in the pregnancy.

Dental plaque present at the gingival margin results in an exaggerated inflammatory response of the gingiva. Tissue inflammation and enlargement seen in pregnancy is not caused by the pregnancy itself but rather by the shifts in the hormonal levels, which aggravate the inflammation. Hormonal changes during pregnancy are due to elevated progesterone and estrogen levels, which in the final gestational month are 10 to 30 times greater than that seen during the normal menstrual cycle (Amar & Chung, 1994). Elevations in these steroids, especially progesterone, cause an increased permeability of the blood vessels (microvasculature) (Lindhe & Bränemark, 1968) within the lamina propria, resulting in gingival redness, edema, and increased flow of gingival crevicular fluid (Amar & Chung, 1994; Lindhe, Lindhe, Attström, & Björn, 1968). Subgingival growth of *Prevotella intermedia* is enhanced because this bacterium can substitute progesterone, as well as testosterone and estradiol, as growth factors. Elevated levels of *Prevotella intermedia* are also seen in puberty gingivitis (Kornman & Loesche, 1980). Clinically, it presents as a painless protuberant, mushroom-like exophytic mass that is attached to a base at the gingival margin. It will regress or completely disappear postpartum.

Pregnancy gingivitis is not synonymous with a pregnancy tumor. A pregnancy tumor is a non-neoplasm, pyogenic granuloma occurring in a pregnant patient. It arises from an analogue of a dormant (inactive) tumor and is stimulated during pregnancy.

Diabetes Mellitus–Associated Gingivitis   Diabetes mellitus is one of the important risk factors for periodontal diseases. Type 1 diabetes is not as common as type 2 diabetes, which is caused by the development of either resistance to insulin in muscle (insulin is not working to bring glucose into cells), impaired secretion of insulin from the pancreas, or increased glucose production by the liver. All causes result in an elevation of blood glucose levels or hyperglycemia, which causes complications related to accelerated artherosclerosis, retinopathy (blindness), renal (kidney) failure, neuropathy (diseases of the nervous system), altered wound healing, and periodontal conditions.

Diabetes mellitus-associated gingivitis is characterized by inflammation of the gingiva, especially where plaque is present without clinical attachment loss or bone loss. It is similar to plaque-induced gingivitis and is more commonly seen in children with poorly controlled type 1 diabetes.

Gingivitis Associated with Blood Dyscrasias

Leukemia-Associated Gingivitis   Leukemia is a disease characterized by an abnormal proliferation of leukocytes (white blood cells) in the blood and bone marrow. Oral manifestations are seen as gingival inflammation and enlargement starting at the interdental papilla and spreading to the attached gingiva.

Gingivitis Associated with Medications

Drug-Influenced Enlargements   Commonly used drugs can lead to the appearance of gingivitis. There are many types of medications (Table 9–3■) that can cause gingival overgrowth or enlargement.

There are no specific bacteria associated with this type of gingivitis and no specific risk factors other than poor oral hygiene and use of the medication.

Based on current histological and ultrastructural findings, drug-influenced gingival changes are more accurately referred to as "gingival overgrowth" or "enlargement," rather than "gingival hypertrophy," which is defined as an increase in connective tissue volume, or gingival hyperplasia, which is defined as an abnormal increase in the number of fibroblasts (Hallmon & Rossmann, 1999).

The etiology of drug-induced gingival overgrowth is not exactly known. Either there is an excessive production of collagen by gingival fibroblasts, making the gingiva appear thickened or enlarged (Brown, Beaver, & Bottomley, 1991), or the action of collagenase, which breaks down collagen, is reduced (Hallmon & Rossmann, 1999). The highly active fibroblasts become sensitive to these medications in the presence of inflammation (Brown et al., 1991).

Enlargement often occurs within 1 to 3 months after the start of the medication (Nishikawa et al., 1991). Although the amount of the drug used daily and duration

---

Table 9–3   Classification of Medications Associated with Gingival Enlargement

- Phenytoin (incidence 50%): used to control convulsive or seizure disorders (Angelopoulos & Goaz, 1972; Dongari, McDonnell, & Langlais, 1993; Steinberg & Steinberg, 1982)
- Cyclosporine (incidence about 30%): used for immunosuppressive or antirejection therapy when an individual receives an organ transplant (Seymour & Jacobs, 1992; Thomason et al., 1995)
- Sodium valproate (Depakene®): used as an antidepressant and anticonvulsant (rare occurrence)
- Calcium channel blockers: used for the treatment of cardiovascular conditions such as hypertension, angina, and arrhythmias. Although nifedipine was the first calcium channel blocker (Barclay, Thomson, Idle, & Seymour, 1992) and is the one most frequently associated with gingival enlargement (incidence about 15%), the condition can occur with any drug in this class (Nishikawa et al., 1991)

of use may be related to the severity of the overgrowth (Addy, McElnay, Eyre, Campbell, & D'Arcy, 1982), several studies have failed to see any relationship between these factors (Hassell & Hefti, 1991).

While some clinical studies have shown the level of plaque accumulation affects the severity of the overgrowth, others have shown that, although plaque control and the removal of local irritants is of some benefit for gingival health, these measures alone do not prevent gingival overgrowth (Hefti, Eshenaur, Hassel, & Stone, 1994; Seymour & Smith, 1991). It is often difficult to determine whether the increased plaque accumulation preceded the gingival overgrowth or occurred because of ineffective oral hygiene in the presence of enlarged gingiva (Rees, 1998). Since hypertension is an adverse side effect of cyclosporine, patients may also be taking a calcium channel blocker such as nifedipine, which may also induce gingival overgrowth. Other calcium channel blockers associated with gingival enlargement include diltiazem, verampamil, and amlodipine. Thus, it is difficult to assess the actual frequency of gingival overgrowth related to the use of cyclosporine (Lundergan, 1989).

Drug-Influenced Gingivitis

ORAL CONTRACEPTIVE–ASSOCIATED GINGIVITIS   The etiology of oral contraceptive-induced gingival inflammation is similar to that seen in pregnancy (Pearlman, 1974), since the drugs used contain combinations of estrogen and progesterone that simulate pregnancy. Therefore, the same gingival changes observed during pregnancy are seen with oral contraceptive use (Mealey, 1996). *However, much lower concentrations of hormones are used in today's oral contraceptive pills, thus reducing the incidence of gingival diseases* (Preshaw, Knutsen, & Mariotti, 2001).

Non-Plaque-Induced Gingival Diseases (Holmstrup, 1999)

Gingival Diseases of Specific Bacteria Origin

This category includes gingival lesions caused by infections with *Neisseria gonorrhea, Treponema pallidum, Streptococci,* or other microorganisms. The gingival lesions appear as either erythematous (red), edematous (fluid-filled) ulcers, or inflamed, nonulcerated gingiva.

Gingival Diseases of Viral Origin

This section is associated with gingivitis caused by viral infections such as herpes viruses (herpes simplex virus type 1 and 2, primary herpetic gingivostomatitis and varicella-zoster virus). These viruses primarily affect babies and then become latent or dormant until adulthood at which time it appears as recurrent herpes labialis. Primary gingivostomatitis may also be seen during adolescence or adulthood.

Gingival Diseases of Fungal Origin

This section is associated with gingivitis caused by fungal infections such as candidosis, coccidioidomycosis, cryptococcosis, histoplasmosis, and others. Oral candidosis (*C. albicans*) is usually seen in HIV-seropositive and other immunocompromised patients. The lesions appear as a band of erythema of the attached gingiva, which is termed linear gingival erythema (LGE).

Gingival Lesions of Genetic Origin

Hereditary gingival fibromatosis clinically appears as a fibrotic gingival enlargement that is genetically derived and has a rare occurrence. The enlargement of the gingiva may cover the entire tooth surface.

Gingival Manifestations of Systemic Conditions

Mucocutaneous diseases are lesions involving the mucous membranes including the mouth and/or the skin. Oral manifestations of mucocutaneous diseases are seen in erosive lichen planus, benign mucous membrane pemphigoid, bullous pemphigoid, and pemphigus vulgaris. More adult women than men have been documented with the disease. Oral lesions may involve all or part of the gingiva and other mucous membranes of the oral cavity. Gingival involvement may manifest as desquamative gingivitis characterized by desquamation or sloughing (peeling) of the epithelium, leaving a red, painful underlying connective tissue surface. No specific bacteria have been identified. The cause of these mucocutaneous diseases is multifactoral, with some of the diseases being autoimmune in nature whereby the body attacks and destroys its own tissue (Weinberg, Insler, & Campen, 1997).

Allergic reactions due to ingredients or contents of dentifrices, mouth rinses, chewing gum are relatively rare and are usually attributed to chemical additives.

Traumatic Lesions

Physical injury to the gingival tissues may be due to thermal (e.g., burns from hot beverages), chemical (e.g., chemical products such as sloughing of tissues from oral rinses or dentifrices, aspirin burn), or physical (e.g., aggressive tooth brushing, incorrect use of dental floss, fingernails, or toothpicks) injury.

Pathogenesis of Gingivitis

The Gingival Pocket

In early periodontal lesions a gingival pocket (Figure 9–7■), which is also referred to as a pseudopocket, is formed. A gingival pocket is formed by gingival enlargement and coronal migration of the gingival margin. There is no loss of clinical connective tissue attachment (the gingival fibers remain attached to the root surface and the junctional epithelium has not migrated apically onto the root surface). Additionally, there is no alveolar and supporting bone loss. Gingival pockets are not true pockets, they are false or "pseudo," which means that the increased height of the gingiva creates an impression that a deep pocket has been formed when probing instruments are used around a tooth (Ranney, 1986). There is no attachment of gingival connective tissue above the cementoenamel junction, and since there is no loss of clinical connective tissue attachment to the root surface, it is not a true pocket. The pocket epithelium extends laterally and detaches from the tooth surface, permitting apical movement of the bacteria in plaque between the tooth

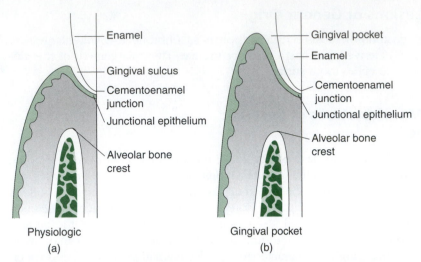

Figure 9–7   (a) Physiologic periodontium. (b) A gingival pocket. The gingival margin has migrated coronally, but there is no attachment loss or bone loss. There is a deepened pocket but it is not a true pocket because the depth is due to the coronal position of the gingiva. This type of pocket is seen in gingivitis.

and epithelium. A pseudopocket is often seen in drug-induced gingivitis (e.g., gingivitis produced by the use of phenytoin, cyclosporine, and certain calcium channel blockers), severe gingival inflammation, and hormone-induced gingivitis (e.g., during pregnancy or puberty).

Host Response to Gingival Inflammation

The gingiva reacts to the presence of microorganisms within dental plaque by alterations in the gingival vascular (blood) supply. The initial response from the gingival tissue is vasodilation of the blood vessels in the lamina propria (gingival connective tissue) in close proximity to the junctional epithelium. With this, there is an increased permeability (increased opening) of the vessels allowing the exchange of fluid and cells between the blood and lamina propria. This allows for the increased migration of neutrophils (leukocytes) from the blood vessels into the lamina propria and junctional epithelium.

These changes in the underlying lamina propria and epithelium cause the clinical features of edema (fluid filled) and redness in the gingival tissues. The ulceration of the junctional epithelium (due to the vascular changes) allows for a communication into the underlying lamina propria where there are an increased number of blood vessels. Thus, when a periodontal probe is placed in the gingival sulcus of inflamed gingiva, bleeding occurs. There is no loss of gingival connective tissue attachment (gingival fibers) and no alveolar and supporting bone loss. Gingivitis is reversible if the irritant is removed below the threshold of causing a host response.

Summary

Gingivitis is a type of inflammatory periodontal disease that is defined as a microbial infection that is confined to the gingival unit. Gingivitis is the result of the outcome of host-bacterial interactions and are modified by systemic factors including medical conditions and medications. Gingivitis is characterized by the presence of a gingival pocket in which there is neither loss of attachment nor bone loss.

Key Points

- Inflammatory periodontal diseases are broadly classified into gingivitis and periodontitis.
- Gingivitis is defined as inflammation confined to the gingiva.
- Gingivitis is reversible.
- Dental plaque is the major risk factor for gingivitis; there are other contributory risk factors such as medications, hormones, and systemic diseases.

Web Sites

www.perio.org

www.emedicine.com

www.agd.org

Self-Quiz

1. Which one of the following features describes gingivitis? (pp. 136, 139)
   a. occurs primarily in children
   b. extensive attachment loss
   c. bone loss does not occur
   d. primary risk factors include pathogenic bacteria and calculus

2. All of the following medications are contributing risk factors in causing gingival enlargement except one. Which one is the exception? (pp. 141–142)
   a. phenytoin
   b. cyclosporine
   c. ibuprofen
   d. nifedipine
   e. valproic acid

3. Which one of the following periodontal diseases is described by having inflammation of the gingiva without loss of clinical connective tissue attachment? (pp. 136, 139)
   a. dental plaque-induced gingivitis
   b. chronic periodontitis
   c. aggressive periodontitis
   d. refractory periodontitis
   e. necrotizing ulcerative periodontitis

4. Which one of the following bacteria is found in high numbers in pregnancy gingivitis? (p. 140)
   a. *Porphyromonas gingivalis*
   b. *Prevotella intermedia*
   c. *Actinomyces viscosus*
   d. *Actinobacillus actinomycetemcomitans*
   e. *Streptococcus sanguis*

5. Which one of the following conditions features gingival involvement due to elevated glucose levels? (p. 140)
   a. pregnancy
   b. puberty
   c. diabetes
   d. leukemia

References

Addy, V., J. McElnay, D. Eyre, N. Campbell, and P. D'Arcy. 1982. Risk factors in phenytoin-induced gingival overgrowth. *J. Periodontol.* 54:373–377.

Amar, S., and K. M. Chung. 1994. Influence of hormonal variation on the periodontium in women. *Periodontology 2000* 6:79–87.

American Academy of Periodontology. 1992. *The etiology and pathogenesis of periodontal diseases* (Position Paper), 1–9. Chicago: Author.

American Academy of Periodontology. 2003. *Glossary of periodontal terms* (4th ed.). Chicago: Author.

Angelopoulos, A. P., and P. W. Goaz. 1972. Incidence of diphenylhydantoin gingival hyperplasia. *Oral Surg. Oral Med. Oral Path.* 34:898–906.

Barclay, S., J. M. Thomason, J. R. Idle, and R. A. Seymour. 1992. The incidence and severity of nifedipine-induced gingival overgrowth. *J. Clin. Periodontol.* 19:311–314.

Brown, R. S., W. T. Beaver, and W. K. Bottomley. 1991. On the mechanisms of drug-induced gingival hyperplasia. *J. Oral Pathol. Med.* 20:201–209.

Cohen, D. W., J. Shapiro, L. Friedman, G. C. Kyle, and S. Franklin. 1971. A longitudinal investigation of the periodontal changes during pregnancy and fifteen months post-partum. Part III. *J. Periodontol.* 42:653–657.

Dongari, A., H. T. McDonnell, and R. P. Langlais. 1993. Drug-induced gingival overgrowth. *Oral Surg. Oral Med. Oral Pathol.* 76:543–548.

Hallmon, W. W., and J. A. Rossmann. 1999. The role of drugs in the pathogenesis of gingival overgrowth. *Periodontology 2000* 21:176–196.

Hassell, T., and A. F. Hefti. 1991. Drug-induced gingival overgrowth: Old problem, new problem. *Crit. Rev. Oral Pathol. Med.* 2:103–137.

Hefti, A. F., A. E. Eshenaur, T. M. Hassell, and C. Stone. 1994. Gingival overgrowth in cyclosporine A treated multiple sclerosis patients. *J. Periodontol.* 65:744–749.

Holmstrup P. 1999. Non-plaque-induced gingival lesions. *Ann. Periodontol.* 4:20–29.

Kornman, K. S., and W. J. Loesche. 1980. The subgingival microflora during pregnancy. *J. Periodontol. Res.* 5:111–122.

Lindhe, J., and P. I. Brånemark. 1968. Experimental studies on the etiology of pregnancy gingivitis. *Perio. Abst.* 16:50–51.

Lindhe, J., J. Lindhe, R. Attström, and A. Björn. 1968. Influence of sex hormones on gingival exudation in dogs with chronic gingivitis. *J. Periodont. Res.* 3:279–283.

Löe, H. 1965. Periodontol changes in pregnancy. *J. Periodontol.* 36:209–217.

Löe, H., E. Theilade, and S. B. Jensen. 1965. Experimental gingivitis in man. *J. Periodontol.* 36:177–187.

Lundergan, W. P. 1989. Drug-induced gingival enlargements. Dilantin hyperplasia and beyond. *J. Calif. Dent. Assoc.* 17:48–52.

Mariotti, A. 1999. Dental plaque-induced gingival diseases. *Annals of Periodontology* 4:7–19.

Mealey, B. L. 1996. Periodontal implications: Medically compromised patients. *Ann. Periodontol.* 1:256–321.

Moore, L. V. H., W. E. C. Moore, and E. P. Cato. 1987. Bacteriology of gingivitis. *J. Dent. Res.* 66:989–995.

Nishikawa, S., H. Tada, A. Hamasaki, S. Kasahara, J. Kido, et al. 1991. Nifedipine-induced gingival hyperplasia: A clinical and in vitro study. *J. Periodontol.* 62:30–35.

Page, R. C. 1985. Oral health status in the United States. Prevalence of inflammatory periodontal diseases. *J. Dent. Educ.* 49:354–364.

Page, R. C. 1986. Gingivitis. *J. Clin. Periodontol.* 13:245–255.

Pearlman, B. A. 1974. An oral contraceptive drug and gingival enlargement: The relationship between local and systemic factors. *J. Clin. Periodontol.* 1:47–57.

Preshaw P.M., M.A. Knutsen, and A. Mariotti 2001. Experimental gingivitis in women using oral contraceptives. *J Dent Res* 80:2011–2015.

Ranney, R. R. 1986. Discussion: pathogenesis of gingivitis. *J. Clin. Periodontol.* 13:356–359.

Ranney, R. R. 1993. Classification of periodontal diseases. *Periodontology 2000* 2:13–25.

Rees, T. D. 1998. Drugs and oral disorders. *Periodontology 2000* 18:21–36.

Seymour, R. A., and D. J. Jacobs. 1992. Cyclosporin and the gingival tissues. *J. Clin. Periodontol.* 19:1–11.

Seymour, R. A., and D. G. Smith. 1991. The effect of a plaque control programme on the incidence and severity of cyclosporin-induced gingival changes. *J. Clin. Periodontol.* 18:107–110.

Silness, J., and H. Löe. 1963. Periodontal disease in pregnancy. *Acta Odontol. Scand.* 21:533–551.

Stamm, J. W. 1986. Epidemiology of gingivitis. *J. Clin. Periodontol.* 13:360–370.

Steinberg, S. C., and A. D. Steinberg. 1982. Phenytoin-induced gingival overgrowth in severely retarded children. *J. Periodontol.* 53:429–433.

Suzuki, J. B. 1988. Diagnosis and classification of periodontal diseases. *Dent. Clin. North America* 32:195–216.

Thomason, J. M., R. A. Seymour, J. S. Ellis, P. J. Kelly, G. Parry, et al. 1995. Iatrogenic gingival overgrowth in cardiac transplantation. *J. Periodontol.* 66:742–746.

Weinberg, M. A., M. S. Insler, and R. B. Campen. 1997. Mucocutaneous features of autoimmune blistering diseases. *Oral Surg. Oral Med. Oral Pathol. Oral Radiol. Endod.* 84:517–534.

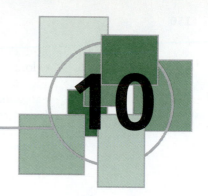

The Periodontitis Lesion

Surendra Singh, D.D.S., M.S.

Outline

Inflammatory
  Periodontal Diseases
Progression of
  Gingivitis into
  Periodontitis
Chronic Periodontitis
Aggressive
  Periodontitis
Periodontitis as a
  Manifestation of
  Systemic Diseases

Peri-Implant Diseases
Pathogenesis of the
  Periodontitis Lesion
Summary
Key Points
Web Sites
Self-Quiz
References

Goal

To provide an understanding of the features of periodontitis.

Educational Objectives

Upon completion of this chapter, the dental hygiene student should be able to:

Explain changes in the 1999 classification of periodontitis.
Define the course of the progression of periodontitis.
Explain the different features of the various types of periodontitis.
Explain the pathogenesis of periodontitis.

Periodontitis is widespread in the population, afflicting children and adults. Periodontitis is defined as clinical attachment loss with subsequent bone loss. According to the 1999 classification of the periodontal diseases, periodontitis is categorized into chronic and aggressive forms. Diagnosis of periodontitis is not based on the age of the patient but rather on clinical and radiographic findings. Dental biofilms are the primary risk factor for periodontitis. Modifying contributory factors such as systemic diseases are also involved in the development and progression of the periodontitis lesion.

Chronic Periodontitis

The new classification system (Armitage, 1999) refers to adult periodontitis as chronic periodontitis (Table 10–1■) and does not rely on the age of the patient to make a diagnosis. Chronic periodontitis is the most common form of periodontal disease affecting both adults and adolescents and has a slow rate of progression (Löe, Anerud, Boysen, & Morrison, 1986). It is directly related to the presence of plaque. Recently, researchers have documented that genetics may play an important noncontrollable risk factor linked to periodontitis (Newman, 1998). Chronic periodontitis may be modified by and/or associated with systemic diseases (e.g., diabetes mellitus, HIV infection). Also, other nonsystemic factors such as smoking and stress may modify the progression of periodontitis.

In order for a person to develop periodontitis, gingivitis must have been present. Even though specific bacteria have been identified as related to the disease, it is still considered a nonspecific bacterial infection. Detection of *Porphyromonas gingivalis* indicates a high probability that periodontitis is present (Christersson, Zambon, Dunford, Grossi, & Genco, 1989). Other local risk factors include calculus, overhanging restorations and other retentive conditions that favor microbial growth, smoking, systemic conditions, hormonal factors, and stress (American Academy of Periodontology, 1992).

Features of chronic periodontitis include pocket formation and alveolar and supporting bone destruction (see Fig. 10–1). Tooth mobility may not necessarily be evident.

Established risk factors for chronic periodontitis include bacteria within dental plaque, smoking, and diabetes mellitus. Smoking causes both gingivitis and chronic periodontitis. Clinical features seen in smokers with periodontitis include deeper probing depths, enhanced gingival recession, more supragingival dental plaque, and more bone loss and attachment loss. There is little clinical gingival inflammation and bleeding because the tissues become less vascular and more fibrotic (thicker gingival tissue), which in a way masks the clinical appearance of inflammation. The nicotine present in tobacco appears to cause constriction of the blood vessels. Smokers also appear to have a decreased PMN migration into the oral cavity and depressed phagocytic function resulting in a diminished immune host response to bacteria and impaired healing response.

Aggressive Periodontitis

At the 1999 International Workshop for a Classification of Periodontal Diseases and Conditions, the American Academy of Periodontology suggested to eliminate the old term "early-onset periodontitis" because it was too restrictive in terms of age.

Table 10–1 Common Features of the Periodontal Diseases

Disease	Patient Population	Clinical Features	Causes of the Disease	Microbiologic Features	
Chronic periodontitis (Figure 10–1■)	Most prevalent in adults but can occur in children and adolescents	Pocket information; bone loss: inflammation	Primary etiologic factor is dental plaque (poor oral hygiene); many other risk factors (e.g., smoking, systemic diseases)	High numbers of *Porphyromonas gingivalis, Bacteroides forsythus, Prevotella intermedia,* and *Eikenella corrodens*	**Figure 10–1** Chronic periodontitis
Generalized aggressive periodontitis (Figure 10–2■)	Usually affects persons under 30 years of age	Generalized: Severe gingival inflammation rapid bone destruction affecting at least three permanent teeth other than first molars and incisors	Defect in polymorphonuclear (PMN) and/or macrophage function	Some predominant bacteria include *Prevotella intermedia, Actinobacillus actinomycetemcomitans*	**Figure 10–2** Aggressive periodontitis in an adolescent (Courtesy of Procter & Gamble, Cincinnati, OH)
Localized aggressive periodontitis (Figure 10–3■)	Except for the presence of periodontitis patients are otherwise clinically healthy; circumpubital onset	Sparse amount of plaque and calculus; little inflammation Localized: Incisor and first molar sites	Defect in PMN chemotaxis	*Actinobacillus actinomycetemcomitans Capnocytophaga* species	**Figure 10–3** Localized aggressive periodontitis (Courtesy of Procter & Gamble, Cincinnati, OH)

151

Early-onset periodontitis included prepubertal periodontitis, juvenile periodontitis, and rapidly progressive periodontitis. Aggressive periodontitis (AgP) can occur at any age and the disease is not necessarily confined to individuals under age 35 and is considered to have a rare occurrence. The term "aggressive periodontitis" was chosen since it is a *rapidly progressive form of periodontitis* and is less dependent on the age of the individual than "early-onset periodontitis" (Tonetti & Mombelli, 1999) (see Figs. 10–2 and 10–3).

Aggressive periodontitis (AgP) is divided into localized and generalized. Localized aggressive periodontitis (LAgP) replaces the older term localized juvenile periodontitis (LJP) and generalized aggressive periodontitis (GAgP) replaces the older term generalized juvenile periodontitis (GLP). Individuals with aggressive periodontitis have specific clinical and laboratory findings that make it distinctively different from chronic periodontitis. The common features of localized and generalized aggressive periodontitis are (Tonetti & Mombelli, 1999):

1. except for the presence of periodontitis, patients are otherwise clinically healthy;
2. rapid attachment loss and bone destruction; and
3. familial disposition.

Secondary features that may be present include:

1. amounts of microbial deposits are inconsistent with the severity of the periodontal tissue destruction;
2. elevated levels of *Actinobacillus actinomycetemcomitans* and, in some populations, *Porphyromonas gingivalis;*
3. progression of attachment loss and bone loss may be self-arresting; and
4. Phagocyte abnormalities.

Features of localized aggressive periodontitis include:

1. circumpubertal onset;
2. serum antibody response to the bacteria; and
3. localized first molar/incisor presentation with interproximal attachment loss on at least two permanent teeth, one of which is a first molar, and involving no more than two teeth other than first molars and incisors.

Features of generalized aggressive periodontitis include:

1. usually affecting individuals under 30 years of age, but can be older;
2. pronounced episodic nature of the destruction of attachment and bone;
3. poor antibody response to the bacteria; and
4. generalized interproximal attachment loss and bone destruction affecting at least three permanent teeth other than first molars and incisors.

To these primary classifications, secondary descriptors may be added. For example, risk factors that modify the disease progression include cigarette smoking, emotional stress, drugs, and sex hormones.

Etiology

A distinguishing feature found in AgP that is not seen in chronic periodontitis is the presence of polymorphonuclear (PMN) and macrophage defects (Page et al., 1983). These white blood cells do not function properly in eliminating the bacteria. Thus, there is a strong genetic or heredity component to this disease, which means that genetic factors may be important in the development of AgP. Children with GAgP are more prone to ear, skin, and upper respiratory tract infections (Suzuki, 1988).

Plaque accumulation is minimal in LAgP, there is slight gingival inflammation, and bone loss is not as rapid as in the generalized form. There is usually no accompanying infection. Patients may have either defective PMNs or macrophages, but not both. There is a defect in PMN chemotaxis and impaired phagocytosis in 70 to 80% of patients (Suzuki, Collison, Falkner, & Nauman, 1984). The PMNs are not working properly and arrive late to the diseased site (depressed chemotaxis), so they cannot properly devour the foreign material including bacteria (impaired phagocytosis).

Predominant bacteria in LAgP include *Actinobacillus actinomycetemcomitans, Prevotella intermedia, Eikenella corrodens, Campylobacter rectus,* and *Capnocytophaga* species (American Academy of Periodontology, 1989). High numbers of *Actinobacillus actinomycetemcomitans* in the subgingival pocket are associated with the localized form and they may invade the soft tissue rather than just staying in the pocket.

Refractory Periodontitis

Refractory periodontitis is a type of periodontitis wherein periodontitis patients previously treated conventionally (periodontal debridement, periodontal surgery, oral hygiene instructions) do not respond favorably to therapy and are considered resistant to treatment. Persistent periodontitis in patients with poor compliance with home care or heavy tobacco use precludes the use of the term refractory. These patients more likely have recurrent periodontitis. High numbers of *Prevotella intermedia, Bacteroides forsythus* (new name: *Tannerella forsythensis*), *Fusobacterium nucleatum,* and *Porphyromonas gingivalis* are found in subgingival refractory sites.

Under the new classification system (Armitage, 1999), periodontitis associated with refractory conditions has been eliminated as a separate disease category. It was concluded that only a small percentage of periodontitis cases are actually nonresponsive to treatment. Instead, the refractory designation could be applied to all forms of periodontitis (e.g., refractory chronic periodontitis, refractory aggressive periodontitis).

Periodontitis as a Manefestation of Systemic Diseases

Dental plaque initiates periodontal diseases but the form of disease and its progression is dependent on the host defenses to this challenge. Systemic conditions and environmental exposures may modify the normal defenses and influence the outcome of periodontal disease (Kinane, 1999). A reduction in the number of function of polymorphonuclear leukocytes (PMNs) usually results in increased rate and severity of periodontal tissue destruction. Additionally, numerous drugs such as phenytoin, nifedipine, and cyclosporine predispose to gingival overgrowth in response to plaque and thus may be an effect in modifying preexisting periodontitis (Kinane, 1999). Several systemic diseases such as diabetes mellitus, Down syndrome, Papillon-Lefévre syndrome, hyphophosphatasia, Chediak-Higashi syndrome, and HIV infection also appear to predispose individuals to periodontitis. These patients also have compromised host responses. Certain environmental conditions or exposures including cigarette smoking and emotional stress may modify periodontitis.

Peri-Implant Diseases

Inflammatory conditions surrounding dental implants are becoming more common today, as more implants are being placed. Periodontal disease around implants is not listed in the original or new classification from the American Academy of Periodontology; however, inflammation and periodontal destruction around implants is clinically recognized. Loss of an implant after successful placement is often due to a bacterial infection. Gram-negative anaerobes, primarily the *Fusobacterium* species and *Prevotella intermedia,* are found in the subgingival pockets. Peri-implant disease is a collective term for soft-tissue inflammation surrounding an implant. Peri-implant mucositis is the term used to describe reversible inflammation in the gingiva around a functioning implant (Albrektsson & Isidor, 1994). Peri-implantitis is the term used for inflammatory changes in the soft tissues leading to loss of supporting bone around a functioning implant (Albrektsson & Isidor, 1994). The primary risk factor for peri-implant diseases is the presence of certain bacteria (Mombelli & Lang, 1998).

Treatment of peri-implant diseases is based on proper clinical and radiographic assessment. It may include periodontal debridement, oral hygiene instruction, mouthrinses, systemic antibiotics, periodontal surgery, or removal of the implant.

Pathogenesis of the Periodontitis Lesion

Sequence of Events in Pocket Formation

A pocket is defined as a pathologically deepened gingival sulcus (American Academy of Periodontology, 2001). The development of a periodontal pocket between the root surface and the gingiva includes the transformation of a thin junctional epithelium into a pocket epithelium with the development of microulcerations and epithelial ridges (Müller-Glauser & Schroeder, 1982) (Fig. 10–4■).

The Periodontal Pocket

As the inflammatory infiltrate progresses from the coronal gingival connective tissue subjacent to the junctional epithelium into the underlying connective tissue, an extensive amount of collagen is destroyed. The detachment of the gingival clinical connective tissue attachment (gingival fibers) to the tooth allows apical migration of the junctional epithelium onto the root surface. Apical migration of the junctional epithelium continues, and as this epithelium separates from the root surface, a periodontal pocket is formed. The junctional epithelium migrates apically only as a result of the destruction of the gingival collagen fibers. With increasing periodon-

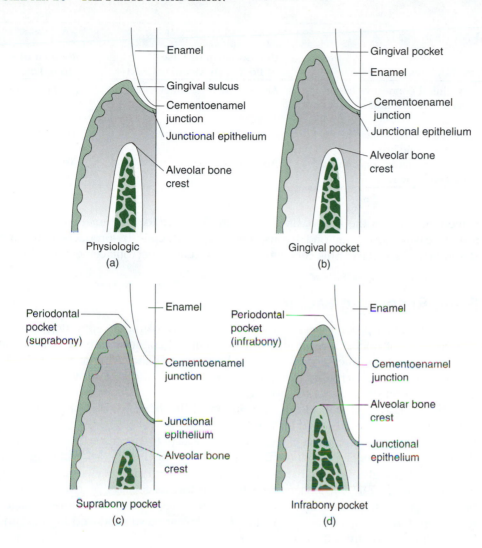

Physiologic
(a)

- Enamel
- Gingival sulcus
- Cementoenamel junction
- Junctional epithelium
- Alveolar bone crest

Gingival pocket
(b)

- Gingival pocket
- Enamel
- Cementoenamel junction
- Junctional epithelium
- Alveolar bone crest

Suprabony pocket
(c)

- Periodontal pocket (suprabony)
- Enamel
- Cementoenamel junction
- Junctional epithelium
- Alveolar bone crest

Infrabony pocket
(d)

- Periodontal pocket (infrabony)
- Enamel
- Cementoenamel junction
- Alveolar bone crest
- Junctional epithelium

Figure 10–4 (a) Healthy periodontium. (b) Gingivitis pocket seen in gingivitis. Note that the junctional epithelium is located at the CEJ. (c) A suprabony pocket is a type of periodontal pocket. The deepened pocket is caused by attachment loss. There is also bone loss. The base of the pocket is coronal to the crest of alveolar bone. This type of pocket is a result of the tissue destruction that occurs in periodontitis. (d) An infrabony pocket is another type of periodontal pocket. The base of the pocket is apical to the crest of bone. This type of pocket is seen in periodontitis.

tal pocket depths, it becomes an ideal environment for plaque accumulation, making it difficult to clean.

There are two types of periodontal pockets: suprabony and infrabony. The difference between the two kinds of pockets lies in the relationship of the base of the pocket or the coronal extent of the junctional epithelium to the alveolar crest and the type of bone destruction (Table 10–2■). Bone destruction occurs as the inflammatory infiltrate extends into the alveolar crest and then into the trabecular bone.

The base of a suprabony pocket (junctional epithelium) is coronal to the crest of bone (see Fig. 10–4b), while the base of an infrabony pocket (junctional epithelium) is apical to the crest of bone (see Fig. 10–4c). This can be identified on a radiograph when a dense object such as a periodontal probe is placed at the base of the pocket as the radiograph is taken.

Root Surface   The areas of cementum that no longer have gingival or periodontal ligament fibers attached undergo changes. The surface of the cementum is rough because of the detachment of the previously inserting connective tissue. Cementoblasts within the periodontal ligament are no longer present to lay down

Table 10–2 Classification of Pockets

Type of Pocket	Pathogenesis	Relationship of Base of Pocket to Alveolar Crest	Pattern of Bone Loss
Gingival (pseudopocket) pocket	No clinical connective tissue attachment loss and no bone loss	At the cementoenamel junction	No bone loss
Periodontal pockets:			
Suprabony pocket	Connective tissue attachment loss and bone loss	Coronal to alveolar crest	Horizontal
Infrabony pocket	Connective tissue attachment loss and bone loss	Apical to alveolar crest	Vertical or angular

cementum due to the endotoxin deposition. The surface of cementum becomes rough, easily absorbing endotoxins, bacteria, and their by-products onto and slightly into its surface. This cementum is referred to as necrotic cementum.

Bone Resorbing Factors

The inflammatory process causes the resorption of alveolar and supporting bone. A consequence of pocket formation and loss of clinical connective tissue attachment is bone resorption. The process of bone loss involves the inflammatory cells including PMNs and macrophages. As the inflammatory infiltrate destroys more collagen in the connective tissue, the bone is approached.

Three classes of substances are involved in bone resorption: (1) prostaglandins, (2) endotoxins, and (3) cytokines.

Numerous factors can act directly on osteoclasts to stimulate their activity to destroy bone. One of the main mechanisms of bone resorption is through the release of prostaglandins (PGE$_2$) from macrophages or PMNs (Offenbacher, Heasman, & Collins, 1993). Prostaglandins activate resting osteoclasts, increase the number of osteoclasts, increase the number of macrophages, and inhibit bone collagen formation (Offenbacher et al., 1993). Protaglandins are also produced in bone and have a direct resorptive effect on bone.

Bone resorption can also occur when bacteria release endotoxins, which activate inflammatory cells such as macrophages resulting in the production and release of cytokines such as IL-1 (Schwartz, Goultschin, Dean, & Boyan, 1997). IL-1 is most important in periodontal destruction (Ishikawa, Nakashima, & Koseki, 1997). IL-1 can also stimulate PGE$_2$ production. Another theory of bone resorption is explained by the role of cytokines and prostaglandins in stimulating collagenase production by PMNs (Reynolds & Meikle, 1997). Collagenase is an enzyme that destroys collagen, which is a component of bone.

Site Specificity

An important feature of inflammatory periodontal diseases is the site-specific localization of periodontal destruction. Pocket formation and bone loss does not occur in all areas of the dentition at the same time, but it could occur on a few teeth at a time or even on only some aspects of some teeth at any given time, while other teeth are healthy. The composition of subgingival plaque samples from different sites in the oral cavity of the same mouth has been shown to be different. These differences have presented a problem for research analysis and treatment response to therapy (Socransky & Haffajee, 1997).

Relationship of Bone Loss and Pocket Formation

Alveolar and supporting bone is destroyed as the pocket develops. Since the level of bone corresponds to previous periodontal destruction and changes in the soft tissue of the pocket wall reflects the present inflammatory condition, the degree of bone loss is not necessarily correlated with the depth of periodontal pockets. Radiographically, extensive bone loss can be associated with shallow pocket depths and vice versa. For example, a patient may have had severe periodontitis at one time, but had periodontal treatment that stopped the progression of the disease. Clinically the probing depths are shallow, but radiographically bone loss is evident.

Pattern of Bone Loss

The types of pockets that form and the pattern of bone loss depend on the route the inflammation takes from the gingiva to the underlying supporting structures. The route of extension of the inflammatory infiltrate from the gingiva into the interdental bone is by way of the blood vessels. The interdental bone is resorbed more rapidly than the bundle bone because it is more vascular and less resistant to resorption. Interproximally (between adjacent teeth), inflammation usually spreads along the interdental blood vessels from the gingiva through the crestal bone into the bone marrow spaces extending out to the periodontal ligament fibers (Fig. 10–5a■). On the facial and lingual surfaces of teeth, the inflammatory infiltrate follows along the supraperiosteal blood vessels located in the periosteum on the outer surface of the bone (Fig. 10–5b■). Usually, the principal fibers are the most resistant to destruction and are the last to be resorbed.

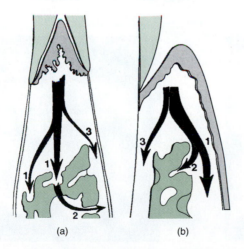

(a)   (b)

Figure 10–5   (a) The inflammatory infiltrate spreads from the gingiva through the lamina propria into the bone following the most vascular pathway, which is where most of the blood vessels are located. Sometimes the most vascular area (larger blood vessels) is on the side of the alveolar crest, allowing the inflammation to directly enter the periodontal ligament. (b) On the direct facial surface, inflammation extends along the supraperiosteal artery before entering bone. (From Fedi P. R., Jr., and A. R. Vernino, *The Periodontic Syllabus.* Copyright © 2000 by Williams & Wilkins.)

The penetration of the inflammatory infiltrate into the marrow spaces and on the bone surfaces is associated with a loss of the equilibrium (balance) between bone formation and bone resorption, leading to loss of alveolar bone. The pattern of bone loss varies among individual teeth and on different surfaces of the same tooth. Bone destruction can occur on any surface of the tooth. The pattern of bone loss can occur in two different ways:

1. Horizontal bone loss when bone resorption occurs from its outer aspect. Bone is lost equally on the surfaces of two adjacent teeth with the interproximal bone level remaining flat (Fig. 10–6a■) and the deepest portion of the pocket is located coronal to the alveolar crest.

2. Vertical or angular bone loss occurs when the inflammation travels directly from the gingiva into the periodontal ligament and then the bone. The interproximal bone level is not flat and even as in horizontal bone loss. Bone loss occurs at different rates around the tooth and is more rapid on

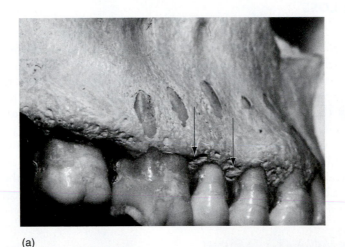

(a)

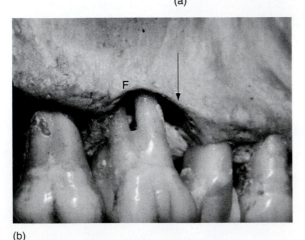

(b)

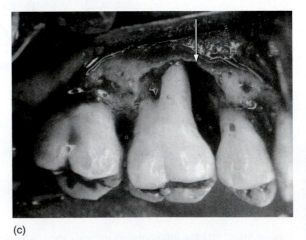

(c)

Figure 10–6   (a) Horizontal pattern of bone loss between the premolars and second premolar and first molar. Interproximal bone (arrows) is destroyed on both sides of adjacent teeth equally. (b) *Left side:* Dry skull specimen showing furcation involvement (F) and vertical pattern of bone loss on the mesial aspect of the first molar. Note that the interproximal bone is not flat as with horizontal bone loss. (c) *Right side:* After the gingiva has been reflected from the tooth and bone, a vertical defect is seen on the mesial aspect of the first molar.

one side of the tooth than the other. The base or the deepest portion of the bony defect is apical to the alveolar bone crest creating an infrabony defect (Fig. 10–6b,c■). The terms infrabony and intrabony have been used interchangeably to describe all vertical bony defects; however, these terms are frequently misused in the periodontal literature (Weinberg & Eskow, 2000). The term intra- translates to mean "within or inside the bone" and infra- to mean "below the crest of bone." An infrabony defect is a "generic" term to describe any periodontal vertical bony defect.

Periodontal infrabony defects are classified according to the number of osseous (bony) walls surrounding the pocket (Fig. 10–7■). There are four bony interproximal walls surrounding the tooth: the mesial, facial (buccal), distal, and lingual. Most vertical bone loss occurs interproximally, although vertical bone loss does occur on the direct facial and lingual walls. Types of defects include:

1. Three-wall bony defect. The three-wall defect has three bony walls remaining interproximally or facially or lingually, with the tooth forming the fourth wall. An intrabony defect is a type of three-wall bony defect with specific characteristics (Prichard, 1979). As a result of the disease process, the bone lining the infrabony defect is usually composed of cortical bone. In an intrabony defect, the walls have cancellous bone behind them. The only way to determine if the defect is intrabony is during the surgical procedure when the bone is exposed. Thus, it is incorrect to refer to all infrabony defects as intrabony. A three-wall defect that wraps around the tooth and involves two or more adjacent root surfaces is referred to as a circumferential defect.

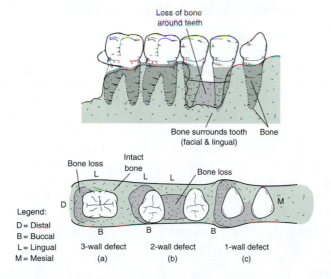

Figure 10–7 Vertical bone destruction is classified according to the number of bony walls surrounding the defect. In health there are four bony walls surrounding a tooth: mesial (M), buccal (B) or facial, distal (D), and lingual (L). In periodontitis one or more of the bony walls is destroyed. If three bony walls remain, it is called a three-wall defect (a). If the buccal and lingual bony walls remain, it is called a two-wall defect or crater (b). If one bony wall remains (e.g., buccal/lingual cortical plate or proximal [mesial, distal] wall of bone), it is called a one-wall defect or hemiseptum (c).

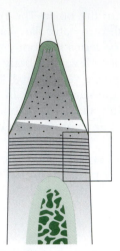

Figure 10–8   The range of bone destruction determines the pattern of bone loss. The area of bone destruction radiates from the plaque mass about 2 mm. (Copyright © 1997 by J. Lindhe and T. Karring, Anatomy of the periodontium, in *Clinical periodontology and implant dentistry*, ed. J. Lindhe. Copenhagen: Munksgaard.)

2. Two-wall bony defect. The two-wall defect has two bony walls remaining. An interdental crater is the most common angular bony defect. It is a two-wall osseous defect with a buccal and lingual wall remaining.
3. One-wall bony defect. The one-wall defect has one bony wall remaining and usually occurs interdentally. If the remaining wall is the proximal wall, the defect is referred to as a hemiseptum.

Factors Related to Pattern of Bone Loss

The bone destructive process radiates from the plaque mass, at the base of the periodontal pocket, 1.5 to 2.5 mm circumferentially (Tal, 1984) (Fig. 10–8■). Within this 2-mm "circle," bone destruction does not occur. Outside this 2-mm "circle," bone destruction occurs. Thus, the width and thickness of the interdental septum primarily determines if the pattern of bone destruction is horizontal or vertical. Bone destruction occurring where there is a wide interdental septum (> 2 mm in width) will most likely not occur across the entire septum and results in a vertical pattern of bone loss. Bone destruction occurring where the interdental septum is narrow (< 2 mm) can be total and results in a horizontal pattern of bone loss.

Teeth such as lower incisors, which have thin facial or lingual cortical plates of bone with little to no cancellous bone between the alveolar bone proper and the outer plate, will usually show a horizontal pattern of bone loss. Molars that have a thick facial cortical plate of bone will usually show a vertical pattern of bone loss.

Summary

Periodontitis is classified based on clinical presentation rather than age, as was done in previous classification systems. Periodontitis is a microbial infection that is the result of host–bacteria interactions. Periodontitis is characterized by attachment loss with subsequent bone loss. Different patterns of bone loss are evident on radiographs. Periodontitis can be modified by systemic factors wherein the host has a reduced capacity to resist infection.

Key Points

- Periodontitis is inflammation that extends from the gingiva into the supporting periodontal structures.
- Periodontitis is most common in adults, although it does occur in a smaller number of children and adolescents.
- Dental plaque (biofilms) is the major risk factor for periodontal diseases; there are other contributory risk factors such as medications, hormones, and systemic diseases.
- Inflammatory periodontal disease is also seen around dental implants.

Web Sites

www.perio.org

www.dental.ucla.edu

www.merck.com

Self-Quiz

1. Which one of the following features describes chronic periodontitis? (p. 150)
   a. occurs primarily in children
   b. no connective tissue attachment loss occurs
   c. bone loss does not occur
   d. risk factors include pathogenic bacteria and smoking

2. The latest classification of periodontitis is based on all of the following factors except one. Which one is the exception? (p. 150)
   a. age of patient
   b. clinical presentation
   c. radiographic survey
   d. historical data
   e. microbial profile

3. Which one of the following forms of periodontitis is associated with a chemotactic defective in the polymorphonuclear leukocytes? (pp. 150–153)
   a. dental plaque-induced gingivitis
   b. chronic periodontitis
   c. puberty gingivitis
   d. localized aggressive periodontitis
   e. drug-influenced gingivitis

4. Which one of the following bacteria is found in high numbers in localized aggressive periodontitis? (p. 153)
   a. *Prophyromonas gingivalis*
   b. *Prevotella intermedia*
   c. *Actinomyces viscosus*
   d. *Actinobacillus actinomycetemcomitans*
   e. *Streptococcus sanguis*

5. Which one of the following types of pocket has its base located apical to the alveolar crest as evidenced on a radiograph? (p. 155)
   a. gingival
   b. psuedo
   c. suprabony
   d. infrabony

References

Albrektsson, T., and F. Isidor. 1994. Consensus report of session IV. In eds. N. P. Lang and T. Karring, *Proceedings of the First European Workshop on Periodontology,* 365–369. London: Quintessence.

American Academy of Periodontology. 1989. *Proceedings of the World Workshop in Clinical Periodontics,* I-2–I-4. Chicago: Author.

American Academy of Periodontology. 1992. *The etiology and pathogenesis of periodontal diseases* (Position Paper), 1–9. Chicago: Author.

American Academy of Periodontology. 2001. *Glossary of periodontal terms* (4th ed.). Chicago: Author.

Armitage, G. C. 1999. Development of a classification system for periodontal diseases and conditions. *Ann. Periodontol.* 4:1–6.

Brown, L. J., and H. Löe. 1993. Prevalence, extent, severity and progression of periodontal disease. *Periodontology 2000* 2:57–71.

Christersson, L. A., J. J. Zambon, R. G. Dunford, S. G. Grossi, and R. J. Genco. 1989. Specific subgingival bacteria and diagnosis of gingivitis and periodontitis. *J. Dent. Res.* 68:1633–1639.

Ishikawa, I., K. Nakashima, T. Koseki, et al. 1997. Induction of the immune response to periodontopathic bacteria and its role in the pathogenesis of periodontitis. *Periodontology 2000* 14:79–111.

Kinane, D. F. 1999. Periodontitis modified by systemic factors. *Ann. Periodontal.* 4:54–63.

Löe, H., A. Anerud, H. Boysen, and E. Morrison. 1986. Natural history of periodontal disease in man. Rapid, moderate and no loss of attachment in Sri Lankan Laborers 14 to 46 years of age. *J. Clin. Periodontol.* 13:431–440.

Mombelli, A., and N. P. Lang. 1998. The diagnosis and treatment of periimplantitis. *Periodontology 2000* 17:63–76.

Müller-Glauser, W., and H. H. Schroeder. 1982. The pocket epithelium: A light- and electron-microscopic study. *J. Periodontol.* 53:133–144.

Newman, M. 1998. Genetic, environmental, and behavioral influences on periodontal infections. *Compendium* (special issue) 19:25–31.

Offenbacher, S., P. A. Heasman, and J. G. Collins. 1993. Modulation of host PGE_2 secretion as a determinant of periodontal disease expression. *J. Periodontol.* 64:432–444.

Page, R. C., T. Bowen, L. Altman, E. Vandesteen, H. Ochs, et al. 1983. Prepubertal periodontitis I. Definition of a clinical disease entity. *J. Periodontol.* 54:257–271.

Prichard, J. F. 1979. Management of intrabony defects. In ed. J. F. Prichard, *The diagnosis and treatment of periodontal disease,* 358–361. Philadelphia: W. B. Saunders.

Reynolds, J. J., and M. C. Meikle. 1997. Mechanisms of connective tissue matrix destruction in periodontitis. *Periodontology 2000* 14:144–157.

Schwartz, Z., J. Goultschin, D. D. Dean, and B. D. Boyan. 1997. Mechanisms of alveolar bone destruction in periodontitis. *Periodontology 2000* 14:158–172.

Socransky, S. S., and A. D. Haffajee. 1997. The nature of periodontal diseases. *Ann. Periodontol.* 2:3–10.

Suzuki, J. B. 1988. Diagnosis and classification of periodontal diseases. *Dent. Clin. North America* 32:195–216.

Suzuki, J. B., B. C. Collison, W. A. Falkler, and R. R. Nauman. 1984. Immunologic profile of juvenile periodontitis. II. Neutrophil chemotaxis, phagocytosis and spore germination. *J. Periodontol.* 55:461–467.

Tal, H. 1984. Relationship between the interproximal distance of roots and the prevalence of intrabony pockets. *J. Periodontol.* 55:604–607.

Tonetti, M. S., A. Mombelli. 1999. Early-onset periodontitis. *Ann. Periodontol.* 4:39–52.

Weinberg, M.A., and R.N. Eskow. 2000. Osseous effects: proper terminology revisited. *J. Periodontol.* 71:1928.

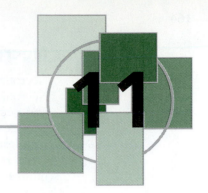

Necrotizing Periodontal Diseases

Surendra Singh, D.D.S., M.S.

Outline

Necrotizing
   Periodontal Diseases
Summary
Key Points

Web Sites
Self-Quiz
References

Goal

To provide an understanding of ulcerative periodontal diseases.

Educational Objectives

Upon completion of this chapter, the dental hygiene student should be able to:

Explain the 1999 classification of ulcerative periodontal diseases.
Discuss periodontal disease associated with HIV-positive patients.
Describe the features of periodontal ulcerative gingivitis.
Explain the features of periodontal ulcerative periodontitis.

KEY WORDS
• necrotizing ulcerative gingivitis
• necrotizing ulcerative periodontitis
• immuno-suppression

Necrotizing Periodontal Diseases

Necrotizing periodontal diseases are unique from other periodontal diseases. Necrotizing periodontal diseases include necrotizing ulcerative gingivitis (NUG) and necrotizing ulcerative periodontitis (NUP). Even though necrotizing periodontal diseases are classified as a separate entity, these conditions may actually be manifestations of underlying systemic problems (e.g., HIV infection). Additionally, other risk factors include tobacco smoking, preexisting periodontal disease, and trauma.

Necrotizing Ulcerative Gingivitis (NUG)

Clinical features of necrotizing ulcerative gingivitis (NUG) are different from other periodontal diseases (e.g., gingivitis). Necrotizing ulcerative gingivitis is a rapidly destructive, recurring, noncommunicable gingival infection. Under the new classification (Armitage, 1999), NUG is considered a type of necrotizing periodontal disease limited to the gingival tissues. Additionally, the term "acute" in ANUG is a clinical descriptive term and should not be used as a diagnostic classification (Rowland, 1999). NUG is relatively uncommon (incidence 0.1 to 10%) and mostly affects young adults 18 to 30 years old. It has also been known as "trench mouth" or "Vincent's infection." During World War I, NUG reached very high levels of incidence and was called "trench mouth," referring to the trenches soldiers inhabited during the war. In addition to bacteria, other predisposing factors are emotional stress, cigarette smoking, decreased nutritional intake, or systemic conditions (e.g., HIV, AIDS). During stressful periods, oral hygiene measures may decrease, smoking may increase, and immune function may be suppressed.

NUG is clinically characterized by small, gray, ulcerative lesions that begin at the tips of the interdental papillae and spread to the gingival margin to form punched-out or cratered lesions. A grayish-white pseudomembrane covering the affected areas may be present. A prominent sign of NUG is "punched out," necrotic interdental papillae, which is caused by ulcer formation on the tip of the papillae. The marginal gingiva is bright red and inflamed and extremely painful. Patients complain of difficulty eating and a burning sensation in the mouth. There is spontaneous gingival bleeding (i.e., the gingiva bleeds when touched or during eating). There are usually heavy deposits of plaque. These signs and symptoms are sudden in onset, localized, and recurrent. If left untreated, the infection may spread to the underlying periodontal structures. Lymphadenopathy (lymph nodes that are abnormal in size, consistency, or number), fever, and fetid oral odor (foul mouth odor) are variable findings and not always present. The signs and symptoms of NUG usually resolve a few days after adequate treatment, however.

This condition is usually recognized on the basis of clinical signs and symptoms. It has a bacterial origin. It is confirmed to be an infectious disease because reduction of dental biofilms either by mechanical debridement or the use of antibiotics will resolve clinical signs and symptoms. Microbiological samples of the affected areas show specific bacteria. High numbers of *Prevotella intermedia,* spirochetes (*Treponema* sp.), and *Fusobacterium* sp. have been isolated (Loesche, Syed, Laughon, & Stoll, 1982). Spirochetes have been shown to penetrate deep into the connective tissue (Listgarten & Lewis, 1967). Normally bacteria stay in the pocket and do not invade the underlying tissues. Thus, NUG is a manifestation of a mixed bacterial infection modified by particular systemic determinants. Necrotizing ulcerative gingivitis may also be the first clinical sign of underlying systemic disease, such as in human immunodeficiency virus (HIV) infection (Murayama, Kurihara, Nagai, Dompkowski, & Van Dyke, 1994).

A complete laboratory work-up is indicated in the management of patients with NUG, especially if a systemic disease is suspected or if the patient does not respond to conventional therapy (Murayama et al., 1994).

Primary herpetic gingivostomatitis must be differentiated (differential diagnosis) from NUG. The primary distinctions are that in primary herpes the patient is usually much younger, elevated temperature is more common, and the patient appears more ill and shows a general malaise. The oral lesions in primary herpes are vesicles that coalesce into ulcers, which occur on the attached gingival and oral mucosa, and the papillae are not "punched out" as in NUG.

Thus, primary herpetic gingivostomatitis is a differential diagnosis of necrotizing ulcerative gingivitis. Actually, NUG can be easily recognized when interproximal papillae necrosis, bleeding, and pain are all seen. If these three features are not present, a diagnosis of NUG cannot be made.

Immunosuppression

Depressed PMN function (chemotactic, phagocytic) is suppressed in patients with NUG. NUG may be the first sign of HIV infection. HIV-infected patients may present with severe forms of periodontal diseases. These patients are immunodeficient with a specific decrease in CD4+ lymphocytes. Conflicting reports concerning the classification system of HIV-associated periodontal lesions exist. New terminology was proposed in the early 1990s that are recognized by the United States and the rest of the world (EEC-Clearinghouse, 1993). Linear gingival erythema (LGE) replaces the older term HIV-gingivitis, and necrotizing ulcerative periodontitis (NUP) replaces HIV-periodontitis (the latter is discussed later in this chapter). A third subdivision of HIV-associated periodontal diseases was also added, necrotizing ulcerative gingivitis (NUG). In the newest classification system (Armitage, 1999) all periodontal conditions related to HIV infections are grouped together with Necrotizing Periodontal Diseases.

The prevalence of LGE in HIV-infected populations is relatively unknown since the stage of HIV disease varies among the population (Mealey, 1996) and more structured studies need to be conducted. Linear gingival erythema is characterized by a distinct band of intense redness along the marginal gingiva extending apically into the attached gingival and alveolar mucosa (Table 11–1■; Figs. 11–1■ & 11–2■).

Necrotizing ulcerative gingivitis in HIV-infected patients is characterized by the destruction of one or more interdental papillae that became ulcerated, cratered, and necrotic (Murray, 1994), but there is no bone loss. NUG may represent an early form of NUP (Mealey, 1996).

These oral findings do not seem to correspond to supragingival plaque accumulation (Mealey, 1996) since removal of dental plaque does not improve the gingival condition as typically seen in chronic, plaque-associated gingivitis. The lesion is confined to the gingiva and does not involve bone loss. Pain is not a prominent feature with this lesion, as it is in NUG (Winkler & Robertson, 1992).

It is important for dental practitioners to recognize soft tissue lesions early, since they may be the first signs of HIV infection (Mealey, 1996; Winkler, Grassi, & Murray, 1988; Winkler & Robertson, 1992). Subtle lesions may go unnoticed by the examiner because pain is not a common symptom.

Table 11–1	Common Features of Necrotizing Periodontal Diseases			
Disease	Patient Population	Clinical Features	Causes of the Disease	Microbiologic Features
Necrotizing periodontal diseases (NUG)	Young adults	Punched out interdental papillae, pain, and free bleeding	Inadequate oral hygiene; stress; cigarette smoking	Specific bacteria: spirochetes, *Prevotella intermedia, Fusobacterium nucleatum*	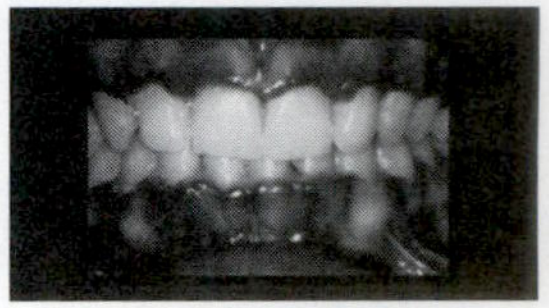
Necrotizing periodontal diseases (NUG)	HIV-infected individuals	Distinct red band around marginal gingiva	Immunodeficiency (decrease in CD4+ lymphocytes)	Similar to chronic periodontitis; bacteria: *Porphyromonas gingivalis, Prevotella intermedia, F. nucleatum, Candida albicans* (fungus)	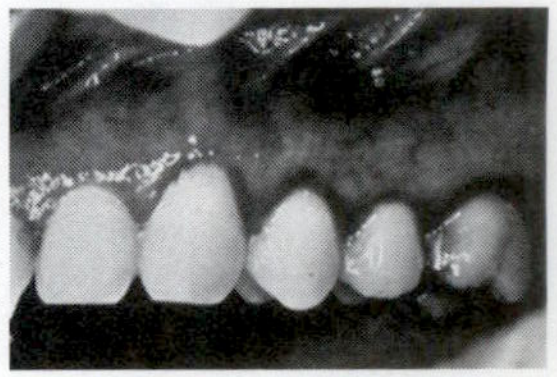
Necrotizing periodontal diseases (NUP)	Patients with HIV infection	Periodontal involvement of deeper structures; rapid loss of bone and spontaneous gingival bleeding	Immunodeficiency	Similar to adult periodontitis; bacteria: *Porphyromonas gingivalis, P. intermedia, F. nucleatum, Candida albicans* (fungus)	

Figure 11–1 NUG (Courtesy of Procter & Gamble, Cincinnati, OH)

Figure 11–2 NUG (Courtesy of Procter & Gamble, Cincinnati, OH)

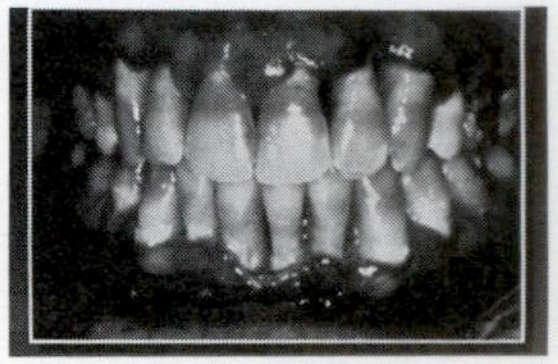

Figure 11–3 NUP (Courtesy of Procter & Gamble, Cincinnati, OH)

The microorganisms present in the gingival lesions of HIV-positive patients are not similar to the microorganisms found in the gingival lesions of HIV-negative individuals but may be similar to those found in HIV-negative individuals who have chronic periodontitis (Mealey, 1996; Murray, Winkler, Peros, French, & Lippke, 1991). Implicating pathogens include *Porphyromonas gingivalis* (Pg), *Prevotella intermedia* (Pi), *Actinobacillus actinomycetemcomitans* (Aa), *Fusobacterium nucleatum,* spirochetes, and *Candida albicans* (fungus) (American Academy of Periodontology, 1994).

Necrotizing Ulcerative Periodontitis (NUP)

Necrotizing ulcerative periodontitis (NUP) previously replaced the term "HIV-periodontitis." Under the new system (Armitage, 1999) NUP is included with necrotizing periodontal diseases. Necrotizing ulcerative periodontitis is not limited to HIV infections and is often seen in patients that have severe malnutrition and are immunosuppressed. However, this form of periodontal disease in the HIV-positive patient may coexist with other forms of periodontitis such as aggressive or chronic periodontitis. NUP is characterized by the extensive necrosis of the gingiva with exposure and rapid destruction of the underlying bone extending past the mucogingival junction (Fig. 11–3■). If not successfully treated, NUP can spread into the adjacent maxilla and mandible (Mealey, 1996). Compared with NUG, severe pain is a prominent feature (Murray, 1994). Essentially all NUP sites bleed on probing, and about 50% of sites show spontaneous bleeding (American Academy of Periodontology, 1992). Extensive clinical attachment loss is common, but deep periodontal pocket formation is not evident (American Academy of Periodontology, 1992).

The microbial population of subgingival sites with NUP is similar to that of chronic periodontitis, which is also similar to NUG. This may prove that NUG may be a precursor to the tissue and bone destruction seen in NUP (Murray, 1994).

Summary

The American Academy of Periodontology refers collectively to necrotizing ulcerative gingivitis (NUG) and necrotizing ulcerative periodontitis (NUP) as ulcerative periodontal diseases (Rowland, 1999). The reason for this is that both NUG and NUP may be considered the same disease but at different stages. Thus, they may not be separate diseases but named under the Necrotizing Ulcerative Diseases. Both NUG and NUP are diseases related to a decreased systemic resistance, as seen in HIV-infected patients, to bacteria present in the periodontal tissues and that NUG is confined to the gingival unit and NUP involves the attachment apparatus (bone, cementum, periodontal ligament). Three criteria (pain, bleeding, and papillae necrosis) must be present for a diagnosis of NUG.

Key Points

- NUG and NUP are ulcerative inflammatory periodontal diseases.
- Pain is the hallmark of NUG.
- NUG involves the gingival unit.
- NUP involves the attachment apparatus.
  Prevotella intermedia and spirochetes are associated with gingival lesions.
- NUG and NUP are involved in HIV infections.

Web Sites

www.perio.org

www.who.int/en/

www.nidcr.nih.gov/health/pubs/mouth_hiv

www.hivdent.org

Self-Quiz

1. Which one of the following statements describes an HIV-positive patient with necrotizing periodontal disease? (p. 164)

   a. Higher prevalence in females than males

   b. Higher incidence of skin lesions

   c. Microbial profile is similar in noninfected periodontally involved patients

   d. Geographic distribution shows a higher prevalence in the eastern United States

2. Which of the following bacterium present in NUG patients may penetrate periodontal tissues? (pp. 164–166)

   a. spriochetes

   b. *Prevotella intermedia*

   c. *Fusobacterium species*

   d. *Porphyromonas gingivalis*

3. Both necrotizing ulcerative gingivitis and necrotizing ulcerative periodontitis are currently categorized under the title: (p. 164)

   a. acute necrotizing diseases

   b. necrotizing ulcerative diseases

   c. chronic periodontitis

   d. aggressive periodontitis

4. Necrotizing ulcerative gingivitis may be the first clinical sign of an underlying systemic disease such as: (pp. 164–165)

   a. human immunodeficiency virus infection

   b. diabetes mellitus

   c. osteoporosis

   d. kidney failure

5. Which of the following diseases must be differentiated from NUG? (pp. 164–166)

   a. herpes simplex type 2

   b. primary herpetic gingivostomatitis

   c. acute necrotizing ulcerative gingivitis

   d. acquired immunodeficiency syndrome

References

American Academy of Periodontology. 1992. *The etiology and pathogenesis of periodontal diseases* (Position Paper), 1–9. Chicago: Author.

Armitage, G. C. 1999. Development of a classification system for Periodontal diseases and conditions. *Ann. Periodontol.* 4:1–6.

EEC-Clearinghouse on Oral Problems Related to HIV Infections and WHO Collaborating Centre on Oral Manifestations for the Human Immunodeficiency Virus. 1993. Classification and diagnostic criteria for oral lesions in HIV infection. *J. Oral Pathol. Med.* 22: 289–291.

Listgarten, M. A., and D. W. Lewis. 1967. The distribution of spirochetes in the lesion of acute necrotizing ulcerative gingivitis: An electron microscopic and statistical survey. *J. Periodontol.* 38:379–386.

Loesche, W. J., S. A. Syed, B. E. Laughon, and J. Stoll. 1982. The bacteriology of acute necrotizing ulcerative gingivitis. *J. Periodontol.* 53:223–230.

Mealey, B. L. 1996. Periodontal implications: Medically compromised patients. *Ann. Periodontol.* 1:256–321.

Murayama, Y., H. Kurihara, A. Nagai, D. Dompkowski, and T. Van Dyke. 1994. Acute necrotizing ulcerative gingivitis: Risk factors involving host defense mechanisms. *Periodontology 2000* 6:116–124.

Murray, P. A. 1994. Periodontal diseases in patients infected by human immunodeficiency virus. *Periodontology 2000* 6:50–67.

Murray, P. A., J. R. Winkler, W. J. Peros, C. K. French, and J. A. Lippke. 1991. DNA probe detection of periodontal pathogens in HIV-associated periodontal lesions. *Oral Microbiol. Immunol.* 6:34–40.

Rowland, R. W. 1999. Necrotizing ulcerative gingivitis. *Ann Periodontol.* 4:65–73.

Winkler, J. R., M. Grassi, and P. A. Murray. 1988. Clinical description and etiology of HIV-associated periodontal diseases. In eds. P. B. Robertson and J. S. Greenspan, *Perspectives on oral manifestations of AIDS,* 49–70. Littleton, MA: PSG Publishing.

Winkler, J. R., and P. B. Robertson. 1992. Periodontal disease associated with HIV infection. *Oral Surg. Oral Med. Oral Pathol.* 73:145–150.

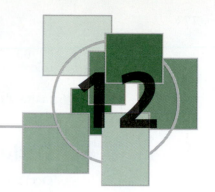

The Occlusal Lesion

Mea A. Weinberg, D.M.D., M.S.D., R.Ph.
Stuart J. Froum, D.D.S.

Outline

Occlusion

Pathogenesis of
Occlusal Trauma

Classification of
Occlusal Trauma

Clinical Findings in
Occlusal Trauma

Radiographic Findings
in Occlusal Trauma

Outcomes of
Treatment of
Occlusal Trauma

Occlusal Therapy

Summary

Key Points

Web Site

Self-Quiz

References

Goal

To provide information about the etiology, clinical manifestations, and therapy of occlusal trauma.

Educational Objectives

Upon completion of this chapter, the dental hygiene student should be able to:

List the classification of malocclusion.

Identify and distinguish between the two types of occlusal trauma.

Identify and describe the clinical and radiographic signs of occlusal trauma.

Define the interrelationship between occlusal trauma and periodontitis.

KEY WORDS

- occlusion
- malocclusion
- tooth wear
- parafunctional habits
- occlusal trauma
- traumatogenic occlusion
- parafunctional habits
- occlusal therapy
- primary occlusal trauma
- secondary occlusal trauma

Soon after the identification of microorganisms as a risk factor for periodontitis, the role of occlusion in periodontal diseases was considered. Although numerous studies using human and animal models have been published on this subject, it still remains a controversial issue.

Occlusion

Occlusion describes the contact relationship of teeth in function and dysfunction and is defined as any contact between the incisal or occlusal surfaces of the maxillary and mandibular teeth. It consists of all tooth contacts during swallowing and chewing. Centric occlusion (CO) is defined as maximal intercuspation or contact of the maxillary and mandibular teeth. The centric relation (CR) is the most retruded (posterior) position of the mandible in relation to the maxilla from which lateral movements of the jaw can be made.

An "ideal" or normal occlusion occurs where the arrangement of teeth is considered to be most correct. This is to say, upon closing the mouth, all upper and lower teeth come together at the same time and there are no crowded, malpositioned, or tipped teeth. Few patients have an ideal or normal occlusion. Usually, there are deviations from normal. Any deviation from the ideal or normal occlusion, for example, crowding, malpositioned, or tipped teeth, is referred to as malocclusion. However, malocclusion does not necessarily indicate occlusal disease. Classification of the various forms of malocclusion is done with Edward H. Angle's principles of defining occlusion. This classification is based on the interdigitation of the maxillary and mandibular teeth. Malpositioning is described in terms of crowding of individual teeth or groups of teeth. Figure 12–1■ describes the three classes of malocclusion. If the maxillary first molar is missing, the maxillary canine is used. The use of study casts to provide a better indication of occlusion is sometimes required. The main purpose for using this classification is for diagnostic consistency and treatment planning because malocclusion is a contributing risk factor for inflammatory periodontal diseases.

Functional occlusion consists of teeth that are in function when the mandible moves in lateral and protrusive excursions or movements. Lateral movements are defined by the direction in which the mandible is moving (Fig. 12–2■). If the mandible moves to the left, the movement is called a left working movement, and the left side of the arch is known as the working side. In a left working movement, the right side is known as the nonworking (balancing) side. If the mandible moves to the right, the movement is called a right working movement, and the right side of the arch is then referred to as the working side. The left side is referred to as the nonworking (balancing) side. For some patients, a lateral movement results in contacts between the posterior teeth on the working side. This is called group function (Fig. 12–3■). For other patients, a lateral movement results in contact only between the maxillary and mandibular canines on the working side. This is called canine protection or canine guidance (see Fig. 12–3). It is generally believed that during lateral movements there should be no tooth contact on the nonworking side. However, balancing side contacts are probably prevalent in most patients. Denture wearers need tooth-to-tooth contacts on both the working and nonworking sides for the dentures to function effectively.

Protrusive occlusion is movement of the mandible in a direction anterior to centric occlusion (Fig. 12–4■). Guidance for this movement should be on the ante-

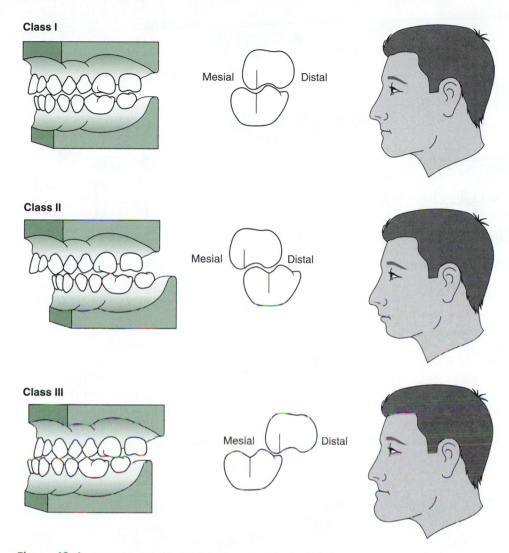

Class I

Mesial   Distal

Class II

Mesial   Distal

Class III

Mesial   Distal

Figure 12–1   Classification of malocclusion: Angle's classification.

rior teeth, and edge-to-edge contact of the incisors should be possible. Any posterior contact during protrusive occlusion is considered undesirable. Prematurity, or premature contact (also called an occlusal interference), occurs when there are interferences to closure of opposing teeth. In other words, individual teeth touch the opposing teeth before full closure in centric occlusion and prevent the other teeth in the arch from achieving contact. Premature contact also can occur during lateral movements, either on the working side or on the nonworking side. Posterior interference is seen frequently with an extruded or tipped tooth. A classic example of a prematurity occurs when an amalgam filling is too high (placed above the line of occlusion), and upon biting down, the patient feels as though that particular area is touching first. Therefore, in this situation, one or more teeth are touching the occlusal surface rather than all the teeth touching simultaneously.

Cases where patients have occlusions that are not ideal but are symptom-free and their dentition "survives" or "adapts" to this deviated occlusion are referred to

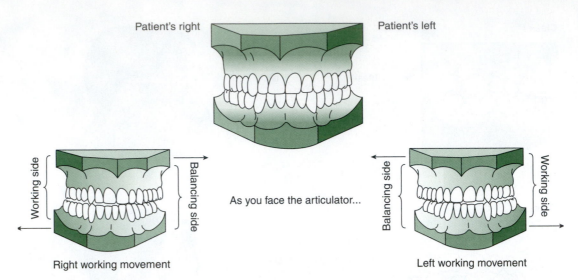

Patient's right   Patient's left

Working side   Balancing side   As you face the articulator...   Balancing side   Working side

Right working movement   Left working movement

Figure 12–2 Illustration of centric occlusion (*center*). Teeth close together with even pressure on both sides of the mouth. In right working movement (*left*), the mandible moves to the right. In left working movement (*right*), the mandible moves to the left.

as physiologic occlusion. Pathologic occlusion occurs when patients show evidence or signs and have symptoms of occlusal disease (Goldman & Cohen, 1980).

Overbite (amount of vertical overlap of anterior teeth) and overjet (horizontal protrusion of upper teeth beyond the lower) are measured with a periodontal probe. Normally, the incisal edges of the lower incisors and the cingulum of the upper incisors establish the stops necessary to maintain tooth position. A deep

Figure 12–3 Group function: Lateral movement results in contact of all posterior teeth (*top*). Canine guidance: Lateral movement results in contact between the maxillary and mandibular canines (*bottom*).

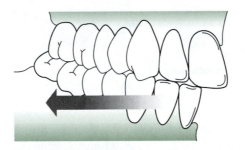

Right working movement
All posterior teeth are in contact: group function

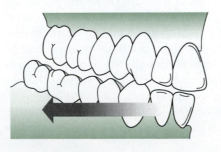

Right working movement
Only the canines are in contact: canine protection

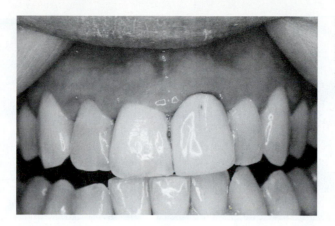

Figure 12–4 Protrusive occlusion (movement): Mandible moves forward from centric occlusion so that there is contact of the incisors.

overbite can occur as a result of skeletal relationship, extrusion or migration of teeth, or if posterior teeth are missing causing the anterior teeth to handle the occlusal load. Overclosure of anterior teeth can cause trauma to the gingiva of the maxillary and/or mandibular anterior teeth (Fig. 12–5■). This is referred to as a traumatic overbite. An open bite occurs when anterior and/or posterior maxillary and mandibular teeth do not occlude.

Conditions of Tooth Wear

Conditions and situations that may account for loss of tooth structure include dental attrition, abrasion, and erosion. Usually, the intraoral examination coupled with a patient interview will reveal the type of tooth wear and its causes.

Attrition is the loss of tooth structure as a result of tooth-to-tooth contact. Causes include unconscious clenching or grinding of teeth, constant chewing of abrasive foods, the normal wear of tooth structure by physiologic masticatory (chewing) forces, or the mesial drifting of teeth due to the normal aging process. It is important to recognize a bruxing habit in patients who are undergoing restorative care. Contact between a natural tooth and a porcelain crown surface results in rapid wear of the tooth because porcelain is a very hard material. It is best to have

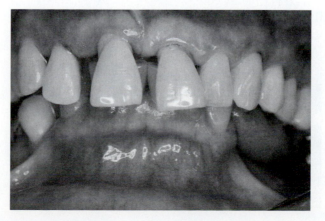

Figure 12–5 A deep overbite causes the mandibular incisors to touch the palatal gingiva of the maxillary anterior area.

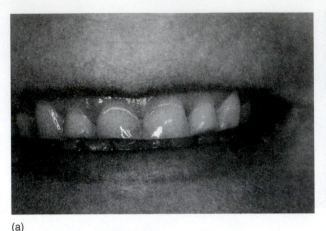

(a)

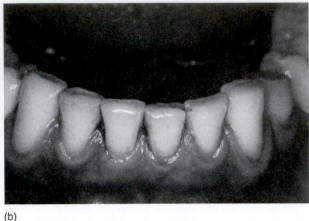

(b)

Figure 12–6 (a) Attrition of the maxillary teeth due to bruxism. (b) Note that the brownish dentin is exposed as a result of enamel loss.

tooth-to-artificial-crown contacts on a metallic surface or a highly polished porcelain surface. Attrition is found most often on the incisal/occlusal surfaces of teeth (Fig. 12–6■) but also is found on proximal tooth surfaces that are flat, as seen with mesial drifting. Attrition also occurs as wear facets, which are small, smooth, polished, flat surfaces on the enamel where there is heavy tooth contact. Usually wear facets are seen on the side of a tooth cusp.

Abrasion is the abnormal mechanical wearing-away of tooth structure for reasons other than mastication. Frequently, it is evident on exposed cementum as a notch apical to the cementoenamel junction (Fig. 12–7■). Examples of abrasion include excessive force from improper toothbrushing techniques (Dyer, Addy, & Newcombe, 2000), use of a hard-bristle toothbrush, and very abrasive dentifrices. Abrasion also can occur on the incisal/occlusal surfaces when an object such as a pin or pipe is held between the teeth for many years.

Abfractions (cervical erosions) are classified as a noncarious dental lesion. Numerous theories are found in dental literature concerning the etiology of abfraction including tooth fatigue, flexure (stress), and biomechanical loading of the tooth especially at the cervical area of the tooth. These lesions are usually wedge shaped with sharp line angles. Dental abfractions can occur alone or associated with tooth-

Figure 12–7 V- or U-shaped notching at the exposed cervical root surface just apical to the cementoenamel junction. This pattern of tooth wear (abrasion) may be associated with improper toothbrushing technique.

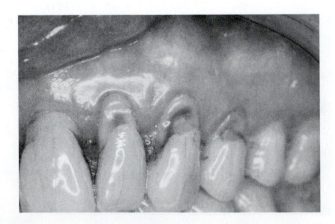

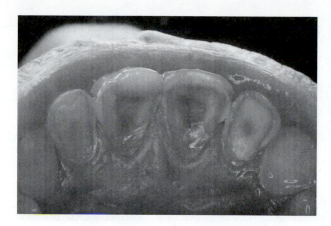

Figure 12–8   Erosion in a 35-year-old woman who was bulimic. Chronic vomiting wore away the enamel on the palatal surfaces of the maxillary anterior teeth, creating a shiny, smooth surface.

brush abrasion. Treatment involves observation or placement of a restoration (Owens & Gallien, 1995).

Erosion is the chemical wearing-away of tooth structure, usually enamel (Fig. 12–8■). It is caused by dietary acids (e.g., acidic beverages, lemons) and gastric juices coming from regurgitation or vomiting, as seen in bulimia. Location of the erosion cannot be considered pathognomonic (a direct cause) for certain etiologic factors, although if erosion is present on the palatal surfaces of maxillary incisors, it is most likely due to gastric juices. Traditionally, erosion is proportionally greater in younger patients, but erosion may increase with age as the salivary flow rate decreases.

Terminology

Occlusal trauma (also termed trauma from occlusion, periodontal traumatism, or occlusal disease) is defined as injury to the attachment apparatus (bone, periodontal ligament, and cementum) as a consequence of normal or excessive occlusal force(s) applied to a tooth or teeth (American Academy of Periodontology, 2001). In addition to periodontal tissue damage, excessive occlusal force also can affect the temporomandibular joint, muscles of mastication, pulp tissue, and integrity of the restoration. Occlusal force is a force (or energy) transmitted to the teeth and their supporting structures by tooth-to-tooth contacts or through food substances or any other intervening material. When the magnitude (size), direction, frequency, and/or duration of these forces exceeds the reparative capacity of the attachment apparatus, the result is occlusal disease. This is determined clinically by signs and symptoms. Traumatogenic occlusion is defined as any occlusion that produces forces that directly or indirectly cause injury to the attachment apparatus.

Premature occlusal contact (also called occlusal interference) occurs when there are interferences to closure of opposing teeth (Fig. 12–9■). That is, a tooth that occludes with an opposing tooth before full closure is achieved in centric occlusion. This premature contact prevents the other teeth in the arch from achieving contact simultaneously. Premature contacts also can occur during lateral movements when the mandible moves from one side to the other. In addition, an extruded (also termed supererupted) or a tipped tooth may cause posterior occlusal interferences. Premature contacts should be eliminated if there is evidence of damage to the attachment apparatus or increasing tooth mobility.

Figure 12–9 In protrusion (anterior teeth edge to edge), note that the initial interference is on the maxillary incisors, which prevents the left lateral incisor from occluding.

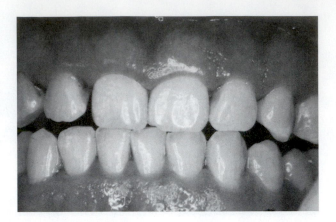

Parafunctional habits are activities of the masticatory (chewing) system that are beyond the normal range of function. Chewing and swallowing are normal, whereas grinding and clenching are abnormal or parafunctional activities. Parafunctional activities often occur during sleep or stressful situations. Involuntary or unconscious clenching or grinding of teeth, when the patient is not intentionally chewing or swallowing, is termed bruxism. Premature contacts also may predispose to parafunctional habits. Physiologic occlusion is defined as survival of the dentition despite its deviation from a preconceived hypothetical normal. Most people have some occlusal discrepancies, but in most cases, the dentition has "adapted" to the discrepancies and shows no signs of occlusal trauma. On the other hand, the dentition in a pathologic occlusion generally shows evidence of occlusal disease.

Occlusal therapy is designed to control the forces generated by tooth-to-tooth contact so they are tolerated by the attachment apparatus.

Parafunctional Habits

Bruxism, a type of parafunctional habit, is the unconscious grinding and/or clenching of the teeth when the patient is not swallowing or chewing. During sleep, it is called nocturnal bruxism and is often associated with stressful situations. While most patients show signs of bruxism, only 5 to 20% are consciously aware of it (Hallmon et al., 1999). The early signs of bruxism may go undetected, but with increased duration, intensity, and direction of the habit, wear facets will be visible on tooth surfaces and tooth mobility may be seen. Initially, this increase in functional demand will be accommodated by the periodontium. Other changes include cusp fractures, increased thermal sensitivity, and increased tooth mobility, which can resolve when the parafunctional action is discontinued. Other examples of parafunctional habits include nail biting, tongue thrusting, and chewing of foreign objects between the teeth such as bobby pins, nails, pipes, and pencils.

Tongue thrusting or thumb sucking often creates a class II, division I malocclusion with an anterior and posterior open bite (Fig. 12–10■). During swallowing, the tongue is placed between the maxillary and mandibular anterior teeth and on the sides rather than on the hard palate near the rugae. The lips and chin muscles contract, visualized as a massive grimace. Tongue thrusting eventually can lead to a mouth-breathing habit, which may cause a localized gingival inflammation of the maxillary and mandibular incisor region that is unrelated to plaque accumulation.

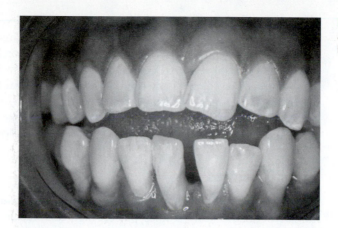

Figure 12–10 An anterior open bite caused by tongue thrusting.

In addition, the lips will be dry and parted at rest. Parafunctional activity can produce symptoms from the musculature or TMJ. Palpation of the muscles of mastication can detect muscle spasms or pain. Parafunctional habits may lead to occlusal trauma. Occlusal trauma is defined as injury to the attachment apparatus as a result of excessive occlusal force.

The Role of Occlusal Trauma in the Initiation and Progression of Periodontal Diseases

Research has concluded that occlusal trauma alone does not cause gingivitis, periodontitis, pocket formation, or gingival recession (Ramfjord & Ash, 1981; Svanberg, King, & Gibbs, 1995). The gingival unit is independent, having its own blood supply, and is not affected by occlusal trauma (Keller & Cohen, 1955). In healthy conditions, the structure and adaptive nature of the attachment apparatus to occlusal forces permit a certain degree of physiologic mobility. Adaptation refers to alterations or adjustments that the body develops to accommodate to its environment. However, when occlusal forces are excessive, beyond the capability of the attachment apparatus to repair itself, tissue injury occurs, resulting in occlusal trauma.

A more complex and controversial issue is the interrelationship between periodontal inflammation and trauma from occlusion. Numerous human and animal models were developed to determine the effects of occlusal forces on the progression of periodontitis. It is also debatable whether these factors interfere with wound healing in the treatment of periodontal diseases. The conflicting results of different studies may be due to differences in animal species, the procedures used for producing occlusal trauma, and inherent measurement inaccuracies.

Human Studies

Glickman (1963) introduced the concept of codestruction, whereby inflammation and trauma from occlusion are synergistic factors in periodontal destruction. He suggested that while occlusion does not cause gingival inflammation or pocket formation, inflammation of the supporting tissues in the presence of occlusal trauma alters the pathway of inflammation. Subsequently, the inflammatory infiltrate will spread more rapidly through tissue damaged by excessive occlusal forces and move directly into the periodontal ligament space, causing the development of angular bone defects and infrabony pockets. Thus, according to Glickman, inflammation and occlusal trauma become codestructive, whereby the progression of periodontitis is accelerated by the presence of occlusal trauma.

However, other investigators (Shefter & McFall, 1984) reported no relationship between occlusal disharmonies and pathoses associated with inflammatory periodontal disease in patients with mild to moderate periodontitis.

Animal Studies

In an attempt to reproduce the kind of occlusal trauma that might occur in the human dentition, early studies placed high restorations on teeth to reproduce the jiggling forces caused by premature tooth contacts. Jiggling or reciprocating forces were applied in opposite directions on a tooth at the same time. This prevented the tooth from moving away from the force. Unilateral forces would have allowed the traumatized teeth to migrate away from the occlusal forces. In many studies, tissue inflammation was induced using silk ligatures placed around the teeth near the gingival margin to enhance plaque retention.

Primate Model　Meitner (1975) examined the effects of jiggling forces on marginal periodontitis in squirrel monkeys by forcing wedges into the embrasure between teeth. The wedges were moved every 48 hours, allowing the teeth to be subjected to reciprocating forces every other day. Although this type of trauma is quite different from that caused by premature contacts, there was no accelerated loss of connective tissue attachment.

Polson (1974) also found that there was no difference in loss of connective tissue attachment and bone destruction in periodontally involved teeth of squirrel monkeys subjected to a single episode of trauma.

Beagle Model　The results of several beagle dog studies (Ericsson & Lindhe, 1982; Lindhe & Svanberg, 1974) showed that when heavy occlusal forces were combined with plaque-induced periodontitis, the rate of clinical attachment loss was accelerated; but this model system also showed that trauma from occlusion does not aggravate gingival inflammation or cause loss of clinical attachment in chronic gingivitis (Ericsson & Lindhe, 1977). In the beagle, when jiggling forces were applied to a periodontally healthy tooth or a tooth with chronic gingivitis, the tooth became hypermobile.

Pathogenesis of Occlusal Trauma

The pathologic features of occlusal trauma are different from those of inflammation. With occlusal trauma, healing of traumatized tissue need not be considered an inflammatory process because no inflammatory/immune cells such as leukocytes, lymphocytes, or plasma cells are present. Thus repair is initiated after the trauma is removed, without the tissue exhibiting the classic signs of inflammation. The lesion of occlusal trauma in the normal, healthy periodontium usually develops following compression and tension of the periodontal ligament (PDL) fibers and resorption and deposition of bone. Compression of the PDL fibers results in obstruction of blood flow to the fibers, which in turn results in bone resorption. If the destructive process is greater than the repair potential of the periodontal tissue, injury may result. The alveolar bone undergoes osteoclastic resorption in areas of pressure, which results in the widening of the periodontal ligament space (Svanberg, et al., 1995). Clinically, increased tooth mobility may result to accommodate for the widened PDL. Regardless of the status of the original attachment apparatus, there will be increasing tooth mobility until the PDL can adapt to the applied force. When adaptation is complete, new lamina dura may be seen radiographically, even though the increased PDL space of hypermobile teeth will remain. When the occlusal trauma is eliminated, bone repair will occur, and a functional width of the PDL will be reestablished. If, however, the trauma continues, excessive widening of the PDL results to accommodate the bone loss. This results in increasing tooth mobility.

The gingival connective tissue attachment is not affected, nor is there apical migration of the junctional epithelium. This same tissue reaction that occurs in a patient with a healthy periodontium also occurs in a patient with a reduced bony support who also has a healthy periodontium.

If the codestructive theory was correct, then the pathway of inflammation would be seen as proceeding not from the gingiva to the bone and finally to the PDL but rather from the gingiva directly into the PDL, inducing the formation of an infrabony pocket with associated vertical bone loss (Glickman & Smulow, 1965). Removal of the trauma but not the inflammation does not decrease tooth mobility, and the crestal bone does not repair (Polson, Meitner, & Zander, 1976). Kantor, Polson, and Zander (1976) removed both jiggling forces and inflammation, resulting in new bone formation without an increase in alveolar bone height. Collectively, these studies show that occlusal trauma does not initiate gingivitis or periodontitis. Although the importance of the role of dental plaque in inflammatory periodontal diseases is undisputed, the influence of occlusal trauma on the attachment level remains controversial (Hallmon, 1999).

Classification of Occlusal Trauma

Occusal trauma can be classified as either primary or secondary and either can be localized to a single tooth or generalized, affecting several teeth (Table 12–1■).

Primary occlusal trauma is defined as injury to the supporting structures (PDL, cementum, and bone) caused by excessive occlusal forces (forces greater than experienced during normal chewing function) placed on a tooth or teeth with normal

Table 12–1	Periodontal Occlusal Traumatic Lesions				
Type of Occlusal Trauma	**Etiology**	**Pocket Formation**	**Bone Height**	**Mobility**	**Treatment Options**
Primary	Excessive occlusal force(s)	No	Normal height or slight bone loss	Adapted	Selective grinding, appliances, monitoring without treatment
Secondary	Normal or excessive occlusal force(s)	No/Yes Periodontal pockets may be present, but due to periodontal destruction rather than the occlusal trauma	Reduced height (moderate/severe)	Progressive	Splinting if necessary, selective grinding, extraction, orthodontic movement, appliances, monitoring

Figure 12–11   Primary occlusal trauma. A tooth with normal periodontal tissues is exposed to excessive occlusal load (arrow). As a result of bone resorption, the periodontal ligament space gradually increases in size on both sides of the teeth as well as in the periapical region.

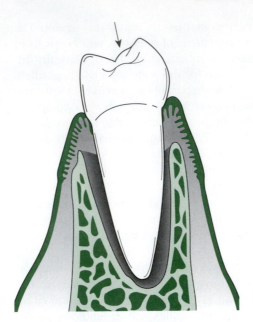

periodontal tissue support (Fig. 12–11■). Examples of causes of primary occlusal trauma include

1. a "high" restoration, where, on biting, the restored tooth creates a premature contact with the opposing tooth;
2. parafunctional habits involving tooth-to-tooth contact such as bruxism, clenching, or object-to-tooth contact such as biting on pencils or nail biting;
3. a malpositioned or maligned tooth, including teeth that are extruded (moved occlusally) or tipped;
4. a periapical (around the apex of the root) abscess or infection causing a tooth to be extruded;
5. physical "blow" to a tooth or teeth;
6. a removable partial denture clasp around an abutment tooth; and
7. orthodontic movement of teeth.

Secondary occlusal trauma occurs when normal (e.g., chewing) or excessive occlusal forces cause injury in a periodontium with reduced bone support (Fig. 12–12■). Bone levels around the tooth are inadequate to support these forces, and the tooth is less resistant to occlusal loading. In other words, a tooth in secondary occlusal trauma has insufficient bone support, and normal chewing and swallowing forces are excessive, causing injury to the attachment apparatus. This can occur even when the periodontal tissues are healthy, but there is a reduced bone height. Therefore, the distinguishing feature between primary and secondary occlusal trauma is the amount of bony support surrounding the tooth.

Parafunctional Activity

Parafunctional activity may result in primary occlusal trauma. This occurs when a tooth is subjected to greater forces over a longer period of time than what normally occurs in chewing and swallowing. Food chewing is not a cause of primary occlusal trauma because the forces are most likely not long-standing or severe enough to affect the attachment apparatus.

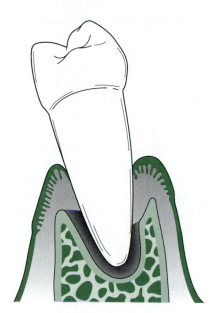

Figure 12–12
Secondary occlusal trauma. If a tooth with reduced periodontal tissue support has been exposed to excessive occlusal forces, a widened periodontal ligament space and increased mobility result.

Bruxism usually occurs unconsciously, whether the patient is awake or asleep. Thus many patients are not aware of their habit. When the forces generated during bruxism exceed the adaptive capacity of the periodontium on a regular basis, occlusal trauma is initiated (Caffesse & Fleszar, 1992).

Other parafunctional habits such as lip, nail, or cheek biting, tongue thrusting, or the placement of foreign objects between the teeth (e.g., pipe clenching and chewing, pencil biting, playing a wind musical instrument, and clenching fingernails or bobby pins) may affect the attachment apparatus. However, these do not appear to occur as frequently as tooth-to-tooth contact habits. A less common cause of primary occlusal trauma is occupational bruxism, which occurs in certain stressful occupations.

Clinical Findings in Occlusal Trauma

Tooth Mobility

The most common sign of occlusal trauma is increasing tooth mobility over a period of time. However, excessive occlusal forces may not always cause tooth hypermobility (Svanberg et al., 1995). Since mobility due to occlusal trauma is an adaptive function, it may not be considered pathologic (resulting in disease). A tooth with excessive occlusal load may adapt to the forces by exhibiting increased but not increasing mobility. However, if there is progressive tooth mobility over a period of several days or weeks, it may then be considered pathologic (Green & Levine, 1996). Consequently, for the proper recognition of occlusal disease, tooth mobility has to be assessed on two or more separate occasions (Svanberg et al., 1995).

A tooth in primary occlusal trauma may show mobility. In this case, the tooth becomes mobile so that it can adapt to the abnormal force placed on it. Thus the mobility of the tooth could be classified as an adapted mobility (Tarnow & Fletcher, 1986). For example, mobility of a tooth caused by a high restoration will come to a plateau and no longer increase; this is adapted mobility. Tooth mobility in absence of supporting alveolar bone may be characteristic of a parafunctional habit. However, tooth mobility does not occur in all patients who grind and clench their teeth. In some cases tooth wear accommodates for the bruxing habit.

Tooth hypermobility, produced by excessive occlusal forces, does not cause gingival inflammation, worsen the severity of chronic gingivitis, or act as a primary cause for connective tissue attachment loss (Svanberg et al., 1995).

Besides excessive occlusal forces, tooth mobility may result from severe gingival inflammation extending into the connective tissue attachment, the loss of supporting alveolar bone, pregnancy, and orthodontic movement, or may occur following surgical therapy. Tooth mobility will usually decrease by the fourth week after surgery. The cause and progression of the mobility must be determined because treatment options differ.

Fremitus

Fremitus is the vibrational movement of a tooth under occlusal function. Fremitus is detected by placing the index finger on the gingival-tooth interfaces (Fig. 12–13■) of the maxillary teeth and asking the patient to tap the teeth up and down, grind from side to side, and move the jaw into an edge-to-edge (protrusive) occlusion. Centric prematurities are detected by the presence of fremitus.

Pain

Pain from percussion, pain upon biting, and the pain of tooth hypersensitivity are symptoms of primary and secondary occlusal trauma. For example, after receiving a restoration, a patient may call to report tooth pain. An evaluation will reveal that the restoration is high, causing pain and mobility upon biting or chewing. Once the restoration is reduced in height, the pain and mobility will disappear.

Figure 12–13 A technique for detecting fremitus. The index finger is placed partly on the facial tooth surfaces and the gingiva. Tooth movements can be detected when the patient taps the teeth together and grinds side to side.

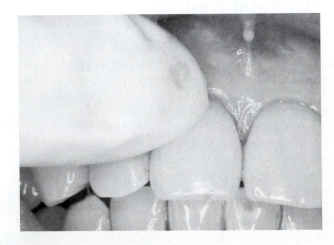

Tooth Migration

Pathologic tooth migration usually is indicative of moderate to severe periodontitis and secondary occlusal trauma (Towfighi et al., 1997). Pathologic migration is defined as a change in tooth position resulting from disruption of the forces that maintain teeth in a normal position (Chasens, 1979). Excessive occlusal forces, which include the normal forces of chewing or swallowing applied to teeth, and extensive bone loss, may cause teeth to migrate (Towfighi et al., 1997). Clinically, pathologic tooth migration results in widened spaces between teeth (diastemas), flaring or fanning of anterior teeth, and/or extrusion of teeth (Fig. 12–14■). Although it is a common sign of secondary occlusal trauma, pathologic tooth migration may be caused by periodontal surgery or extensive inflammation extending into the PDL.

Attrition

Forces generated during bruxism frequently are greater than the adaptive capacity of the periodontium. Consequently, the contoured surface of a tooth may be ground flat, to the point where the dentin may be exposed (Figs. 12–15■ and 12–16■). Cracks and pits form on the worn edges and may become plaque traps. Clinical features of attrition include flattened occlusal or incisal surfaces of teeth. The canines and central and lateral incisors most commonly receive the heaviest and earliest lateral wear (Lytle, 1990). Exposed dentin may cause a tooth to become sensitive. Wear facets frequently are seen as a flat, shiny, worn spot on the side of a cusp of a tooth (Fig. 12–16). The presence of attrition and wear facets does not necessarily indicate occlusal habits. Wear on teeth also may be due to the patient's age or diet. Once a facet has developed, it remains. If a patient has wear facets for many years with no changes, it is probably not an active process.

Muscle/Temporomandibular Joint

Occlusal trauma may cause the muscles that work the jaw, the largest being the temporalis and the masseter, to become chronically sore, resulting in headaches and muscle pain. Pain usually occurs during chewing or upon waking in the morning. This type of pain may be emanating from the temporomandibular joint (TMJ).

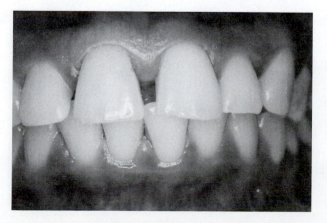

Figure 12–14 A 45-year-old patient with advanced periodontitis. Patient complaints of recently widened spaces, flaring of the maxillary incisors, and extrusion of the maxillary right central incisor are often an indication that the reduced attachment apparatus is reacting to occlusal forces.

Figure 12–15   Anterior view of a 55-year-old woman who was unaware she was a bruxer. Note the generalized heavy wear such that all teeth appear flat and on the same plane.

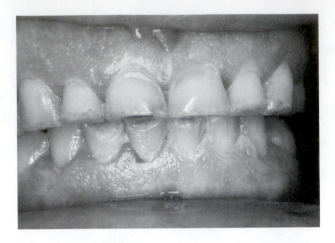

The patient may report muscle spasms in the head, neck, and ear area. Pathology must be ruled out when a patient complains of any type of facial pain, including TMJ pain.

Tooth Structure

Tooth fractures and long-term chipping of enamel are additional signs of occlusal trauma related to the magnitude of forces that the teeth endure.

Radiographic Findings in Occlusal Trauma

Along with the clinical examination, radiographs are useful for recognizing the signs of occlusal trauma and/or the signs of adaptation to significant occlusal forces (Caffesse & Fleszar, 1992).

Widening of the PDL occurs as an adaptation response to accommodate excessive occlusal loading and also may result in the resorption of alveolar bone. Radiographically, when the PDL space is wider at the coronal third of the root, it is referred to as crestal funneling.

Figure 12–16   View of mandibular anterior teeth showing heavy wear through the enamel contributed to by the abrasive quality of the porcelain crown on the maxillary teeth. Note wear facet on the mandibular left canine.

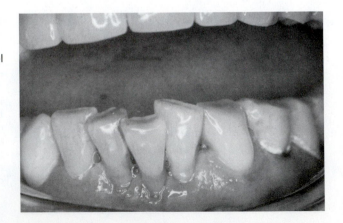

Radiographically, a tooth in primary occlusal trauma may or may not show vertical bone loss as a result of widening of the PDL space. However, this should not be confused with bone loss related to periodontitis (Ricchetti, 1998; Figs. 12–17■ and 12–18■) because primary occlusal trauma does not show loss of connective tissue attachment, increased probing depth, and related infrabony pockets (Polson & Zander, 1983). The presence of angular bony defects is not necessarily a sign of occlusal trauma. If a widened PDL space is present but no tooth mobility exists, occlusal trauma is not necessarily present. The findings may be a functional adaptation to the occlusal forces.

Radiographically, a tooth in secondary occlusal trauma shows reduced bone levels that are inadequate to support the tooth under a normal load without increasing mobility, migration, or fremitus (Ricchetti, 1998). Vertical bone loss is accompanied by widening of the PDL. Occasionally, root resorption may occur.

If the codestructive theory were correct, occlusal forces will accelerate the rate of destruction and result in vertical or angular bone defects, in the presence of pre-existing inflammation. However, there are still some questions of whether this occurs.

Outcomes of Treatment of Occlusal Trauma

The desired outcome of treatment of occlusal trauma is that the patient remains comfortable during chewing and is able to maintain the dentition in a state of health. The dental hygienist can determine if the reversal of signs and symptoms of occlusal trauma has achieved the following outcomes (American Academy of Periodontology, 1996). These include:

1. elimination or significant reduction of tooth mobility (the patient should be comfortable when in function);
2. elimination of occlusal prematurities and fremitus;

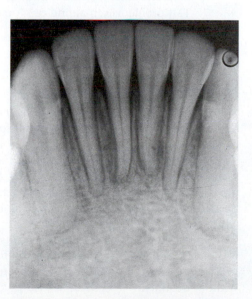

Figure 12–17   A radiograph showing a typical lesion of primary occlusal trauma. Widening of the periodontal ligament space has occurred due to a heavy occlusal force placed on the tooth. Note that there is no alveolar crestal bone loss and no increased probing depths.

Figure 12–18 A radiograph showing a typical lesion of secondary occlusal trauma. The tooth has a reduced bony support and increasing tooth mobility. The tooth has an adverse crown-to-root ratio.

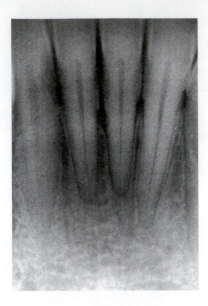

3. elimination of parafunctional habits;
4. prevention of further tooth migration; and
5. decrease or stability of radiographic changes.

Inadequate resolution of occlusal trauma is identified by

1. increasing tooth mobility;
2. progressive tooth migration;
3. patient continuing to complain of discomfort with pain and tooth mobility;
4. premature contacts remaining;
5. radiographic signs remaining, including widening of the PDL space;
6. parafunctional habits continuing; and
7. TMJ problems remaining or worsening.

Occlusal Therapy

The objective of occlusal therapy is to control the direction, duration, magnitude, and/or frequency of excessive occlusal forces. Practitioners have different views as to whether occlusal therapy is necessary in the overall periodontal treatment plan.

Table 12–2■ lists the most common approaches to treating trauma from occlusion. The key to treatment of occlusal trauma lies in the ability to determine if physiologic or pathologic occlusion exists. Physiologic occlusion does not need to be treated, whereas pathologic occlusion that shows signs and symptoms of occlusal problems requires treatment.

Since primary occlusal trauma is caused by excessive occlusal forces, treatment is aimed at eliminating or reducing the forces. Treatment options include selective grinding, control of habits, orthodontic movement, or monitoring of the condition without treatment.

Table 12–2	Approaches to Treating Occlusal Trauma

- Selective grinding
- Control of habits
- Orthodontic tooth movement
- Splinting
- Restorative procedures
- Monitoring without treatment

In contrast to the primary occlusal traumatic lesion, the secondary occlusal traumatic lesion is not reversible, since its cause is loss of bony support around a tooth or teeth. Treatment options for secondary occlusal trauma include splinting, selective grinding, orthodontic movement, extraction, or monitoring of the condition without treatment. Reductions in tooth mobility are limited, because the mobility is due to a reduced periodontal support rather than to excessive occlusal force. Premature contacts on mobile teeth are detected and eliminated by selective grinding.

Selective Grinding

Selective grinding is defined as the reshaping of the occlusal or incisal surfaces of teeth to create harmonious contacts between the upper and lower dentition. The goal of selective grinding is to eliminate premature contacts in primary or secondary occlusal trauma. Correction of prematurities should be done in centric occlusion, centric relation, and protrusive and lateral movements so that a traumatic contact of teeth occurs during movements of the mandible (Burgett, 1995). Prematurities are detected by the use of wax, articulating paper, or dental floss.

Selective grinding always should be completed after inflammation has been controlled. Once the inflammation is eliminated by periodontal debridement and oral hygiene self-care, the tooth mobility may decrease because the fibers of the connective tissue attachment repair and a tooth with an intact connective tissue attachment has additional rigidity. Once periodontal health is reestablished, the occlusal condition is reevaluated. A decision to perform selective grinding depends on the degree of patient discomfort and function rather than on the assumption that selective grinding is necessary to halt the progression of disease (Gher, 1996).

Primary occlusal trauma caused by a high restoration is treated by selective grinding. However, severe discrepancies may be resolved best by replacing the restoration. Selective grinding reshapes the occlusal surfaces of teeth to create harmonious contact relationships between the opposing teeth. This is accomplished with hand instruments or a high-speed handpiece and a bur. Tooth surfaces should be smooth so that patients do not develop secondary occlusal habits by "playing" with a rough surface. Selective grinding also can be performed on teeth in secondary occlusal trauma.

Control of Parafunctional Habits

Appliances

If the cause of the occlusal trauma is bruxism, selective grinding usually will not correct the problem; however, counseling the patient may alleviate the psychological component of clenching and grinding. Because such problems are difficult to resolve, a bite plane or Hawley appliance may be fabricated from an orthodontic resin material that discoccludes the posterior teeth. This does not allow the opposing arches to contact and permit the attachment apparatus to heal. The appliance also can be used as an adjunct to selective grinding to stabilize the occlusion and allow the attachment apparatus to rest.

During sleep, a night guard can be worn to control occlusal habits. A night guard serves to protect the teeth from abnormal occlusal wear due to bruxism. Occlusal contacts between the upper and lower teeth are eliminated, thus stabilizing the occlusion and negating the effects of grinding and clenching at night (Chasens, 1990). The night guard is made of either hard or soft acrylic, usually covering the occlusal surfaces of all teeth in the maxillary arch (Fig. 12–19■). The night guard is adjusted so that all mandibular teeth make simultaneous contact in centric occlusion.

Exercise

Besides using appliances to alter or control occlusal habits, exercise is important as well, especially if the patient clenches. An exercise to follow includes clenching for 5 seconds, then releasing, and repeating this five times in a row (for a total of 60 seconds). This should be done five times a day for 14 consecutive days. If one day is missed, the exercise must be started again.

Orthodontics

Orthodontic treatment may be indicated in periodontal patients exhibiting drifting, migration, extrusion, or flared anterior teeth. The goal is to move a tooth or teeth into a more functional, less traumatic position.

Restorative Procedures

To establish a stable posterior occlusion, restorations may be placed if other treatment options, including orthodontics or selective grinding, are not possible. For example, if a patient has anterior teeth and some or all of the posterior teeth on both sides are missing, the anterior teeth may become overloaded. Thus restorations (e.g., removal partial dentures [RPDs] or crowns) will restore the posterior occlusion and distribute the load to protect the anterior teeth.

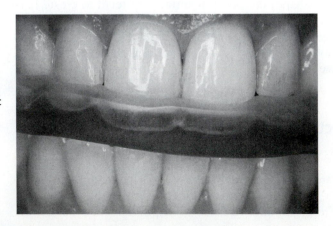

Figure 12–19 A hard acrylic night guard was made for this 35-year-old bruxer. It is used to protect the teeth during the night and help eliminate the habit. Night guards have full occlusal coverage and usually are made for the maxillary arch.

Splinting

Splinting of teeth is considered the treatment of choice for patients who complain of discomfort or if the examination reveals that the mobility interferes with chewing (mastication). Although tooth mobility that develops after periodontal surgery usually will subside within a few months, temporary splinting may be necessary to prevent secondary occlusal trauma. Splinting is also done on teeth in primary occlusal trauma if the mobility was caused by avulsion of the tooth or if the patient received a blow to the mouth resulting in loosening of a tooth or teeth.

Splinting permits healing of the attachment apparatus by holding a tooth in a totally fixed position. This allows the PDL to become narrower and the mobility to be reduced (Ricchetti, 1998). Instead of one tooth experiencing the brunt of forces, the forces are distributed and spread over several teeth, which are better able to absorb the trauma. If mobility is not increasing over time, it may not be necessary to splint. The attachment apparatus may have adapted to the excessive forces and is in a stage of repair (Chasens, 1990). Unfortunately, it is difficult to determine at any given point in time if a patient's attachment apparatus is in a state of repair. That is why monitoring mobility is so important.

Temporary splinting uses wires and composite material, acid etching nylon mesh, or fixed bridges or crowns that are joined or soldered together (Fig. 12–20■). A night guard is considered a type of occlusal splint.

Disadvantages of splinting include compromised aesthetics, reduced plaque-control efficacy, and a changed stable occlusion. Because of these disadvantages, splinting is not done routinely, and if it is selected, it should be considered with the preceding problems in mind.

Summary

Overall, the periodontal response to occlusal trauma can be considered a physiologic adaptation. This adaptation can result in permanently increased tooth mobility if the trauma continues. However, if plaque control is adequate, connective tissue attachment loss should not occur. Removal of the injurious occlusal forces allows the lesion to repair itself, but this may be compromised by the presence of dental plaque. Therefore, maintenance of adequate plaque control is of utmost importance in preventing and reversing the problem. The question of increased

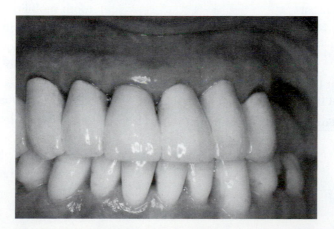

Figure 12–20 The fixed prosthesis consists of multiple crowns on the maxillary teeth that have been soldered. This represents a form of permanent splinting.

periodontal tissue destruction when periodontitis coexists with occlusal trauma remains unresolved.

Occlusal trauma alone does not cause gingivitis, loss of connective tissue attachment, or pocket formation. Unless there is compromised periodontal support, there is little or no damage to the teeth or the attachment apparatus from normal masticatory (chewing) forces. Normal forces are only traumatogenic in secondary occlusal trauma, when the periodontal support is reduced by disease.

The role of the dental hygienist in the identification of occlusal trauma is important for the overall treatment of the patient. Treatment differs depending on the type of occlusal trauma and its etiology. To help distinguish between primary and secondary occlusal trauma, the dental hygienist can use radiographs and present and past dental history. The occlusal forces required to produce occlusal trauma generally are related to the remaining bony support for a given tooth.

Key Points

- Occlusal trauma does not initiate gingivitis or periodontitis.
- Parafunctional habits may cause occlusal trauma.
- The most common clinical sign of occlusal trauma is increasing tooth mobility.
- Pathologic tooth migration is usually indicative of moderate to severe periodontitis and secondary occlusal trauma.
- Different treatments are available for occlusal trauma.

Web Sites

www.perio.org
www.dentalarticles.com

Self-Quiz

1. All the following parts of the periodontium are affected by occlusal trauma except one. Which one is the exception? (pp. 180–181)
   a. periodontal ligament
   b. alveolar bone
   c. gingiva
   d. cementum

2. Which one of the following definitions pertains to primary occlusal trauma? (p. 181)

Type of Occlusal Force	Bone Support
a. Normal	Adequate
b. Excessive	Adequate
c. Normal	Reduced
d. Excessive	Reduced

3. All the following signs and symptoms are found in occlusal trauma except one. Which one is the exception? (pp. 183–186)
   a. tooth mobility
   b. tooth migration
   c. pain upon chewing
   d. occlusal erosion

4. Which one of the following radiographic signs is evident in occlusal trauma? (pp. 186–187)
   a. widening of the periodontal ligament space
   b. deposition of acellular cementum
   c. deposition of alveolar bone
   d. receding pulp tissue

5. Occlusal trauma in combination with chronic inflammatory periodontitis may result in greater tooth mobility and alveolar bone loss because occlusal trauma causes periodontal pocket formation. (pp. 179–180)

   a. Both the statement and the reason are correct and related.

   b. Both the statement and the reason are correct but not related.

   c. The statement is correct, but the reason is not.

   d. The statement is not correct, but the reason is correct.

   e. Neither the statement nor the reason is correct.

6. Two days after a patient receives an amalgam restoration, he reports back to the office complaining of pain and looseness of the tooth. Which one of the following treatments would be most appropriate? (p. 189)

   a. Replace the amalgam with composite.

   b. Reduce the height of the restoration.

   c. Polish the restoration.

   d. Maintain the restoration as is.

7. Which one of the following factors is the primary cause of secondary occlusal trauma? (pp. 181–182)

   a. tooth with severe bone loss

   b. night and daytime bruxism

   c. tongue thrusting

   d. pipe chewing

8. A patient complains of soreness in the jaw upon wakening in the morning. She is having stressful problems at work. She complains that some of her lower teeth are "wearing down." Which one of the following conditions does this patient most likely have? (pp. 178–179, 185)

   a. fractured jaw

   b. parafunctional habit

   c. severe periodontitis

   d. necrotizing ulcerative gingivitis

9. A patient has returned for a 2-week follow-up visit after periodontal surgery complaining of tooth mobility. There was no mobility before the surgery was done. Which one of the following should be explained to the patient? (pp. 183–184)

   a. Teeth must be splinted immediately.

   b. Mobility will decrease in time.

   c. Additional surgery will be needed.

   d. Systemic antibiotics are indicated.

10. Which one of the following conditions is best treated with a night guard? (pp. 189–190)

    a. tooth with severe bone loss

    b. tongue-thrusting habit

    c. teeth with severe abrasion

    d. clenching and grinding

References

American Academy of Periodontology. 1996. *Parameters of care*. Chicago: American Academy of Periodontology, Scientific and Educational Affairs Department.

American Academy of Periodontology. 2001. *Glossary of periodontal terms* (4th ed.). Chicago: Author.

Burgett, F. G. 1995. Trauma from occlusion. *Dent. Clin. North Am.* 39:301–311.

Caffesse, R. G., and T. J. Fleszar. 1992. Occlusal trauma. In eds. T. G. Wilson, K. S. Komman, and M. G. Newman, *Advances in periodontics,* 205–225. Chicago: Quintessence.

Chasens, A. I. 1990. Controversies in occlusion. *Dent. Clin. North Am.* 34:11–123.

Chasens, A. I. 1979. Periodontal disease, pathologic tooth migration and adult orthodontics. *N.Y. J. Dent.* 49:40–43.

Dyer D., M. Addy, and R. Newcombe. 2000. Studies invitro of Abrasion by different manual toothbrush heads and a standard toothpaste. *J Clin Periodontal.* 27:99–103.

Ericsson, I., and J. Lindhe. 1977. Lack of effect of trauma from occlusion on the recurrence of experimental periodontitis. *J. Clin. Periodontol.* 4:115–127.

Ericsson, I., and J. Lindhe. 1982. Effect of long-standing jiggling on experimental marginal periodontitis in the beagle dog. *J. Clin. Periodontol.* 9:497–503.

Gher, M. E. 1996. Nonsurgical pocket therapy: Dental occlusion. *Ann. Periodontol.* 1:567–580.

Glickman, I. 1963. Inflammation and trauma from occlusion: Codestructive factors in chronic periodontal disease. *J. Periodontol.* 34:5–10.

Glickman, I. 1967. Occlusion and the periodontium. *J. Dent. Res.* 46(Suppl 53):53.

Glickman, I., and J. B. Smulow. 1965. Effect of excessive occlusal forces upon the pathway of gingival inflammation in humans. *J. Periodontol.* 36:141–147.

Goldman, H. M., and W. D. Cohen (eds.). 1980. Occulsal adjustment. In *Periodontal therapy,* 6th ed. 1065–1111 St. Louis MO: Mosby.

Green, M. S., and D. F. Levine. 1996. Occlusion and the periodontium: A review and rationale for treatment. *J. Calif. Dent. Assoc.* 24:19–27.

Hallmon, W. W. 1999. Occlusal trauma: Effect and impact on the periodontium. *Ann. Periodontol.* 4:102–107.

Kantor, J., A. M. Polson, and H. A. Zander. 1976. Alveolar bone regeneration after removal of inflammatory and traumatic factors. *J. Periodontol.* 47:687–695.

Keller, G., and W. Cohen. 1955. India ink perfusions of the vascular plexus of oral tissues. *Oral Surg.* 8:539–542.

Lindhe, J., and G. Svanberg. 1974. Influence of trauma from occlusion on progression of experimental periodontitis in the beagle dog. *J. Clin. Periodontol.* 1:3–14.

Lytle, J. D. 1990. The clinician's index of occlusal disease: Definition, recognition, and management. *Int. J. Periodontic Restorative Dent.* 10:103–123.

Meitner, S. 1975. Codestructive factors of marginal periodontitis and repetitive mechanical injury. *J. Dent. Res.* 54:78–85.

Owens, B. M., and G.S. Gallien. 1995. Noncarious dental "abfraction" lesions in an aging population. *Compend. Contin. Educ. Dent.* 16(6):552–554.

Polson, A. M. 1974. Trauma and progression of marginal periodontitis in squirrel monkeys. II. Codestructive factors of periodontitis and mechanically produced injury. *J. Periodontol. Res.* 9:108–113.

Polson, A. M., S. W. Meitner, and H. A. Zander. 1976. Trauma and progression of marginal periodontitis in squirrel monkeys: IV. Reversibility of bone loss due to trauma alone and trauma superimposed upon periodontitis. *J. Periodontol. Res.* 11:290–298.

Polson, A. M., and H. A. Zander. 1983. Effect of periodontal trauma upon intrabony pockets. *J. Periodontol.* 54:586–591.

Ramfjord, S. P., and M. M. Ash. 1981. Significance of occlusion in the etiology and treatment of early, moderate and advanced periodontitis. *J. Periodontol.* 52:511–517.

Ricchetti, P. A. 1998. Treatment of the periodontium affected by occlusal traumatism. In M. Nevins and J. T. Mellonig, eds. *Periodontal therapy: Clinical approaches and evidence of success,* Vol. 1, 132–133. Chicago. Quintessence.

Shefter, G. J., and W. T. McFall. 1984. Occlusal relations and periodontal status in human adults. *J. Periodontol.* 55:368–374.

Svanberg, G. K., G. J. King, and C. H. Gibbs. 1995. Occlusal considerations in periodontology. *Periodontology 2000* 9:106–117.

Tarnow, D. P., and P. Fletcher. 1986. Splinting of periodontally involved teeth: Indications and contraindications. *N.Y. State Dent. J.* (May):24–25.

Towfighi, P. P., M. A. Brunsvold, A. T. Storey, B. M. Arnold, D. E. Willman, and C. A. McMahan. 1997. Pathologic migration of anterior teeth in patients with moderate to severe periodontitis. *J. Periodontol.* 68:967–972.

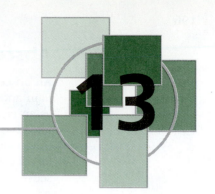

Abscesses of the Periodontium

Surendra Singh, D.D.S., M.S.

Outline

Abscesses of the
   Periodontium

Summary

Key Points

Web Site

Self-Quiz

References

Goal

To educate about the etiology, clinical manifestations, and therapy of different types of abscesses.

Educational Objectives

Upon completion of this chapter, the reader should be able to:

List the classification of abscesses of the periodontium.

Identify and describe the clinical and radiographic findings of three types of abscesses of the periodontium.

KEY WORDS

- gingival abscess
- periodontal abscess
- pericoronal abscess

Abscesses of the Periodontium

An abscess is defined as an infection originating from the tooth or periodontium. Pain and swelling from an abscess usually brings the patient into the dental office as an emergency visit. Classification of abscesses is based upon the location of the infection. For example, a gingival abscess is an infection located in the gingival unit, usually the free (marginal) gingiva; a periodontal abscess is an infection located within the tissues adjacent to the periodontal pocket; and a pericoronal abscess is an infection located within the tissue around the crown of a partially erupted tooth, usually the last tooth in the arch.

The 1999 American Academy of Periodontology Classification of Periodontal Diseases added abscesses of the periodontium. It was a consensus that gingival/periodontal abscesses are part of the clinical course of gingivitis and periodontitis and thus a specific diagnosis and treatment challenges are required (Armitage, 1999). This chapter reviews the classification and definitions of abscesses of the periodontium, while Chapter 29 (treatment section) reviews the treatment of these abscesses.

Gingival Abscess

A gingival abscess is an acute infection characterized by a localized, painful edema at the free gingival margin or interdental papilla (Fig. 13–1■). Usually there are no signs of periodontitis in the patient's mouth. Foreign objects such as popcorn kernels, fish bones, or seeds that become lodged in the gingival crevice are responsible for many gingival abscesses. Calculus is usually not the cause. Since the abscess develops fairly rapidly, the patient often will know the cause. The infection usually is rapidly expanding from the gingival margin or interdental papilla. Within 24 to 48 hours, the lesion will appear fluctuant (soft and moveable). Purulent exudate (pus) may be exuding from the surface. If treatment is not immediately given, the abscess will usually rupture on its own.

Periodontal Abscess

A periodontal abscess, also called a lateral abscess, is the most common type of abscess involving the periodontium. It is a localized purulent nidus of acute inflammation within the periodontal tissues, specifically within the gingival wall of a

Figure 13–1 Gingival abscess involving the mandibular central incisor. (Courtesy Ann Goodwin, formerly NYU College of Dentistry.)

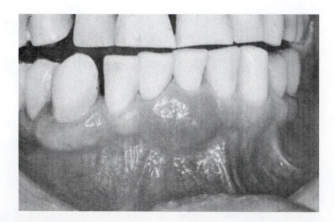

periodontal pocket. The furcation area of molars is a common site for periodontal abscess formation, probably because of anatomical limitations, which makes oral hygiene and professional instrumentation difficult. A periodontal abscess develops as a result of a bacterial infection that eventually leads to the formation of pus (suppuration) and often associated with preexisting periodontitis. Usually, pus will exude from the gingival margin with gentle digital pressure or when probing with a periodontal probe. Microorganisms found in the periodontal abscess resemble the microbiota of chronic periodontitis lesions. Microorganisms that colonize and are found in the exudate of the periodontal abscesses are primarily Gram-negative anaerobic rods (Meng, 1999). Other bacteria associated with and found with high frequency in periodontal abscesses include *Porphyromonas gingivalis, Prevotella intermedia, Fusobacterium nucleatum, Campylobacter retus,* and *Capnocytophaga* sp. The eradication of *Porphyromonas gingivalis* from abscessed sites after treatment indicates that this bacterium is highly associated with abscess formation. *Actinobacillus actinomycetemocomitans* is usually not found in the exudate. Periodontal abscess formation is often seen in deep periodontal pockets and in furcation sites. Such patients often have a number of sites with chronic periodontitis; however, there an abscess can develop at nonperiodontitis sites. For instance, periodontal abscesses can occur as a result of inadvertent embedding of a foreign body subgingivally (calculus fragment) that obstructs the normal sulcular drainage of gingival crevicular fluid and inflammatory by-products of chronic periodontitis. A periodontal abscess may cause destruction of the periodontal ligament and alveolar and supporting bone (Meng, 1999). Postscaling periodontal abscess occurs after scaling/root planing when calculus remains in the pocket (or on the tooth/root surface) causing an obstruction to the pocket entrance. To reestablish drainage, a fistula may form that drains pus through the otherwise intact surface of the gingiva or mucosa. Patients with diabetes mellitus are more susceptible to periodontal abscess formation. Periodontal abscesses sometimes are seen following scaling and root planing at sites with deeper probing pocket depths.

Periodontal abscesses can present as acute or chronic. A common chief complaint when a periodontal abscess is developing is that "I have pressure in my gums." The acute periodontal abscess presents as a shiny, swollen, discolored mass on the gingiva or mucosa at the lateral aspect of the root, but not at the free gingival margin as is the gingival abscess. It is usually located on the lateral aspect of the tooth surface where the periodontal pocket is. Finger pressure may produce purulent drainage. The involved tooth is often tender to percussion (especially upon chewing or mastication), mobile, has deep probing depths, edematous gingiva, and may feel "high" to the patient because of the inflammation in the supporting tissues that extrudes the tooth. Patients usually complain of pain and "pressure" in the gums. Occasionally, patients may demonstrate localized lymphadenopathy (palpable lymph nodes) and fever.

A chronic (long-standing) periodontal abscess occurs if the acute abscess is not resolved or treated. A draining fistulous tract, in which purulent exudate originates from deep within the periodontal tissues and opens and drains onto the gingiva, is usually present. The patient does not usually display symptoms as in an acute periodontal abscess, but some symptoms such as a deep, dull pain or elevation of the tooth may be present. Clinicians often must be able to differentiate between a periodontal abscess and a periapical (endodontic) abscess. An endodontic abscess usually occurs adjacent to the apex of a necrotic tooth. It often heals following endodontic therapy. Table 13–1■ shows the usual characteristics of periapical and periodontal abscesses.

Table 13–1	Differences between a Periodontal and Periapical Abscess	
Periodontal Abscess	**Periapical Abscess**	
Vital tooth	Nonvital tooth	
No tooth caries	Tooth caries present	
Deep pocket	No pocket	
Tooth mobility	No or minimal mobility	
Draining fistula usually located at lateral aspect of tooth	Draining fistula usually located in apical area	
Lateral radiolucency	Apical radiolucency	

Pericoronal Abscess

Pericoronal abscess, also referred to as pericoronitis, is a localized infection involving the gingiva adjacent to a partially erupted tooth, usually the mandibular third molar region (Fig. 13–2■). The gingival flap (or operculum) overlying the erupting tooth is usually red and edematous with food and debris collecting under the operculum. The operculum will disappear once the tooth fully erupts, but many of these teeth remain partially erupted indefinitely because of inadequate arch space for complete eruption or when the tooth is extracted. The offending microorganisms are Gram-negative anaerobes. The infection may spread posteriorly into the oropharyngeal area and medially to the base of the tongue and involve the regional lymph nodes (Meng, 1999). Patients may experience difficulty in swallowing and complain of a dull ache and may demonstrate limited jaw opening (trismus).

Summary

An abscess is an infection originating from the tooth or periodontium. It is important to determine the point of origin so that proper treatment is given.

The patient's chief complaint and a review of the dental history will help to determine the type of abscess. For instance, the patient should be asked if he/she recently had anything to eat that would cause a gingival abscess. The gingival abscess is confined to the marginal gingival or interdental papilla. If the patient has moderate to advanced periodontitis, then most likely it will be a periodontal

Figure 13–2
Pericoronitis. The third molar is partially covered by a "gingival flap." (Courtesy: Ann Goodwin, formerly NYU College of Dentistry.)

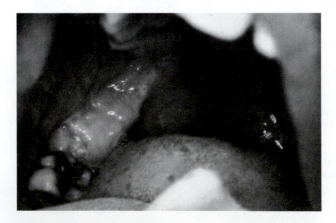

abscess. Periodontal abscesses are part of the clinical course of the progression of periodontitis. Upon probing these sites, pus will usually come out of the pocket. The microbiota of a periodontal abscess is Gram-negative anaerobic rods, which are similar to that found in deep periodontal pockets (Meng, 1999) This is a form of drainage that is necessary to eliminate the infection. A periapical abscess differs from a periodontal abscess in that the abscessed tooth is usually nonvital and will require endodontics (root canal).

Oral examination of a patient complaining of pain and trouble opening his/her mouth will most likely reveal an operculum around a partially erupted mandibular third molar.

The location of the infection will give a good indication on the type of abscess.

Key Points

- Periodontal abscesses are bacterial infections.
- It is important to determine the origin of the abscess.
- The location of the abscess is important.

Web Site

www.perio.org

Self-Quiz

1. Which of the following is the most common bacterium found in the purulent exudate of a tooth with a periodontal abscess? (p. 197)
   a. *Porphyromas gingivalis*
   b. *Candida albican*
   c. *Staphlococcus sp.*
   d. *Actinobacillus actinomycetemcomitans (Aa)*

2. A gingival abscess is localized to the (p. 196)
   a. periapical area
   b. interdental papilla
   c. periodontal pocket
   d. pericoronal area

3. Which of the following is a clinical feature of a periodontal abscess? (p. 197)
   a. fibrotic gingiva
   b. edematous gingiva
   c. gingival recess
   d. firm gingiva

4. Which of the following is a complication from a pericoronal abscess? (p. 197)
   a. gingival recession
   b. trismus
   c. attrition
   d. furcation defect
   e. fibrotic gingiva

5. Which of the following is occurring when a pocket is probed on a tooth with an acute periodontal abscess? (p. 198)
   a. transformation of the epithelium into connective tissue
   b. conversion of the acute abscess into a gingival abscess
   c. incision and drainage
   d. laceration of the fistula tract

References

Armitage, G. C. 1999. Development of a classification system for periodontal diseases and conditions. *Ann. Periodontol.* 4:1–6.

Meng, H. X. 1999. Periodontal abscess. *Ann. Periodontol.* 4:79–82.

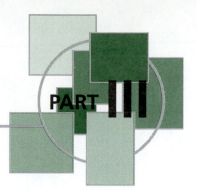

PART III

The Periodontal Diseases: The Assessment Phase

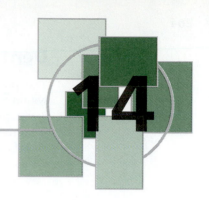

Dental Hygiene Process of Care for the Periodontal Patient

Cheryl Westphal, R.D.H., M.S.

Outline

Dental Hygiene: Procedures for Patient Care

Social, Economic, and Cultural Considerations

Technology and Documentation

Key Points

Web Site

Self-Quiz

References

Goal

To provide information on the procedures of patient care.

Educational Objectives

Upon completion of this chapter, the reader should be able to:

List and explain five phases of the dental hygiene process for periodontal patient care.

Explain the importance of stating the goals for periodontal patient care.

Compare the differences between a dental diagnosis and a dental hygiene diagnosis.

KEY WORDS

- assessment
- subjective data
- objective data
- dental hygiene diagnosis
- treatment plan
- implementation
- evaluation
- documentation

Dental Hygiene: Procedures for Patient Care

The purpose of the dental hygiene process of care is to provide a framework within which the individualized needs of the patient can be met. The dental hygiene process of care is an assessment process involving five phases (Mueller-Joseph & Petersen, 1995) of a search for clues leading up to the identification and classification of the nature of the disease and the steps in patient care needed to alleviate the problem (Bates, Bickley, & Hoekelman, 1995; DeGowin, 1994):

1. assessment
2. dental hygiene diagnosis
3. planning
4. implementation
5. evaluation

Assessment

Assessment is the gathering of all relevant information concerning the patient including medical/dental history, vital signs, extraoral and intraoral examination, periodontal and dental examination, radiographs, indices, and risk assessments (e.g., patient use of tobacco, presence of systemic caries). In the patient history assessment, clues are symptoms, which are abnormalities experienced by the patient. Information obtained by observations of and statements made by the patient are termed subjective data. In the clinical examination, on the other hand, clues are signs, which are abnormalities perceived by the practitioner. Information obtained from observations of the patient and statements made by the practitioner are termed objective data.

Data collection starts with taking down the medical/dental history, followed by the intra/extraoral examination, restorative charting, gingival assessment, periodontal assessment, oral hygiene evaluation, radiographs, and additional diagnostic laboratory tests if required.

Dental Hygiene Diagnosis

After the data are collected, the dental hygienist reviews and analyzes the information. A dental hygiene diagnosis differs from a dental diagnosis, since a dental diagnosis gives a name to the disease and the dental hygiene diagnosis identifies the patient's actual or potential response to the disease process (Mueller-Joseph & Petersen, 1995). The purpose of a dental hygiene diagnosis is to keep the planning of patient care centered on problems or conditions that are responsive to dental hygiene intervention (Mueller-Joseph & Petersen, 1995). For example, a patient has inflamed gingiva, but no bone loss is shown on the radiographs. The dentist will make a dental diagnosis of gingivitis, whereas the dental hygiene diagnosis focuses on educating the patient on the need and benefit (Mueller-Joseph & Petersen, 1995) of proper plaque control to reduce supragingival plaque accumulation. The dental hygienist should also understand the need to disrupt the pathogenic bacteria so that a more beneficial microflora will populate the tooth/soft tissue area.

After the disease is diagnosed, the practitioner should determine the cause so that a treatment plan can be established that will eliminate or control the condition. The dental hygienist should know why the patient developed the condition in order for appropriate treatment to be rendered. For example, a patient complains of tooth pain. The dental hygienist assesses the situation and asks questions of the patient to determine whether the pain occurs with cold or hot foods or liquids. The dental hygienist can then determine the etiologic factor for this condition and develop a plan to eliminate the pain.

Planning

Planning is the establishment of realistic goals and treatment strategies to facilitate optimal oral health. A treatment plan involves the development of a written treatment plan for the patient's individual needs based on data collection and assessment. Alternative options should be included in the plan that may be implemented instead of the ideal plan if the patient is in poor health, if the patient is not compliant or motivated to follow the ideal plan, or if the patient cannot afford the ideal treatment. The treatment plan must be presented to the patient and agreed upon before any treatment is started. An appropriate sequence of treatments must be stated. Developing a plan involves knowledge from a variety of disciplines besides dental hygiene, including behavioral sciences, pharmacology, anatomy and physiology, chemistry, and microbiology. Critical thinking and decision-making skills are necessary to provide effective and efficient dental hygiene services.

When developing a dental care plan, the goal or end result of treatment must be stated (Mueller-Joseph & Petersen, 1995). The goal is a statement that addresses and identifies the purpose for implementing dental care. The individualized plan also identifies the interventions necessary to meet the health care goals of the patient. Interventions are procedures carried out by the dental hygienist to help the patient reach the desired goal. For example, let us say that a dental diagnosis is pregnancy gingivitis. The dental hygiene diagnosis is gingival inflammation related to the elevated hormonal levels and inadequate home care of the teeth and gums by the patient. The aims of dental hygiene treatment are to reduce plaque levels by oral hygiene instruction and educate the patient on the influence of plaque and hormones on overall dental health. Dental hygiene intervention deals with the disruption of plaque by mechanical debridement.

Implementation

Once the care plan is presented to the patient and an informed consent form is signed by the patient and dentist, treatment commences. This implementation phase includes (1) preparing the operatory for the patient; (2) using proper infection control procedures; (3) carrying out periodontal debridement procedures; (4) implementing pain management procedures; (5) applying chemotherapeutic agents; (6) carrying out fluoride therapy; (7) undertaking coronal polishing; (8) teaching the patient proper care of oral prostheses; (9) teaching the patient proper care and maintenance of restorations; (10) providing the patient with health education and preventive counseling; (11) providing the patient with nutritional counseling; and (12) documenting the process properly.

Evaluation

The evaluation phase of therapy deals with feedback on the effectiveness of the treatment and procedures. This phase occurs after treatment has been completed, when the patient returns for a follow-up visit a few weeks after the nonsurgical periodontal therapy (initial therapy or Phase I therapy) or surgical therapy has been completed, or for periodontal maintenance (recall) procedures.

Social, Economic, and Cultural Considerations

From the moment the patient enters the care cycle within the practice, the whole person is assessed to understand aspects such as his or her health background, health beliefs, cultural background, social and economic background, educational background, and work-related issues. These factors play an important role when determining a home-care regime for the person that will yield compliance.

A review of the patient's dental and medical history from the viewpoint of social and economic concerns provides insight as to the patient's ability to afford subsequent dental follow-up home-care regimes. Often factors such as people's beliefs about the role they should play in their own health care and the part their bad habits play in causing periodontal disease will impact upon their desire to maintain their oral health after surgery or other extensive dental care. A complete discussion with the patient is crucial to elicit the information instead of a nonverbal form of the medical history questionnaire often done without any review of these factors.

Technology and Documentation

Since data collection is an ongoing process, an appropriate method of written and visual documentation is required. The intraoral camera is a recent technological advance that can be used to document various findings before and after the treatment procedure. The practitioner is able to view and record such conditions as plaque retention sites, gingival conditions, faulty margins or caries, and stain or other deposits. The recordings can then be utilized to explain the condition and create a historical file that can be placed in the patient's file and used to show the patient any progress or degeneration of the periodontal condition being treated at subsequent appointments. Many different manufacturers exist that offer systems of computers and cameras available for chairside use. The intraoral camera can be employed during the charting, oral soft tissue exam, or oral hygiene evaluation to involve the patient in the process and discuss the findings. Currently the great majority of practitioners who use intraoral video cameras do not have those cameras integrated with their computer systems, although the number who do is growing. This involves converting the images to a digital format using specialized software. Although some practitioners do not feel the need to permanently save images after case presentation, doing so is a valuable tool in terms of educating patients and increasing the likelihood that the recommended treatment procedures will be performed.

Computer technology is becoming essential for the treatment record, appointment planning, recare visit booking, and patient documentation parts of running a dental practice. Oral hygiene evaluations as part of the computer record of the patient offer an array of visual presentations, which can enhance treatment planning and patient compliance with the recommended procedures. Patients can be shown a pictorial display of their probing depths, caries, gum and tooth recession, other gingival involvement, or potential treatment outcomes of surgery or prosthetic replacements.

Key Points

- Five components of the dental hygiene process enable the dental hygienist to identify the patient's periodontal problem, to determine the cause of the problem, and then to treat the problem.
- An intraoral camera can be useful to point out areas of recession, plaque-retentive sites, bleeding points, and restorations.
- Documentation is an integral part of the dental hygiene process; good documentation in the patient's chart is of utmost importance.

Web Site

www.adha.org

Self-Quiz

1. All of the following are components of the dental hygiene process except one. Which one is the exception? (p. 204)
   a. assessment
   b. dental diagnosis
   c. treatment planning
   d. implementation
   e. evaluation

2. Which one of the following reasons is important for determining the individual goals for periodontal patient care? (pp. 205–206)
   a. establishes a rapport with the patient
   b. emphasizes the need for prevention in the care of the patient
   c. identifies the purpose for treating the patient
   d. evaluates for treatment needs after the first appointment

3. Which one of the following statements explains the purpose of a dental hygiene diagnosis? (p. 204)
   a. keeps the planning of patient care centered on problems or conditions that are responsive to dental hygiene intervention
   b. helps the dental hygienist determine the need for additional radiographs
   c. identifies the type of periodontal disease
   d. anticipates the effectiveness in achieving the desired outcome of therapy

4. Before undergoing any periodontal treatment, every patient should have his/her mouth and dentition photographed with an intraoral camera because the intraoral camera is an important part of documentation. (p. 206)
   a. Both the statement and the reason are correct and related.
   b. Both the statement and the reason are correct but not related.
   c. The statement is correct, but the reason is not.
   d. The statement is not correct, but the reason is correct.
   e. Neither the statement nor the reason is correct.

5. Which of the following reasons best explains the purpose of evaluation of periodontal therapy? (p. 205)
   a. determines the need for additional periodontal intervention
   b. deals with the feedback on the effectiveness of treatment
   c. identifies the type of disease present
   d. allows the dental hygienist to introduce oral hygiene care products for home use

References

Bates, B., L. S. Bickley, and R. A. Hoekelman. 1995. *A pocket guide to physical examination and history taking,* 2nd ed. Philadelphia: Lippincott.

DeGowin, R. L. 1994. *DeGowin & DeGowin's diagnostic examination,* 3–4. New York: McGraw-Hill.

Mueller-Joseph, L., and M. Petersen. 1995. The dental hygiene process of care. In eds. L. Mueller-Joseph and M. Petersen, *Dental hygiene process: Diagnosis and care planning,* 1–19. Albany, NY: Delmar.

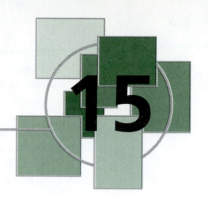

Patient History

Ann M. Goodwin, R.D.H., M.S.
Rosemary DeRosa Hays, R.D.H., M.S.

Outline

Goal

To provide information on the patient history-taking process.

Educational Objectives

Upon completion of this chapter, the reader should be able to:

Explain the importance of data collection.

Illustrate the importance of total health assessment in providing periodontal services.

KEY WORDS

- dental/medical history
- interview process
- chief complaint

The patient's first visit is the time to collect subjective data. A complete dental/ medical history is an essential aspect of the initial evaluation. It is here that the dental hygienist becomes an advantageous partner in the health-care evaluation process. The hygienist interviews the patient for his or her history, which is divided into the personal profile, social history, chief complaint, history of the present illness, medical history, family history, and dental history. The collective diagnostic information developed through this interview provides a basis for future comparisons to evaluate the progress of disease, the efficacy of treatment, and the appearance of new findings. Therefore, taking the patient history is a mandatory first step in the treatment process.

The Interview

The interview process, so critical to the successful completion of the dental and medical history, demands a high level of communication between the patient and the dental hygienist. If done properly, an interview helps establish a rapport between the dental hygienist and the patient. History taking can be accomplished through a questionnaire, a patient interview, or a combination of both. The most practical and successful method for assessing the health status of a patient is a combination questionnaire and interview.

During the interview, open-ended questions such as "What changes in your health or medications have occurred since your last dental visit?" or "What in your mouth bothers you?" open doors to gaining more pertinent information. If good rapport develops, the patient will feel more comfortable, and as the interview progresses, he or she will volunteer more information. Open-ended questions put patients more at ease. Nevertheless, closed-ended questions also are necessary, such as "When was your last dental visit?" These types of questions do not require much responding from the patient; rather, they can be answered usually in one sentence.

Personal Profile

The obvious place to begin the interview is by asking questions concerning the patient's identity. This personal profile consists of the patient's name, age, address, occupation, and telephone number. Some of this information is needed for identification purposes, while the patient's age and sex may be useful in the classification of the periodontal disease. Document the name, address, and telephone number of the patient's physician, which will be useful if consultation is necessary.

Social History

The social history includes the patient's occupation, lifestyle, marital status, diet, and use of alcohol and tobacco, both smoking and chewing tobacco. Habits such as cigarette smoking or use of smokeless tobacco should be noted because they are potential risk factors for periodontal diseases.

Cigarette smoking is reported in pack-years, which is determined by multiplying the number of packs of cigarettes smoked per day by the number of years the patient has smoked. Documenting the amount of smoking in pack-years gives a better understanding of the total exposure of nicotine during the lifetime of an individual. For example, if a person smoked one pack every day for 10 years, this is 10 pack-years.

The patient's lifestyle, including family and social structure, attitudes, and behaviors, is part of the social history. A patient's social perceptions, priorities, amount of stress, and ideas on aesthetics provide clues to compliance with dental care. A dental hygienist can work toward changing a patient's attitudes and behaviors by understanding the patient's cultural differences, motivation, patience, education, and expectations.

Chief Complaint

The next step is to ask the patient to identify his or her chief complaint (CC). The patient should state in his or her own words why he or she is seeking treatment. Determination of the CC assists in the identification of any ongoing disease process. Symptoms of periodontal problems include pressure in the gingiva or jaw or itchy gingiva. Signs of periodontal disease include bleeding, halitosis (bad breath), and/or tooth mobility. Given the insidious nature of periodontal diseases, many patients have no idea there is a problem. If the patient's CC involves something other than periodontal disease, that must be treated first before any other dental treatment is rendered.

History of Present Illness

The history of the CC expands on the patient's awareness of the problem and is also referred to as the history of present illness. The dental hygienist should inquire how long the patient's problem has existed, any previous treatment(s), and if this problem has occurred before. For instance, if the patient's CC is "bleeding from the gums," the dental hygienist should ask about the onset, cause, location, and duration of the bleeding.

Medical History

The current and past status of the patient's general health, or medical history, should be the next area of investigation. A questionnaire, an interview, or a combination of questionnaire and interview can be used to accomplish this. Sometimes, however, a simple telephone call to the patient prior to the first appointment may screen for potential medical problems. A written questionnaire provides a baseline for treatment, whereas an interview provides both personal contact with the patient and supplementary information that may contribute to a more comprehensive evaluation. It is important to listen closely to the patient and have a genuine interest in what is said in order to provide insight, accuracy, and clarity in the history (McDaniel, Miller, Jones, & Davis, 1995). Allowing the patient to describe symptoms or complaints at length encourages trust and fosters a sympathetic professional relationship, but it is only necessary to record the relevant facts and details. A high percentage of dental patients have medical conditions that can have an affect on a clinician's therapeutic decisions (Peacock & Carson, 1995).

Questions concerning current medication use and drug allergies are crucial because the answers may have a direct effect on any treatment the dentist eventually prescribes. Both prescription and over-the-counter medications the patient is taking should be recorded. The name, dosage, and indications also should be written on the form. The hygienist should look especially for any potential drug–drug or drug–food interactions. Adverse side effects (undesirable effects of the drug on the body) of certain medications may be the source of dental problems. For example, antidepressant and antihypertensive medications may cause xerostomia, or dry mouth. Some medications for hypertension or epileptic seizures may cause enlargement of the gingiva, which can result in plaque-control problems. Absorption from the intestines of certain antibiotics such as tetracycline is delayed with food and calcium-containing products including milk and other dairy products. Consultation with the patient's physician may be necessary. If the patient does not know the names of the medications, ask him or her to bring the containers to the next office visit. If a patient is regularly taking medication for diabetes or hypertension, it is extremely important to ask if he or she took the medication as prescribed on that day; if so, the dosage and frequency of usage should be noted on the form. Sometimes a patient may forget to take high blood pressure (antihypertensive) medication and present with uncontrolled blood pressure. If this is the case, the hygienist should contact the patient's physician.

The medical history may uncover other conditions that can have an affect on periodontal health or treatment, such as diabetes mellitus, leukemia, or acquired immunodeficiency syndrome (AIDS) (Neff, 1997). At this time a link between periodontal disease and certain discussed medical conditions that the patient has can be made. If the patient is suspected of being medically compromised, consultation with the patient's physician is indicated, and a written release should be obtained from the patient before treatment begins.

Infective endocarditis is of particular concern in dental care. Infective endocarditis is an infection of the tissue lining of the heart that can result in damage to the heart valves. Any dental procedure that causes bleeding could allow bacteria to enter the bloodstream, resulting in bacteremia. Before initiating any dental treatment that may cause bleeding in patients who are susceptible to developing infective endocarditis, proper antibiotic protection should be administered. The American Heart Association (AHA) recommends a prophylactic antibiotic regimen for such patients (see Chapter 30). Because specific recommendations vary depending on the individual patient's condition, the dental hygienist should collaborate with the dentist and/or patient's physician to determine the appropriate premedication therapy. It is the responsibility of the dental hygienist, however, to screen for susceptible patients by taking a complete health history.

The medical history form is a legal document that provides a past and present profile of the patient's health. After the medical history is complete, the document must be dated and signed by the patient and the dentist, and at each future visit, the form should be updated. The patient should review this information and sign the form again. A new form should be filled out yearly. Indelible ink, preferably black (because it will copy better than blue), should be used. If the patient is a minor, a parent or legal guardian should date and sign the form.

Family History

The family history consists of the present and past medical illnesses of family members. Such a record may help to identify disease trends in the family that are risk factors for dental/periodontal diseases such as diabetes and ischemic heart disease.

Dental History

The dental history includes past and present dental treatments, past dental problems, oral habits, nutritional profile, past response to treatment, and oral hygiene status. This information is collected by way of a written form and an interview with the patient.

The past dental history often provides insight into previous dental experiences, pleasant or unpleasant, in all areas of dentistry, including oral surgery, periodontics, restorative dentistry, endodontics, and orthodontics. Experiences with local anesthetics and nitrous oxide should be recorded. Questions especially pertinent to the dental hygiene visit include those regarding the patient's last dental visit, what was done, and how long since the last prophylaxis.

A nutritional or diet profile of the patient is helpful in assisting the dental hygienist in recognizing a caries-prone diet. During the interview, the dental hygienist can suggest ways in which the patient can alter his or her diet to promote better dental health.

Past dental history also provides information on the patient's dental health values. The periodontal history may be significant. For example, a patient should be asked if previous periodontal surgery was performed (make sure he or she understands what periodontal surgery is). The patient may respond that he or she has had periodontal surgery twice in the past year. Upon further questioning, it may become apparent that the patient returned to the dental office only once for a periodontal maintenance appointment. This information suggests that the patient is noncompliant with oral hygiene self-care and dental visits.

Other areas to explore include the patient's attitude toward dental care and the present surroundings and the level of desire for treatment. Question the patient on what specific oral hygiene regimen he or she follows, including the types of products used. Question the patient on what kind of toothbrush (e.g., soft, medium, or hard bristled), dental floss, and mouthrinse he or she uses. The frequency of product use should be documented, as well as compliance with recommended periodontal maintenance appointments.

Summary

The initial step performed on a periodontal patient is to obtain a complete dental/medical history. Dermination and recording of medications the patient is taking is important since certain drugs affect the periodontium and severe drug interactions can occur. Other risk factors such as the amount of cigarettes smoked should also be recorded.

Key Points

- The interviewing process establishes rapport with the patient.
- Medical diseases and medications can affect conditions in the mouth.
- Update a patient's dental/medical history at every appointment.

Web Site

www.adha.org

Self-Quiz

1. Which one of the following information collected from the patient is subjective? (pp. 210, 211)
   a. medical history
   b. dental examination
   c. periodontal examination
   d. radiographic survey
   e. oral hygiene evaluation

2. Which one of the following statements explains the importance of patient information collected during the interview? (p. 210)
   a. Anticipates patient's attitude about periodontal care.
   b. Determines the number of visits for the patient.
   c. Allows the patient to voice their opinions about treatment.
   d. Provides a basis for future comparison.
   e. Establishes a rapport between patient and hygienist.

3. Which one of the following actions should a dental hygienist take before periodontal treatment is started if the patient cannot remember the names of the medications he or she is taking? (pp. 211, 212)
   a. Call the patient's pharmacist to confirm the medications.
   b. Call the patient's physician to confirm the medications.
   c. Tell the patient to bring the containers to the next appointment.
   d. Tell the patient to call home.

4. On which one of the following parts of the interview does the history of present illness expand? (p. 211)
   a. chief complaint
   b. dietary profile
   c. medical history
   d. social history
   e. dental history

5. All the following types of communications are most appropriate to determine the medical history of a patient except one. Which one is the exception? (p. 211)
   a. telephone
   b. questionnaire
   c. interview
   d. computer

References

McDaniel, T. F., D. Miller, R. Jones, and M. Davis. 1995. Assessing patient willingness to reveal health history information. *J. Am. Dent. Assoc.* 126:375–379.

Neff, L. 1997. Oral health and systemic disease. *Access* 11(3):29–34.

Peacock, M. E., and R. E. Carson. 1995. Frequency of self-reported medical conditions in periodontal patients. *J. Periodontol.* 66:1004–1007.

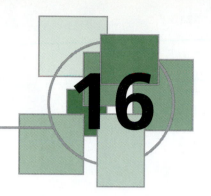

16

Clinical Examination: Extraoral/Intraoral Examination and Dental Evaluation

Ann M. Goodwin, R.D.H., M.S.
Rosemary DeRosa Hays, R.D.H., M.S.
Cheryl M. Westphal, R.D.H., M.S.

Outline

Goal

To explain the clinical components of a dental examination and how it relates to the periodontal condition.

Educational Objectives

Upon completion of this chapter, the reader should be able to:

Discuss the role of the dental hygienist in evaluating the dental and oral hygiene status of a patient.

Describe the importance of performing an intraoral and extraoral examination.

Describe the components of the dental examination.

KEY WORDS
• oral cancer
• dental charting
• caries
• dental implants
• occlusion
• tooth wear
• parafunctional habits
• dental anomalies
• dentinal hypersensitivity

215

Explain how the findings of the dental evaluation relate to the recognition of periodontal diseases.

Discuss the different types of tooth stains and their clinical significance.

After completing the patient history, the next aspect of patient assessment involves the collection of objective data by means of a physical examination of the patient. The dental hygienist's tools for this task include the intraoral/extraoral examination, the dental evaluation, the oral hygiene evaluation, the gingival assessment, and the periodontal examination. This section focuses on the intraoral/extraoral examination and the dental evaluation. The section concludes with a brief discussion of dental hypersensitivity.

Extraoral/Intraoral Examination

There are five steps to an extraoral and intraoral examination: (1) inspection, (2) palpation, (3) percussion, (4) auscultation, and (5) olfaction. Inspection involves using the eyes to observe the patient. Palpation is the action of feeling by the sense of touch. Auscultation is the act of listening to sounds from different parts of the body (e.g., using the stethoscope to hear temporomandibular joint [TMJ] sounds upon opening). Percussion is the process of striking a part of the body (e.g., detection of the source of a painful tooth) to give off a sound. Olfaction involves using the nose to smell odors on the breath such as alcohol or the fruity breath of diabetes mellitus.

In the overall appraisal, the dental hygienist should examine the patient's gait, eyes, lips, skin, and head and neck area. Check for lymphadenopathy or lymph nodes that are abnormal in size, consistency, or number. The TMJ also should be examined.

The overall assessment also includes determination of the patient's vital signs. Vital signs include blood pressure, pulse rate, and respiration rate and provide immediate evidence of the patient's basic physiologic functions. Vital signs should be taken at every dental appointment.

The intraoral examination involves screening for oral cancer by examining the tongue, gingiva, lining mucosa, and hard palate for color, bleeding, enlargements, and the presence of pain. It is not within the scope of this textbook to thoroughly discuss the components of the extraoral/intraoral examination.

Dental Evaluation

Dental evaluation begins with a general assessment of the dentition. Dental charting is done and analyzed not only for existing restorations, periodontal factors, and needed care but also for the impact of each finding on gingival health. The dental hygienist must examine overhangs, food impaction sites, crown contours, bridge abutments (a tooth or implant used for support and retention of a crown or removable partial denture), and pontics (a missing tooth that is replaced with a restoration and for which there are no roots) as possible plaque-retention sites and evaluate the success of the patient in cleansing these areas. Table 16–1■ lists the components of the dental evaluation. Identification of these areas and any resulting dental needs will allow for sequential planning, proper instrumentation, and continual recording and updating of the patient's clinical services.

Evaluate the Number of Teeth

The dental hygienist should begin by determining which teeth are present or missing in the dentition and charting the findings. Information provided by the past dental history, patient interview, and radiographic findings will enable the dental hygienist to determine whether missing teeth were missing at birth, are impacted, or have been extracted due to periodontal, endodontic, or restorative problems. The history of extractions should be discussed to determine the patient's attitude toward dental health and the incidence of dental disease.

Caries

Clinical evidence of dental caries may be detected first visually, through a change in tooth color, and then by tactile instrumentation and radiographs, fiberoptics, or other transilluminating devices. The standard method for classifying dental caries is G. V. Black's classification system. Types of dental caries are described by location. Pit and fissure caries frequently is found in the grooves and crevices of occlusal, lingual, and buccal surfaces. Smooth-surface caries is found on the facial, lingual, and interproximal surfaces of teeth.

Root-surface caries is found on the roots of teeth. This is of particular concern in periodontal therapy because of an increased accumulation of plaque due to loss of anatomic tooth structure and difficulty in removing tooth-accumulated materials (e.g., bacterial plaque, calculus, and stains) from that location. Several risk factors predispose to root caries: (1) gingival recession, which exposes the cementum to the oral environment (causes of gingival recession include periodontal disease and postperiodontal surgery; the number of teeth with gingival recession increases with age only because the teeth have been in the mouth longer); (2) xerostomia, particularly in the

Table 16–1	**Components of the Dental Evaluation**

- Number of teeth present or absent
- Evaluation of the teeth for dental and root caries
- Restorative status: presence and condition of existing restorations
- Dental implants
- Malpositioning and proximal contact relationships
- Occlusion
- Intraoral appliances
- Conditions of tooth wear
- Parafunctional habits
- Dental anomalies
- Dentinal hypersensitivity

elderly due to systemic medication, which may decrease salivary flow; (3) head and neck radiation, resulting in xerostomia; (4) advanced age, because of age-related reduction in salivary gland function; (5) lack of fluoride; and (6) smoking and poor general health status or multiple medication use (smokers and patients on multiple medications had a significantly higher prevalence of root caries than nonsmokers and patients in good health (Page, 1998; Ravald & Birkhed, 1992).

Root caries is detected clinically by visual inspection and/or use of an explorer or periodontal probe. There are two classifications of root caries. Root caries either can be apparent on an exposed root surface (Fig. 16–1■), where the gingival margin has receded onto the root surface below the caries, or has developed in a pocket, with the gingival tissue covering the root area in a way that makes detection of the caries more difficult. Root caries is preventable with rigorous oral self-care and professional care.

Restorative Status

Existing dental restorations should be evaluated for defective or overcontoured surfaces, overhanging margins, and proximal contacts. Ill-fitting removable prosthetic appliances, including clasps, also should be noted. Patients' complaints of floss breaking or shredding may indicate a defective restorative margin. Noting any inadequacies is of particular concern in the periodontal assessment. Any dental restoration should follow the contour of the original tooth, and there should be a tight, firm contact point between the restoration and the adjacent tooth. Overhangs and open margins are conducive to plaque retention, impede oral hygiene, hinder proper scaling and root planing, affect probing accuracy, and can contribute to gingival inflammation and periodontal breakdown. At each appointment, the dental hygienist should update and record any changes that will influence ongoing treatment and continuity of care.

Dental Implants

Dental implants and their prosthetic suprastructures present a vast array of dental configurations conducive to plaque retention. Patient complaints about an implant should be addressed as soon as possible (Wilson, 1996). Methods of examination of dental implants and peri-implant tissues (Fig. 16–2■) are reviewed in Chapter 28.

Figure 16–1 Gingival recession allows for visibility of root caries on the palatal surface of the maxillary first molar.

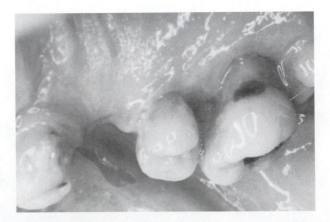

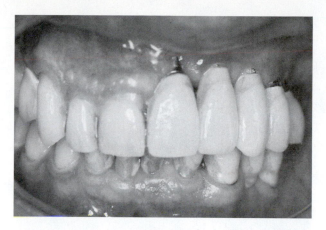

Figure 16–2 Dental implants replacing the maxillary left central and lateral incisor, canine, and first premolar. Check the tissues around implants and implant stability.

Malpositioning and Proximal Contact Relationships

Evaluation of malposed teeth should include teeth that are in facial or lingual version when compared with the normal alignment of existing dentition. Malpositioning can have an effect on oral hygiene and the integrity of a sound periodontium. Tooth crowding can occur anywhere in the dentition. Crowding of teeth may encourage food impaction and plaque accumulation by compromising oral hygiene and consequently exacerbating gingival inflammation (Fig. 16–3■). Crowding of teeth per se does not cause or accelerate periodontal tissue destruction, but crowding does make oral hygiene difficult, resulting in the accumulation of bacterial plaque and calculus, and this can then start the process of tissue destruction.

Often a missing tooth may cause the adjacent tooth to tip mesially. When the crown tips or tilts into the edentulous space, causing the gingival on the mesial surface to bunch up, a plaque trap is created. When proximal contact is lost, for example, after an extraction, teeth can drift or shift physiologically (both crown and root movement) into the edentulous space. Tipped (just the crown moves, whereas the root is stationary) and drifted teeth (the entire tooth has moved) can lead to uneven marginal ridges. If a tooth is missing, the opposing tooth may extrude into the edentulous space (Fig. 16–4■). In such a situation, the tooth will be coronal to the line of occlusion. When a tooth is apical to the occlusal plane, it is

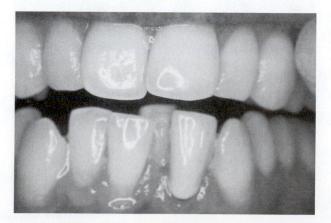

Figure 16–3 Crowding of the mandibular incisors decreases the efficiency of oral hygiene practices.

Figure 16–4 The maxillary first molar is ankylosed and never fully erupted. This tooth is intruded. The mandibular first molar is extruded above the occlusal plane. Uneven marginal ridges result from this occlusal problem.

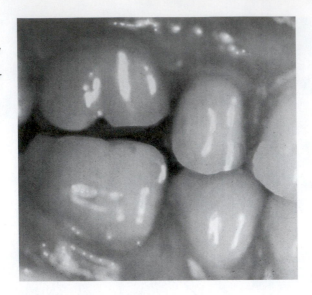

considered to be intruded. Frequently, a tilted or extruded tooth is associated with a plunger cusp, which is a pronounced cusp with steep inclined planes that causes a wedging effect on the interproximal area of the opposite arch. This may lead to food impaction and inflamed tissues.

Contacts between teeth should be checked using dental floss. The patient may complain of food impaction where there is an open contact or disastema between two adjacent teeth. Open contacts develop because of (1) congenital tooth abnormalities, (2) teeth that are extruded beyond the occlusal plane, (3) loss of support from an adjacent tooth, and (4) loss of bone support around a tooth (causing the tooth to move and lose adjacent tooth contact; Fig. 16–5■).

Adjacent marginal ridges should be at the same level. Uneven marginal ridges due to extrusion or intrusion of a tooth produce a poor tooth contact relationship, which results in loss of protection of the interdental papillae from food impaction or trauma.

Figure 16–5 Numerous diastemas in the maxillary arch were caused by loss of bony support.

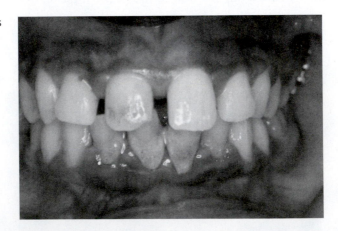

Intraoral Appliances

Orthodontics, retainers, and splinting wires often present difficulty in cleansing the areas through normal toothbrushing and flossing techniques. Once plaque builds around such appliances and the gingival tissue response occurs with edema and gingival overgrowth, the condition becomes even more difficult to manage. Determining the need for altered home care through a complete oral hygiene analysis can prevent future inflammatory responses.

Tooth Stain Evaluation

Development and Significance

Tooth stains are discolorations on or within tooth surfaces. Depending on its origin, the stain can be classified as exogenous or endogenous. Depending on its location, the stain can be intrinsic if it is internal to the hard tissue or extrinsic if it is external to the surface. Exogenous stains are derived from external sources and often are thought to reside on the outer surface of the tooth. They come from chromogenic (producing color or pigment) bacteria, foods, or chemicals. Endogenous stains are incorporated into the structure of the tooth and cannot be removed by surface polishing. Combinations of these classifications can exist, so stains can be exogenous and extrinsic or endogenous and intrinsic (Table 16–2■).

Types of Intrinsic Stains

Endogenous stains are always intrinsic because they come from within the tooth and therefore are incorporated into the tooth structure. Examples include (Goldstein & Garber, 1995):

1. A nonvital tooth where the pulpal contents have discolored the enamel (this could have resulted from deep dental caries);
2. An older patient in whom the teeth appear "yellowish brown" from dentin exposure (with aging, the enamel becomes thinner, exposing the darker color of the underlying dentin).
3. Ingestion of excessive fluoride (fluorosis) between the third month of pregnancy and 8 years of age (the teeth appear as whitish opaque to brownish).
4. Ingestion of the antibiotic tetracycline during calcification of the developing teeth.

Women should not take tetracycline after the second trimester of pregnancy, and children up to 8 years of age also should not be given tetracycline. Minocycline, a semisynthetic derivative of tetracycline, can cause discoloration in adult teeth. Discoloration depends on concentration (the more tetracycline ingested, the more discoloration). Initially, a yellow fluorescent color is seen that changes to a nonfluorescent grayish brown color.

Extrinsic stains may become intrinsic if they are incorporated into the enamel or dentin, as in amalgam leakage or tobacco stain embedded into the enamel surface.

Table 16–2 Classification of Common Tooth Stain

Stain	Origin	Treatment	Figure
Intrinsic stains			
Brownish red, bluish black	Nonvital pulp	Root canal treatment, tooth leaching	Brownish stain
Grayish brown	Tetracycline	Vital tooth bleaching	Grayish-brown stain
Whitish brown Localized	Decalcification	Restore with a restoration; use sodium fluoride (0.05%) rinse	Whitish-brown stain
Generalized	Excessive fluoride ingestion during enamel formation (fluorosis)	Restorative care or no treatment neccessary	
Yellowish brown	Dentin exposure	No treatment necessary	Yellowish-brown stain

Extrinsic stains

Brown	Tobacco (nicotine)	Remove with scaling and tooth polishing
	Coffee or tea (tannins)	Remove with scaling and tooth polishing
	Chlorhexidine oral rinse, stannous fluoride dentifrice or rinse	Remove with scaling and tooth polishing Brush dorsal surface of tongue
Black-line	Gram-positive rods	Remove with scaling and tooth polishing
Green stain	Chromogenic bacteria	No scaling, polish with mild abrasive

Brown (tobacco) stain

Brown (chlorhexidine) stain

Black-line stain

223

Types of Extrinsic Stains

Yellow stain can cause the tooth to appear yellowish or dull. It is associated with the color of the underlying plaque and can be removed by plaque removal. Brown-black stain can be seen in coffee or tea drinkers who do not brush enough to remove the tannin. Plaque does not have to be present, since the pellicle may take on the brown staining alone. Increasing brushing frequency or changing the toothpaste to a more abrasive one may be all that is needed to control the staining. Chewing tobacco often penetrates microcracks in the enamel, resulting in a dark brown-black stain.

Smoking tobacco can produce a stain that is light to dark brown and leathery. It will follow the distribution of the plaque or lodge on the tooth surface most exposed to the tar products of combustion. The stain can cover the cervical third of the tooth or expand to cover the central third as well. It is mostly on the lingual surfaces but can be in the pits and fissures as well. Some tobacco staining can be so severe that it will incorporate in the irregular surfaces of the enamel or exposed dentin. The exogenous, extrinsic stain becomes subsurface and intrinsic, and it increases with neglect. After removal of the extrinsic stain by polishing, increased frequency of plaque removal is required for maintenance. Intrinsic stains may require bleaching for removal.

Black-line stain is a black line that follows in continuous fashion, the facial and lingual gingival margin. It has virtually no thickness and is only 1 mm wide. It usually traverses 1 mm above the gingival margin. This stain is associated with the gram-positive rod of *Actinomyces* species (Slots, 1974). Even though this bacterium is present, the stain is not associated with poor oral hygiene. The microorganisms embed in an adherent matrix and attach to the pellicle. The stain is common in women and children and occurs naturally. Meticulous home care is required to reduce the quantity or frequency of black stain.

Green stain is light or yellowish green to very dark green. The composition comes from chromogenic bacteria and fungi, decomposed hemoglobin (blood), and some inorganic elements. The stain is common in children, occurring on the gingival half of the facial surfaces of the maxillary anterior teeth and extending to the proximal surfaces. The stain can occur as a small curved line following the gingival margin or become a diffused smear covering the facial surface. The enamel under the stain is often rough and demineralized, which encourages plaque retention. Plaque and stain removal through polishing is necessary, yet prevention of recurrence depends on meticulous home care.

Chlorhexidine, used in oral rinses to control plaque and gingivitis, discolors the teeth with a yellow-brown stain on the proximal surfaces, on restorations, and on the tongue (Löe & Schlott, 1970). In approximately 50% of patients, staining occurs within a few days after starting the rinse. The cause of the staining is unclear, but it may be the result of a reaction with foods containing aldehydes or ketones. Although the staining is not permanent, it is a significant side effect that may deter routine compliance. Polishing the enamel or exposed root surfaces removes the stain. Often a patient will have staining only interproximally and not on the direct facial or lingual surfaces. This indicates that the patient practices good oral self-care.

Significance of Stains

The significance of stains relates to the rough surfaces they may create and the resulting plaque retention sites. Stains can adhere directly to a tooth, discolor the pellicle and plaque, or become part of the tooth.

If either of the first two occurs, the tooth surface could have an overlay of stain. This is cosmetic at first until it increases in thickness. If plaque adheres to the stain, the same gingival response occurs. The stain needs to be removed in order to promote oral cleanliness and eliminate possible plaque retention sites.

The key to choosing a removal process is identification of the stain by source and location. Analysis of the color is not always the only determinant of source. Some colors, such as brown, may represent poor hygiene, tobacco use, tea or coffee consumption, or dental fluorosis. The analysis also must determine if the stain resides on the surface and can be removed by polishing or is intrinsic and must be removed by tooth bleaching.

Dentinal Hypersensitivity

Many patients experience dentinal hypersensitivity as a painful response to an irritation where roots are exposed. Dentinal hypersensitivity is a transient, sharp pain arising from exposed dentin in response to a stimulus; it does not last very long. Hypersensitivity will vary in intensity from very mild to excruciatingly painful. Some patients can tolerate the pain, whereas others simply cannot endure it.

Etiology of Dentinal Hypersensitivity

Although not all patients with exposed dentin experience dentinal or root surface hypersensitivity, an estimated 10 to 25% of people in the United States complain of some type of acute or chronic dentinal hypersensitivity resulting from vigorous toothbrushing, tooth whitening, thermal stimulus, mechanical periodontal debridement, or periodontal surgery that exposes the root surfaces.

While there are numerous theories explaining the etiology of hypersensitive tooth surfaces, the most prevalent theory is the hydrodynamic explanation (Paine, Slots, & Rich, 1998). This theory states that the fluid in the exposed dentinal tubules contracts or expands when an external stimulus is applied. The pain experienced is due to this minute fluid movement within the tubules.

The most common situation in which hypersensitivity occurs is as follows: Initially, gingival recession occurs, in which the gingival margin migrates apically as a result of trauma or forceful toothbrushing, and this exposes the underlying cementum. The thin cementum can be worn away easily by the abrasive agents in dentifrices or from mechanical root debridement, which exposes the underlying dentin and the open dentinal tubules. Usually the pain is instigated by thermal changes such as cold air or cold foods (ice cream or a cold drink), a mechanical stimulus such as toothbrushing or touch with an instrument or other object, or a chemical stimulus such as sweets.

Identification

It is important to rule out any dental pathology. The dental hygienist can be among the first practitioners to recognize dentinal hypersensitivity. A patient usually complains of a tooth that hurts but will not say, "I have a hypersensitive tooth." If a patient cannot identify a specific tooth, then the problem probably is not a hypersensitive tooth but rather a root or crown fracture, leaking restorations, or teeth in hyperfunction. If the patient points to a tooth, the dental hygienist should ask further questions pertaining to various risk factors.

Testing for sensitivity should be a part of the initial examination and should include something that can be used as a baseline measurement of sensitivity. The air-blast test is one method of assessing hypersensitivity. The area should be dried before using the air syringe. Most patients who have gingival recession should have sensitivity tests. It also may be important to do pretreatment sensitivity tests before periodontal therapy (e.g., instrumentation, periodontal surgery) so that it can be determined if any posttherapy sensitivity was present before treatment or has resulted from the treatment.

Summary

The dental examination follows the medical/dental history and is an intricate step in assessing baseline data and dental care of the patient. With a thorough and systematic approach to the dental examination, risk factors can be identified that will aid in the appropriate treatment planning needs of the patient.

Key Points

- The dental examination involves identification of contributory local risk factors for periodontal diseases.
- Individual teeth and the entire dentition are examined for deviations.
- Dentinal hypersensitivity is a common complaint; identification causes will help in its treatment.

Web Sites

www.perio.org
www.dentalcare.com

Self-Quiz

1. Which one of the following risk factors is characteristic for root caries? (pp. 217–218)
   a. smoking
   b. xerostomia
   c. parafunctional habit
   d. alcohol consumption

2. Which one of the following methods best detects root caries? (pp. 217–218)
   a. explorer #23
   b. radiographs
   c. rinsing with a disclosing agent
   d. brushing with an abrasive dentifrice

3. Which one of the following terms describes the action of feeling by the sense of touch? (p. 216)
   a. inspection
   b. palpation
   c. percussion
   d. olfaction

4. Which one of the following extrinsic stains is related to chromogenic bacteria? (p. 222, Table 16–2)
   a. black
   b. brown
   c. green
   d. yellow

5. All visible stains have to be removed from the tooth surfaces because stains are harmful to the teeth? (pp. 221–225)

   a. Both the statement and the reason are correct and related.

   b. Both the statement and the reason are correct but not related.

   c. The statement is correct, but the reason is not.

   d. The statement is not correct, but the reason is correct.

   e. Neither the statement nor the reason is correct.

References

Goldstein, R. E., and D. A. Garber. 1995. Complete dental bleaching, 2–13. Chicago: Quintessence.

Löe, H., and C. Schlott. 1970. The effect of mouthrinses and topical application of chlorhexidine on the development of dental plaque and gingivitis in man. *J. Periodont. Res.* 5:79–83.

Page, R. 1998. Risk assessment for root caries in adults. *Oral Care Rep.* 8:7.

Paine, M. L., J. Slots, and S. K. Rich. 1998. Fluoride use in periodontal therapy: A review of the literature. *J. Am. Dent. Assoc.* 129:69–66.

Ravald, N., and D. Birkhed. 1992. Prediction of root caries in periodontally treated patients maintained with different fluoride programmes. *Caries Res.* 26:450–458.

Slots, J. 1974. The microflora of black stain on human primary teeth. *Scand. J. Dent. Res.* 82:484.

Wilson, T. G. 1996. A typical maintenance visit for patients with dental implants. *Periodontology 2000* 12:29.

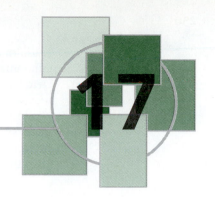

Clinical Examination: Gingival Assessment

Eva M. Lupovici, R.D.H., M.S.

Outline

Objectives of a
  Gingival Assessment
Risk Factors for
  Gingival Diseases
Clinical Assessment
  Procedures

Documentation
Key Points
Web Sites
Self-Quiz
References

Goal

To provide knowledge of the clinical and histologic features of gingival changes in disease.

Educational Objectives

Upon completion of this chapter, the reader should be able to:

Describe the rationale for performing a gingival assessment as part of the patient evaluation.

Describe the clinical features of the gingiva in health and disease.

Evaluate the procedures used in performing a gingival assessment.

Differentiate bleeding at the gingival margin from bleeding on probing.

Recognize and discuss factors found in gingival assessment procedures that may be predictors of future disease activity.

KEY WORDS
• gingival assessment
• inflammatory periodontal diseases
• risk factors

Traditional diagnostic procedures are divided into two components: detection of inflammation and assessment of damage to periodontal tissues (Armitage, 1996). Detection of inflammation will be discussed in this subsection, and the next subsection addresses the resulting damage to the periodontium.

In considering the status of the periodontium, practitioners frequently state that the tissue is either "normal" or "diseased," with no in-between stage. In medicine as well as in dentistry, however, there is a range of normality. Slight deviations from the healthy norm can fall within the range of normality for an individual.

Objectives of a Gingival Assessment

The purpose of performing a gingival assessment is to evaluate the condition of the gingival tissues and to determine inflammatory and noninflammatory changes. Gingival assessment is one of the essential steps in identifying inflammatory periodontal diseases. The accurate recording of initial examination findings is essential in formulating an appropriate treatment plan, as a baseline comparison with future clinical findings after the initial phase of therapy is completed, and in subsequent periodontal maintenance visits.

Risk Factors for Gingival Diseases

The inflammatory process occurs in response to the presence of irritation to the tissues caused by dental plaque. Inflammation is the host's response to the irritation, which stimulates tissue repair. However, as noted in previous chapters, additional risk factors predispose a host to gingival or periodontal diseases. Host susceptibility to periodontal diseases should be considered if inflammation is not resolved after treatment. Having knowledge of all the potential risk factors is important in providing the appropriate treatment.

Risk factors for gingival inflammation or gingival enlargement include the following:

1. changes in hormone levels, as seen in pregnancy, menopause, puberty, or use of oral contraceptives;
2. systemic diseases, such as diabetes mellitus, leukemia, or human immunodeficiency virus (HIV) infection;
3. eruption of the permanent dentition; and
4. certain drugs including phenytoin, valproate, cyclosporine, and calcium channel blockers.

Clinical Assessment Procedures

When examining the interdental papillae and gingival margin, the dental hygienist should compare them with adjacent areas. These are the first areas that are affected clinically by inflammation. In the presence of inflammation, gingival tissue manifests some or all of the following five cardinal signs: redness (rubor), swelling (tumor), and heat (calor). Pain (dolor) and loss of function (functio laesa) may not be present until the advanced stages of periodontal disease. If inflammation is not resolved, then the inflammatory infiltrate progresses into the attached gingiva and alveolar mucosa. Since the alveolar mucosa is composed of loose connective tissue, the inflammatory infiltrate travels through it more quickly than through the attached gingiva, which is composed of dense connective tissue.

Color

The entire mouth should be examined visually, not just the anterior portions of the oral cavity. In health, the color of the gingiva is salmon pink. Color is determined by the degree of vascularity, epithelial keratinization, presence of melanin, and thickness of the epithelium. In the presence of inflammation, the color of the tissues can be various shades of red (erythema) or light to whitish pink, depending on the chronicity of the lesion. Initially, there is a bright red color, which can change to deeper red or bluish red (cyanotic) or pale white in severe periodontal disease. Tissue redness should not be used as the sole indicator of inflammation, nor is it strongly associated with or a predictor for future periodontal disease activity (PDA) (Halazonetis, Haffajee, & Socransky 1989). However, the absence of gingival redness is more indicative of the absence of disease (Lang, Adler, Joss, & Nyman, 1990).

Gingiva color may appear to be healthy superficially at clinical examination and still be diseased because the site of inflammation is deep within the tissues and not seen at the gingival margin until after the disease progresses. Conversely, individuals with thin oral epithelium may have a healthy gingiva that is red in color.

Within the norm range, healthy gingiva varies in color. In certain dark-skinned individuals such as Asians, African descendants, and Mediterranean people, the gingiva will appear to have a light brown to black pigmentation due to the presence of melanin (Table 17–1■). Another cause for variation in gingival color may be an amalgam restoration. The metals from an amalgam restoration may absorb into the gingiva causing a bluish-gray color. This is termed an amalgam tattoo. This condition causes discoloration of the gingiva (Fig. 17–1■) but is not inflammatory in nature, and the gingiva is considered to be healthy.

Contour

Examining the contour of the gingiva is the next phase of the gingival assessment. Gingival contour is determined by the shapes and positions of the teeth, alignment of the teeth, location and size of the contact area, size of the gingival embrasure, and soft-tissue inflammation. Therefore, the contour of the gingiva will vary from anterior to posterior areas and between individual teeth.

Marginal Gingiva and Interdental Papillae

In health, the marginal gingiva (or free gingival margin) is knife-edged in contour. In disease, the margins become rolled or rounded due to destruction of the circular fibers.

Interdental papillae in healthy gingiva are tightly tucked into the gingival embrasures. Papillae of anterior teeth are pyramidal in shape because they follow the cementoenamel junction (CEJ) and contact areas, which are narrow. Papillae of

Figure 17–1 An amalgam tattoo is seen on the lingual surface near the second premolar. This is healthy gingiva.

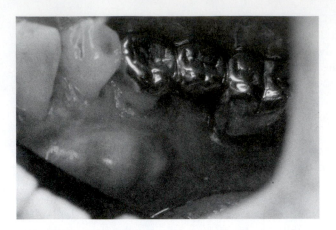

posterior teeth are flatter because the CEJ is flatter and the contact areas are wider. In disease, the papillae become bulbous or enlarged because of edema. The papillae may be cratered where there is a depression between the facial and lingual papillae or blunted where the tip of the papilla is absent and there is an open gingival embrasure. Blunting of the gingiva also may be due to noninflammatory causes such as overuse or misuse of interdental cleaning aids. It may be caused in response to the use of an interdental brush in areas where the interdental papilla completely fills the gingival embrasure. Changes in the contour of the gingiva can reflect current or past periodontal tissue destruction.

Gingival Clefts

In examining gingival contour, the dental hygienist may observe a gingival cleft or a pseudocleft. A gingival cleft is a V-shaped slit that extends apically from the gingival margin. A gingival cleft may be caused by many factors, such as incorrect toothbrushing, improper flossing (flossing cleft), or a break through the gingiva around a tooth as a result of pocket formation. Gingival clefts can resolve spontaneously or may require periodontal surgery.

A pseudocleft is a gingival cleft that occurs when adjacent papillae become enlarged to the point that they join each other at the center of the tooth (see Table 17–1). This is not a true cleft because there is no marginal tissue destruction. Pseudocleft is seen commonly in patients with crowding of teeth or in patients with severely enlarged gingiva who are taking certain medications such as phenytoin, cyclosporine, or nifedipine. Additionally, coronal migration of the gingival margin caused by the gingival overgrowth results in the formation of a pseudopocket or gingival pocket.

Consistency

The consistency of the gingiva is examined by lightly pressing the side of the periodontal probe against the marginal and interdental gingiva. Consistency refers to the firmness of the underlying connective tissue. In health, the gingiva is firm and resilient when pressed. As stated earlier, inflammatory changes occur within the vascular connective tissue of the gingiva, and when edema is present, the tissue will "pit" and not rebound quickly when the periodontal probe is applied lightly.

(text continues on p. 236)

Table 17–1
Clinical and Histologic Changes Seen in Health and Gingivitis

Clinical Features	Histologic Features	Figure

Color

Clinical Features	Histologic Features	Figure
In *health,* the gingiva is salmon pink.	Presence of keratin.	 1 salmon pink gingiva
Pigmentation	Indicates the production of melanin by melanocytes; this does not indicate the presence of inflammation or disease.	 2 pigmented gingiva
In *acute inflammation,* the tissues exhibit various shades of red (fiery red); in *chronic inflammation,* the gingiva may be a bluish red (cyanotic or magenta), or pale white.	Redness is due to increased vasodilation (engorged blood vessels) resulting in locally increased blood flow. As the condition worsens, the bluish red color is due to stagnation of blood in the vessels. The pale white color is due to the repair process with excessive collagen formation.	 3 inflamed gingiva

Contour

Free gingival margin

Clinical Features	Histologic Features	Figure
Knife-edged	Intact gingiva fibers brace the gingiva to the tooth.	 4 knife-edged free gingiva margins
Rolled or rounded	Destruction of gingival fibers.	 5 rolled free gingiva margins
Gingival cleft	Narrow slit in the gingiva starting at the gingival margin; probably associated with tooth position in the arch or the beginning of pocket formation; not related to occlusal forces, as once thought.	 6 gingival cleft

(continued)

Clinical Features	Histologic Features	Figure
Interdental papillae		
Pyramidal or pointed (flatter in posterior)	Papillae completely fill in gingival embrasure; no tissue destruction.	7 pyramidal papillae
Bulbous	Enlarged papillae due to accumulation of fluid in the tissue; the papilla is not tucked in the gingival embrasure but partly covers the enamel.	8 bulbous papillae
Blunted	Destruction of the tip of the papilla.	9 blunted papillae
Absent	Destruction of the entire papilla; occurs where there is a diastema.	10 absent papillae
Cratered	Destruction of the tissue between the papillae; a "concavity."	11 cratered papillae
Consistency		
Firm and resilient	Intact collagen fibers in the lamina propria give the gingiva its firm consistency. Tissues are easily compressed with a blunt instrument.	12 firm gingiva

Table 17–1   Clinical and Histologic Changes Seen in Health and Gingivitis

Clinical Features	Histologic Features	Figure
Edematous	Loss of collagen and vascular permeability resulting in fluid accumulation in the surrounding tissue.	 13 edematous gingiva
Fibrotic	Reparative process whereby the fibroblasts in tissue in an attempt to heal produce and secrete excessive collagen. Tissue becomes hard and nonresilient. Tissue is not compressible.	 14 fibrotic gingiva
Retractable	Loss of collagen fibers. Papillae and margins are easily retracted by a blast of air.	 15 retractable gingiva
Surface Texture		
Stippling	Stippling results from the intersecting epithelial ridges on the undersurface of the epithelium. An excessive amount of stippling is seen in chronic inflammation.	 16 stippling
Shiny and smooth	Can occur in health or disease. In disease, loss of stippling occurs because of accumulation of fluid in the underlying gingival connective tissue.	 17 loss of stippling

Edema causes gingival enlargement, resulting in the formation of a gingival pocket or pseudopocket. Firm, resilient gingiva may not be an indicator of health, however, as seen with fibrotic gingiva. Upon examination, fibrotic gingiva will be hard and will not show a "pit" when tested with a periodontal probe.

Recent studies have found that smokers have the same or less gingival inflammation than nonsmokers (American Academy of Periodontology, 1996; Stafne, 1997). However, the gingival consistency in smokers tends to be fibrotic with rolled gingival margins. Smoking or smokeless tobacco chewing causes the tissue to become hyperkeratinized with an abnormal whitish thickening of the keratin layer of the epithelium. Following smoking cessation, the gingiva returns to its condition prior to smoking (Haber, 1994).

During the disease process, the collagen fibers are destroyed, causing the gingiva to be retractable or flaccid (see Table 17–1). Once the inflammation is eliminated and controlled, the collagen fibers may reform and unite the gingiva to the tooth.

Surface Texture

Surface texture is assessed by drying the attached gingiva with gauze and observing the surface for stippling. Clinically, stippling is described as having an appearance similar to the outside peel of an orange. The presence or absence of stippling does not necessarily indicate the health status of the gingiva. Stippling is present in health and in chronic inflammation when the gingiva becomes fibrotic. In chronic inflammation, the presence of stippling represents tissue scarring. Edematous gingival tissue may retain stippling. In the absence of stippling, the gingiva is described as being smooth or shiny.

Size: Gingival Enlargement

The size of the gingiva is influenced by several factors, such as cellular and intercellular elements and vascular supply. In gingival overgrowth or enlargement, the free gingival margin is located coronal to its normal position at or slightly coronal to the CEJ. Gingival enlargement can be the result of a tissue response to inflammation caused by dental plaque, hormonal imbalance in pregnancy and puberty, side effects of certain medications, mouth breathing, and iatrogenic dentistry such as poorly contoured crowns.

The alternative drying and wetting of the gingiva during mouth breathing promotes an inflammatory response causing gingival enlargement from the maxillary canine to the canine. The appearance of the gingiva, especially the palatal surface, is usually shiny and red in color.

Gingival enlargement of the maxillary tuberosity is not considered to be a disease state. The enlargement is developmental in origin.

Hereditary gingival fibromatosis is a rare form of severe gingival enlargement seen commonly in children beginning with the eruption of either the primary or permanent dentition. The etiology is unknown, but heredity is most likely involved, and many such patients are mentally retarded. Gingival enlargement is generalized throughout the mouth, involving both the papillae and the marginal gingiva. The teeth may be completely covered by tissue overgrowth, preventing eruption.

Hormonal and Drug-Influenced Gingivitis

Hormonal Changes

Clinically, gingivitis in pregnancy is characterized by either generalized or localized inflammation to the gingival papillae, which show a sharp demarcation from the attached gingiva. The inflammation or swelling can spread to involve the marginal gingiva. The gingiva is bright red and edematous, with a shiny, smooth surface. The molars show the most inflammation, followed by the premolars and the incisors (Silness & Löe, 1963).

In more severe cases, pregnancy tumors also may occur, but these are not considered a true neoplasm; they are an inflammatory reaction to the dental plaque. Actually, a pyogenic granuloma occurring in a pregnant patient is called a pregnancy tumor. This swelling appears mainly in the anterior facial areas of the mouth. It is a mass of tissue that protrudes outward. It is deep red and edematous.

Postpartum, these gingival conditions usually regress to their status during the second month of pregnancy. Most of the gingival changes seen during pregnancy can be prevented by removal of plaque and meticulous home care.

Gingival inflammation during pregnancy is not exclusive to pregnancy. Similar gingival changes, except for pregnancy tumors, are seen in adolescents as puberty gingivitis. These patients develop massive gingival enlargement that recurs even in the presence of little plaque. After puberty, the enlargement regresses, but total disappearance only occurs after all local irritants are removed.

Drug-Influenced Gingival Enlargement

Clinically, drug-induced gingivitis is seen as a generalized overgrowth of the gingiva, especially of the interdental papillae on the facial gingiva, of the maxillary and mandibular teeth, particularly the anterior sextent, and does not often occur in edentulous areas (Figs. 17–2■ and 17–3■). Enlargement of the gingiva may result in malpositioning of teeth and interference with normal chewing, speech, and oral hygiene (Pihlstrom, 1990). The gingival tissue in cyclosporine-induced overgrowth tends to be more soft, red or bluish red, and fragile, and it bleeds more easily on probing than tissue undergoing phenytoin-induced overgrowth (Hallmon &

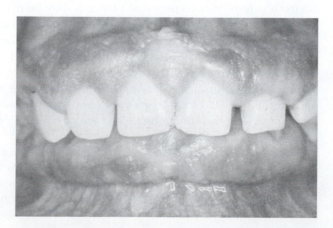

Figure 17–2 A 38-year-old woman taking phenytoin for seizures for the last 3 years. Note the generalized gingival enlargement, especially the interdental papillae.

Figure 17–3   A 56-year-old woman taking nifedipine for hypertension. Note the enlargement of the interdental papillae. The enlarged papillae take on a lobulated or nodular appearance.

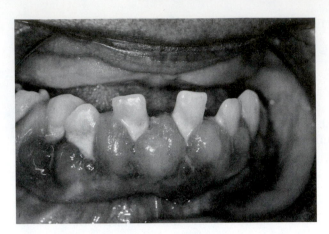

Rossmann, 1999). Other medications that may cause gingival enlargement are the calcium channel blockers (e.g., nifedipine).

In most cases, maintaining strict plaque control can prevent this enlargement, but surgical intervention frequently is required to obtain physiologic gingival contours and aesthetics.

Gingival Bleeding

The next step in the gingival examination is to determine the presence of marginal bleeding. This can be done by several methods, including stroking the lining of the sulcus or inserting a wooden or plastic wedge to assess proximal bleeding (Caton & Polson, 1985). If the stroke method is used, the probe is placed within the gingival crevice and is dragged from one interproximal space to the other interproximal space on the same tooth. Any bleeding seen within 30 seconds is labeled as a bleeding site. Bleeding measured at the gingival margin or crevice is often indicative of gingival inflammation. On the other hand, bleeding on probing (bleeding coming from a pocket during periodontal probing) indicates a deeper inflammatory involvement. In private practice or a clinic setting, bleeding on probing usually is recorded as being either absent or present by placing a red dot over the site that bleeds. For research purposes, a bleeding index is used to standardize measurements. It is important to note that bleeding may be masked if the gingiva is fibrotic.

Bleeding occurs when there is disruption of the sulcular and junctional epithelium allowing for passage of blood or exudate from the lamina propria into the sulcus. The epithelium is avascular and receives its blood supply and nutrients from the underlying vascular lamina propria. When the epithelium becomes inflamed, it reacts by forming microulcerations. Thus, sweeping the lining of the crevice or probing allows for blood to pass through from the engorged and newly formed blood vessels in the lamina propria subjacent to the epithelium.

Bleeding traditionally is accepted as an objective clinical sign of inflammation; however, some visually inflamed gingival sites do not bleed. Therefore, it can be stated that bleeding is not always an early sign of gingival inflammation, and the actual mechanisms responsible for bleeding probably are not truly understood. In addition, the presence of bleeding from a periodontitis site is a poor predictor of future attachment loss (Armitage, 1996). On the other hand, the absence of bleeding is strongly indicative of low levels of inflammation (Lang et al., 1990) and high periodontal stability (Goodson, 1992). Gingival bleeding has been related to increased gingival crevicular fluid flow rate, which is associated with the presence of inflammation (Armitage, 1996). Another limitation of the use of bleeding as an inflammatory parameter is the possibility that healthy tissues may bleed on stimulation or probing (Lang et al., 1990) when excessive probing forces are used or improper toothbrushing methods or improper use of interdental cleaning aids has occurred. Thus the dental hygienist must discriminate between bleeding sites that are inflamed and those that bleed for other reasons. In order to eliminate bleeding, the pathologic process must be changed. Traditionally, altering plaque levels by periodontal debridement and improved oral hygiene has been successful, especially in the reduction of gingivitis.

Documentation

After the gingival assessment is completed, the findings are summarized according to location, distribution, and severity of the gingival changes. The findings can be either localized or generalized (localized to certain areas such as the mandibular lingual teeth or generalized throughout the entire mouth). Distribution is either marginal, papillary, or diffuse. If the marginal gingiva is affected, it is called marginal inflammation. If the interdental papillae is affected, it is called papillary inflammation. If the free, attached, and/or alveolar mucosa is affected, it is referred to as diffuse. Severity is classified as mild, moderate, or severe.

Key Points

- The purpose of performing a gingival evaluation is to determine the status of the gingiva and the presence or absence of gingival inflammation and/or gingival enlargement.
- Gingival enlargement can be due to an inflammatory response to dental plaque or to certain drugs.
- The steps involved in a gingival evaluation include assessing for gingival color, contour, consistency, surface texture, size, and bleeding.
- The absence of bleeding indicates periodontal stability.

Web Sites

www.perio.org

www.ncbi.nlm.nih.gov

www.dent.ucla.edu

www.blackwell-synergy.com

www.cda-adc.ca/jcda

Self-Quiz

1. Which one of the following features describes the gingival appearance in a patient who is a 30 pack-years smoker? (p. 236)

   a. red gingiva and cratered interdental papillae

   b. red gingiva and bulbous gingival margins

   c. whitish gingiva and absent interdental papillae

   d. whitish gingiva and rolled, receded gingival margins

2. Which one of the following considerations must be addressed by the dental hygienist when performing a gingival assessment? (pp. 230–231)

   a. Determine inflammatory gingival changes.

   b. Evaluate periodontal disease activity.

   c. Assess destruction of supporting and alveolar bone.

   d. Evaluate probing depth changes.

3. Which one of the following statements is related to bleeding on probing or sulcular stimulation? (p. 238)

   a. The absence of bleeding is strongly indicative of low levels of inflammation.

   b. The presence of bleeding from a periodontitis site is a good predictor for future attachment loss.

   c. All visually inflamed gingival sites bleed.

   d. Bleeding occurs when there is disruption of the oral epithelium.

4. All of the following factors are related to gingival enlargement except one. Which one is the exception? (pp. 236–237)

   a. gingival inflammation

   b. hormonal changes

   c. cigarette smoking

   d. mouth breathing

   e. nifedipine

5. Tissue redness should be used as the primary indicator of inflammation because it is strongly associated with future periodontal disease activity. (p. 231)

   a. Both the statement and the reason are correct and related.

   b. Both the statement and the reason are correct but not related.

   c. The statement is correct, but the reason is not.

   d. The statement is not correct, but the reason is correct.

   e. Neither the statement nor the reason is correct.

References

American Academy of Periodontology. 1996. Tobacco use and the periodontal patient. *J. Periodontol.* 67:51–56.

Armitage, G. C. 1996. Periodontal diseases: Diagnosis. *Ann. Periodontol.* 1:37–215.

Caton, J., and A. Polson. 1985. The interdental bleeding index: A simplified procedure for monitoring gingival health. *Compend. Contin. Educ. Dent.* 6:88–92.

Goodson, J. M. 1992. Diagnosis of periodontitis by physical measurement: Interpretation from episodic disease hypothesis. *J. Periodontol.* 63:373–382.

Haber, J. 1994. Cigarette smoking: A major risk factor for periodontitis. *Compend. Contin. Educ. Dent.* 15:1002, 1004–1008, 1014.

Hallmon, W. W., and J. A. Rossmann. 1999. The role of drugs in the pathogenesis of gingival overgrowth. *Periodontology 2000* 21:176–196.

Halazonetis, T. D., A. D. Haffajee, and S. S. Socransky. 1989. Relationship of clinical parameters to attachment loss in subsets of subjects with destructive periodontal diseases. *J. Clin. Periodontol.* 16:563–568.

Lang, N. P., R. Adler, A. Joss, and S. Nyman. 1990. Absence of bleeding on probing: An indicator of periodontal stability. *J. Clin. Periodontol.* 17:714–721.

Pihlstrom, B. L. 1990. Prevention and treatment of Dilantin®-associated gingival enlargement. *Compend. Contin. Educ. Dent.* *11*(Suppl. 14):S506–S510.

Silness, J., and H. Löe. 1963. Periodontal disease in pregnancy. *Acta Odontol. Scand.* 21:533–551.

Stafne, E. E. 1997. Cigarette smoking and periodontal disease: The benefits of smoking cessation. *Northwest Dent.* (Sept.–Oct.): 25–29.

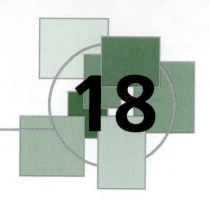

Clinical Examination: Periodontal Assessment

Theodore L. West, D.D.S., M.D.S.

Outline

Rationale for
    Periodontal
    Assessment
Periodontal
    Terminology
Examination
    Techniques

Documentation
Key Points
Web Sites
Self-Quiz
References

Goal

To provide the basic elements for performing a periodontal examination.

Educational Objectives

Upon completion of this chapter, the reader should be able to:

Describe the components of a periodontal assessment.

Explain the clinical significance of each component of a periodontal assessment.

Differentiate the significance of measuring clinical attachment loss from probing depths.

List several factors that can affect the accuracy of probe readings.

KEY WORDS

- screening
- periodontal assessment
- monitoring
- outcome measure
- periodontal disease severity
- periodontal disease activity
- clinical attachment level
- clinical attachment loss

The periodontal examination performed by a dental hygienist has many purposes. First, large population groups in health fairs, schools, hospitals, clinics, and other institutions may need to be examined rapidly for periodontal diseases requiring further evaluation and subsequent treatment—the periodontal screening. For visual detection of periodontal diseases, rapid screening can be performed with as little instrumentation as two disposable wooden tongue blades and a flashlight to evaluate tooth loss, migration, and mobility; gingival recession, redness, suppuration, and swelling; and calculus and plaque levels. Essentially, screening is done in a single visit to differentiate between health and disease.

Rationale for Periodontal Assessment

A more thorough examination requires a mouth mirror, a periodontal probe, and radiographs. The periodontal assessment includes complete medical and dental histories, and the recording of gingival findings, probing depths, clinical attachment levels, tooth mobility, tooth malposition, level of oral hygiene, occlusal relationships, and bone levels.

This periodontal assessment provides the baseline for the long-term monitoring of periodontal disease activity. Such monitoring is often performed by the dental hygienist from one to four times a year at the periodontal maintenance visit. Such monitoring for increases in clinical attachment loss, gingival recession, swelling, bleeding, tooth mobility, and so on, because of the episodic and recurrent nature of periodontal diseases, is vitally necessary if the patient is to be maintained in a state of periodontal health. It often becomes the dental hygienist's responsibility to find and point out areas of recurrent periodontal disease activity in a patient's mouth.

Finally, the periodontal assessment examination should be used by the practitioner as an outcome measure to evaluate the success of periodontal treatment and the need for and frequency of periodontal maintenance visits.

It seems likely that some general dental practices do not adequately assess periodontal diseases (McFall, Bader, Rozier, & Ramsey, 1988). In a study of almost 2,500 patient records from 36 general practices, radiographic bone loss was seen in over half the film sets. However, in only one in five records was there a periodontal diagnostic entry or a notation about pocket formation. This random sample of adult patient records had very infrequent recordings of bleeding, recession, furcation invasions, pocketing, tooth mobility, and so on. These findings can be compared with an epidemiologic study in the same state of North Carolina (Bawden & DeFriese, 1981) that indicated that 55 to 75% of the adult population was affected by periodontal disease.

If periodontal disease assessment in the general dental practice is inadequate, then it certainly must follow that the monitoring of periodontal disease progression becomes an impossibility. It seems probable that the burden for assessing and monitoring periodontal diseases in a general practice may fall, to a greater or lesser extent, on the shoulders of the dental hygienist.

Although periodontal diseases occur primarily in the adult population, they also can occur in young people, occasionally in a very severe form. Therefore, a periodontal evaluation should be performed for all patients regardless of their age. A national survey of over 2,600 individuals 19 years of age and older, using a mouth mirror, explorer, and periodontal probe, showed 28% with periodontitis,

53.9% with gingivitis, and only 17.3% free of periodontal disease in the youngest group (19–44 years). In the 45- to 64-year age group, only 8.3% were free of periodontal disease, and 47.6% had pocket depths of 4 mm or more (Brown, Oliver, & Löe, 1989). Periodontal diseases have now been associated with increased risk for heart disease, stroke, diabetic complications, and premature, low-birth-weight babies. Since race, socioeconomic factors, nutrition, tobacco use, and various systemic diseases can further increase the prevalence of periodontal diseases at any age, the importance of the periodontal examination is obvious.

Periodontal disease severity represents the total destruction and healing that occur during the lifetime of a tooth (Jeffcoat, 1994). It is the status of the periodontium or extent of tissue damage at the time of the examination (Lamster, Celenti, Jans, Fine, & Grbic, 1993) and is determined by visual inspection, single measurements of probing depths, and evaluating radiographs for bone loss.

Periodontal disease activity, which is different from periodontal disease severity, is defined as the current or ongoing (at the time of the examination) loss of soft-tissue attachment, specifically destruction of the gingival fibers and apical migration of the junctional epithelium with subsequent alveolar bone loss. Periodontal disease activity is usually seen as episodic periods of exacerbation or active periodontal tissue destruction (loss of connective tissue attachment and alveolar bone) with intervening periods of quiescence or disease inactivity (Greenstein & Caton, 1990; Jeffcoat, 1994; Lamster et al., 1993). Periodontal disease activity is difficult to determine because it is a measurement of the continued breakdown of periodontal pockets between two points in time (separated by several weeks to months). Destruction must have occurred at some time between these two measurements.

While periodontal probing and radiographic assessment are retrospective views of disease activity and cannot identify an active disease site from an inactive one (nor accurately predict future destruction), they are still the foundation on which the classification of the disease and its treatment is made (Haffajee, Socransky, & Goodson, 1983). The clinical importance of distinguishing between a progressive or active periodontal lesion and a stable or inactive lesion is apparent. Therefore, more sophisticated techniques and assessments have been introduced recently that are designed to determine current periodontal disease activity and/or if a site will break down in the future (Williams, Beck, & Offenbacher, 1996). For a review of these adjunctive assessment tests, see Chapter 20.

Periodontal Terminology

Periodontal Probing Depths

Screening Method

Periodontal probing is the most commonly used physical screening method for measuring the depth of the gingival crevice and the clinical attachment level. Periodontal probing is a clinical approximation of the depth of a gingival sulcus or periodontal pocket (Armitage, 1995). Measurement of probing depths allows the practitioner to make certain presumptions about the state of health of the periodontium. Periodontal pockets are the result of the destruction of the coronal part

Figure 18–1 Probing depth measurement. (a) Deep pocket with apical migration of the junctional epithelium and bone loss. Probing depth is 6 mm. (b) Shallow probing depth (2 mm). There is no attachment loss or bone loss.

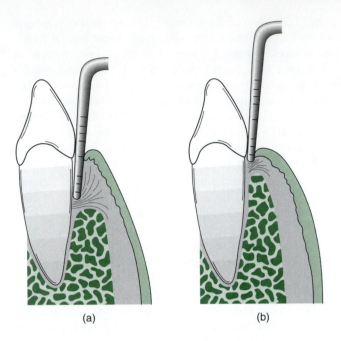

(a)   (b)

of the junctional epithelium and the connective tissue attachment to the tooth surface at the apical aspect of the junctional epithelium (Fig. 18–1■). The clinical significance of having pockets greater than 5 mm in depth is that such pockets may be difficult or impossible for the dental team to maintain in a state of health even with a patient's best oral hygiene self-care efforts and frequent professional cleanings.

Clinically, probing depth is defined as the distance from the gingival margin to the most apical extent of the probe or where physical resistance of the probe is met. This approximates the level of soft tissue attachment (junctional epithelium) to the tooth. In healthy gingiva the free gingival margin is approximately 0.5 to 2 mm coronal to the cementoenamel junction (CEJ).

It should be noted that here we are using the term probing depth rather than pocket depth because what is being probed could be a pocket or a sulcus. This text will continue to use the term probing depth unless otherwise indicated.

Limitations of Probing   In health, the apical extent of the periodontal probe routinely penetrates the coronal to middle portion of the junctional epithelium (Listgarten, Mao, & Robinson, 1976; Robinson & Vitaek, 1979; Spray, Garnick Doles, & Klawitter, 1978). When the gingiva is inflamed, the probe can transverse the junctional epithelium to deeper levels within the tissue. It can stop at, enter, or go through the lamina propria to the alveolar bone crest. Thus this measurement may be greater than the actual tissue destruction. Therefore, the clinical probing depth noted may be greater than the histologic probing depth due to probe penetration of inflamed tissue (Armitage, Svanberg, & Löe, 1977).

Probing depth measurements have several inherent limitations besides the degree of gingival inflammation (Robinson & Vitaek, 1979). The apical extent of probe penetration depends on the force used to probe (van der Velden, 1979), variations in placement and angulation of the probe, the site being probed, the type of probe used, the size of the probe (Keagle et al., 1989), and tooth anatomy.

Other factors that influence the accuracy of probing include the presence of calculus, the visibility of the area, and the level of patient sensitivity. Despite these limitations, periodontal probing remains the most accurate and widely used method of assessing periodontal destruction. When done carefully, a probing difference of 2 mm or more can be clinically meaningful.

Disease Progression   Periodontal probing is important in determining past periodontal disease activity and is used to evaluate the results of periodontal treatment. Single probing measurements do not adequately reflect periodontal disease progression; they only signify past disease activity or the severity of attachment or bone loss at one point in time. Therefore, serial probing measurements must be done (e.g., at periodontal maintenance visits) and compared with previous measurements to determine whether the disease is progressing (Jeffcoat, 1994).

Probing depth measurements therefore are good for identifying areas that are potential therapeutic problems on a site-by-site basis (Armitage, 1995) and to determine the type of treatment needed. However, in longitudinal monitoring (e.g., at periodontal maintenance visits) for disease progression, probing depths are not reliable in determining the amount of detachment of the soft tissues from the root surface because the gingival margin may change its position over time due to gingival recession or gingival enlargement. This was first described in 1961 by Garguilo, Wentz, and Orban (Fig. 18–2■).

Level of Attachment

Clinical attachment level (CAL) is the distance from the CEJ to the most apical extent of the periodontal probe or where resistance is met. Clinical attachment level is a clinical approximation of the loss of connective tissue attachment from the root surface (Armitage, 1996). Measuring the level of attachment of the base of the pocket on the tooth surface gives a better indication of the severity of periodontal disease.

Since the position of the gingival margin changes over time, probing depth measurements are not reliable for determining the extent of detachment of soft tissue from the root surfaces. Measurement of the clinical attachment level is the reference method used to establish disease progression. The CEJ is a stable reference point that does not move over time. If the stationary point used is a part of the tooth other than the CEJ (e.g., cusp tip or restoration), the term used is relative attachment level. Although probing depth measurements are considered to be less valid for monitoring disease progression, they still should be considered as a clinical measure (Carlos, Brunelle, & Wolfe, 1987; Reddy, 1997).

When performing a periodontal charting, it is advisable to measure probing depths and to record the location of the free gingival margin. Future comparisons can then determine disease activity. In addition, the position of the gingival margin relative to the CEJ should be drawn on the chart.

Connective Tissue Attachment Loss   Attachment level measurements determine the amount of attachment loss if it has occurred on a tooth. Clinical attachment loss is defined as the pathologic detachment of the gingival collagen fibers from the root surface with the concomitant apical migration of the junctional epithelium along the root surface. Supporting and alveolar bone resorption also occurs as a result of the inflammatory events, but is a consequence of the attachment loss.

A. Sulcus depth
B. Attached epithelium
C. Apical point of
   epithelial attachment
   below cementoenamel
   junction
D. Bottom of sulcus from
   cementoenamel
   junction
E. Cementoenamel
   junction to alveolar
   bone
F. Deepest point of
   epithelial attachment
   to alveolar bone

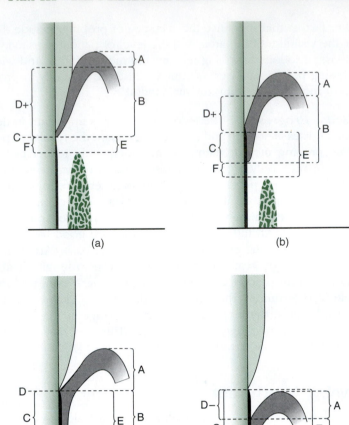

Figure 18–2   Schematic illustrations showing the different positions of the gingival margin. (a) Periodontal health. (b–d) The junctional epithelium has migrated onto the root surface. (Dimensions and relations of the dentogingival junction in humans. Gargiulo, A. W., F. M., Wentz, B. Orban. Copyright by the American Academy of Periodontology, Chicago; reprinted with permission of the *Journal of Periodontology* 1961; 32:261–267.)

A significant increase in CALs is the gold standard for measurement of periodontal disease activity or a site that is actively losing connective tissue attachment at a given site (Goodson, 1986). Currently, a change in clinical attachment level of between 2 and 3 mm, measured at different examination visits, must occur before a site can be labeled disease-active (with attachment loss). Clinical attachment level measurements are important because over time it will determine if a site has experienced further connective tissue attachment loss or gain.

Individuals who have extensive attachment loss also may have gingival recession, but if they have shallow probing depths and no bleeding, they are considered to have a healthy periodontium and not periodontitis at that point in time. Such patients could have been treated successfully and the disease progression stopped, or they may be in remission with no disease activity present.

Other Uses of the Periodontal Probe

The periodontal probe can be used not only to determine the level of the soft tissue attachment to a tooth but also to establish the presence of bleeding, the location of the mucogingival junction, the amount of gingival recession, the width of keratinized/attached gingiva, and the consistency of the gingiva.

Controlled-Force Probes

Within the past decade, automated pressure-sensitive or controlled-force probes have been developed that provide a fixed 20- to 25-g probing force in order to reduce examiner error and to make changes of less than 2 mm clinically meaningful. Examples of these probes include the Florida probe (Florida Probe® Corporation, Gainesville, FL) and the Interprobe™ (The Dental Probe Inc., Richmond, VA). Most such probes are connected to a computer for storage of data (see Fig. 18–3■). Automated recording of the CEJ also has been developed.

With automated probing, the loss of tactile sense inherent in manual probing has been shown to increase rather than decrease probing errors. This is especially true in probing the patient with untreated periodontitis in whom subgingival calculus deposits are present. In the treated patient, controlled-force probing has been shown to be more accurate in some studies but not in others (Armitage, 1996).

Although the Florida probe has been used in a number of research studies to reduce the interexaminer error and the Interprobe was designed for routine clinical practice, their use has not been widely accepted. The automated probing examination may be more time consuming when compared with manual probing with no clear advantage of increased accuracy. It seems likely, however, that rapid, accurate, and easy-to-use automated probes will be available in the near future.

Examination Techniques

Periodontal Probing Depths

To assess the probing depth, six measurements are recorded for each tooth: three on the facial surface (mesiofacial, facial, distofacial) and three on the lingual surface (mesiolingual, lingual, distolingual). It is best to develop a standardized sequence when probing. For instance, probing should start on the facial tooth surfaces of the maxillary right quadrant, proceeding to the maxillary left quadrant, then to the palatal surfaces of the maxillary right quadrant, then to the maxillary left quadrant, and finally to the mandibular quadrants in the same sequence. The probe is "walked" in approximately 1-mm increments to follow the level of attachment (Fig. 18–4■). Spot probing is not adequate for a thorough periodontal examination. When a reading is between two millimeter marks on the probe, the higher reading is used.

Most errors occur in interproximal readings. When probing interproximal sites on posterior teeth, the probe is angled slightly so that the tip of the probe reaches the col area, just under the contact area of the tooth (Fig. 18–5■). When probing interproximal sites on anterior teeth, the probe needs to be parallel to the long axis of the tooth but at the same time should be as close to the interproximal area and

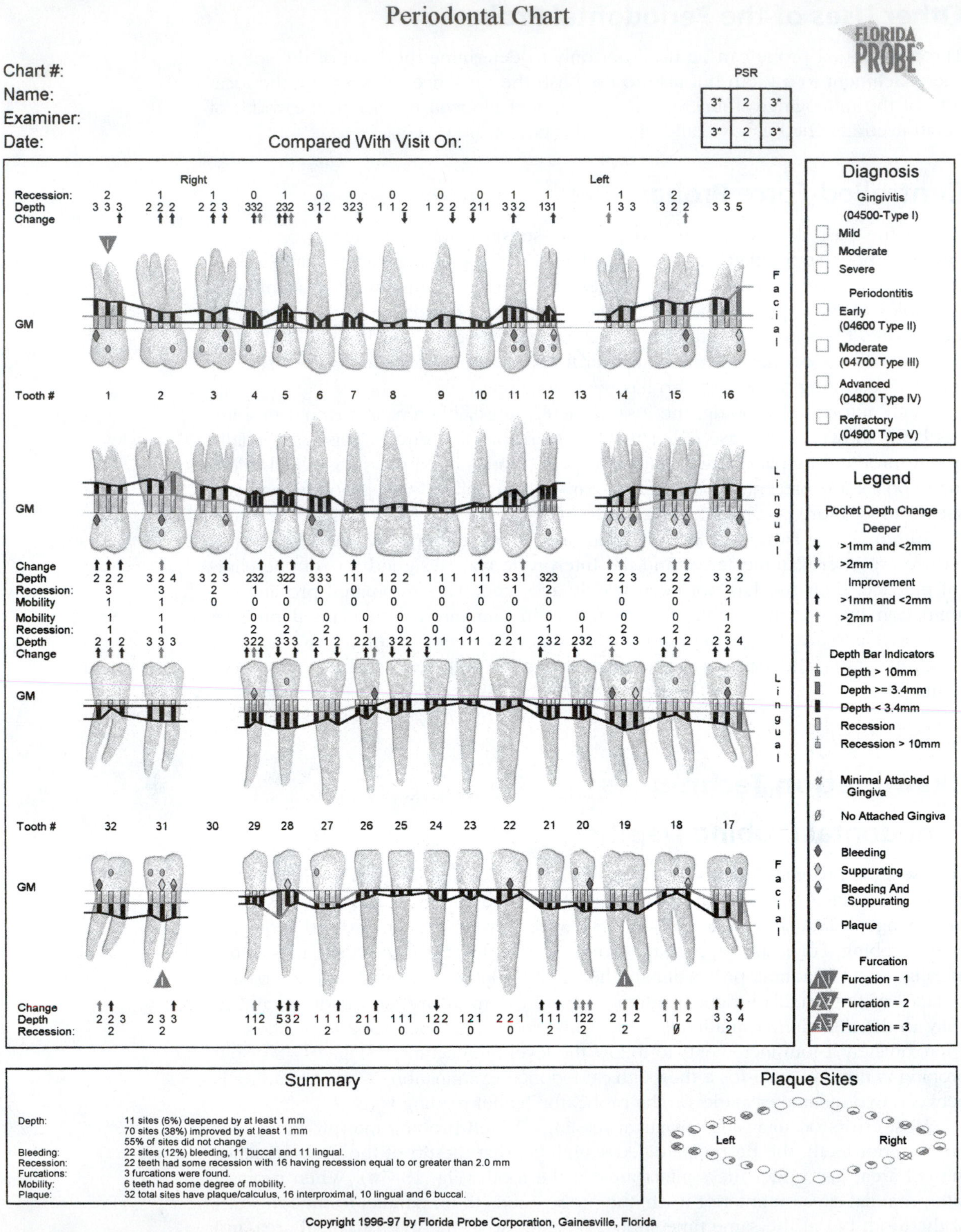

Periodontal Chart

Figure 18–3a   Example of a periodontal chart generated from a controlled-force probe. (Courtesy of Florida Probe Corporation, Gainesville, FL, www.floridaprobe.com)

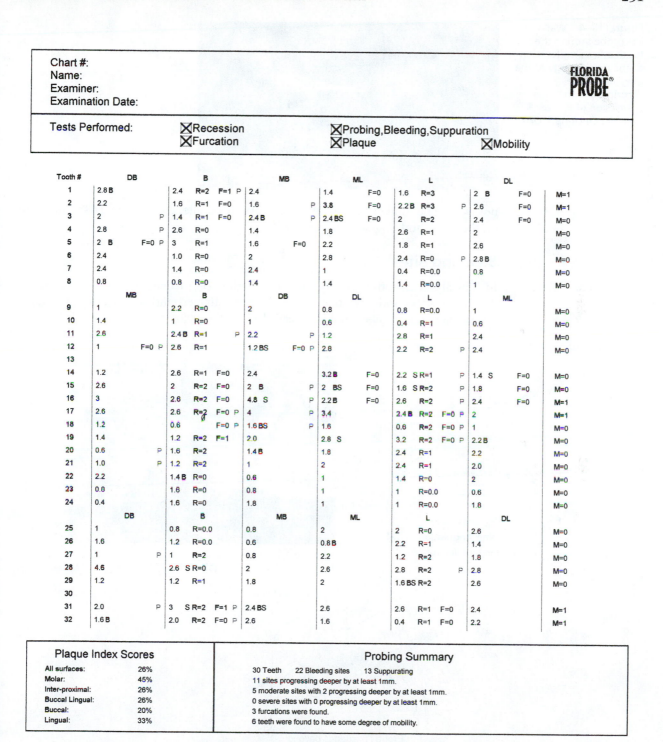

Chart #:											
Name:											
Examiner:											
Examination Date:											

FLORIDA PROBE®

Tests Performed: ☒Recession ☒Probing,Bleeding,Suppuration
☒Furcation ☒Plaque ☒Mobility

Tooth #	DB		B			MB		ML		L		DL		
1	2.8 B		2.4	R=2	F=1 P	2.4		1.4	F=0	1.6	R=3	2 B	F=0	M=1
2	2.2		1.6	R=1	F=0	1.6	P	3.8	F=0	2.2 B R=3	P	2.6	F=0	M=1
3	2	P	1.4	R=1	F=0	2.4 B	P	2.4 BS	F=0	2	R=2	2.4	F=0	M=0
4	2.8	P	2.6	R=0		1.4		1.8		2.6	R=1	2		M=0
5	2 B	F=0 P	3	R=1		1.6	F=0	2.2		1.8	R=1	2.6		M=0
6	2.4		1.0	R=0		2		2.8		2.4	R=0 P	2.8 B		M=0
7	2.4		1.4	R=0		2.4		1		0.4	R=0.0	0.8		M=0
8	0.8		0.8	R=0		1.4		1.4		1.4	R=0.0	1		M=0
	MB		B			DB		DL		L		ML		
9	1		2.2	R=0		2		0.8		0.8	R=0.0	1		M=0
10	1.4		1	R=0		1		0.6		0.4	R=1	0.6		M=0
11	2.6		2.4 B R=1	P	2.2		P	1.2		2.8	R=1	2.4		M=0
12	1	F=0 P	2.6	R=1		1.2 BS	F=0 P	2.8		2.2	R=2 P	2.4		M=0
13														
14	1.2		2.6	R=1	F=0	2.4		3.2 B	F=0	2.2 S R=1	P	1.4 S	F=0	M=0
15	2.6		2	R=2	F=0	2 B	P	2 BS	F=0	1.6 S R=2	P	1.8	F=0	M=0
16	3		2.6	R=2	F=0	4.8 S	P	2.2 B	F=0	2.6	R=2 P	2.4	F=0	M=1
17	2.6		2.6	R=2	F=0 P	4	P	3,4		2.4 B R=2	F=0 P	2		M=1
18	1.2		0.6		F=0 P	1.6 BS	P	1.6		0.6	R=2	F=0 P	1		M=0
19	1.4		1.2	R=2	F=1	2.0		2.8 S		3.2	R=2	F=0 P	2.2 B		M=0
20	0.6	P	1.6	R=2		1.4 B		1.8		2.4	R=1	2.2		M=0
21	1.0	P	1.2	R=2		1		2		2.4	R=1	2.0		M=0
22	2.2		1.4 B R=0		0.6		1		1.4	R=0	2		M=0
23	0.8		1.6	R=0		0.8		1		1	R=0.0	0.6		M=0
24	0.4		1.6	R=0		1.8		1		1	R=0.0	1.8		M=0
	DB		B			MB		ML		L		DL		
25	1		0.8	R=0.0		0.8		2		2	R=0	2.6		M=0
26	1.6		1.2	R=0.0		0.6		0.8 B		2.2	R=1	1.4		M=0
27	1	P	1	R=2		0.8		2.2		1.2	R=2	1.8		M=0
28	4.6		2.6 S R=0		2		2.6		2.8	R=2 P	2.8		M=0
29	1.2		1.2	R=1		1.8		2		1.6 BS R=2	2.6		M=0
30														
31	2.0	P	3	S R=2	F=1 P	2.4 BS		2.6		2.6	R=1	F=0	2.4		M=1
32	1.6 B		2.0	R=2	F=0 P	2.6		1.6		0.4	R=1	F=0	2.2		M=1

Plaque Index Scores		Probing Summary
All surfaces:	26%	30 Teeth 22 Bleeding sites 13 Suppurating
Molar:	45%	11 sites progressing deeper by at least 1mm.
Inter-proximal:	26%	5 moderate sites with 2 progressing deeper by at least 1mm.
Buccal Lingual:	26%	0 severe sites with 0 progressing deeper by at least 1mm.
Buccal:	20%	3 furcations were found.
Lingual:	33%	6 teeth were found to have some degree of mobility.

Figure 18–3b Example of a periodontal chart generated from a controlled-force probe. (Courtesy of Florida Probe Corporation, Gainesville, FL, www.floridaprobe.com)

Figure 18–4 Walking the probe around the tooth allows exploration of the morphology of the gingival crevice. (Reprinted with permission of Procter & Gamble, Cincinnati, OH)

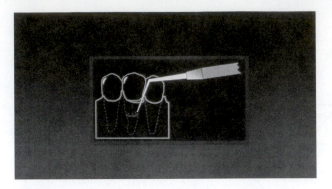

not at the line angle (Fig. 18–6■). The probe is parallel to the long axis of all teeth on the facial and lingual surfaces.

Bleeding Sites

In clinical practice, the primary value of bleeding on probing as a diagnostic sign is that its presence indicates that the tissues are inflamed and not healthy (Armitage, 1995). Bleeding points should be recorded on the chart with a small red dot over

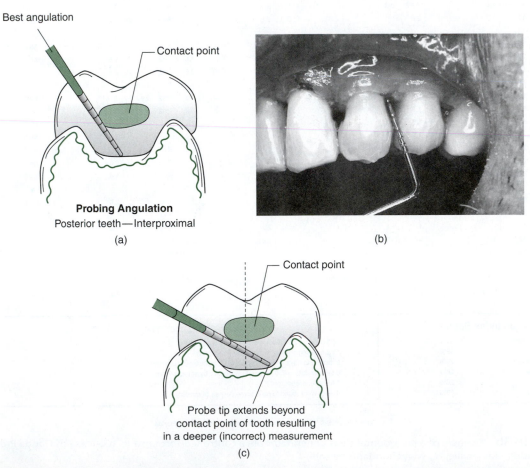

Figure 18–5 (a) Correct probe angulation on a posterior tooth. Probe inserts under the contact area into the col. (b) Clinically, the probe is angled to reach the col. (c) Incorrect probe angulation.

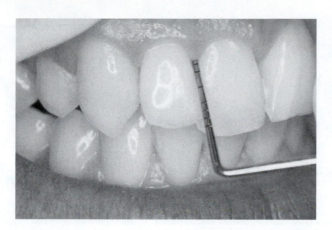

Figure 18–6 Correct probe placement on an anterior tooth. Probe is not angled, but it must reach interproximally with the shank against the teeth.

the probing depth measurement. Bleeding on probing indicates inflammation in the deeper tissues, whereas bleeding or stroking the gingival crevice indicates gingivitis. Sites that bleed with deep pockets and clinical attachment loss are at greater risk for future tissue destruction and should be monitored (Lang, Joss, & Nyman, 1990; Lang & Löe, 1993). Sites that do not bleed on probing are likely not breaking down.

Clinical Attachment Level

The CAL must take into account the probing depth and location of the gingival margin. To assess the CALs, two measurements are needed: probing depth and the distance of the gingival margin from the CEJ at each of the six sites around the tooth. If gingival recession is present (Fig. 18–7a■), the CAL is determined by adding the gingival recession value and the probing depth. If there is gingival overgrowth or a pseudopocket (see Fig. 18–7b■), the CAL is determined by subtracting the amount of gingiva (in millimeters) coronal to the CEJ from the probing depth. If the free gingival margin is located at the CEJ (see Fig. 18–7c■), the CAL is equal to the probing depth. There is more tissue destruction or loss of attachment when gingival recession is present. When the attachment loss is 5 mm or greater with deep periodontal pockets, the patient should be referred to a specialist.

Another method to determine the CAL is to give a negative number to the amount of recession and then subtract it from the probing depth. A positive number is given to the amount of gingival overgrowth and then subtracted from the probing depth.

Repeated measurements, when done in this manner, have been shown in numerous studies to be reproducible to within 61 mm 90% of the time and within 62 mm 99% of the time (Armitage, 1996). Attachment loss of more than 2 mm has become the gold standard for the assessment of periodontal disease progression (Armitage, 1996). This change is necessary to take into consideration the inherent errors, as mentioned earlier, in periodontal probing.

A patient has clinical attachment loss when there is periodontitis with apical migration of the junctional epithelium. Determination of attachment loss is part of the calculation of clinical attachment levels.

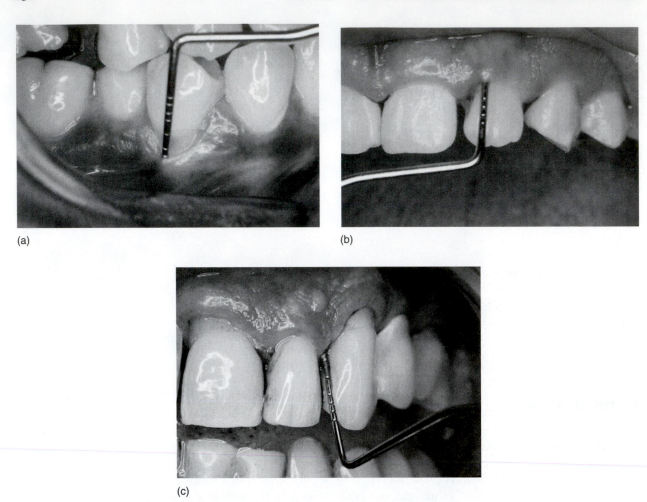

(a)

(b)

(c)

Figure 18–7   Probing depth versus clinical attachment level. Probing depth is the distance from the free gingival margin to the attached gingival tissues. Clinical attachment level is the distance from the CEJ to the attached gingival tissues. When the free gingival margin is apical to the CEJ (a), add the amount of recession to the probing depth (3 mm + probing depth [2 mm] = 5 mm clinical attachment level). When the free gingival margin is coronal to the CEJ (b), the distance to the CEJ is measured and subtracted from the probing depth (5 mm probing depth − 2 mm gingival enlargement = 3 mm clinical attachment level). (c) When the free gingival margin is at the CEJ, the probing depth equals the clinical attachment level (2 mm probing depth = 2 mm clinical attachment level).

Periodontal Screening and Recording

The Periodontal Screening and Recording (PSR) system provides a rapid, 2- to 3-minute periodontal screening examination to be performed by a dentist or hygienist for the detection of periodontal diseases and monitoring of the periodontal patient. This system was developed by the American Dental Association and the American Academy of Periodontology with financial support from the Procter & Gamble Company. PSR indicates when a more comprehensive full-mouth periodontal examination should be done. Implants are examined in the same way as natural teeth.

The key component of the system is a thin, plastic or metal, ball-end periodontal probe. The ball tip enhances patient comfort and aids in detecting overhanging margins and subgingival calculus. The probe has a colored band extending from 3.5 to 5.5 mm for classifying pocket depth. The mouth is divided into six sextants or sections. Although six sites are probed on each tooth as in a conventional periodontal examination, only the deepest site in each sextant is scored and recorded in the patient's chart. The PSR code score is determined by how much of the colored band is visible when the PSR probe is placed in the gingival crevice (Fig. 18–8a■).

The following are the codes used:

Code 0: Colored probe area completely visible; no bleeding; no calculus or roughness

Code 1: Colored probe area completely visible; bleeding; no calculus or roughness

Code 2: Colored probe area completely visible; bleeding; calculus and/or roughness

Code 3: Colored probe area partially visible (4–5 mm depth)

Code 4: Colored probe area submerged completely (5.5 mm depth)

An asterisk is used to denote a furcation defect, tooth mobility, mucogingival involvement, or soft tissue recession.

The treatment of patients is based on their sextant scores (see Fig. 18–8b,c■). A code 3 or code 4 indicates that a more comprehensive periodontal examination and charting of the affected sextant is required to determine the treatment. When this system is used in the long-term monitoring of periodontal patients whose deep probing sites are being maintained nonsurgically, recording the tooth number and attachment level alongside the PSR coding box facilitates rapid monitoring of these sites at each periodontal maintenance visit.

Suppuration

Suppuration, also referred to as purulent exudate or pus, is a clinical feature of inflammation. Pus is composed of dead cells, polymorphonuclear leukocytes (PMNs or neutrophils), and tissue fluids. The presence of suppuration indicates an ongoing infection in the periodontal pocket. Pus can be detected visually coming from the pocket by either probing the gingival crevice or using digital pressure from the base of the crevice on the outer surface of the gingiva moving in a coronal direction.

Tooth Mobility

Tooth mobility is classified as either physiologic or pathologic. Physiologic movement of a tooth is limited to the width of the periodontal ligament space. All teeth have some degree of physiologic mobility that occurs with normal function. The range of physiologic mobility varies according to the time of the day and the tooth. It is most evident on teeth with short roots, such as mandibular incisors, and early in the morning. Increased tooth mobility in the hours just after awakening is due to slight extrusion of the tooth as a result of limited occlusal contact during sleep.

Pathologic mobility of teeth results from bone loss, gingival inflammation, periapical pathology, hormonal imbalance (e.g., pregnancy gingivitis), or occlusal

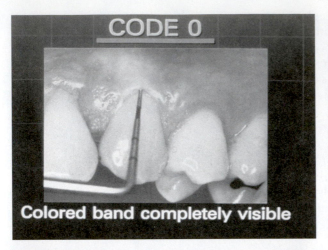

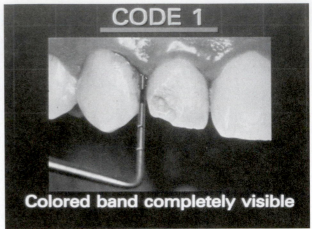

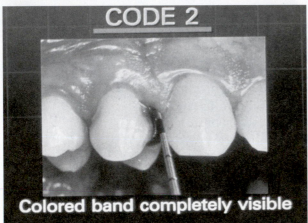

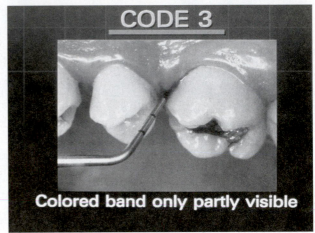

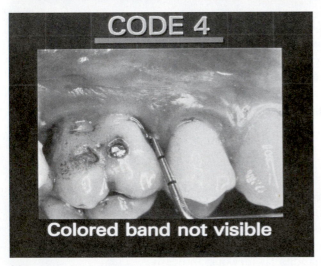

(a)

Figure 18–8   PSR system. (a) Code 0, code 1, code 2, code 3, code 4. (Courtesy of the American Dental Association, Chicago)

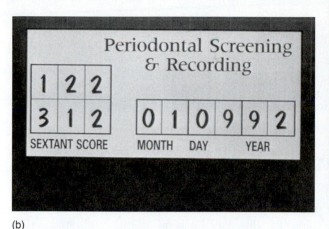

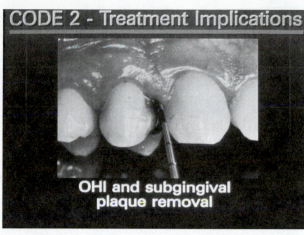

(b)   (c)

Figure 18–8, cont.   PSR system. (b) A box chart is used to record the scores for each sextant. (c) Treatment implication for code 2 involves oral hygiene instructions and subgingival plaque removal. (Courtesy of the American Dental Association, Chicago)

trauma, where excessive occlusal forces are placed on a tooth. Periodontal disease can be advanced without any evidence of increased tooth mobility. Therefore, the severity of tooth mobility is not always due to the amount of bone loss. Since tooth mobility may not result from periodontal problems, identification of the cause is important so that the appropriate treatment can be rendered.

Measurement of Tooth Mobility

The degree of mobility can be measured either manually or with electronic devices. Although the most common classification for measuring pathologic tooth mobility is the Miller classification, it remains very subjective. Mobility is assessed by using the handles of two hand instruments on the facial and lingual aspects of the crown and applying force. The Miller classification is summarized in Table 18–1■ (Miller, 1950). Mobility requires treatment when the patient feels discomfort or when the mobility increases over time.

Fremitus

Fremitus is the vibrational movement of a tooth under occlusal forces. Fremitus is determined by gently placing the index finger on the facial surfaces of the maxillary teeth while instructing the patient to tap the teeth together and grind them side to side. Only the maxillary teeth are checked for fremitus because the arch is fixed whereas the mandibular arch is moving.

Table 18–1	Classification of Pathologic Mobility (Miller's Classification)

I. First distinguishable sign of tooth movement in a facial/lingual direction
II. Movement of the crown in a facial/lingual direction up to 1 mm
III. Movement of the crown in a facial/lingual direction more than 1 mm and/or depressed in a vertical direction

The amount of fremitus is subjective, but the following guide can be used:

+ (slight vibrations can be felt);

++ (obvious, palpable vibrations can be felt, but movement of the tooth is barely visible); or

+++ (visible movement is seen).

Fremitus should be eliminated by occlusal adjustment by means of, say, selective grinding.

Pathologic Tooth Migration

Pathologic tooth migration is defined as the movement of teeth due to the disruption of forces that normally maintain physiologic tooth position. Tooth movement can occur in any direction. Clinically, this may be seen as increased spacing between teeth, dramatic overjet of anterior teeth (anterior flaring), rotation of teeth, or extrusion where tooth migration occurs in an occlusal or incisal direction (Fig. 18–9■). Usually tooth mobility is also present. Any of these symptoms is a common chief complaint of a patient that may prompt a professional evaluation. As part of the clinical examination, it is important to ask the patient if spaces between the teeth have increased over time or if they have always been present. It is important to recognize signs and symptoms of pathologic migration and determine the cause of the problem in order to render appropriate treatment.

Periodontal disease destruction of the attachment apparatus plays a major role in the etiology of pathologic migration (Towfighi et al., 1997). Other contributing factors include parafunctional habits such as tongue thrusting or bruxism, teeth adjacent to edentulous areas, and drug-induced gingival enlargement.

Furcation Involvement

A furcation or furca is the area of root division on multirooted teeth, including the maxillary first and second molars, maxillary first premolar, and mandibular first and second molars. The third molars usually have fused conical roots. Since the maxillary molars have three roots (mesiobuccal, distofacial, palatal), they are tirfurcated. There are three furcation entrances: mesial, distal, and buccal. The mandibular

Figure 18–9
Pathologic tooth migration in a 26-year-old woman with rapidly progressive periodontitis. The patient complained of flaring and increasing space between the maxillary central incisors.

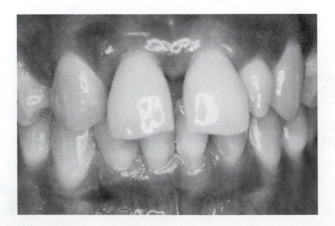

molars are bifurcated; that is, they have two roots (mesial and distal). There are two furcation entrances: buccal and lingual. The maxillary first premolar is also bifurcated, having a buccal and lingual root. There are two furcation entrances: mesial and distal.

Furcation involvement occurs when interradicular bone (bone between the root branches of the same tooth) destruction occurs. Furcation involvement is affected by factors such as the length of the root trunk and the presence of root concavities, which create a plaque trap. The root trunk is the area on the tooth from the CEJ to the roof or entrance of the furca (Fig. 18–10■). As seen radiographically, high furcation with a short root trunk will have a greater chance of interradicular bone destruction early in the disease process than a low furcation with a long root trunk. The average root trunk length on a maxillary molar is about 4 mm at the mesial, 5 mm at the distal, and 4 mm at the buccal furcation. The root trunk length of the mandibular molar is 3 mm on the buccal aspect and 4 mm on the lingual aspect (Dunlap & Gher, 1985; Gher & Dunlap, 1985). This suggests that a minimum of 5 mm of attachment loss on a molar may result in early furcation involvement.

Classification of Furcation Involvement

The clinical detection of furcation involvements is important because it is difficult for both the patient and the dental hygienist to effectively clean these areas. Radiographic interpretation does not allow sufficient detection of furcation involvement. The anatomy of the tooth and location of the furca are determined from both the radiograph and clinical examination. The pattern of interradicular bone loss is both horizontal and vertical. Although many classifications of horizontal furcation involvement have been suggested, Glickman's classification is described in Table 18–2■. Classification of vertical bone loss (Tarnow & Fletcher, 1984) is described in Fig. 18–11■.

Technique for Locating Furcation Involvements

A calibrated curved Nabers probe is used to clinically locate the furcation entrances and degree of horizontal pattern of bone destruction (Fig. 18–12a■). In the maxillary molar, the mesial furcation is not centered. The entrance is usually located about two-thirds of the buccal-lingual width toward the palatal aspect of the tooth

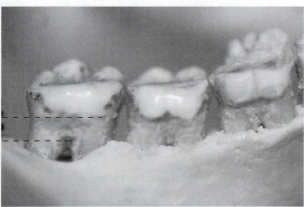

ROOT TRUNK

ROOF
OF FURCA

Figure 18–10   Dry-skull specimen of a furcation involvement on the mandibular molars. Root trunk length is the distance from the CEJ to the entrance (roof) of the furca.

Table 18–2	Glickman's Classification of Furcation Involvement (Horizontal Pattern of Bone Destruction)

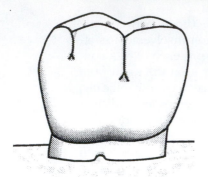

Grade I Involvement: Pocket formation into the fluting of the furca, but the interradicualr bone is intact. No gross or radiographic evidence of bone loss. This is recorded on the periodontal chart as ∧

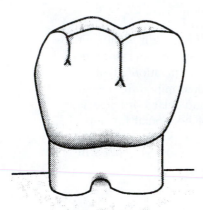

Grade II Involvement: Interradicular bone is destroyed on one or more aspects of the furcation, but a portion of alveolar bone and periodontal ligament remains intact. This is recorded on the periodontal chart as △

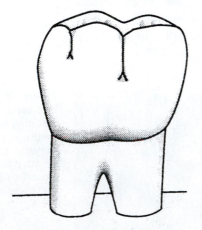

Grade III Involvement: The furcation is occluded by gingiva but the interradicular bone has been destroyed so that a probe can be passed through from one surface to the other. This is recorded on the periodontal chart as ▲

Grade IV Involvement: The periodontium is destroyed to such a degree that the furcation is open and exposed and clinically visible. ▲

Source: From Carranza, F. A., and H. H. Takei. 1996. Treatment of furcation involvement and combined periodontal-endodontic therapy. In F. A. Carranza and M. G. Newman (eds.), *Clinical periodontology,* 640. Philadelphia: W. B. Saunders. Illustrations courtesy of James A. Simonds, D.D.S., Copyright 1991 Practical Periodontics. Continental Education. Santa Rosa, CA.

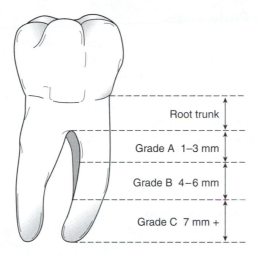

Root trunk

Grade A 1–3 mm

Grade B 4–6 mm

Grade C 7 mm +

Figure 18–11   Schematic drawing of a mandibular molar demonstrating the vertical classification of furcation involvement. The amount of vertical bone loss is determined from the roof of the furca apically. (Reprinted with permission from the American Academy of Periodontology. Copyright 1984. Tarnow D., and P. Fletcher. Classification of the vertical component of furcation involvement. *J. Periodontol.* 1983;55:283–284.)

(see Fig. 18–12b■). Thus the mesial furcation is approached from the palatal side. The distal furcation is centered equally from the buccal and palatal aspects of the tooth (in the interproximal area), and thus the Nabers probe can be positioned from either the buccal or palatal side. The instrument handle is placed parallel to the long axis of the tooth. When a furcation defect is found, it is noted in the chart on the involved root. Furcations thus can be classified according to their horizontal and vertical component of bone loss, for example, IIA.

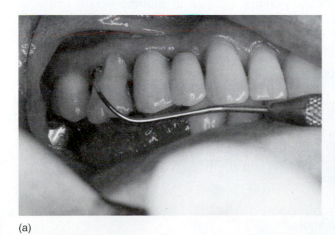

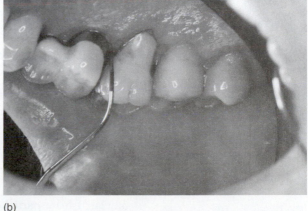

(a)   (b)

Figure 18–12   (a) Placement of the Nabers probe in determining the presence of a buccal furcation. Note that the handle is parallel to the occlusal plane. (b) Nabers probe placed to determine the presence of a mesial furcation of a maxillary molar. Note that the handle is parallel to the long axis of the tooth when probing interproximal furcations.

Cervical Enamel Projections

Cervical enamel projections (CEPs) are extensions of enamel toward and often into the furcation area. This area is thought to be a plaque trap, enhancing plaque accumulation. This area may be more prone to attachment loss because instead of a connective tissue attachment, the periodontal attachment on enamel will be via a junctional epithelium, which may not be as strong (Easly & Drennan, 1969). However, it has been demonstrated that an epithelial attachment may be just as resistant as a connective tissue attachment to inflammatory disease.

Gingival Position

In health, the free gingival margin is located approximately 0.5 to 2 mm coronal to the CEJ. Gingival recession (also called gingival atrophy) is defined as a shift in the gingival margin apical to the CEJ with exposure of the root surface to the oral environment. Actually, since the soft tissue margin may not always be composed of gingiva, the term soft tissue recession rather than gingival recession may be more appropriate. However, since this is currently not universally accepted, this text will continue to use gingival recession (Wennström, 1996). Gingival recession may be localized to one tooth or generalized throughout the mouth. Usually the facial surface is involved, but all other tooth surfaces could be involved as well.

Measurement of Gingival Recession

Visible recession, which is seen clinically, is measured from the CEJ to the gingival margin and represents the apparent position of the gingiva. Hidden recession, which is covered by the gingiva and therefore not visible, can only be measured by placing a periodontal probe at the level of attachment. This represents the actual position of the gingiva or the level of soft tissue attachment (junctional epithelium) to the tooth surface (Carranza, 1996; Fig. 18–13■). The visible recession added to the hidden recession equals the clinical attachment level. The clinical importance of measuring recession is often overlooked. There can be loss of attachment or gingival recession without a corresponding increase in probing depth. This often can be misleading, and it could be assumed that there is no tissue destruction occurring when actually there is.

Etiology of Gingival Recession

The principal predisposing factor that determines whether recession occurs is the anatomy of the area, specifically the thickness of the alveolar bone and overlying gingiva. The etiology of gingival recession is multifactoral. Etiologic factors include:

1. mechanical trauma: soft tissue trauma from overzealous toothbrushing;
2. orthodontic movement;
3. dental procedures;
4. crown margins;
5. clasps from partial dentures;
6. destructive inflammatory periodontal disease, where there is loss of attachment (destruction of gingival fibers and apical migration of the junctional epithelium; Fig. 18–14■);

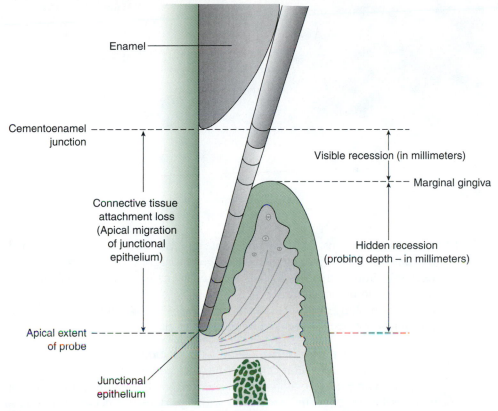

Enamel

Cementoenamel
junction

Visible recession (in millimeters)

Marginal gingiva

Connective tissue
attachment loss
(Apical migration
of junctional
epithelium)

Hidden recession
(probing depth – in millimeters)

Apical extent
of probe

Junctional
epithelium

Figure 18–13 Diagram showing visible and hidden recession. Clinically, visible recession is determined by measuring with a periodontal probe from the CEJ to the free gingival margin. Hidden recession corresponds to the probing depth. The visible recession measurement added to the hidden recession measurement equals the clinical attachment level (CAL).

7. tooth malposition (rotated, lingually or facially displaced teeth), where the alveolar bone over a prominent root such as a maxillary canine is thin or absent;
8. periodontal therapy (periodontal debridement or surgery), where tissue shrinkage has occurred;
9. oral habits causing injury to the gingiva such as fingernail biting;

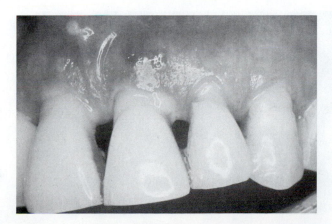

Figure 18–14 Gingival recession in a refractory periodontitis patient. Note the presence of inflammation and suppuration. Gingival recession is due to the disease process.

Figure 18–15
Recession on the mandibular incisors caused by the high frenum attachment pulling on the free gingival margin. Note the heavy accumulation of plaque and calculus.

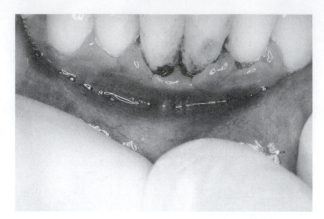

10. anatomic variations that may accelerate gingival recession include a high frenum attachment pulling the free gingival margin (Fig. 18–15■);
11. occlusal trauma (this has been suggested to cause gingival recession but has not been demonstrated; and
12. cigarette smoking and chewing tobacco (Fig. 18–16■), but the exact mechanism has not been elucidated (Gunsolley et al., 1998).

It is imperative that the cause be determined in individual cases so that the progressive nature of the recession can be controlled and interceptive therapy initiated if necessary. Gingival recession can be seen in healthy gingiva; inflammation may or may not be present. The association with age does not necessarily suggest a physiologic effect of aging on recession. It may just reflect the fact that older people have been subject to the force of brushing for longer periods of time (Joshipura, Kent, & DePaola, 1994).

Clinical Significance of Gingival Recession

Identification of gingival recession has clinical significance. Root surfaces exposed to the oral environment are more vulnerable to the development of root caries. The thin layer of cementum on the exposed root surface may wear away easily, exposing the underlying dental tubules to the oral environment. Fluid in the exposed

Figure 18–16 A 45-year-old man who placed chewing tobacco in the facial vestibule of the anterior teeth. Note the gingival recession on the anterior teeth.

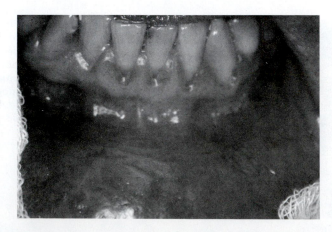

dentinal tubules contracts or expands when an external stimulus such as cold or touch is applied. This may stimulate nerves to produce pain. In addition, the col shape changes when gingival recession is present. If the interdental area is open so that no col exists, the facial and palatal gingiva become continuous and keratinized. Thus interproximal recession may create areas of food impaction.

Pathogenesis

The pathogenesis of gingival recession is debatable. As mentioned earlier, it has been considered perhaps to be a normal physiologic process that occurs with increasing age, but there is limited documentation to uphold this concept. Others consider it to be a pathologic condition. When the free gingiva is thin, the inflammatory lesion will occupy and degrade the entire connective tissue portion, resulting in collapse of the free gingiva (Wennström, 1994). If there is less than 1 mm or more of attached gingiva, the free gingival margin may be movable, which allows microorganisms to enter into the crevice, initiating an inflammatory response.

The amount of attached gingiva needed for gingival health is controversial. Experimental studies (Wennström & Lindhe, 1983a, 1983b) have failed to consistently support the concept of a minimal width of gingiva for maintenance of periodontal health.

Mucogingival Considerations

A mucogingival involvement or defect is defined as a discrepancy in the relationship between the free gingival margin and the mucogingival junction. Pathology or loss of attachment may not be involved. Common mucogingival conditions may be the result of

1. gingival recession resulting in inadequate or diminished attached gingiva;
2. probing depths extending to or beyond the mucogingival junction into the alveolar mucosa (Fig. 18–17■); and
3. anatomical variations that may complicate the management of these conditions, including a high frenum attachment pulling the gingival margin away from the tooth surface (see Fig. 18–15) (surgical intervention may be

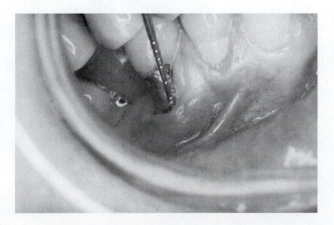

Figure 18–17   There is no attached gingiva present on this tooth. This is a mucogingival defect.

necessary to augment the amount of attached gingiva and correct the mucogingival problem).

Mucogingival Examination

A thorough mucogingival examination using appropriate screening techniques and recording the free gingival margin and mucogingival junction on the chart is necessary to detect these conditions. This also enables the practitioner to monitor the progressive nature at future periodontal maintenance visits so that appropriate treatment can be rendered. While radiographs are not used in the identification of mucogingival problems, appropriate radiographs may be used as part of a preoperative appraisal.

Recording the free gingival margin on the chart will identify the presence or absence of gingival recession or overgrowth. Recession on all six tooth surfaces should be recorded. It is important to measure the amount of recession (in millimeters) because it provides information for determining total attachment loss.

The next step in the mucogingival examination is to determine the total width or height of keratinized gingiva. The width of keratinized gingiva is determined by measuring with a periodontal probe the distance from the gingival margin to the mucogingival junction. The width of attached gingiva is determined by subtracting the probing depth (free gingiva) from the amount of keratinized gingiva (Fig. 18–18■). Mucogingival involvement exists when no attached gingiva is present on a tooth. To establish the position of the mucogingival junction, move the side of the periodontal probe gently across the alveolar mucosa in an apical-coronal direction until the tissue stops moving (Fig. 18–19■). At this point, elastic fibers are not present, and attached gingiva is coronal to the mucogingival junction. Other methods include the visual method. The problem with this technique is that with inflammation, the gingiva is red, and it will be difficult to differentiate between the red alveolar mucosa and the gingiva. Another method is to pull the lip outward, and the mucogingival junction is seen at the point of tension. This is sometimes misleading, and the actual location of the mucogingival junction is not always distinguished.

To determine if any frenal attachments are encroaching on the gingival margin, retract the cheeks and lips laterally by pulling with the thumb and index finger, and watch for movement of the gingival margin in the frenal attachment area.

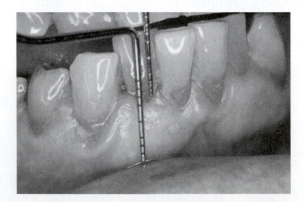

Figure 18–18   (*Left probe*) Determination of the amount of gingiva (free + attached) by measuring from the free gingival margin to the mucogingival junction. (*Right probe*) Determination of the amount of attached gingiva by subtracting the probing depth (right probe measurement) from the total width of gingiva (left probe measurement).

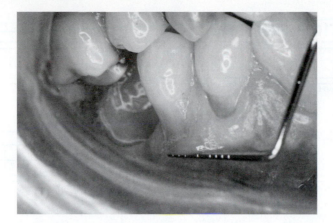

Figure 18–19   The periodontal probe is gently placed on the alveolar mucosa and moved coronally until the tissue does not move. This is the mucogingival junction.

Delayed Passive Eruption

Delayed passive eruption occurs in adults when the free gingival margin failed to migrate apically toward the CEJ and still remains on or near the cervical bulge of the enamel, creating a "gummy smile" (Fig. 18–20■). This condition is also seen in children up to the time of completed eruption of permanent teeth. This is a normal situation, and the process of passive eruption ultimately will move the free gingival margin apically.

Documentation

Documentation of clinical findings is done on a periodontal chart. Many types of charts are available. An example of a chart is given in Figure 18–21■. It is important to accurately date and record all clinical findings for legal reasons and to permit the comparison of pretreatment measurements with posttreatment values. Documentation includes the medical and dental histories, chief complaint, oral hygiene evaluation (plaque index), and gingival and periodontal evaluations.

Findings from the periodontal examination should be interpreted together with the medical, dental, oral hygiene, gingival, and radiographic assessments. Recording of clinical attachment level is important for long-term monitoring of patients for periodontal destruction.

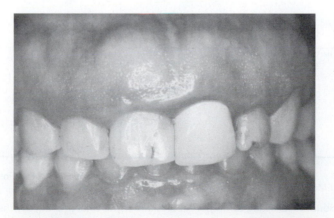

Figure 18–20   A 40-year-old patient exhibiting delayed passive eruption. Note that the gingival margin is located on the cervical bulge of the enamel.

PERIODONTICS RECORD

FILE NO. ☐☐☐☐☐☐

NAME	BIRTHDATE	CLINICIAN	EXAM DATE

CHIEF PERIODONTAL COMPLAINT

ORAL HYGIENE METHODS
  Current:

  Rx:

HISTORY OF PERIODONTAL ILLNESS

PLAQUE INDEX (P.I.)

Date								
P.I.								

PREVIOUS PERIO (prophylaxis, other perio, inc. dates)

HABIT HISTORY

OCCLUSAL OBSERVATIONS

  Arch Rel. (angle):   Overbite: Overjet:

  Teeth in fremitus:

  C.R. ⟶ C.O.:

  C.O. ⟶ P.:

  P.:

  R.L. working:

    non-working:

  L.L. working:

    non-working:

  TMD:

RADIOGRAPHIC FINDINGS

SOFT TISSUE EXAM

ETIOLOGY

  Local Factors:

GINGIVAL EXAM (color, form, density, bleeding on probing, etc.)

  Microbiological Findings:

  Occlusal Factors:

  Systemic Factors:

DIAGNOSIS

TREATMENT PLAN

PRE-TREATMENT PROGNOSIS

SYSTEMIC FACTORS OF IMPORTANCE IN TREATMENT

(Courtesy Department of Oral Biology, School of
Dental Medicine, State University of New York at Buffalo, Buffalo, NY)

Figure 18–21   A periodontal charting form that records initial and final probing depths, clinical attachment levels, tooth mobility, bleeding points, furcation involvement, and gingival recession.

PERIODONTAL EXAMINATION

PATIENT'S NAME:_____   DATE:_____

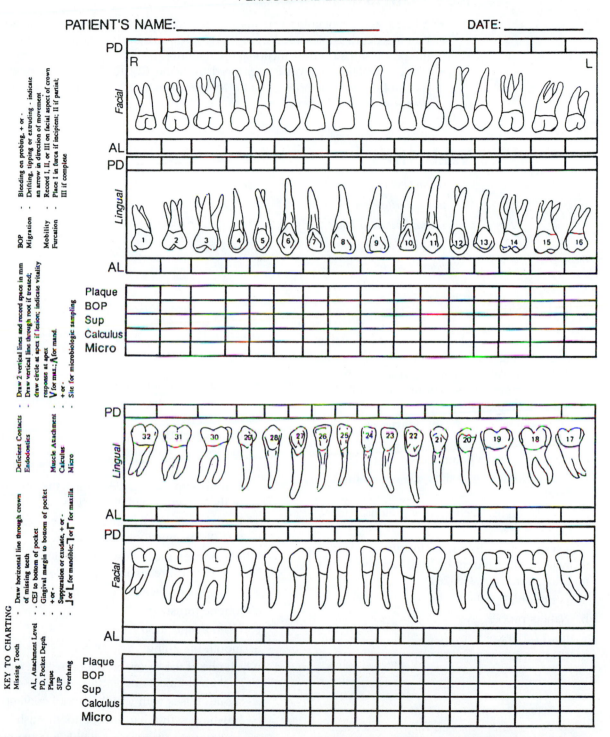

Figure 18–21, cont.   A periodontal charting form that records initial and final probing depths, clinical attachment levels, tooth mobility, bleeding points, furcation involvement, and gingival recession.

Key Points

- All new and maintaining patients should receive a periodontal examination.
- Probing depth is measured from the gingival margin to wherever the tip of the probe stops (in the junctional epithelium).
- Clinical attachment level is measured from the CEJ to the apical extent of the probe and is a more accurate long-term measurement for disease progression than probing depths.

Web Sites

www.perio.org

www.dentalcare.com

www.dent.ucla.edu

www.guideline.gov

www.colgate.com

Self-Quiz

1. Which one of the following reasons explains why measuring the clinical attachment levels (CALs) is a more reliable method for determing clinical attachment loss over time than probing depth measurements? (p. 253)

   a. Less penetration into the junctional epithelium occurs.

   b. Stable reference point is used (e.g., CEJ).

   c. More measuring points are used on the tooth.

   d. Less bleeding occurs at periodontal active sites.

2. Which one of the following instruments is best to measure the amount of horizontal bone loss in a furcation? (pp. 258–261)

   a. periodontal probe

   b. Nabers probe

   c. no. 11/12 explorer

   d. CH3 explorer

3. Which one of the following techniques describes how visible recession is recorded? (p. 262)

   a. Use a periodontal probe to measure from the cementoenamel junction to the free gingival margin.

   b. Use a periodontal probe to measure from the free gingival margin to the base of the pocket.

   c. Use an explorer to determine the location of the cementoenamel junction.

   d. Use an explorer to determine the apical extent of the junctional epithelium.

4. Which one of the following conditions is related to gingival recession? (pp. 262–263)

   a. grinding and clenching of teeth

   b. tongue thrusting

   c. tooth malposition

   d. mouth breathing

5. Which one of the following is a cause of a mucogingival involvement or defect? (pp. 265–266)

   a. mouth rinses with a high alcohol content

   b. brushing with a hard-bristle toothbrush

   c. inadequate amount or width of attached gingiva

   d. inadequate amount or width of alveolar mucosa

References

Armitage, G. C. 1995. Clinical evaluation of periodontal diseases. *Periodontology 2000* 7:39–52.

Armitage, G. C. 1996. Periodontal diseases: diagnosis. *Ann. Periodontol.* 1:37–215.

Armitage, G. C., G. K. Svanberg, and H. Löe. 1977. Microscopic evaluation of clinical measurements of connective tissue attachment levels. *J. Clin. Peridontol.* 4:173–190.

Bawden, J. W., and G. H. DeFriese. (eds.). 1981. *Planning for dental care on a statewide basis: The North Carolina Dental Manpower Project.* Chapel Hill: The Dental Foundation of North Carolina.

Brown, L. J., R. C. Oliver, and H. Löe. 1989. Periodontal diseases in the U.S. in 1981: Prevalence, severity, extent, and role in tooth mortality. *J. Periodontol.* 60:363–380.

Carlos, J. P., J. A. Brunelle, and M. D. Wolfe. 1987. Attachment loss versus pocket depth as indicators of periodontal disease: A methodologic note. *J. Periodont. Res.* 22:524–525.

Dunlap, R. M., and M. E. Gher. 1985. Root surface measurements of the mandibular first molar. *J. Periodontol.* 56:234–238.

Easly, J. R., and G. A. Drennan. 1969. Morphological classification of the furca. *J. Can. Dent. Assoc.* 35:105–107.

Garguilo, A. W., F. M. Wentz, and B. Orban. 1961. Dimensions and relations of the dentogingival junction in humans. *J. Periodontol.* 32:261–267.

Gher, M. E., and R. W. Dunlap. 1985. Linear variation of the root surface area of the maxillary first molar. *J. Periodontol.* 56:39–43.

Goodson, J. M. 1986. Clinical measurements of periodontitis. *J. Clin. Periodontol.* 13:446–455.

Greenstein, G., and J. Caton. 1990. Periodontal disease activity: A critical assessment. *J. Periodontol.* 61:543–552.

Gunsolley, J. C., S. M. Quinn, J. Tew, C. M. Gooss, C. M. Brooks, and H. A. Schenkein. 1998. The effect of smoking on individuals with minimal periodontal destruction. *J. Periodontol.* 69:165–170.

Haffajee, A. D., S. S. Socransky, and J. M. Goodson. 1983. Clinical parameters as predictors of destructive periodontal disease activity. *J. Clin. Periodontol.* 10:257–265.

Jeffcoat, M. K. 1994. Current concepts in periodontal disease testing. *J. Am. Dent. Assoc.* 125:1071–1078.

Joshipura, K. J., R. L. Kent, and P. F. DePaola. 1994. Gingival recession: Intra-oral distribution and associated factors. *J. Periodontol.* 65:864–871.

Keagle, J. G., J. J. Garnick, J. R. Searle, G. E. King, and P. K. Morse. 1989. Gingival resistance to probing forces: I. Determination of optimal probe diameter. *J. Periodontol.* 60:167–171.

Lamster, I. B., R. S. Celenti, H. H. Jans, J. B. Fine, and J. T. Grbic. 1993. Current status of tests for periodontal disease. *Adv. Dent. Res.* 7:182–190.

Lang, N. P., A. R. Joss, and S. Nyman. 1990. Absence of bleeding on probing: An indicator of periodontal stability. *J. Clin. Periodontol.* 17:714–721.

Lang, N. P., and H. Löe. 1993. Clinical management of periodontal diseases. *Periodontology 2000* 2:128–139.

Listgarten, M. A., R. Mao, and P. J. Robinson. 1976. Periodontal probing and the relationship of the probe tip to periodontal tissues. *J. Periodontol.* 47:511–513.

McFall, W. T., Jr., J. D. Bader, G. R. Rozier, and D. Ramsey. 1988. Presence of periodontal data in patient records of general practitioners. *J. Periodontol.* 59:445–449.

Miller, S. C. 1950. *Textbook of periodontia,* 3rd ed., 125. Philadelphia: Blakiston.

Reddy, M. S. 1997. The use of periodontal probes and radiographs in clinical trials of diagnostic tests. *Ann. Periodontol.* 2:113–122.

Robinson, P. J., and R. M. Vitaek. 1979. The relationship between gingival inflammation and resistance to probe penetration. *J. Periodont. Res.* 14:230–243.

Spray, J. R., J. J. Garnick, L. R. Doles, and J. J. Klawitter. 1978. Microscopic demonstration of the position of periodontal probes. *J. Periodontol.* 49:148–152.

Tarnow, D., and P. Fletcher. 1984. Classification of the vertical component of furcation involvement. *J. Periodontol.* 55:283–284.

Towfighi, P. P., M. A. Brunsvold, A. T. Storey, R. M. Arnold, D. E. Willman, and C. A. McMahan. 1997. Pathologic migration of anterior teeth in patients with moderate to severe periodontitis. *J. Periodontol.* 68:967–972.

van der Velden, U. 1979. Probing force and the relationship of the probe tip to the periodontal tissues. *J. Clin. Periodontol.* 6:106–114.

Wennström, J. L. 1994. Mucogingival surgery. In eds. N. P. Lang and T. Karring, *Proceedings of the 1st European Workshop on Periodontology,* 193–199. London: Quintessence.

Wennström, J. L. 1996. Mucogingival therapy. *Ann. Periodontol.* 1:671–701.

Wennström, J. L., and J. Lindhe. 1983a. Plaque-induced gingival inflammation in the absence of attached gingiva in dogs. *J. Clin. Periodontol.* 10:266–276.

Wennström, J. L., and J. Lindhe. 1983b. The role of attached gingiva for maintenance of periodontal health: Healing following excisional and grafting procedures in dogs. *J. Clin. Periodontol.* 10:206–221.

Williams, R. C., J. D. Beck, and S. N. Offenbacher. 1996. The impact of new technologies on the diagnosis and treatment of periodontal disease: A look to the future. *J. Clin. Periodontol.* 23:299–305.

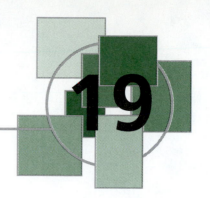

Radiographic Assessment

Herbert Frommer, D.D.S.

Outline

Goal

To provide a radiology background that is used in conjunction with clinical data to recognize and classify periodontal diseases.

Educational Objectives

Upon completion of this chapter, the reader should be able to:

Identify and discuss the periodontal structures seen on a radiograph.

Discuss the rationale for radiographs in periodontics.

KEY WORDS

- full-mouth survey
- conventional radiographs
- exposure time
- paralleling technique
- direct digital radiography
- computed tomographic (CT) scans

Explain the features of conventional and computer-based digital imaging.

List and discuss the benefits and limitations of radiographs used in periodontics.

Explain the radiographic improvements aimed at decreasing patient radiation exposure.

Discuss the types of radiographs used in the treatment planning and evaluation of implants.

Introduction

The proper classification, evaluation, and treatment of the periodontal diseases can be accomplished only with a combination of radiographic and clinical examinations (Fig. 19–1■). One must be aware of the diagnostic limitations of radiographs because periodontal diseases have both soft tissue and bony components. Soft-tissue changes such as inflammation, gingival enlargement, and recession cannot be seen on radiographs because such tissues are radiolucent and therefore appear black. Owing to the superimposition of the buccal and lingual alveolar bone plates, bone loss in some areas also may not be seen. Radiographs essentially portray a three-dimensional disease process in two planes. This point must be kept in mind when viewing radiographs because the appearance can be very misleading.

Despite these limitations, a proper periodontal classification cannot be made without a full-mouth survey. Radiographs serve to (1) identify predisposing factors, (2) detect early to moderate bone changes where treatment can preserve the dentition, (3) approximate the amount of bone loss and its location, (4) help in evaluating the prognosis of affected teeth and the restorative needs of these teeth, and (5) serve as baseline data and as a means to evaluate posttreatment results.

This chapter will discuss the role of conventional radiographs (i.e., radiographs taken on film with an x-ray machine) and computer-based image processing (i.e., the use of a computer to display and enhance images of teeth and bone).

Figure 19–1
Radiographs are used to obtain a visual image of the bone and teeth or dental implants. (Courtesy of Procter & Gamble, Cincinnati, OH)

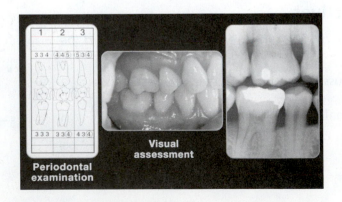

Conventional Radiographs: Intraoral Technique

Parameters

The three parameters, or choices, that the dental professional selects at the control panel of an x-ray machine are kilovoltage, milliamperage, and exposure time. Understanding the effect of each of these parameters on the diagnostic x-ray beam is important and will help in making a correct classification of the disease process (i.e., dental hygiene diagnosis).

Kilovoltage The amount of penetration of the x-ray beam is controlled by the kilovoltage. The suitable range for dental radiography is 65 to 100 kilovolt peak (kVp). This range is determined by the density of the objects to be radiographed (e.g., teeth, bone). Kilovoltage settings above 100 kVp result in overpenetration, and settings below 45 kVp would result in underpenetration. Kilovoltage settings in the range of 45 to 65 kVp, although producing a diagnostic beam, are never used because of the excess secondary radiation that results.

The question to be answered is: "Within the acceptable kilovoltage range, what kilovoltage is most appropriate for periodontal diagnosis?" The answer is determined by the degree of density and contrast that is most diagnostic for the clinician. Density is the degree of blackness on a film, and contrast is the difference in the degrees of blackness between adjacent areas.

Radiographs have a high degree of (short scale) contrast when low kilovolt-peak settings are used. The x-ray photons either penetrate the tissue or are absorbed—a sort of yes or no, black or white reaction. When higher kilovolt-peak settings are used, there is less contrast, and the overall tone of the radiograph is gray (Fig. 19–2■). This occurs because there is much more partial penetration with the resulting long-scale contrast. Such low contrast is not as satisfying visually as high contrast, but early changes in object density such as early bone loss may be seen in the gradations of gray as a result of more selective penetration, which is not present in high-contrast films. Theoretically, therefore, higher kilovolt-peak settings with their resulting long-scale contrast produce better results in terms of periodontal diagnosis. A number of clinicians, however, feel that the human eye is not capable of seeing these very subtle gray changes and recommend using 75 kVp, where bony changes are distinguished more easily.

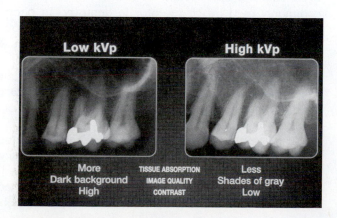

Figure 19–2
Selection of settings. (Courtesy of Procter & Gamble, Cincinnati, OH)

Milliamperage   The milliamperage setting controls the number of x-rays generated in a given exposure time. As noted above, the kilovoltage determines the quality (penetration) of the x-rays produced, but the milliamperage determines the quantity of x-rays produced.

It is more precise, however, to consider the concept of milliampere seconds (mAs) than milliamperage alone because the milliamperage setting and duration of exposure are interdependent values. In order to make a diagnostic exposure, different types of film need different milliamperage-second settings, and this is determined by the sensitivity of the film and the focal distance of the film. If the milliamperage setting is increased, then the exposure time can be reduced. For example, an exposure, at a given kilovolt-peak setting, of 1 s using 10 mA is 10 mAs. A 2-s exposure at the same kilovolt-peak setting using 5 mA would produce an identical film because the resulting exposure is again 10 mAs (10 1 = 10 and 5 $\times$ 2 = 10). Both patients would receive the same amount of radiation. The only advantage of the higher milliamperage is the decrease in exposure time, which lessens the chance of patient movement. Common practice today is to use short exposure times at a magnitude of 6 impulses (1/10 s), so patient movement is less of a factor (see below). This reduction in exposure time to 1/10 s alone, however, will not prevent patient movement or gagging; it just facilitates obtaining the radiograph before such movement occurs. Thus it is apparent that it makes no diagnostic and little technical difference if we work at 5, 6, 7, 10, or 15 mA. It should be pointed out that conventional dental x-ray machines do not have milliamperage settings higher than 15 because of heat limitations within the tube.

Dental x-ray machines do not emit a continuous stream of radiation when an exposure is made; rather, they emit a series of radiation impulses. The number of impulses depends on the number of cycles per second in the electric current being used. With 60-cycle alternating current, which is standard, there are 60 x-ray pulses per second. Newer-generation x-ray machines have timer dials calibrated in impulses, not in seconds. On the timer dial, 15 would mean 15 impulses or 15/60-s exposure. These extremely short exposure times can only be controlled by an electric timer. The old mechanical timers are not this precise, and all x-ray machines should have electronic timers that are capable of delivering short, accurate exposure times.

Film Type

Even with the introduction of digital radiographs, film remains by far the most commonly used image receptor in dentistry. In periodontal diagnostic radiology, the most commonly used sizes are number 1 (narrow anterior), number 2 (adult size), and number 3 (long bitewing). Number 2 film with either loops or stick-on tabs can be converted into a bitewing film.

The film sensitivity, or speed, determines how much radiation for how long (e.g., milliampere seconds) is necessary to produce an image on the film. The speed of the film is determined mainly by the size of the silver halide crystals in the film emulsion.

Films are designated by American National Standards Institute (ANSI) categories, with category A film being the slowest and category F film being the fastest. At present, only category E and D films are available for use. The category E film speed is twice as fast as category D film and thus needs half the radiation exposure. Both films are equally diagnostic. The early objections to category E film based on decreased definition and lack of contrast have not been supported by studies in the literature. Thus, because it has the same diagnostic capability and results in 50% less radiation exposure than category D film, category E speed film generally should be used.

Paralleling versus the Bisecting Technique

In periodontal radiographic diagnosis, use of the paralleling technique with a 16-inch film focal distance for periapical radiographs is the method of choice. In this technique, the teeth and the film are parallel to each other, and the central ray of the x-ray beam is directed perpendicular (right angle) to both. With this technique, there will be no dimensional distortion or false and misleading indications of bone levels. The 16-inch focal distance, the so-called long cone, is used to compensate for the image enlargement caused by the increase in tooth-to-film distance necessary to achieve the parallelism between the teeth and the film.

In the bisecting technique, the film is placed as close to the tooth as possible, and the central ray of the x-ray beam is directed perpendicular to an imaginary line between the angle formed by the long axis of the tooth and the plane of the film. This technique is not recommended for periodontal diagnosis because it results in a distortion and exaggeration of the alveolar bone level. Excess vertical angulation (i.e., distortion of the length of the roots, either foreshortening or elongation) may lead to a perception of early furcation involvement when there is actually no interradicular bone loss (Fig. 19–3■).

Conventional Radiographs Used in Periodontics

Table 19–1■ reviews the different types of conventional intraoral and extraoral radiographs used in conjunction with clinical data to recognize and classify periodontal diseases (Hodges, 1997). Many radiographs are available, but periapical, bitewing, and panoramic radiographs are used most commonly in periodontics to evaluate periodontal structures.

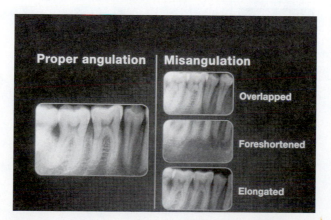

Figure 19–3 Diagnostic quality. (Courtesy of Procter & Gamble, Cincinnati, OH)

Table 19–1	Selection Criteria of Conventional Radiographs for Periodontics	
Type of Film	**Indications**	**Limitations**
Periapical	Viewing the apex of the root for any pathology (i.e., periapical radiolucency) Determining morphology (shape) of roots and root length Recognizing horizontal and vertical patterns of bone loss Evaluating implants Viewing interproximal dental caries	Technique errors may reduce the ability to detect crestal bone loss. Detection of incipient interproximal dental caries. Detection of pathologic lesions in the mandible and maxilla. Evaluation of other structures such as sinuses and the mandibular canal.
Bitewing	Viewing the alveolar crest bone height (use vertical bitewings) Evaluation of defective restorations (i.e., overhang)	Cannot view the apical area of a tooth. Evaluation of the morphology and length of roots.
Panoramic	Viewing the area of the maxilla and mandibular arches (i.e., impacted teeth, sinuses, and pathologic lesions)	Not used for recognizing periodontal diseases or dental caries.

Conventional radiographs give a history of past periodontal disease destruction but do not provide information on current periodontal disease status. As mentioned earlier, radiographs represent a two-dimensional view of three-dimensional objects, so it is difficult to recognize the slight changes in alveolar bone that would indicate early or mild periodontal disease. Other limitations and benefits of radiographs are discussed in Table 19–2■. As a result, radiographs are used primarily in periodontics to determine the severity and pattern of bone loss, the morphology (i.e., length and shape) of roots, root proximity, pathologic lesions such as a cyst or an abscess, and the effects of occlusion.

Just as a single periodontal probing recording only provides information on past disease activity, it is important to compare several sets of full-mouth radiographs over a period of time to evaluate for periodontal disease progression (Hol-

Table 19–2	Benefits and Limitations of Conventional Radiographs

Radiographs *do* show:
   crestal alveolar bone levels
   clinical crown-to-root ratio
   calculus on proximal tooth surfaces
   metallic restorations
   morphology of roots (i.e., root length, root shape)

Radiographs *do not* show:
   periodontal pockets
   buccal and lingual plates of bone
   hard-to-soft-tissue relationship
   a successfully treated patient
   bone loss until about 30 to 50% of loss of mineralization occurs

lender, 1992; Jeffcoat & Reddy, 1991). In addition, radiographic findings always should be correlated with the corresponding probing depth measurements.

Periapical Radiographs

A periapical radiograph shows the entire area around a tooth, including the apex of the root. Periapical radiographs are part of the full-mouth survey and are taken of anterior and posterior teeth. The number of periapical films taken for a full-mouth survey varies from 14 to 20.

Film technique errors occur quite often with periapical radiographs as a result of improper alignment of the film with the tooth and the x-ray beam with the film. Excessive vertical angulation causes foreshortening (roots appear shorter and the alveolar crest appears to be closer to the cementoenamel junction than it truly is) and occlusal surfaces to be cut off. This can result in inaccurate recording of the crestal alveolar bone level. Insufficient vertical angulation causes elongation and roots to be cut off from the x-ray. Overlapping of proximal tooth surfaces is caused by improper horizontal angulation of the radiographic beam.

Bitewing Radiographs

The bitewing radiograph is by far the best radiograph to interpret posterior alveolar bone levels and bone loss with the least amount of distortion or technique error. Bitewing radiographs show the crowns of the maxillary and mandibular teeth and the alveolar crest. Identification of carious lesions is best with bitewing radiographs. Posterior bitewing radiographs are part of the full-mouth survey and can include up to four views. Bitewing films can be placed either horizontally or vertically (Fig. 19–4■). Vertical bitewing radiographs are especially useful in periodontal patients with moderate to severe bone loss (this is determined by periodontal probing and previous radiographs, if available) in order to evaluate crestal bone. Horizontal bitewing radiographs do not show the entire bone height. Two posterior vertical bitewing radiographs may be sufficient, however, for visualization of both maxillary and mandibular teeth. The radiographs are taken perpendicular to the alveolar crest so that the crestal bone is depicted accurately. Anterior vertical bitewing radiographs also can be taken.

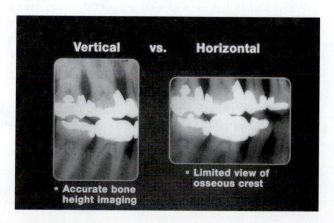

Figure 19–4   View selection—bitewing. (Courtesy of Procter & Gamble, Cincinnati, OH)

Figure 19–5 View selection—panoramic. (Courtesy of Procter & Gamble, Cincinnati, OH)

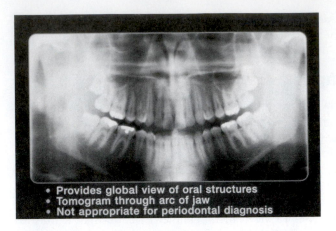

- Provides global view of oral structures
- Tomogram through arc of jaw
- Not appropriate for periodontal diagnosis

Panoramic Radiology

The image on a panoramic film shows the entire dentition and supporting bone structure from condyle to condyle on one film (Fig. 19–5■). The resulting image, however, does not have the same degree of definition seen on an intraoral periapical or bitewing radiograph. This shortcoming is inherent to the pantomographic process and is also caused by the use of intensifying screens.

Many diagnostic problems in dentistry require a high degree of radiographic definition. Early detection of such conditions as disruption of the periodontal ligament, loss of crestal alveolar bone, a thickened periodontal ligament, and ongoing caries requires the maximum amount of radiographic definition. Because of this, panoramic films have very limited value in the diagnosis of periodontal disease. If a panoramic film is used instead of a full-mouth survey, it must be augmented with both anterior and posterior bitewing radiographs and selected periapical films where indicated. Many technique errors can occur with panoramic radiographs, including improper patient positioning and operator errors.

Periodontal Structures

In order to recognize disease, the normal anatomy must be understood. Periodontal anatomy identified on radiographs includes the supporting structures such as the alveolar bone, periodontal ligament space, and cementum (Fig. 19–6■). Since gingiva is a noncalcified soft tissue structure, the x-rays go completely through it and are not absorbed, and thus the gingiva is not seen as a radiopaque structure.

Interdental Septum

The normal crest of interproximal bone runs parallel to a line drawn between the cementoenamel junctions on adjoining teeth at a level approximately 2.0 mm apical to the cementoenamel junction (Fig. 19–7■). The shape of the alveolar crest is determined primarily by the contact area of adjacent teeth and the shape of the cementoenamel junction. The alveolar crest is flatter in posterior areas and more convex and pointed anteriorly. The width of the interdental septum can be determined by viewing a radiograph. The interdental septum can be narrow in cases of close

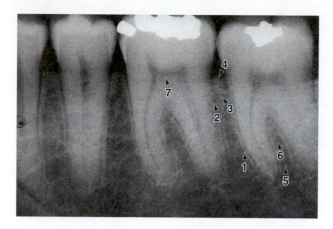

Figure 19–6
Radiograph of the periodontal structures (1 = lamina dura; 2 = periodontal ligament space; 3 = interproximal bone; 4 = alveolar bone crest; 5 = trabecular bone; 6 = interradicular bone; 7 = pulp).

root proximity. In some instances, the roots of adjacent teeth are so close that there may be little to no cancellous bone. Teeth that frequently show close root proximity include the distobuccal root of the maxillary first molar and the mesiobuccal root of the maxillary second molar and the mandibular anteriors.

Radiographically, a thin radiopaque line surrounds the entire tooth and is continuous with the alveolar crest (see Fig. 19–6). This is referred to as the lamina dura. Clinically, it represents the alveolar bone that lines the tooth socket.

Periodontal Ligament Space

The periodontal ligament fibers (or principal fibers) transverse from the cementum to the alveolar bone. Since these fibers are soft tissue, they are not evident on radiographs. Instead, the space where the fibers are located appears as a radiolucent area surrounding the entire tooth (see Fig. 19–6). On one side of the space is the cementum, and the other border is the lamina dura. Evaluating the width of the periodontal ligament (space) is important during the occlusal examination. If a tooth has excessive occlusal loads placed on it, the periodontal ligament compensates for the resulting tooth mobility by becoming thicker. This shows up on a radiograph as a widened periodontal ligament (Fig. 19–8■).

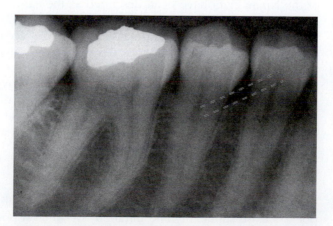

Figure 19–7
Radiograph showing the normal relationship of the crestal bone level being parallel with the cementoenamel junctions of adjacent teeth. No bone loss is depicted in this radiograph.

Figure 19–8 The maxillary second premolar shows a widened periodontal ligament space due to an excessive occlusal load placed on it.

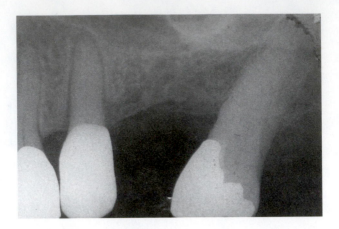

Periodontal Interpretation

Using radiographs as an evaluation tool in the recognition of periodontitis has several limitations that are listed in Table 19–2. It is difficult to determine changes in bone simply by viewing radiographs. For this reason, clinical data must be incorporated with radiographic findings in an assessment of periodontal status. For example, a patient's radiographs may show moderate bone loss, but previously the patient may have had periodontal surgery for pocket reduction. Thus the radiographs still show bone loss, but the periodontal charting shows probing depths from 1 to 3 mm without bleeding on probing. At this time the patient does not have periodontitis. The radiographs show past disease activity, not what is occurring presently.

Bone Loss

Conventional radiographs represent an insensitive technique in detecting early, small bony defects (bone loss). Before bone loss is identified on a radiograph, approximately 30 to 50% loss of mineralization must occur (Jeffcoat, 1992; Jeffcoat & Reddy, 1991). In addition, radiographically, the cortical bone plates may hide slight bone loss.

Radiographic evaluation of alveolar bone loss associated with periodontitis is based on the status of the interdental septum. Fuzziness or breaks in the continuity of the lamina dura have been described as the earliest radiographic signs of bone loss (Carranza, 1996). However, the radiographic observation that the loss of crestal lamina dura is a sign of periodontitis is not totally accurate (Armitage, 1996). Clinical studies have shown that sites did not break down even though there was a break in the lamina dura. Moreover, absence of crestal lamina dura is a common radiographic finding in normal, nondiseased interproximal sites (Rams, Listgarten, & Slots, 1994). Thus it is more accurate to state that the presence of an intact crestal lamina dura represents a stable site than that the absence of a crestal lamina dura indicates a disease site (Armitage, 1996; Rams et al., 1994).

Patterns of Bone Loss

The severity, distribution, and pattern of bone loss can be determined from radiographs. Clinically, as measured with a periodontal probe, two types of bony pockets exist: suprabony and infrabony. A gingival pocket or pseudopocket is not associated with bone loss. These bony pockets are associated with two patterns of bone loss: horizontal and vertical. In horizontal bone loss, interdental bone is destroyed equally along the surfaces of adjacent teeth (Fig. 19–9a■). Suprabony pockets, where the base of the pocket is coronal to the alveolar bone crest, are characterized by horizontal bone loss. In vertical (angular) bone loss, the resorption on one tooth sharing the septum is greater than on the other tooth (Fig. 19–9b■). Infrabony pockets, where the base of the pocket is apical to the alveolar crest, are associated with vertical bone loss.

Severity of Bone Loss

The severity, or amount, of bone loss is classified as mild, moderate, or severe. One way to determine the amount of bone loss is to determine the percentage of bone loss. This is done by measuring the length from the cementoenamel junction to the tip of the root and the distance from the cementoenamel junction to the alveolar crest. The percentage of bone loss is calculated by dividing this number by the root length and multiplying by 100 (Hodges, 1997). Bone loss of less than 20% is usually classified as mild; bone loss between 20 and 50% is moderate; and bone loss of more than 50% is severe. It also should be remembered that 30 to 50% bone loss must be present before it is evident radiographically.

Determination of Bone Loss

The first step in determining if there is radiographic bone loss is to draw an imaginary line connecting the cementoenamel junction of adjacent teeth and then a line on the alveolar crest. If the alveolar crest is more than approximately 2 mm apical to the cementoenamel junction, there is bone loss. The next step is to determine if the pattern of bone loss is horizontal or vertical. In vertical bone loss, the bone

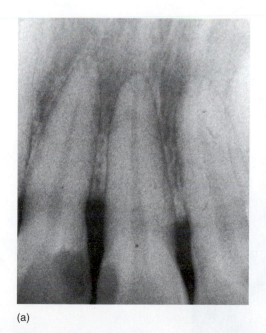

(a)

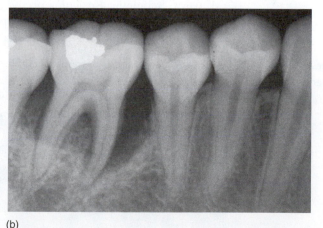

(b)

Figure 19–9   (a) A periapical radiograph showing a horizontal pattern of bone loss. (b) Vertical or angular bone loss on the mesial surface of the first molar with furcation involvement.

Figure 19–10   The area between the premolar and molar shows uneven crestal alveolar bone that parallels the uneven cementoenamel junctions. There is horizontal bone loss but not angular bone loss.

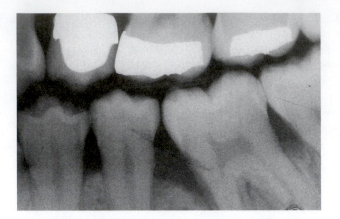

level is not parallel to the cementoenamel junctions of adjacent teeth. In horizontal bone loss, the bone level is parallel to the cementoenamel junctions of adjacent teeth. If a tooth is not in the normal occlusal plane (e.g., extruded, intruded, or tipped), the bone level will not be in a straight line, but neither will the cementoenamel junctions, so the lines will still be parallel to each other (Fig. 19–10■).

Despite these limitations, conventional radiographs are still mandatory in the recognition and treatment of periodontal diseases. They provide an excellent measurement of the history of periodontal disease in a patient and provide important information about the interproximal bone changes that occur over time (Douglass, Levine, Otomo-Corgel, Sims, & Taggart, 1991). The detection of predisposing factors is one of the most important roles of radiography in periodontal diseases, and the detection and elimination of local irritants are essential steps in prevention or actual periodontal therapy.

Calculus

Early deposits, small and not fully calcified, are not seen radiographically. Even calcified supragingival calculus, which is seen most often on the lingual surfaces of lower anterior teeth and the buccal surfaces of upper molars, is not seen clearly in its early stage because of superimposition of tooth structure (e.g., roots) and cortical plates. Subgingival calculus on the proximal surfaces is more easily detected in the early calcified stages. Calculus appears as an irregularly pointed radiographic projection from the proximal root surface (Fig. 19–11■).

Figure 19–11   Calculus spurs evident on all tooth surfaces.

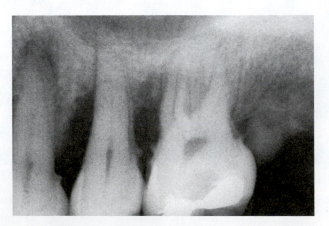

Anatomic Configurations

Only through radiographic examination can information about the size, shape, and positions of the roots of periodontally involved teeth be obtained. It is important to document the lengths of the root trunks of multirooted teeth to ensure tooth survival. A tooth with a short root trunk has "higher" furcation entrances and longer roots. A tooth with a long root trunk has shorter roots, but the furcation entrance is more apical. Therefore, more bone has to be destroyed in the development of a furcation involvement.

Another important factor in the overall periodontal prognosis is the shape of the roots. The space between the roots is important. Roots of multirooted teeth can be diverging, converging, or conical. Diverging roots have a larger surface area for periodontal attachment including bone. Teeth with thicker, diverging, longer roots have a better prognosis than conical or converging roots. Roots also can be long and tapered or short, bulbous, and conical. These factors are important in evaluating the present condition and planning periodontal and restorative therapy.

In restorative case planning, the crown-to-root ratio is an important factor. This ratio is the relationship of the length of the root embedded in bone compared with the length of the rest of the tooth. The greater the length of the tooth embedded in bone, the better is the prognosis for support of a fixed or removable prosthesis. A 2:1 crown-to-root ratio is desirable. Teeth with bulbous roots have more area for attachment than those with fine tapered roots.

Radiographically Detectable Periodontal Changes

Gingivitis

Because gingivitis is a soft-tissue change, there are no radiographic findings other than the presence of predisposing or contributing factors (e.g., condition of restorations).

Slight (Mild) Periodontitis

This stage of periodontal disease is characterized radiographically by changes in the crest of the interproximal bone septum and triangulation of the periodontal ligament space (Fig. 19–12■). Triangulation is widening of the periodontal ligament space at the crest of the interproximal septum that gives the appearance of a radiolucent triangle to what is normally a radiolucent band. Fading of the density of the crest with cup-shaped defects appears in the early stages of periodontitis.

Moderate Periodontitis

In this stage, bone loss may be apparent in both horizontal and vertical planes. Radiolucencies appear in the furcations of multirooted teeth, indicating interradicular bone loss. This is a furcation involvement and is confirmed clinically using a Nabers probe. In this stage, horizontal bone loss on the buccal or lingual surface

Figure 19–12   Slight (mild) chronic periodontitis. Generalized slight horizontal bone loss of less than 20%.

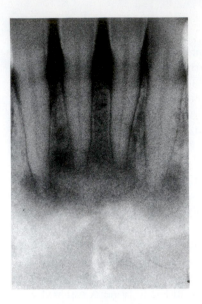

may go undetected because of superimposition. Careful examination of the radiograph in most cases reveals a difference in density indicating different levels of bone on the buccal and lingual surfaces (Fig. 19–13■).

Severe Periodontitis

This stage of periodontal disease is easily identified radiographically by the advanced vertical and horizontal patterns of bone loss, furcation involvement, thickened periodontal ligament, and indications of changes in tooth position (Fig. 19–14■).

Periodontal Abscess

The radiographic signs of a periodontal abscess may vary greatly. Such a diagnosis is dictated by an acute clinical manifestation. Clinically, a deep periodontal pocket is usually found. The periodontal abscess is caused by the occlusion of an existing pocket; therefore, the radiograph of the acute episode may not vary greatly from previous radiographs of the existing condition that produced the pocket. In other instances, there may be signs of rapid and extensive bone destruction.

Figure 19–13
Moderate chronic periodontitis. Localized furcation involvement on the mandibular molar.

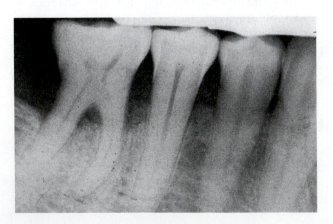

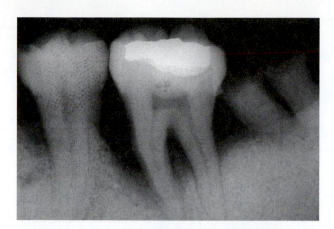

Figure 19–14 Severe chronic periodontitis. Generalized extensive horizontal and vertical bone loss of more than 50% and numerous furcation involvements.

Frequency of Radiographs (Selection Criteria)

Among the many methods of reducing a patient's radiation exposure (e.g., collimation, filtration, and fast film), selection criteria also are very important and are the responsibility of the dentist. Selection criteria are descriptions of clinical conditions and historical data that identify patients who are most likely to benefit from a particular radiographic examination. These guidelines help the practitioner select which patient needs radiographs and determine which radiographs are needed. The final decision rests with the individual dentist and is determined by professional judgment.

The practice of taking radiographs based on a time interval rather than patient needs, as determined by clinical examination and dental history, is not considered the appropriate way to practice dental radiology. In relation to periodontal care, there should never be a policy, for example, that mandates a new full-mouth survey every 2 years or bitewing radiographs every 6 months. The radiographic needs of each patient are different and should not be based on the calendar but rather on a complete clinical examination and the history of previous periodontal therapy or signs and symptoms of the disease.

An expert panel of dentists under the auspices of the Public Health Service (U.S. Department of Health and Human Services, 1987) has developed guidelines for the prescription of dental radiographs. One of the patient categories is "Periodontal disease or a history of periodontal treatment." The recommendations call for a full-mouth survey for every new patient, comprised of periapical and bitewing films. For the recall examination, radiographs should be taken for evaluation of previous periodontal therapy (e.g., surgery, bone grafting, implants, or when there is a dramatic change in the probing depth measurement). In any patient, radiographs should never be taken before there is a complete clinical examination. Based on this examination, a radiographic prescription is formulated, the films are taken, and a final classification and treatment plan are determined.

Digital Imaging

Radiographic improvements are designed to reduce patient radiation exposure and to simplify identification and measurement of changes in alveolar bone height. The most recent addition to dental radiology is direct digital radiography. Presently, about fifteen systems are available on the market, each with its own variations. Many clinicians are converting from film to digital imaging. With digital imaging, there is an up to 90% reduction in radiation exposure compared with conventional radiographs (Jeffcoat, 1998). Direct digital radiography replaces the film used in a conventional intraoral radiograph with an electronic sensor. This sensor, the approximate size of intraoral film, is placed in the patient's mouth in the same manner as one would place film. The exposure is made, and the sensor sends impulses based on the penetration of the object by the x-ray photons to a computer. These impulses are then digitized and formed into an image by the computer. The image can be stored, printed in hard copy, darkened or lightened, reversed, colorized, magnified, measured, or transmitted to a remote sight.

A computer monitor creates an image using pixels or tiny dots that become a recognizable form when projected on the screen. Viewing the digital radiograph allows the clinician to determine bone loss through the percentage of lightness and darkness of pixels. White, the lightest shade, indicates the maximum amount of bone mineral, whereas black, the darkest shade, indicates absence of bone mineral (Fig. 19–15■).

From a periodontal standpoint, all the diagnostic criteria mentioned previously in terms of conventional radiographs stay the same. The instant imaging is a time advantage and the substantial reduction in patient exposure is desirable, but the periodontal diagnostic capabilities, when compared with film, are about equal. There may be some advantage in determining bone levels by image reversal or colorization, but this varies among practitioners. These systems are available for commercial in-office use.

Digital Subtraction Radiology

Digital subtraction radiology (DSR) magnifies images, allowing detection of osseous changes (bone loss) that are too small to be seen in a visual examination of conventional film. As mentioned earlier, comparing radiographs from different time periods is important in detecting progressive bone loss. Because of the superimpo-

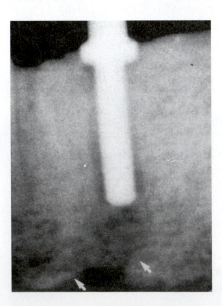

Figure 19–15 An example of a direct digital radiograph. This radiograph was taken during implant surgery to guide in the placement of the implant. Digital images can be changed electronically to improve contrast and density and can magnify the image. The mandibular canal (arrows) is well visualized. (Courtesy of Procter & Gamble, Cincinnati, OH)

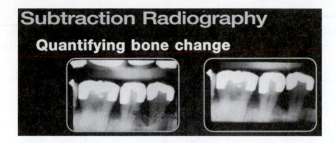

Figure 19–16   Computerized digital radiography is used to quantify the change in bone mineral. A baseline radiograph was taken (*left*). The shaded area indicates 0.84 mm of bone loss between examinations taken over a 6-month period (*right*). This shading allows the area of change to be readily seen. (Courtesy of Procter & Gamble, Cincinnati, OH)

sition of cortical plates and roots of teeth, it is almost impossible to detect changes in the bone level unless there was a dramatic loss of bone (Jeffcoat, 1994). In digital subtraction radiology, two images taken at two different visits are compared, and all structures that do not change, such as cortical plates and roots of teeth, are not shown on (subtracted from) the image. Any changes in bone level are indicated by a color-shaded area; red is for bone loss, and green is for bone gain (Fig. 19–16■). DSR has not been used much in clinical practice because it is a difficult technique to master, but it is used frequently in clinical research.

Radiographs in Implantology

At the present time, the basic diagnostic radiographs used in screening implant patients are conventional radiographs such as periapical, occlusal, and panoramic films. In addition, computed tomographic (CT) scans are used for a three-dimentional view of the bone. It is most important to realize that to diagnose and plan for implant placement, one must be able to view the implant site in three dimensions or planes. As dental professionals, we are used to seeing objects in two planes, mesiodistal and incisoapically. We do not see objects in a three-dimentional view except with occlusal films in the buccolingual plane, and this information is critical in implant planning. Of the techniques used, only CT images can supply this information.

Periapical/Occlusal Films

If the film can be placed parallel to the ridge and the field size allows for visualization of the entire proposed alveolar area, then periapical films can be used. Unfortunately, there are very few patients who fit this criterion, and thus periapical views are of limited value. Occlusal films, if they can be positioned, can augment the periapical film to view the third dimension.

Pantomograms (Panoramic Films)

The panoramic film is currently the most commonly used radiograph in treatment planning for an implant patient. Pantomograms are ideal for showing the structures of the mandible and maxilla, including the locations of nerves. Although the field size is large enough in panoramic films, there is still no cross-sectional visualization. There is also an uneven amount of magnification (27%) in different areas of the mouth, and this can be very misleading in interpreting the radiograph. The exact location of the mandibular canal is difficult to determine on a pantomogram. Thus pantomograms should not be used as the only method for evaluating osseous structures.

Conventional Tomograms

Cross-sectional tomograms are an excellent way to obtain the necessary field visualization. Tomograms are cross-sectional images perpendicular to the edentulous ridge. Images are often blurry or indistinct, and this procedure is time consuming. Since very few offices have tomographic units, referral to medical radiologists or hospitals is necessary. If one is to refer a patient to this type of facility, it is probably better to refer for CT imaging.

Computed Tomography (CT Scanning)

Three-dimensional computed tomography (CT) imaging is essentially digitized tomography that results in an enhanced image in all dimensions or planes that is much easier to read than a conventional tomogram. The CT scanner makes a 1.0 to 1.5 mm thick slice or cut of the edentulous area (Fig. 19–17■). The tomogram measures the amount of energy transmitted through the object. The information is transmitted to a computer, which displays the image on a monitor.

CT scans are ideal for locating the amount and quality of bone available for implant placement above the mandibular canal (this is where the mandibular nerve is located) in the posterior area of the mandible. When maxillary areas are being used as implant sites, CT scans should be used to locate the sinuses and determine the amount and quality of available bone.

Figure 19–17 Axial CT at the level of the maxillary sinus.

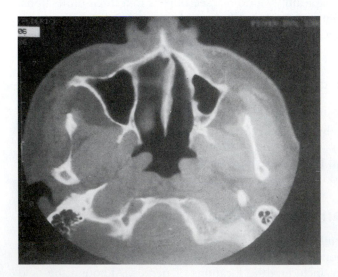

Postoperative Implant Evaluation

Baseline radiographs are taken to verify the fit of the abutment to the fixture head and document bone levels around an implant. After placement of implants, clinical and radiographic evaluations are necessary at continuing care or supportive periodontal therapy visits. Periapical and panoramic films are used for posttreatment evaluation. The primary reason for taking radiographs postoperatively is to help monitor the bone level around the implant. Periapical films are best for this purpose. For the edentulous patient, follow-up radiographs should be taken annually for 3 years and then once every other year. Pantomograms are also used to determine bone changes and the status of the abutment and fixture. Alveolar bone loss of less than 0.2 mm per year after the first year of placement is considered acceptable for a successful implant (Albrektsson, Zarb, Worthington, & Eriksson, 1986). CT scans cannot be used because the metallic implants produce image "noise" that interferes with proper interpretation.

Summary

Adequate radiographs and imaging systems are necessary for a complete periodontal and implant examination. Many techniques and systems are available. Conventional radiographs are adequate for visualizing the tooth and surrounding tissues. Conventional radiographs are also used to determine the amount and quality of bone available for implant placement in the anterior sextant of the mandible and maxilla. However, CT scans are necessary to evaluate the implant site in the maxilla and posterior areas of the mandible for its osseous status and proximity to vital structures (e.g., sinuses and mandibular canal).

Key Points

- Radiographic interpretation is used to supplement clinical findings from the periodontal assessment (e.g., probing depths, clinical attachment levels).
- Posterior vertical bitewing radiographs are ideal for visualizing the level of the alveolar bone crest.
- Radiographs do not show gingival and periodontal pockets or mobile teeth.
- The CT scan is the most commonly used imaging system for visualizing implant sites in the maxilla and posterior areas of the mandible.

Web Sites

www.perio.org
www.ada.org

Self-Quiz

1. The radiographic evaluation of alveolar bone loss associated with periodontitis is based on the status of which one of the following structures? (p. 280)

   a. interdental septum

   b. cementoenamel junction

   c. periapical bone

   d. periodontal ligament fibers

2. Which one of the following radiographic structures is described as a thin radiopaque line surrounding the entire tooth and is continuous with the alveolar crest? (p. 281)

   a. dentin

   b. cementum

   c. lamina dura

   d. periodontal ligament fibers

   e. gingival fibers

3. Which one of the following types of radiographs has nearly 90% reduction in radiation exposure? (pp. 288–289)

   a. panoramic

   b. periapical

   c. computed tomography

   d. digital imaging

   e. vertical bitewing

4. Which one of the following types of radiographs is best to evaluate the alveolar bone crest for moderate to severe bone loss? (p. 279)

   a. periapical

   b. horizontal bitewing

   c. vertical bitewing

   d. panoramic

   e. computed tomography

5. Which one of the following predisposing factors of periodontal diseases can be seen on radiographs? (pp. 282–285)

   a. gingival recession

   b. periodontal pockets

   c. furcation involvement

   d. tooth mobility

6. All the following types of radiographs are currently used in the treatment planning of implants except one. Which one is the exception? (p. 289)

   a. periapicals

   b. bitewings

   c. panoramic

   d. CT scan

7. Which one of the following features does the computed tomographic process provide? (p. 290)

   a. a three-dimensional view of the area of interest

   b. a two-dimensional view of the area of interest

   c. a global view of all oral structures

   d. a close-up view of the periapical structures

8. All the following are reasons for using radiographs in periodontics except one. Which one is the exception? (p. 278)

   a. Identify predisposing factors.

   b. Detect early to moderate bone changes.

   c. Determine the shape and depth of periodontal pockets.

   d. Serve as baseline data and as a means of evaluating posttreatment results

9. The normal crest of interproximal bone is located at a level (p. 280)

   a. 2 mm apical to the cementoenamel junction

   b. 3.0 mm coronal to the cementoenamel junction

   c. 2.0 to 3.0 mm coronal to the cusp tip of the crown

   d. 3.5 mm apical to the cusp tip of the crown

10. Which one of the following types of radiographs is used primarily in clinical research rather than clinical practice? (p. 290)

    a. panoramic films

    b. direct digital radiography

    c. digital subtraction radiography

    d. computed tomography

References

Albrektsson, T. G., Zarb, P. Worthington, and A. R. Eriksson. 1986. The long-term efficacy of currently used dental implants: A review and proposed criteria of success. *Int. J. Oral Maxillofac. Implants* 1:11–25.

Armitage, G. C. 1996. Periodontal diseases: *Diagnosis. Ann. Periodontol.* 1:37–215.

Douglass, G. L., S. M. Levine, J. Otomo-Corgel, T. N. Sims, and E. J. Taggart. 1991. Periodontal examination, diagnosis and treatment. *Can. Dent. Assoc. J.* 19:16–30.

Hodges, K. O. 1997. Recommendations for radiographs. In ed. K. O. Hodges, *Concepts in nonsurgical periodontal therapy,* 118–149. Albany NY: Delmar.

Hollender, L. 1992. Decision making in radiographic imaging. *J. Dent. Educ.* 56:834–843.

Jeffcoat, M. K. 1992. Imaging techniques for the periodontium. In eds. T. J. Wilson, K. S. Kornnan, and M. G. Newman, *Advances in periodontics,* 47–57. Chicago: Quintessence.

Jeffcoat, M. K. 1994. Current concepts in periodontal disease testing. *J. Am. Dent. Assoc.* 125:1071–1078.

Jeffcoat, M. K. 1998. Periodontal diseases: Epidemiology and diagnosis. Consensus reports from the 1996 world workshop in periodontics. *J. Am. Dent. Assoc.* 129:9S–14S.

Jeffcoat, M., and M. S. Reddy. 1991. A comparison of probing and radiographic methods for detection of periodontal disease progression. *Curr. Opin. Dentistry* 1:45–51.

Rams, T. E., M. A. Listgarten, and J. Slots. 1994. Utility of radiographic crestal lamina dura for predicting periodontitis disease activity. *J. Clin. Periodontol.* 21:571–576.

U.S. Department of Health and Human Services. 1987. *The selection of patients for x-ray examinations* (HHS Publication FDA 88-8273). Washington: U.S. Government Printing Office.

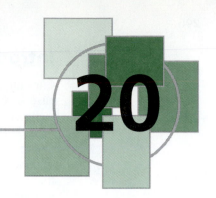

20

Advances in Detecting and Monitoring Periodontal Diseases

Denise Estafan, D.D.S., M.S.

Outline

Introduction

Gingival Crevicular
  Fluid Assays

Microbial Tests

Immunologic Assays

Enzyme-Based Assays

Genetic Assays

Clinical Applications

Summary

Key Points

Web Site

Self-Quiz

References

Goal

To introduce diagnostic methods that can be used as a supplement to conventional periodontal assessments for recognizing and monitoring periodontal diseases.

Education Objectives

Upon completion of this chapter, the reader should be able to:

Evaluate the role of using adjunctive diagnostic aids as a predictor for periodontal breakdown.

Explain the advantages and disadvantages of the various adjunctive diagnostic methods for detecting periodontal disease activity.

Distinguish the type of patient that may benefit from adjunctive diagnostic testing.

KEY WORDS

- periodontal diseases
- periodontal disease activity
- gingival crevicular fluid
- host-derived enzymes
- periodontal pathogens
- genetics

Introduction

Currently, identifying inflammatory periodontal diseases involves recognizing disease severity. Such traditional tests as visual inspection, probing depths, clinical attachment levels, and radiographs have not changed in the last 40 years and are considered the foundation for a periodontal examination. However, newer examination techniques may provide additional information beyond that which can be obtained from a clinical examination. Such information may offer predictions about the future of periodontal disease progression and patient evaluation. Approximately 30% of periodontal diseases are recurrent, so it is necessary to monitor the patient to identify problem sites before further tissue damage occurs. Research is ongoing to determine the overall plausibility and effectiveness of these tests. Ultimately, the screening of at-risk patients may allow for improved treatment and prevention of periodontal diseases.

The past decade has seen the evolution of several diagnostic methods designed to be used as an adjunct or in combination with the clinical examination. These methods help in identifying periodontal disease activity or patients at risk for an episode of active disease and are designed to help determine the most appropriate mode of treatment. The present standard for periodontal disease activity is a change in clinical attachment level of 2 to 3 mm. Various methods are used to analyze the products of the host response to dental plaque and to identify specific microbial (bacterial) species. The greatest value of diagnostic testing may lie in the ability to monitor patients after treatment, as well as those in the supportive periodontal therapy phase. Hopefully, appropriate testing will allow the practitioner to make therapeutic decisions before the onset of disease activity or at an early stage in its development. The initial determination of the need for active periodontal therapy still depends on use of a periodontal probe, gingival inspection, and radiographs (Bader, 1995). Therefore, these new assessment methods shift the focus from determining disease severity to evaluating disease progression or the risk of future periodontal breakdown—in essence, quantifying ongoing disease activity.

Adjunctive tests for the evaluation of periodontal diseases are divided into three main groups: gingival crevicular fluid assays, microbial tests, and genetic assays (Table 20–1■). Only a few of the tests are available in the United States for in-office use. Table 20–2■ reviews the advantages and disadvantages of various tests.

Table 20–1	Supplemental Diagnostic Tests in Periodontics

Methods of detecting bacteria:
    Culture and sensitivity techniques (an outside laboratory is used)
    DNA probes (DMDx®; MicroDenteX, Fort Meyers, FL)
    Dark-field or phase-contrast microscopy (available commercially)
    Immunologic assays (not available commercially)
    Enzyme-based assays (not available commercially)
Methods of detecting sites actively breaking down or at risk for future destruction:
    Gingival crevicular fluid assays (not commercially available)
      Collagenase
      Aspartate aminotransferase
Genetic susceptibility test:
    Interleukin-1 genotype (PST™ Genetic Test; Medical Science Systems, Flagstaff, AZ)

Table 20–2	Advantages and Limitations of Selective Adjunctive Tests	
Test	**Advantages**	**Limitations**
Culture	• Identifies specific microorganisms • Only test available that determines antibiotic sensitivity	• Expensive and time-consuming • Technique sensitive; diverse data from different labs (use of different media, sampling, transport) • Cell vitality must be preserved during transportation to lab • Some organisms may be lost through sampling
DNA probe assays	• Highly sensitive and specific for targeted periodontal pathogens • Viable organisms not needed • Samples sent by mail after collection chairside • Rapid identification (18 hours)	• Need special disposal procedures for radioactive waste • Does not determine antibiotic sensitivity of the bacteria being tested • Certain bacterial species may not be detected due to highly sensitive nature of the test • Performed in a lab
Microscopic test (phase-contrast microscopy)	• Good for chairside patient awareness of the importance of bacteria in periodontal disease • Motivational tool for patient's plaque-control habits	• Does not specifically identify bacterial species, only shape, size, and mobility • Not suitable to monitor disease activity
GCF enzyme assays	• Rapid and inexpensive • Technique insensitive, so easy to perform chairside • Good for screening purposes • In-office use	• Cannot identify specific bacteria, but allows for rapid assessment of bacterial enzymatic activity • Need sufficient amount of enzymes

Gingival Crevicular Fluid Assays

Of the three most common fluids found within the oral cavity (gingival crevicular fluid [GCF], serum, and saliva), GCF has been the focus of most research in recent years. GCF is a fluid that originates from the gingival connective tissue (lamina propria) and flows into the gingival crevice. As a result of inflammation, GCF is formed when fluids leak from dilated blood vessels within the lamina propria. As this fluid flows through the inflamed connective tissue, it picks up tissue breakdown products, enzymes, and other substances involved in the immune response. In this regard, it is an "inflammatory soup" containing subgingival bacteria, inflammatory cells, and a vast array of other substances (mediators) produced by bacteria and host cells. GCF is relatively easy to collect by placing paper strips into selected pockets (Fig. 20–1■). It is these features that make GCF a good source of potential markers of periodontal destruction.

In areas affected by periodontal disease, GCF is an abundant source of substances (e.g., inflammatory mediators) that appear to play a central role in the tissue breakdown processes associated with periodontitis. This idea has led to the investigation of certain inflammatory mediators and their possible role as markers for active periodontitis (Armitage, 1992). Although these investigations have, over the past 20 years, resulted in the evolution of many techniques for assessing various aspects of disease, currently none are commercially available. Among the

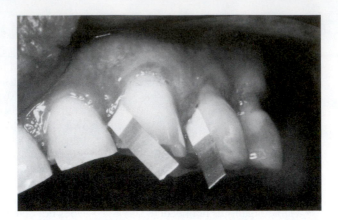

mediators that have been looked at most closely are host-derived enzymes (enzymes produced by host cells), inflammatory mediators, and tissue breakdown products.

Host-Derived Enzymes

During the disease process, certain host cells found in the body, such as polymorphonuclear leukocytes (neutrophils), release certain enzymes, including b-glucuronidase and elastase. These host-derived enzymes are components of GCF and have been reported to be associated with an increased risk of clinical attachment loss and bone loss (Lamster, Oshrain, et al., 1988; Lamster, Holmes, et al., 1995). Elevated levels of these enzymes in the GCF, which can be used as markers for periodontitis, are most evident 6 months before the occurrence of disease (Palcanis et al., 1992).

Aspartate aminotransferase (AST) is an intracellular enzyme (e.g., it stays inside the cell) that indicates cell death when it is present extracelluarly (e.g., outside the cell). Cell death leads to the release of the contents of the cell into the extracellular fluid. When AST is present at elevated levels in GCF, it has been shown to predict clinical attachment loss (Persson, DeRouen, & Page 1990), but over a shorter period than beta-glucuronidase and elastase. Evidence from studies on AST in the GCF of patients at risk for periodontal disease indicates that elevated levels of the enzyme can predict clinical attachment loss an average of 3 months in advance (Chambers et al., 1991). Currently, however, no test is available commercially.

Collagenase is an enzyme that breaks down collagen and is responsible for normal collagen remodeling. In the presence of inflammation, however, excessive amounts of collagenase are produced that cause periodontal tissue destruction during periodontal inflammation. Collagenase is produced by and released from host cells such as neutrophils (Overall, Sodek, McCulloch, & Birek, 1991). Fibroblasts also produce and release collagen and collagenase, but this occurs during normal tissue remodeling. Currently, however, no test is available commercially to detect "high" collagenase levels in the GCF.

Prostaglandin E$_2$

Prostaglandin E$_2$ (PGE$_2$) is a metabolite of arachidonic acid that is associated with many inflammatory effects, including bone loss. PGE$_2$ concentrations in the GCF of patients with clinical attachment loss of 3 mm or more have been shown to be significantly higher than in patients without this level of attachment loss (Offenbacher, Odler, & van Dyke, 1986). Identification of high levels of PGE_2 in GCF can indicate an increased risk of periodontal disease up to 6 months prior to its appearance clinically. Currently, however, no test is available commercially in the United States.

Microbial Tests

Bacterial plaque is the primary cause of the initiation and progression of inflammatory periodontal diseases. Suggested periodontal pathogens include *Actinobacillus actinomycetemcomitans, Porphyromonas gingivalis, Bacteriodes forsythus, Prevotella intermedia, Campylobacter rectus, Eikinella corrodens, Fusobacterium nucleatum, Capnocytophaga sputigena, Peptostreptococcus mitis, Selenomonas spp., Eubacterium spp.,* and *Haemophilus spp.* (Socransky & Haffajee, 1991; Tanner, 1992).

Over the past few decades, the understanding of periodontal diseases has changed dramatically. Since specific bacterial types have been well documented to cause periodontal diseases, including localized and generalized aggressive periodontitis, and refractory cases, treatment of periodontal diseases is best aimed at identification of the periodontal pathogens responsible. While no single one of these pathogens has been indicated as the organism responsible for disease progression, all the preceding bacteria are considered potential periodontal pathogens when identified in subgingival plaque samples. Identification of these pathogens allows for faster and better treatment aimed at eliminating or reducing bacterial levels.

Since gingivitis and chronic periodontitis are not commonly associated with specific bacteria, identification of these diseases probably would not benefit from the use of microbial testing.

Many methods for bacterial testing are available for research and clinical use. These include culturing, microscopic DNA and probe, and immunologic techniques.

Culture Techniques

Culturing allows for the growth of certain microorganisms found in periodontal pockets. Specific in-office procedures must be followed. After removal of supragingival plaque, samples of subgingival bacteria are taken from the plaque with a curet and are placed in a transport fluid and sent to a licensed clinical laboratory within a day or two to maintain bacterial viability (bacteria must be alive on reaching the laboratory). The laboratory then disperses the sample, dilutes it, and plates it on selective and nonselective media. The most common pathogens are identified, and antibiotic susceptibility is determined. A detailed report of the findings is then sent back to the dental office, including the systemic antibiotics to which the cultured bacteria are sensitive. Knowing the susceptibility or resistance of specific microorganisms to these antibiotics provides important guidelines for antibiotic use in conjunction with periodontal therapy.

Cost and time constraints limit the use of such a process, so it is not appropriate for all patients. However, culture analysis may be useful for patients who do not respond to conventional therapy, especially if they have taken antibiotics previously (Armitage, 1993). Culturing is the only test that can determine the antimicrobial sensitivity of cultured bacteria. In addition, culturing is limited in that it can only detect living bacteria; some bacteria may not survive transportation to the laboratory. Only a few dental schools offer this service, including the University of Pennsylvania and the University of Southern California.

Microscopic Techniques

Identification of subgingival biota also may be accomplished through various microscopic techniques such as phase-contrast and dark-field microscopy. Rather than identifying specific bacteria, phase-contrast microscopy categorizes bacteria by motility (motile), and dark-field microscopy identifies the morphology or shape (e.g., cocci, rods). Bacterial shifts from nonmotile to motile species often indicate a change from health to disease (Listgarten & Levin, 1981). Genus and species determination, as well as antibiotic susceptibility, is not possible using these techniques. Many dental offices use microscopic techniques solely for patient education. Clinically, a digital camera and monitor are attached to the microscope.

Nucleic Acid (DNA) Probe Analysis

All living organisms contain DNA (deoxyribonucleic acid), which carries all genetic information needed for the coding for proteins, the basic building blocks of life (Papapanou, Engelbretson, & Lamster, 1999). The DNA of each species consists of a specific sequence that is unique to that organism. Nucleic acid probe analysis identifies DNA sequences specific for certain subgingival periodontal pathogens. In the dental office, plaque samples are collected by inserting a special sterile paper point into the base of a pocket. This paper point is then placed in an air-filled vial and mailed to a testing service. Bacterial DNA is so stable that no special transport fluid is required before mailing the sample, and the bacteria do not have to be living. This is a key advantage to using DNA as a biochemical marker in the identification of periodontal pathogens. The microorganism's DNA is cut into single-strand fragments. The DNA probe is made in the laboratory and labeled with either a radioactive or enzyme marker. If binding of the labeled DNA probe strands occurs, the test organism is thus identified. DNA probe reports are rapid, relatively inexpensive, and can detect nonviable species (Loesche, 1992; Sonnier, 1996). This test (DMDx® Test) is available through a few laboratories, including MicroDenteX in Fort Meyers, Florida. Currently, there are eight pathogens that can be identified: *Actinobacillus actinomycetemcomitans* (Aa), *Prevotella intermedia* (Pi), *Porphyromonas gingivalis* (Pg), *Eikenella corrodens* (Ec), *Campylobacter rectus* (Cr), *Bacteriodes forsythus* (Bf) (new name *Tannerella forsythensis*), *Treponema denticola* (Td), and *Fusobacterium nucleatum* (Fn).

Currently, there is no reason to use DNA probes routinely in every patient. DNA probes should be reserved for difficult refractory cases where previous treatments have failed to control disease progression. It can also be used to monitor therapy outcome and to evaluate implant sites. Susceptibility testing should only be done when usual antibiotic regimens have failed or when unusual pathogens are present. Since certain antibiotics are almost always effective against anaerobic pathogens (infections), these infections are usually treated empirically or hypothetically. However, sometimes this does not work and testing for antibiotic sensitivity is necessary.

Immunologic Assays

The enzyme-linked immunosorbent assay (ELIZA) is based on the specific binding of an antibody to an antigen on the surface of a microorganism. The primary antibody is detected by labeling with a fluorescent secondary antibody. ELIZA is able to identify specific bacteria. It is an expensive test and currently used only in research.

Enzyme-Based Assays

The enzymatic approach is based on the ability to screen for the presence of an enzyme unique to one or more bacterial species. In this assay, a plaque sample is exposed to a substance that is degraded by the specific enzyme in question. For example, *Treponema denticola*, *Porphyromonas gingivalis*, and *Bacteroides forsythus* (proposed new name is *Tannerella forsythensis*) produce a trypsin-like enzyme that degrades a substance called BANA (benzoyldi-arginine-2-naphthy-lamide). A positive test indirectly indicates the presence of one or more of the three bacteria (Papapanou, et al., 1999).

Genetic Assays

Numerous established and potential risk factors are associated with periodontal diseases, including smoking, smokeless tobacco, systemic diseases, age, medications, stress, and genetics (heredity). All these factors, except for genetics and age, are acquired or environmental and can be controlled or eliminated. Genetics is an innate risk factor that one is born with and cannot be altered or modified. Kornman and Colleagues (1997) addressed the first association between genetics and periodontal diseases. Interleukin-1 (IL-1) is a cytokine produced and secreted by inflammatory cells such as macrophages as a result of accumulation of bacterial plaque. IL-1 is responsible for inflammation and bone loss. Some individuals produce too much IL-1 in response to bacterial challenge. These individuals are more susceptible to the onset and rapid progression of periodontal diseases than individuals who do not show an IL-1 genotype (gene). IL-1 does not cause periodontal disease directly, but it predisposes the patient to the disease process by increasing inflammation when bacteria are present (Newman, 1998). This information allows the patient to be monitored more closely and helps dental practitioners recommend optimal preventive therapy and supportive care programs (Newman, 1998).

A test is available that determines if a patient has an IL-1 genotype in his or her blood. This test is called PST™ (Periodontal Susceptibility Testing; Medical Science Systems, Inc., Flagstaff, AZ). The test is performed by taking a finger-stick blood sample from the patient. The sample is analyzed in a licensed medical laboratory to determine if the patient is positive or negative for the IL-1 genotype. An IL-1 gene-positive patient is about seven times more likely to develop or have advanced periodontal disease than a gene-negative patient, and this genotype occurs in approximately 30% of the population.

Clinical Applications

Although at present a good clinical judgment as to the presence of periodontal disease can be made using existing diagnostic procedures, this decision may be very subjective and sometimes unreliable. Therefore, there is a need for more precise decision making, and care should be taken in evaluating and using these new systems. However, presently, there are no completely validated assessment procedures that can identify progressing or active periodontitis.

Since the etiology of and risk factors for periodontal diseases are multifaceted, the most important steps for patient evaluation include a comprehensive clinical and radiographic analysis and identification of modifying systemic risk factors, including cigarette smoking and diabetes mellitus. Additionally, the host response contributes to the development and progression of the disease. Therefore, no microbial or host response test will definitively determine the initiation or progression of disease.

It is without foundation to use these tests on all periodontal patients. A critical factor that needs to be considered when a practitioner chooses to introduce diagnostic testing as part of patient care is when to use the tests. At a time when there is great pressure to reduce health care costs, judicious application is critical (Lamster, 1996).

Culture and sensitivity testing can provide guidelines for antibiotic selection in certain cases, including periodontitis patients who are refractory to previous treatment. Such patients probably have been treated previously with numerous antibiotics, and bacterial resistance could have developed. DNA probe analysis can be helpful in these patients, providing rapid results within 24 hours. Assessment of the genetic susceptibility of a patient or of children of parents with advanced periodontal disease may soon prove to be an important tool in the initiation of preventive measures.

Summary

Traditional clinical assessments usually will detect inflammatory lesions and direct practitioners to areas requiring therapy and possible additional testing (Greenstein & Rethman, 1998). Presently, microbial assays and host-response diagnostic tests appear to have meager use and limited applicability in routine diagnosis in periodontics. These adjunctive diagnostic tests may improve clinical decision making but require further confirmation followed by controlled clinical studies. Additional testing may be beneficial at specific sites or for individual patients when there is diagnostic uncertainty regarding the absence or presence of diseases or when the medical or dental history suggests that a patient is at risk of developing periodontitis (Greenstein & Rethman, 1998). Currently, however, few of these tests are available commercially, and no test is available that will definitively determine if a site is actively losing attachment and bone or will lose attachment in the future. There are no specific guidelines to follow, but some factors to consider include cost of testing, age of the patient, patient motivation, and systemic health of the patient.

Key Points

- No clinical test is available that will currently determine if a site is actively breaking down or predict periodontal breakdown; more research is needed.
- A combination of traditional and new diagnostic testing can, in some cases, provide more complete information for treatment planning.
- Additional bacterial tests are used for site-specific treatment, additional information to assist treatment, and to rule out other causes of disease.

Web Site

www.perio.org

Self-Quiz

1. Which one of the following tests is used to determine the susceptibility of bacteria to certain antibiotics? (pp. 297, 299)

   a. phase-contrast microscopy

   b. DNA probe

   c. culture

   d. temperature

2. All the following types of patients may require adjunctive periodontal diagnostic testing except one. Which one is the exception? (p. 302)

   a. new patients who have not received therapy previously

   b. treated patients who initially present with advanced periodontal disease

   c. patients not responding to periodontal treatment

   d. patients with previously treated gingivitis

3. Which one of the following is the role of genetics as a risk factor for periodontal diseases? (p. 301)

   a. destruction of bone early in life

   b. production of excessive amounts of interleukin-1

   c. demonstration of high levels of bacteria in childhood

   d. presentation with highly inflamed soft tissues

4. Which one of the following is a goal for using host-based diagnostic periodontal tests? (p. 298)

   a. determines the need for future maintenance care

   b. identifies periodontal sites that are bleeding

   c. evaluates the need for more aggressive periodontal treatment

   d. distinguishes between active and inactive disease sites

5. Which one of the following tests is highly sensitive for specific periodontal pathogens present in a subgingival sample of plaque? (pp. 299–300)

   a. culture

   b. DNA probe

   c. GCF enzyme assay

   d. microscopic technique

6. In which one of the following secretions are high levels of host-derived enzymes found? (p. 297)

   a. whole saliva

   b. crevicular fluid

   c. sweat

   d. serum

7. Which one of the following statements is related to adjunctive periodontal tests. (pp. 296, 302)

    a. Eventually they will replace conventional periodontal assessment techniques.

    b. They are used on all periodontal patients presenting in the office.

    c. Established guidelines need to be determined.

    d. They are cost-effective and easy to perform.

8. Which one of the following tests identifies the motility of bacteria? (p. 297)

    a. enzyme-linked immunosorbent assay (ELIZA)

    b. phase-contrast microscopy

    c. DNA probe

    d. GCF enzyme

    e. temperature

9. Which one of the following host cells synthesize and release beta-glucuronidase and elastase? (p. 298)

    a. mast cells

    b. lymphocytes

    c. neutrophils

    d. eosinophils

    e. fibroblasts

10. All of the following statements are correct concerning the use of DNA probe assays except one. Which one is the exception? (p. 300)

    a. They are highly sensitive and specific for targeted periodontal pathogens.

    b. Samples are sent to an outside laboratory.

    c. They require viable microorganisms.

    d. They provide rapid identification.

References

Armitage, G. C. 1992. Diagnostic tests for periodontal diseases. *Curr. Opin. Dent.* 21(1): 53–62.

Armitage, G. C. 1993. Periodontal diagnostic aids. *Calif. Dent. Assoc. J.* 21(11):35–46.

Bader, H. I. 1995. Contemporary periodontics and a vision for the future: Diagnostics and monitoring the treated case. *Dentistry Today* 1:42–45.

Chambers, D. A., P. B. Imrey, R. L. Cohen, J. M. Crawford, M. E. Alves, and T. A. McSwiggin. 1991. A longitudinal study of aspartate aminotransferase in human gingival cervical fluid. *J. Periodont. Res.* 26:65–74.

Greenstein, G. S., and M. P. Rethman. 1998. Diagnosing destructive periodontal diseases. In eds. M. Nevins and J. T. Mellonig, *Periodontal therapy: Clinical approaches and evidence of success,* Vol. 1. Chicago: Quintessence.

Kornman, K. S., A. Crane, H.-Y. Wang, et al. 1997. The interleukin-1 genotype as a severity factor in adult periodontal disease. *J. Clin. Periodontol.* 24:72–77.

Lamster, I. B. 1996. In-office diagnostic tests and their role in supportive periodontal treatment. *Periodontology 2000* 12:49–55.

Lamster, I. B., L. G. Holmes, K. B. Gross, R. L. Oshrain, D. W. Cohen, et al. 1995. The relationship of β-glucuronidase activity in crevicular fluid to probing attachment loss in patients with adult periodontitis: Findings from a multicenter study. *J. Clin. Periodontol.* 22:36–44.

Lamster, I. B., R. L. Oshrain, D. S. Harper, R. S. Celenti, C. A. Hovliaras, and J. M. Gordon. 1988. Enzyme activity in crevicular fluid for detection and prediction of clinical attachment loss in patients with chronic adult periodontitis: Six-month results. *J. Periodontol.* 59:516–523.

Listgarten, M. A., and S. Levin. 1981. Positive correlation between the proportions of subgingival spirochetes and motile bacteria and susceptibility of human subjects to periodontal deterioration. *J. Clin. Periodontol.* 8:122–138.

Loesche, W. J. 1992. DNA probe and enzyme analysis in periodontal diagnostics. *J. Periodontol.* 63:1102–1109.

Newman, M. 1998. Genetic, environmental, and behavioral influences on periodontal infections. *Compend. Contin. Educ.* (special issue) 19(1):25–31.

Offenbacher, S., B. M. Odle, and T. E. van Dyke. 1986. The use of crevicular fluid prostaglandin E_2 as a predictor of periodontol attachment loss. *J. Periodont. Res.* 21:101–112.

Overall, C. M., J. Sodek, C. A. G. McCulloch, and P. Birek. 1991. Evidence for polymophonuclear leukocyte collagenase and 92-kilodalton gelatinase in gingival crevicular fluid. *Infect. Immun.* 59:4687–4692.

Palcanis, K. G., I. K. Larjara, B. R. Wells, K. A. Suggs, J. P. Landis, et al. 1992. Elastase as an indicator of periodontal disease progression. *J. Periodontol.* 63:237–242.

Papapanou, P. N., S. P. Engelbretson, and I. B. Lamster. 1999. Current and future approaches for diagnosis of periodontal diseases. *N.Y. State Dent. J.* (April):32–38.

Persson, G. R., T. A. DeRouen, and R. C. Page. 1990. Relationship between gingival crevicular fluid levels of aspartate aminotransferase and active tissue destruction in treated chronic periodontitis patients. *J. Periodont. Res.* 25:81–87.

Socransky, S. S., and A. D. Haffajee. 1991. Microbial mechanisms in the pathogenesis of destructive periodontal diseases: A critical assessment. *J. Periodont. Res.* 26:195–212.

Sonnier, K. E. 1996. Microbial testing: Present and future. *Clin. Update* 18(4):7.

Tanner, A. 1992. Microbial etiology of periodontal diseases: Where are we? Where are we going? *Curr. Opin. Dent.* 2(1):12–24.

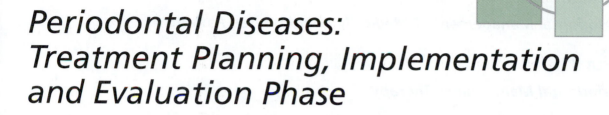

PART IV

Periodontal Diseases: Treatment Planning, Implementation and Evaluation Phase

Problem/Evidence-Based Treatment Planning

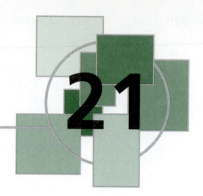

Jill Rethman, R.D.H., B.A.
Michael P. Rethman, D.D.S., M.S.

Outline

Goals

To provide an understanding of problem-based learning (PBL) in developing a periodontal treatment plan.

Educational Objectives

Upon completion of this chapter, the reader should be able to:

Describe the problem-based approach to treatment planning.

Formulate a problem list for each patient.

Formulate an action plan for each problem listed.

Describe treatment guidelines for periodontal patients.

Explain when more aggressive forms of therapy are needed and thus appropriate times for referral to a periodontist.

Describe periodontal prognostic signs.

KEY WORDS

- treatment planning
- evidence-based
- problem-based
- informed consent
- prognosis

Controlling inflammation is the initial treatment objective of therapies aimed at the periodontal diseases. The key to controlling inflammation is to eliminate, reduce, or change the makeup of microbes residing in the mouth. Elimination of deeper periodontal pocket depths is not always necessary, but it is usually desirable to obtain probing depths that are shallow enough for the practitioner and the patient to keep free of pathogenic dental plaque. This is also the goal of many of the periodontal surgical procedures. Of course, once inflammation is brought under control, the prevention of recurrent periodontitis is essential (Hancock, 1996).

Research findings have definitively shown that *plaque microbes and its byproducts are entirely responsible* for the initiation and progression of the periodontal diseases (Ismail, Morrison, Burt, Caffesse, & Kavanagh, 1990). Additional research has found that the *host's immune response to infection plays an important role in determining how the periodontal destruction manifests itself by producing chemical modulators that actually may accelerate periodontal destruction* (Grossi et al., 1994, 1995). Therefore, comprehensive periodontal therapy may soon include tactics to modulate the host's immune response in addition to traditional efforts to suppress periodontal pathogens.

This chapter explores current concepts of periodontal treatment planning based on problem-based learning.

Problem-Based Learning (PBL) Approach to Treatment

A problem-based recording system is designed to introduce the student to a technique for developing an individualized treatment plan for each patient. This problem-based learning (PBL) initially identifies significant problems from the patient's medical/dental history from which a differential dental hygiene diagnosis (or interpretation) will be made for each sign and/or symptom on the problem list. This problem list will be used as a guide to develop a treatment plan and referral system. A decision-making tree can be also be used to help decide on the proper treatment in each case.

Tables 21–1■ through 21–3■ provide an overall concept of therapeutic decision making when treatment planning a periodontal case.

The American Academy of Periodontology has developed practice parameters on the diagnosis and treatment of periodontal diseases. These parameters of care (American Academy of Periodontology, 2000) are strategies to assist dental practitioners in making clinical decisions from a range of treatment options to achieve a desired outcome.

For many years, periodontitis was thought to be the inevitable result of poor oral hygiene along with uncontrolled dental plaque and calculus accumulation. This was termed the nonspecific plaque hypothesis (Loesche, 1976). In recent decades, research has suggested instead that there are microbial species whose presence tends to signal a greater likelihood of progressive periodontal destruction (Haffajee et al., 1991). Furthermore, for most patients, evidence suggests that procedures aimed at suppressing these species will improve clinical outcomes. However, for adults, front-line periodontal therapy remains largely nonspecific in design—because conventional clinical and self-care procedures often succeed among this predominating group of periodontitis patients. For periodontal diseases

(text continues on p. 315)

Table 21–1 Consensus Findings: Diagnosis of Periodontitis

Test	Application	Strengths	Weaknesses	Type of Evidence
Periodontal screening and recording	All patients in every practice	Cost-effective, quick, easy, detects patients with periodontal disease	Does not provide a tooth-by-tooth assessment for later comparison during maintenance therapy; a full periodontal examination is needed for this purpose	Epidemiologic studies
Probing pocket depths	All patients	Shallow probing depths associated with a lack of future disease progression	Moderate to deep pockets in a single probing depth examination will not distinguish with certainty which teeth will undergo progressive periodontal destruction	Longitudinal studies
Gingival inflammation assessment	All patients	Absence of inflammation is associated with a lack of future disease progression; in treated patients, bleeding on probing is associated with an increased risk of progressive loss of attachment	Presence of inflammation will not distinguish with certainty which teeth will undergo progressive periodontal destruction	Longitudinal studies
Radiographic evidence of bone loss	At-risk patients as determined by PSR screening or periodontal examination	Absence of bone loss is associated with a lower risk of future disease progression	Presence of bone loss on a single radiograph will not distinguish with certainty which teeth will undergo progressive periodontal destruction	Longitudinal studies
Microbial plaque tests	High-risk or refractory patients	Absence of supragingival plaque is associated with a lack of disease progression In compromised or refractory patients, may be useful in determining the presence of pathogens	Routine testing offers limited benefit in adult periodontitis	Cross-sectional and longitudinal studies Case reports
Biochemical profiles in gingival crevicular fluid	Not yet determined	A number of biochemical markers may identify individuals at risk	At present, there are no specific biochemical profiles that characterize specific periodontal diseases	Cross-sectional and longitudinal studies

Source: From M. K. Jeffcoat, M. McGuire, and M. G. Newman. 1997. Evidence-based periodontal treatment: Highlights from the 1996 World Workshop in Periodontics. *J. Am. Dent. Assoc.* 128:713–724. Copyright 1997 by the American Dental Association. Reprinted by permission of ADA Publishing Co., Inc.

Table 21–2 Consensus Findings: Nonsurgical Treatment of Gingivitis and Periodontitis

Treatment Category	Treatment	Strengths	Weaknesses	Type of Evidence
Professional mechanical therapy—used in the treatment of gingivitis and periodontitis	Scaling and root planing with manual instrument	Decreases gingival inflammation by 40% to 60%; decreases probing depth; facilitates gain in clinical attachment level	Requires attention to detail	Many longitudinal, cohort, and randomized clinical trials
	Ultrasonic and sonic scaling and root planing	Results are similar to those for manual scaling and root planing		Longitudinal, cohort, and randomized clinical trials
Chemical plaque control with mouthrinses and toothpastes	Chlorhexidine; triclosan with copolymer or triclosan with zinc citrate; essential oils; stannous fluoride	Significant reduction in gingival inflammation	No clear evidence that there is a substantial long-term benefit in periodontitis except to control coexisting inflammation	Randomized, double-blind clinical trials
Irrigation	Supragingival and subgingival irrigation used as an adjunct to brushing	Aids in the reduction of gingivitis	No clear evidence that there is a substantial long-term benefit for periodontitis	Randomized, double-blind clinical trials
Sustained-release antimicrobials	Intrapocket resorbable or nonresorbable delivery systems containing a tetracycline antibiotic	When used as an adjunct to scaling and root planing, gains in clinical attachment level and decreases in probing depth and bleeding	A few reported side effects include transient discomfort, erythema, recession, allergy and, rarely, *Candida*	Randomized, double-blind clinical trials
Systemic antibiotics	Tetracyclines, metronidazole, spiramycin, clindamycin, and combinations such as metronidazole and amoxicillin	May be useful to treat aggressive, destructive periodontitis	Not indicated for gingivitis; not indicated for most adult patients with periodontitis	Assessment of risk-benefit ratio; randomized, double-blind clinical trials; longitudinal assessment of patients' conditions

Source: From M. K. Jeffcoat, M. McGuire, and M. G. Newman. 1997. Evidence-based periodontal treatment: Highlights from the 1996 World Workshop in Periodontics. *J. Am. Dent. Assoc.* 128:713–724. Copyright 1997 by the American Dental Association. Reprinted by permission of ADA Publishing Co., Inc.

Table 21–3 Consensus Findings: Surgical Periodontal Therapy—Selected Procedures

Category and Goal	Treatment	Strengths	Weaknesses	Type of Evidence
Pocket therapy provides access to root surfaces and bony defects, reduces probing depths, facilitates plaque control, and enhances restorative and cosmetic dentistry	Modified Widman flap to provide access to roots and bony defects for debridement; apically repositioned flap with or without bony recontouring; gingivectomy	All procedures decrease pocket depth; with the exception of gingivectomy, all increase clinical attachment level; after 5 years, greatest reduction in probing depth with osseous recontouring; apically repositioned flap with or without bony recontouring used in crown-lengthening procedures to provide biologic width	Procedures designed to reduce probing depths may increase recession; lack of professional maintenance and patient compliance can be detrimental to the long-term success	Randomized clinical trials; longitudinal studies
Regenerative procedures to facilitate growth of new periodontal ligament, cementum and bone over previously diseased root surfaces	Extraoral autogenous bone grafts	High potential for bone growth	Second surgical site (such as iliac crest); root resorption may be associated with fresh grafts	Limited case report data
	Intraoral autogenous grafts (such as maxillary tuberosity, healing extraction sites, osseous coagulum)	Case reports indicate bone gain of more than 50%; controlled studies comparing grafts with nongrafted bone show improved clinical attachment levels and bone, but not as great as those in case reports		Case reports; comparative controlled clinical studies
	Allografts—tissues transferred from one person to another; freeze-dried bone allograft	Bone fill has been reported in a high proportion of defects involving freeze-dried bone allograft		
	Alloplasts—synthetic grafts • Absorbable: plaster, calcium carbonates, ceramics such as tricalcium phosphate and absorbable hydroxyapatite (HA) • Nonabsorbable: dense HA, porous HA, bioglass • Calcium-coated polymer polymethylmethacrylate and hydroxymethyl methacrylate	Improved probing depth and attachment level Some evidence of histologic regeneration in calcium-coated polymer polymethylmethacrylate and hydroxy-methylmethacrylate	Osteogenic potential may vary from vial to vial; patient differences; clinician variability Histologic findings indicate that synthetic grafts primarily act as fillers, with little if any regeneration	Field test; controlled clinical trials Controlled clinical trials

(continued)

313

Table 21–3 Consensus Findings: Surgical Periodontal Therapy—Selected Procedures (cont.)

Category and Goal	Treatment	Strengths	Weaknesses	Type of Evidence
Guided tissue regeneration—physical barriers are used to facilitate selective cell population of the root surface after periodontal surgery to promote regeneration	Nonresorbable membranes	Significant improvement in clinical attachment level compared with debridement alone; most favorable results are in Class II furcations in the mandible and infrabony defects; no need for second-stage surgery (resorbable only)	Less favorable results in maxillary molar and Class III defects; nonresorbable membrane requires a second surgery to remove the membrane	Randomized, controlled clinical trials; uncontrolled studies; and case reports
	Resorbable materials		Clinical results similar to those for nonresorbable membranes but less evidence available to allow a comparison of predictability with respect to nonresorbable membranes	
Gingival augmentation to promote root coverage	Pedicle grafts Free soft tissue grafts (epithelialized or connective-tissue graft) Combination grafts • Connective tissue or biodegradable membrane barrier plus pedicle graft • Coronally positioned, previously placed soft tissue graft • Nonbiodegradable membrane barrier plus pedicle graft	Improve aesthetics/cosmetic results; decrease root sensitivity; manage defects resulting from root caries removal or cervical abrasion; manage mucogingival defects		Case reports; comparison studies
Endosseous dental implants	Two-stage and one-stage implants; titanium; titanium alloy; hydroxyapatite-coated implants	Dental implants are predictable replacements for missing teeth in fully and partially edentulous patients	While there are few studies in the literature, the clinician should use caution in the following cases: smoking, untreated periodontal disease, poor oral hygiene, uncontrolled systemic disease, history of radiation therapy, active skeletal growth	Longitudinal studies

Source: From M. K. Jeffcoat, M. McGuire, and M. G. Newman. 1997. Evidence-based periodontal treatment: Highlights from the 1996 World Workshop in Periodontics. *J. Am. Dent. Assoc.* 128:713–724. Copyright 1997 by the American Dental Association. Reprinted by permission of ADA Publishing Co., Inc.

in young people, for refractory disease in adults, and in special situations, periodontal therapy may include procedures aimed at specific putative periodontal pathogens.

Goals of Periodontal Therapy

The ideal goal of periodontal therapy is to restore the periodontium to an attractive, comfortable, and functional state of health for the balance of the patient's life. Therefore, most periodontal therapy aims to prevent the initiation, progression, or recurrence of periodontal diseases. This can be termed arrestive periodontal therapy. However, where periodontal destruction has occurred, regeneration of the specialized periodontal tissue is often worth pursuing when possible. This is termed regenerative periodontal therapy. Successful regenerative periodontal therapy usually includes an arrestive component. The first step in developing a treatment plan should be to determine individual treatment goals for each patient.

Periodontal Therapy: Ongoing Care

The management of most periodontal patients demands continued reassessments and adjustments to ongoing care. This is so because periodontal care is not permanent in the sense that many other highly successful dental therapies are considered. For most cases of chronic periodontitis, the only permanent periodontal end point is tooth (or implant) loss. Furthermore, no single periodontal treatment produces ideal outcomes for all patients.

Once a patient is practicing thorough daily oral hygiene self-care, the ideal interval between patient appointments—even for patients in periodontal maintenance programs—may be as brief as every 2 to 3 months (Axelsson & Lindhe, 1981). Frequent reexaminations, reevaluations, and adjustments to therapy often are necessary for many years. Given this context, practitioners need to comply with their ethical and medical/legal responsibilities to refer periodontitis patients to specialists, provide comparable periodontal care in the general practice, or partner with a specialist to share responsibilities for periodontal patients. Suggestions governing what, when, and why to refer are made where appropriate throughout this chapter.

Problem List

A problem list should be set up for individual periodontal patients (Table 21–4■). The problem list will identify the patient's problems through reviewing the patient's chief complaint and medical, social (habit), and dental histories. For each problem identified a solution must be written and expected outcomes (the result of taking care of the problem), prognosis (predication of recovery), and any major concerns must be addressed. Identified problems may have multiple solutions.

Table 21–4 Periodontal Problem List

Problems	Solutions (Plan)	Expected Outcome/Prognosis/Major Concerns
Chief Complaint	1. Address chief complaint	1. Treat the chief complaint first
Risk Factors		
Medical History (e.g., diabetes, HIV)	1. Detailed assessment 2. Consultations required 3. Advise patient of relationship between systemic diseases and periodontal disease	1. Concern with possible delayed healing
Dental History (e.g., previous periodontal care)	1. Detailed assessment 2. Previous periodontal surgery 3. How often maintenance care	1. Compliance is deciding factor in prognosis
Genetics	1. Blood test determines susceptibility to periodontal diseases	1. If determined to be susceptible, patient must be compliant with periodontal care
Smoking	1. Smoking cessation program	1. Concerned with periodontal disease 2. Good prognosis if patient is willing to quit
Iatrogenic dentistry	1. Look for open margins, overhangs, open contacts, and replace or modify exisiting restorations	1. Concerned with food impaction and plaque traps
Poor oral hygiene	1. Patient education	1. Noncompliance will increase incidence or progression of periodontal disease
Soft Tissues		
Gingival inflammation	Eliminate/reduce gingival inflammation with mechanical debridement and oral hygiene	Concerned with development/ progression of gingivitis
Soft tissue recession	Determine etiology; may need periodontal surgery (mucogingival)	Future attachment loss
Abnormal tissue architecture Gingival overgrowth	Determine etiology: drug-induced or hereditary or plaque-induced inflammation; may need periodontal surgery to correct	Difficulty with oral hygiene
Lack of attached gingiva	Determine etiology; determine if prosthetics will be done; may need gingival plastic surgery to correct	Increase incidence of inflammation
Probing depths	Deep probing depths: mechanical debridement followed by reevaluation and if needed periodontal surgery	Deep probing depths difficult to perform oral hygiene and mechanical debridement; future attachment loss and periodontal disease
Hard Tissue		
Ridge defects	Surgical intervention; planning for implants	Implant placement/esthetics
Teeth		
Missing teeth	Replacement of missing teeth	Concerned with movement of teeth, function, and comfort

(continued)

Table 21–4	Periodontal Problem List	
Problems	Solutions (Plan)	Expected Outcome/Prognosis/Major Concerns
Mobility	Determine etiology: bone loss, occlusal trauma, inflammation and treat accordingly	Concerned with increasing mobility and patient comfort
Fremitus	Determine etiology: bone loss, occlusal interferences and treat accordingly to eliminate fremitus	Concern with patient comfort and continued occlusal trauma
Parafunctional habits	Eliminate parafunctional habits; counseling or appliances	Concerned with occlusal trauma/good prognosis if eliminated
Radiographic Findings		
Horizontal bone loss	With deep probing depths surgery is needed	Prognosis depends on several factors including amount of bone remaining, mobility, furcation involvement
Vertical bone loss	Surgical intervention	Prognosis depends on several factors including amount of bone remaining, mobility, furcation involvement
Root proximity	Identify teeth and monitor for periodontal breakdown	Concerned with amount of interproximal bone remaining
Pathology		
Mucosal lesions	Determine size, shape, color, and location; refer to specialist; brush biopsy; excisional biopsy	Concerned with oral cancer
TMD/pain	Excercises/appliances/referral to specialist	Reduced function

Adapted from New York University College of Dentistry Problem List) (this list is filled out to show an example)

Treatment Planning

Once the examination is completed, the data must be analyzed. Data include the patient's medical and dental history, complete radiographs, detailed periodontal data, tooth conditions (including vitality, caries, and morphologic abnormalities), and dental awareness.

In addition to developing a "best case" treatment plan, reasonable alternatives should be considered and presented to the patient. Flowcharts may help delineate the general route a patient takes during treatment (Tables 21–5■ through 21–10■).

Phases of Treatment

Ideal treatment planning incorporates a logical interplay between periodontal and nonperiodontal procedures. This is so because successful management of the periodontal diseases is a multifaceted discipline that can be affected by other dental conditions and treatments. Table 21–11■ depicts four sequential phases that are guidelines for overall case management.

Phase I: Nonsurgical/Initial Preparation   The goal of Phase I therapy is to reduce all etiologic and risk factors to the maximum extent possible—short of surgical intervention. Conditions associated with pain, such as a periodontal abscess, necrotizing ulcerative gingivitis, or traumatic injury, should be treated at this time. Nonrestorable teeth should be identified and extracted. Teeth needing endodontic therapy should be treated.

Table 21–5	Periodontal Health

Gingival tissues are healthy when there is no bleeding after gentle probing
First appointment: 45 minutes to 1 hour

- Comprehensive oral evaluation (new patients) or periodic oral evaluation (existing patients)—consisting of a medical and dental history update, vital signs, head and neck examination, and oral cancer screening.
- Complete x-ray series, including vertical bitewings (new patients) or indicated radiographs (existing patients).
- Oral hygiene instruction.
- Oral prophylaxis.
- Selective polishing, if needed.
- Nutritional counseling for the control of dental caries.
- Fluoride treatment (caries control).
- Tobacco counseling for the control and prevention of oral disease, if indicated.
- Suitable maintenance interval established (3, 6, or more months).

Table 21–6	Gingivitis

Probing depths of less than 4 mm; plaque and calculus present; no bone loss or mobility
First appointment: 1 hour

- Comprehensive oral evaluation (new patients) or periodic oral evaluation (existing patients)—consisting of a medical and dental history update, head and neck examination, and oral cancer screening. Make referrals if necessary.
- Periodontal examination.
- Complete x-ray series, including vertical bitewings (new patients) or indicated radiographs (existing patients).
- Note and record sites that bleed on gentle probing.
- Oral hygiene instruction after staining for plaque and relating stained areas to bleeding sites.
- Full-mouth debridement.
- Nutritional counseling for the control of dental caries.
- Tobacco counseling for the control and prevention of oral disease, if indicated.

Second appointment: At least 45 minutes, scheduled 7 to 10 days after first appointment.

- Review medical and dental history.
- Stain for plaque.
- Note and record sites that bleed on gentle probing.
- Evaluate tissue response to previous treatment on a site-by-site basis. If inflammation persists, determine the cause. If plaque or calculus are present, debride the area(s) and reinforce oral hygiene. Adjunctive antimicrobial mouthrinses may be recommended.
- Reinforce plaque control instruction.
- Selective polishing, if indicated.
- Nutritional counseling for the control of dental caries, if needed.
- Fluoride treatment (caries control).
- Tobacco counseling for the control of oral disease, if needed.
- If gingival health has been achieved, a suitable maintenance interval is established (3 to 6 months), or after 7 to 10 days, a third appointment is scheduled if needed.
- Referral to periodontist if necessary with alternating maintenance visits planned.

Table 21–7	Slight Chronic Periodontitis

Probing depths of 4 to 5 mm clinical attachment loss (CAL) of 1 to 2 mm; slight horizontal bone loss (up to 20%); no mobility or furcation involvement; supra- and subgingival deposits; bleeding on probing

First appointment: 1 hour

- Comprehensive oral evaluation (new patients) or periodic oral evaluation (existing patients)—consisting of a medical and a dental history update, head and neck examination, and oral cancer screening. Make referrals if necessary.
- Periodontal examination. Sites that bleed on probing should be recorded.
- Complete x-ray series, including vertical bitewings (new patients) or indicated radiographs (existing patients).
- Stain for plaque and relate stained areas to bleeding sites as part of oral hygiene instruction (patient learns cause and effect).
- Periodontal debridement by quadrant (use of local anesthesia is determined by the practitioner).
- Adjunctive antimicrobial irrigation or mouthrinse, if indicated.
- Nutritional counseling for the control of dental caries.
- Tobacco counseling for the control and prevention of oral disease, if indicated.
- Application of desensitizing medicaments, if needed.

Second, third, and fourth appointments: At least 45 minutes (each scheduled 7 to 10 days after previous appointment)

- Review medical and dental history.
- Evaluate tissue response from previous treatment.
- Stain for plaque.
- Chart sites that bleed on gentle probing.
- Relate stained areas to any bleeding sites as part of oral hygiene instruction (patient learns cause and effect).
- Reinforce plaque-control instruction.
- Continue debridement procedures by quadrant.
- Nutritional counseling for the control of dental caries.
- Tobacco counseling for the control and prevention of oral disease, if indicated.
- Sustained, slow-release, local-delivery antimicrobials may be used at sites not fully responsive to self-care and debridement. (Although long-term use is not yet scientifically validated, so long as clinical parameters are promptly reassessed and nonresponders are referred, this tactic should offer little or no risk.)
- Application of desensitizing medicaments, if needed.

Fifth appointment (reevaluation of therapy): At least 45 minutes (scheduled 4 to 6 weeks after previous appointment)

- Review medical and dental history.
- Evaluate tissue response from previous treatment.
- Oral and dental examination.
- Periodontal examination; record sites that bleed on probing.
- Stain for plaque and relate stained areas to any bleeding sites as part of oral hygiene instruction (patient learns cause and effect).
- Selective polishing, if indicated.
- Nutritional counseling, if needed.
- Tobacco counseling, if indicated.
- Application of desensitizing medicaments, if needed.

At this time, the patient may be put on a suitable maintenance interval of every 2 to 4 months if inflammation appears arrested (e.g., no bleeding on probing from deep pockets

(continued)

Table 21–7	Slight Chronic Periodontitis (*cont.*)

at sites that patient is maintaining plaque-free) and there is no other reason to refer to a specialist (e.g., unresolved dentinal hypersensitivity, gingival recession, desire or need for periodontal plastic surgery). Over time, this interval can be increased in patients who remain inflammation-free.

If there are nonresponsive sites characterized by deep (.4 mm) probing depths that bleed on probing or at sites of previous attachment loss, referral to the periodontist is appropriate. Given the potential for rapid loss of attachment at any susceptible site, a decision to engage in "watchful waiting" is ethically and legally problematic.

If bleeding on probing persists at shallower sites (gingivitis), the practitioner should reevaluate the patient's self-care techniques and remove any subgingival calculus from suspect sites. Referral to the periodontist is an option for these patients as well.

Table 21–8	Moderate Chronic Periodontitis

Probing depths of 6 to 7 mm clinical attachment loss (CAL) of 3 to 4 mm; moderate horizontal/vertical bone loss (20 to 50%); mobility and early furcation involvement; supra- and subgingival deposits; bleeding on probing.
First appointment: 1 hour

- Comprehensive oral evaluation (new patients) or periodic oral evaluation (existing patients)—consisting of a medical and dental history update, head and neck examination, and oral cancer screening. Make referrals if necessary.
- Complete x-ray series, including vertical bitewings (new patients) or indicated radiographs (existing patients). Referral to the periodontist depends on the type and amount of bone loss.
- Periodontal examination. Sites that bleed on probing should be recorded.
- Stain for plaque and relate stained areas to bleeding sites as part of oral hygiene instruction (patient learns cause and effect).
- Nutritional counseling for the control of dental caries.
- Tobacco counseling for the control and prevention of oral disease, if indicated.
- Application of desensitizing medicaments, if needed.

Second, third, and fourth appointments: 1 hour (each scheduled 7 to 10 days after previous appointment)

- Review medical and dental history.
- Evaluate tissue response from previous treatment.
- Chart sites that bleed on gentle probing.
- Stain for plaque and relate stained areas to any bleeding sites as part of oral hygiene instruction (patient learns cause and effect).
- Reinforce plaque-control instruction.
- Periodontal debridement by quadrant (local anesthesia may be indicated).
- Adjunctive antimicrobial irrigation or mouthrinse, if indicated.
- Nutritional counseling for the control of dental caries.
- Tobacco counseling for the control and prevention of oral disease, if indicated.
- Application of desensitizing medicaments, if needed.

Fifth appointment (reevaluation of therapy): 1 hour (scheduled 4 to 6 weeks after previous appointment):

- Review medical and dental history.
- Evaluate tissue response from previous treatment.

Table 21–8	Moderate Chronic Periodontitis (*cont.*)

- Oral and dental examination.
- Periodontal examination; record sites that bleed on probing.
- Stain for plaque and relate stained areas to any bleeding sites as part of oral hygiene instruction (patient learns cause and effect).
- Periodontal debridement by quadrant (local anesthesia may be indicated).
- Adjunctive antimicrobial irrigation or mouth rinse, if indicated.
- Sustained, slow-release, local-delivery antimicrobials may be used at nonresponsive sites. (Long-term use [longer than 9 months] is not currently scientifically validated. However, if clinical parameters are promptly reassessed and nonresponders are referred, this tactic should offer little or no risk.)
- Selective polishing, if indicated.
- Nutritional counseling, if needed.
- Tobacco counseling, if indicated.
- Application of desensitizing medicaments, if needed.

At this time, the patient may be put on a suitable maintenance interval of 2 to 4 months if inflammation appears arrested (e.g., no bleeding on probing from deep pockets at sites that patient is maintaining plaque-free) and there is no other reason to refer to a specialist (e.g., unresolved dentinal hypersensitivity, gingival recession, desire or need for periodontal plastic surgery).

However, if bleeding on probing persists at sites with deeper (.4 mm) probing depths or at sites of previous attachment loss, referral to the periodontist is indicated—probably for periodontal surgery at those sites.

If no bleeding on probing is present but deep pockets persist, referral to the periodontist may be considered. Research suggests that deep pockets will not break down further if they repeatedly fail over time to demonstrate bleeding on probing (Lang, Adler, Joss, & Nyman, 1990). However, this should be viewed in light of other research showing that deeper pockets are more likely than shallower pockets to experience additional attachment loss due to periodontitis (Grbic & Lamster, 1992; Haffajee et al, 1991).

Table 21–9	Severe Chronic Periodontitis

Probing depths of more than 8 mm clinical attachment loss (CAL) of $\geq$ 5 mm; horizontal and vertical bone loss (> 50%); mobility and furcation involvement
First appointment: 1 hour

- Comprehensive oral evaluation (new patients) or periodic oral evaluation (existing patients)—consisting of a medical and dental history update, head and neck examination, and oral cancer screening. Make referrals if necessary. If the patient does not want to be referred to the periodontist, document the refusal in the patient's chart.
- Complete x-ray series, including vertical bitewings (new patients) or indicated radiographs (existing patients). If severe bone loss and heavy deposits exist, consider immediate referral to the periodontist for legal ramifications. If it is decided that initial therapy is to be done in the general practitioner's office, the following steps should be performed.
- Periodontal examination. Sites that bleed on probing should be recorded.
- Stain for plaque and relate stained areas to bleeding sites as part of oral hygiene instruction (patient learns cause and effect).
- Nutritional counseling for the control of dental caries.
- Tobacco counseling for the control and prevention of oral disease.
- Application of desensitizing medicaments, if needed.

(continued)

Table 21–9	Severe Chronic Periodontitis (*cont.*)

Second appointment: 1 hour (scheduled as soon as possible after initial visit)

- Review medical and dental history.
- Stain for plaque and relate stained areas to bleeding sites as part of oral hygiene instruction (patient learns cause and effect).
- Reinforce plaque-control instruction.
- Periodontal debridement by quadrant (use of local anesthesia may be indicated).
- Adjunctive antimicrobial irrigation or mouthrinse, if indicated.
- Nutritional counseling for the control of dental caries.
- Tobacco counseling for the control and prevention of oral disease, if indicated.
- Application of desensitizing medicaments, if needed.

Third, fourth, and fifth appointments: 1 hour (scheduled every 7 to 10 days)

- Review medical and dental history.
- Evaluate tissue response from previous treatment.
- Stain for plaque and relate stained areas to bleeding sites as part of oral hygiene instruction (patient learns cause and effect).
- Reinforce plaque-control instruction.
- Continue debridement procedures by quadrant.
- Adjunctive antimicrobial irrigation or mouthrinse, if indicated.
- Sustained, slow-release, local-delivery antimicrobials may be used at nonresponsive sites. (Long-term use [longer than 9 months] is not currently scientifically validated. However, if clinical parameters are promptly reassessed and nonresponders are referred, this tactic should offer little or no risk.)
- Nutritional counseling for the control of dental caries.
- Tobacco counseling for the control and prevention of oral disease, if indicated.
- Application of desensitizing medicaments, if needed.

Sixth appointment (reevaluation of therapy): 1 hour (scheduled 4 to 6 weeks after previous appointment)

- Review medical and dental history.
- Evaluate tissue response from previous treatment.
- Periodontal examination; record sites that bleed on probing.
- Stain for plaque and relate stained areas to bleeding sites as part of oral hygiene instruction (patient learns cause and effect).
- Reinforce plaque-control instruction.
- Selective polishing, if indicated.
- Sustained, slow-release, local-delivery antimicrobials may be used at nonresponsive sites (Long-term use [longer than 9 months] is not currently scientifically validated. However, if clinical parameters are promptly reassessed and nonresponders are referred, this tactic should offer little or no risk.)
- Nutritional counseling for the control of dental caries.
- Fluoride treatment for root caries control, if indicated.
- Tobacco counseling for the control and prevention of oral disease, if indicated.
- Application of desensitizing medicaments, if needed.
- At this time, referral to the periodontist is necessary for legal ramifications.

Only rarely will the procedures outlined above result in resolution of inflammation in pockets of more than 8 mm. (If this occurs, treat as for moderate chronic periodontitis.) Therefore, these patients are often referred early on to a periodontist.

Table 21–10	Refractory Periodontitis (Nonresponsive Cases)

The patient is biologically resistant to conventional therapy
First appointment: 1 hour

- Comprehensive oral evaluation (new patients) or periodic oral evaluation (existing patients)—consisting of a medical and dental history update, head and neck examination, and oral cancer screening. If this is an existing patient and previous treatment in the office has been ineffective, immediate referral to the periodontist is appropriate.
- If the patient does not want to be referred to the periodontist and wants treatment in the general practitioner's office, document the patient's informed refusal in the chart.
- Complete x-ray series, including vertical bitewings (new patients) or indicated radiographs (existing patients). If severe bone loss and heavy deposits, consider immediate referral to a periodontist for legal ramifications. Even though referral is indicated, if it is decided that therapy is to be done in the general practitioner's office, the following steps should be performed.
- Periodontal examination. Sites that bleed on probing should be recorded.
- Stain for plaque and relate stained areas to bleeding sites as part of oral hygiene instruction (patient learns cause and effect).
- Periodontal debridement by quadrant (use of local anesthesia is determined by the practitioner) in conjunction with systemic antibiotics (4 to 5 appointments).
- Consider adjunctive diagnostic/bacteriologic tests (e.g., genetic test, culture, DNA probe).
- Nutritional counseling for the control of dental caries.
- Tobacco counseling for the control and prevention of oral disease, if indicated.
- Application of desensitizing medicaments, if needed.

Third, fourth, and fifth appointments: 1 hour (scheduled every 7 to 10 days)

- Review medical and dental history.
- Evaluate tissue response from previous treatment.
- Chart sites that bleed on gentle probing.
- Stain for plaque and relate stained areas to bleeding sites as part of oral hygiene instruction (patient learns cause and effect).
- Reinforce plaque-control instruction.
- Continue debridement procedures by quadrant.
- Nutritional counseling for the control of dental caries.
- Tobacco counseling for the control and prevention of oral disease, if indicated.
- Application of desensitizing medicaments, if needed.

These patients are best treated by a periodontist.

Oral hygiene instruction and patient education are performed. Patients need to learn that diligent self-care is the critical foundation for successful periodontal treatment. Tables 21–5 through 21–10 emphasize self-care training, professional analyses, and technique refinement to a degree some may consider excessive. However, failure to provide compulsive clinical emphasis on patient motivation and self-care techniques invites many treatment failures that could be avoided.

Oral prophylaxis and periodontal debridement may be performed. The tissue responses to in-office and improved self-care may be assessed as soon as a week later.

Multiple appointments during this phase help the patient better understand his or her role as cotherapist. They also help build the key concept of a patient–hygienist–dentist team—organized to fight together against periodontitis on a site-by-site basis.

Table 21–11	Phases of Periodontal Treatment

Phase I or initial therapy: Disease control

- Emergency care; relief of acute symptoms*
- Oral hygiene instruction*
- Nutritional counseling*
- Correction of inadequate restorations (e.g., overhang or poorly contoured restorations,* open proximal contacts)
- Periodontal debridement*
- Antimicrobial therapy (oral rinses, oral irrigation, controlled-release products)*
- Systemic antibiotics, if indicated
- Fluoride application for caries control or desensitization, if indicated*
- Smoking cessation*
- Minor orthodontic movement
- Occlusal therapy (including night guards)*
- Extraction of hopeless teeth
- Reevaluation of initial therapy*

Phase II therapy: Surgical correction
Phase III therapy: Restorative/prosthetic care

- Final restorations fabricated

Phase IV therapy: Maintenance care

- Evaluation of patient's oral hygiene*
- Smoking cessation*
- Treatment depends on the condition of the periodontium

*Procedures that may be performed by dental hygienists in some jurisdictions. Check with individual state practice regulations.

As this phase draws to a close, if signs of inflammation persist at deeper probing sites—especially those the patient is keeping free of supragingival plaque—the need for periodontal surgery is often obvious to everyone.

Phase II: Periodontal Surgery Although evidence exists suggesting an approximate equivalence between arrestive outcomes of closed debridement procedures and open (surgical) procedures in many types of periodontal defects, practitioners need to know that the design of these nonsurgical studies (e.g., 20 minutes of root planing per tooth) is clinically unrealistic (Lindhe et al., 1984; Pihlstrom, McHugh, Oliphant, & Ortiz-Campos, 1983; Ramfjord et al., 1987).

Many periodontal surgical procedures are performed to provide the practitioner with better and faster access to deep periodontal pockets. These surgeries may be arrestive or regenerative. A single surgical procedure may incorporate both elements. For example, an osseous (bone) graft may be placed in a deep infrabony defect on one tooth, whereas bone in adjacent areas may be reduced to facilitate the placement of a pocket-eliminating apically positioned surgical flap that establishes a maintainable gingival form.

Other periodontal surgical procedures may be performed to address gingival recession. The indications for such surgery include dentinal sensitivity, aesthetic complaints, or continuing recession. Many times these procedures are both arrestive and regenerative in character.

Other periodontal surgical procedures may be performed to maximize the aesthetic results associated with new restorative dentistry. Examples include ridge augmentation and crown lengthening. Procedures performed for aesthetics alone are usually termed periodontal plastic surgery.

Phase III: Restorative Care   Restorative dentistry is performed in this phase. Ideally, periodontal and prosthetic dentists work together to design restorations that satisfy aesthetic, comfort, and functional needs without compromising future periodontal health.

Phase IV: Maintenance Care   Phase IV consists of periodontal maintenance (also termed recall or continuing care). The goal of periodontal maintenance is to prevent continued periodontal destruction. Maintenance care includes reexamination and assessment of the periodontal condition and patient self-care. It often includes an oral prophylaxis and may include periodontal debridement and other local therapies that target persistently inflamed sites.

The frequency of periodontal maintenance visits is individualized and depends on the patient's periodontal status, medical condition, and self-care motivation and effectiveness.

Referral to a Periodontist

Although patients experiencing periodontal problems may be referred to a periodontist at any time, preliminary phases of periodontal therapy often are performed in the general practice. Sometimes, especially for mild cases, this is all that is necessary to achieve the goal of periodontal therapy. However, even for patients who are ultimately referred, the benefits of the self-care training, motivation, and emphasis on team building in the general practice increase the likelihood of treatment success by the periodontist and beyond. Hygienists, general practitioners, and periodontists who function as a team maximize the likelihood of optimal outcomes.

Although a licensed general practitioner legally may provide comprehensive periodontal therapy to any informed and consenting patient, he or she is ethically and legally required to meet the same standard of care for such therapy as a specialist. Therefore, with the welfare of periodontal patients in mind, the following referral guidelines are proposed—with the knowledge that exceptions occur.

Guidelines for Referral

Any patient who has one or more periodontal sites that show persistent signs of inflammation should be considered for referral. Often these patients fit in one or more of the following categories:

1. Chronic periodontitis with deeper probing depths, furcation involvement, and/or problematic gingival recession
2. Aggressive (localized, generalized) periodontitis
3. Periodontitis associated with systemic diseases (such as diabetes mellitus)
4. Periodontitis with significant or increasing tooth mobility
5. Periodontal lesions adjacent to necrotic (or endodontically treated) teeth
6. Refractory (considered nonresponsive to treatment) or recurrent periodontitis (responsive, but still headed downhill)

7. Patients who have aesthetic concerns about the interplay between teeth, restorations, and the gingiva or alveolar arches
8. Patients with mucocutaneous disorders affecting the oral soft tissues (e.g., pemphigus, lichen planus)

Informed Consent

Before examination and treatment, the patient must give consent. For medicolegal reasons, informed consent is usually recorded using a document signed by the patient and the practitioner, because any treatment provided without consent legally may constitute a battery. Furthermore, a valid consent requires that the patient be made reasonably knowledgeable about the risks and benefits associated with the proposed treatments, alternative treatments, and no treatment. Minor children and the mentally incapacitated ordinarily cannot execute a valid consent.

For periodontal patients, the informed consent form should clearly reflect that the patient understands and accepts the need for periodontal maintenance and oral hygiene self-care.

Treatment Guidelines

The following treatment guidelines were written for new patients but can be adapted for existing patients. Although treatment planning guidelines are helpful, it is important to remember that treatment must be tailored to each patient. Experience and the scientific literature have demonstrated that responses to therapy can vary from one patient to another or even in the same patient at different sites and at different times. Therefore, each patient may respond uniquely to the therapy provided.

This section contains guidelines for treating typical periodontal patients and patients with other periodontal conditions, including medication- and hormone-influenced gingivitis, gingivitis and periodontitis related to systemic conditions, aggressive periodontitis, and acute periodontal conditions.

As discussed previously, these guidelines include intensive and continual emphasis on self-care, self-care assessment (by the practitioner), and professional re-assessments (of tissue status) on a site-by-site basis. For many patients, these are essential for long-term treatment success. Furthermore, the suggested time allowance for each appointment is subject to change based on the patient's response to care. Of course, these are only guidelines. The ultimate decision making and responsibility for how to treat a patient rests with the individual practitioner.

Periodontal Health

Patients presenting with no bleeding on gentle probing and light to no supragingival plaque and calculus only require an oral prophylaxis (see Table 21–5). Subgingival root debridement is contraindicated. Once oral hygiene efficacy is assured, a suitable periodontal maintenance schedule is determined, usually every 6 to 12 months.

The motivated and periodontally healthy patient is often "dentally aware." Indeed, past dental therapy may be responsible for the healthy state the patient now enjoys. Such patients generally enjoy discussing new advancements in dentistry. They usually welcome improvements in professional care and self-care and may question the practitioner about new treatment concepts. Oral hygiene instruction time may be used to discuss new oral hygiene products and their applications. The patient must be reminded of the need for future examinations (since problems may occur even though the patient currently appears healthy).

Gingivitis

Plaque-Induced Gingivitis

Most cases of gingivitis are plaque-related and are best treated by periodontal debridement and oral hygiene instructions (see Table 21–6). The therapeutic goal is to establish gingival health by eliminating the etiologic factors. The ultimate objective is to prevent sites from progressing to periodontitis. Since we are unable to predict which sites will progress, the entire mouth must be treated. Patients need to be aware of the need for adequate toothbrushing and the use of interdental cleaning aids. Supplemental use of antimicrobial agents (e.g., mouth rinses) is recommended in certain patients, such as those with severe bleeding that interferes with debridement procedures or those with poor manual dexterity. Following initial therapy, the patient is placed on a well-monitored periodontal maintenance program.

For all types of gingivitis, initial periodontal debridement and oral hygiene instructions are the key to minimizing microbial plaque accumulation.

Sulcular sites that bleed on gentle probing should be noted and recorded and pointed out to the patient. Plaque staining will reveal areas of plaque accumulation. These should be recorded as well. Bleeding often occurs at these sites. The patient needs to understand this relationship. The patient also needs to appreciate that if a site bleeds as a result of self-care, that site usually needs more self-care attention, not less. This runs counter to the intuition of most patients, whose common response to bleeding is to "leave the area alone."

If the patient is taught to understand that the destructive process is at an early stage and that proper professional care and self-care likely will return the tissues to health, treatment is more likely to succeed. Involve the patient as a "cotherapist."

Gingival Enlargement

Gingival enlargement or overgrowth is sometimes seen in patients with orthodontic appliances or in patients taking certain drugs. Removal of dental plaque and calculus by meticulous oral hygiene and regular professional mechanical debridement may help to prevent or slow gingival overgrowth. Therefore, initial treatment should focus on improved self-care and professional plaque and calculus removal. Unfortunately, gingival enlargement still may occur, making it difficult to perform effective self-care and even interfering with chewing, speech, and appearance.

For orthodontic patients, surgical removal of fibrotic pseudopockets can be performed at any time, but recurrence is likely if orthodontic appliances remain. For patients with drug-induced gingival enlargement, overgrowth usually requires surgical intervention. Recurrence is common if the drug is continued. Therefore, it is important to inform the patient's physician about the oral condition and inquire if an alternative drug could be prescribed.

Hormone-Associated Gingivitis

Pregnancy, oral contraceptives, and puberty can contribute to gingivitis. Treatment of hormone-influenced gingivitis is aimed at lowering plaque levels by maintaining meticulous oral hygiene. Frequent periodontal maintenance also may help.

Periodontitis

Chronic periodontitis (formerly termed adult periodontitis is by far the most common form of periodontitis seen in otherwise healthy patients. Aggressive periodontitis (formerly termed early-onset periodontitis), refractory periodontitis, periodontitis associated with systemic conditions, and peri-implantitis are less common but are more difficult to treat and should be referred.

Chronic Periodontitis

In general, the treatment of patients with chronic periodontitis begins with oral hygiene instructions and periodontal debridement, followed by surgical therapy if needed. Patients are then monitored, and treatment is modified as necessary as part of an ongoing periodontal maintenance program. Repeated surgeries sometimes are necessary.

Periodontal patients who demonstrate attachment loss and probing pocket depths of 4 to 5 mm (slight periodontitis) often respond adequately (e.g., elimination of bleeding on probing) to periodontal debridement and effective oral self-care (see Table 21–7). In moderate periodontitis (attachment loss with probing depths of 6 to 7 mm; see Table 21–8) and severe periodontitis (attachment loss with probing depths of more than 8 mm; see Table 21–9), periodontal debridement is less predictable (Stambaugh, Dragoo, Smith, & Carasali, 1981). Following oral hygiene instruction and periodontal debridement, such patients are usually referred to the periodontist—often for periodontal surgery at nonresponsive sites.

Patients with gingival recession should be evaluated. If the recession causes tooth pain, is progressing, or interferes with aesthetics, gingival grafting may be indicated.

It should be noted that chronic periodontitis is site-specific. Some patients demonstrate clinical attachment loss and/or probing depths that are normal at some sites, suggestive of slight periodontitis at other sites, and indicative of moderate or severe periodontitis at others. Therefore, periodontal debridement and improved self-care may be adequate at some sites but inadequate at others in the same patient. The most problematic sites guide ideal patient management. In other words, the persistence of even one diseased site is sufficient to justify referral for more aggressive therapy.

Refractory periodontal patients who do not respond to proper periodontal treatment (see Table 21–10) despite quality self-care and participation in a well-monitored periodontal maintenance program should be referred to a periodontist.

Aggressive Periodontitis

Apparently healthy young people (younger than 30 years of age) can have underlying immune system irregularities that may manifest as periodontitis with rapid attachment loss and bone destruction (Tonetti & Mombelli, 1999). Treatment of this type of periodontitis is similar to that for chronic forms of periodontitis except that surgical intervention and antibiotic therapy often are used early in therapy. Therefore, these patients should be referred promptly to a periodontist.

Necrotizing Periodontal Diseases

Necrotizing ulcerative gingivitis (NUG) and necrotizing ulcerative periodontitis (NUP) are collectively referred to as necrotizing periodontal diseases. Necrotizing ulcerative gingivitis (NUG) is an infection localized to the gingiva. Contributory risk factors include emotional stress, poor oral hygiene, cigarette smoking, and HIV infections (Rowland, 1999). NUP involves the attachment apparatus and is seen primarily in individuals with systemic conditions including, but not limited to, HIV infection, severe malnutrition, and immunosuppression (Novak, 1999).

Peri-Implantitis

Treatment of peri-implant diseases may include mechanical debridement, oral hygiene instructions, mouthrinses, systemic antibiotics, arrestive and regenerative periodontal surgery, and/or implant removal. Referral to a periodontist is recommended.

Adjunctive Treatment

Antimicrobials

Systemic antibiotics often are prescribed as part of the treatment of aggressive periodontitis or of periodontitis patients with systemic maladies. For example, administration of a systemic antibiotic, debridement, and surgery constitute an appropriate course of therapy for a patient with localized juvenile periodontitis.

In an otherwise healthy chronic periodontitis patient, antibiotics usually are reserved for a specific refractory infection or as an adjunct to certain periodontal surgical procedures. In the case of refractory periodontitis, specific antibiotics are selected based on identification of the suspected pathogens.

The guidelines governing the use of systemic antibiotics in patients with periodontitis are constantly changing. Therefore, practitioners who would use systemic antimicrobials to treat periodontitis must remain very up-to-date with the appropriate biomedical literature.

Controlled-release antimicrobial drug systems as a supplement to periodontal debridement may be indicated when clinical signs of inflammation (bleeding upon probing) persist in pockets of 5 mm or greater at localized sites. However, continuing reassessment is needed to determine if other therapies are indicated, since successful long-term use of these devices has yet to be validated clinically.

Antimicrobial rinses and toothpastes are widely advertised. Chlorhexidine gluconate rinses are prescribed routinely for specified periods when mechanical plaque control is not feasible (e.g., after surgery, after acute infection). Over-the-counter antimicrobial rinses are of limited value but may provide benefits for some patients. Use of mouthrinses should not be a substitute for mechanical self-care.

Prognosis

Prognosis is a prediction of the future course of a malady with or without treatment. All aspects of the patient's history, data from the clinical examination, and the patient's healing capacity are factors.

Common clinical factors used in assigning a prognosis are reviewed in Table 21–12■ (McGuire & Nunn, 1996). This checklist can be reviewed as part of developing a prognosis for each patient. The more unfavorable factors noted, the worse is the prognosis.

Prognosis is usually reported using a graded scale. This may be a simple scale such as good, guarded, or poor or a scale with more intervals such as good, fair, poor, questionable, or hopeless (Table 21–13■; McGuire & Nunn, 1996).

Determination of prognosis is important in treatment planning so that the practitioner and patient can agree on a plan that best satisfies the patient's overall goals while minimizing disappointments if setbacks occur. Realistic prognoses are of amplified importance in complex cases that combine periodontal and restorative therapies. This is so because in these patients, the unexpected loss of a key abutment tooth may necessitate replacement of complicated and expensive crown and bridge prosthetics.

Geriatric Patients

Although the same general guidelines already provided for chronic periodontitis patients apply to the elderly, geriatric patients often have special needs. They may present with uncontrolled dental plaque and/or xerostomia. Other oral pathologies, including oral cancers, are more common among members of this age group.

Table 21–12	Common Clinical Factors Used in Determining a Prognosis

Factors affecting prognosis of individual teeth:
- Amount of bone remaining
- Depth of pockets
- Pattern of bone loss, horizontal or vertical
- Tooth mobility
- Type of infrabony defect: one, two, or three walls
- Root anatomy, favorable or unfavorable
- Furcation involvement
- Crown-to-root ratio, favorable or unfavorable
- Caries or pulpal involvement, yes or no
- Missing teeth and restorative dentistry

Factors affecting overall prognosis:
- Age
- Significant medical history (e.g., diabetes)
- Smoker, yes or no, past smoker
- Family history of periodontal diseases, yes or no
- Oral hygiene: good, fair, or poor
- Compliant with treatment and home care, yes or no

Source: Adapted from McGuire and Nunn, 1996.

Table 21–13	Prognostic Classification for Individual Teeth

- Good prognosis: Adequate periodontal support around the tooth and can be easily maintained by the practitioner and the patient.
- Fair prognosis: About 25% bone loss. Class I furcation involvement present and can be properly maintained.
- Poor prognosis: About 50% bone loss. Class II furcation involvement present and can be maintained but with difficulty.
- Questionable prognosis: Greater than 50% bone loss around the tooth. Class II and III furcation involvements present that cannot be maintained.
- Hopeless prognosis: Not enough bony support around the tooth to maintain it in its socket. Extraction of tooth recommended.

Source: Adapted from McGuire and Nunn, 1996.

Plaque Control

Age-related factors may limit the ability of a patient to perform adequate oral self-care. Visual impairment can diminish an individual's ability to see oral structures and debris. Using a toothbrush or dental floss may be impossible for patients with arthritis or stroke-related impairments. Dementia may affect an individual's ability or motivation to perform daily oral hygiene procedures. Virtually any debilitating systemic illness may predispose patients to periodontitis—and many of these maladies are seen more commonly in aged populations. Most important, periodontal treatment may be complicated by multiple medical conditions.

Xerostomia

Decreased saliva production occurs with advancing age. Furthermore, many of the hundreds of medications known to decrease salivary flow are used by older people. Antidepressants, antihistamines, antihypertensives, antipsychotics, diuretics, antiparkinsonians, and antianxiety agents all may contribute to xerostomia (Brangan, 1994). Older patients, with decreased protective properties of saliva, are at increased risk for dental caries and periodontal diseases.

If a patient complains of xerostomia, or if dryness seems to be contributing to oral problems, relevant systemic medications should be identified and alternatives considered. Saliva substitutes may be recommended, but these have limited effectiveness and can be expensive.

Treatment Considerations

When treating geriatric patients, the practitioner must consider systemic concerns that may complicate the management of periodontal conditions. It may be important for the dentist and hygienist to consult with a patient's physician to review pertinent details of the patient's medical conditions.

Treatment goals for the elderly are the same as for the young, that is, the preservation (or restoration) of an aesthetic, comfortable, and functional dentition. This is not to suggest that age should not be a factor in planning how best to achieve these goals; indeed, conservative therapy may be more appropriate in older patients for a number of reasons. Whatever treatment is planned, it should be flexible and adapted to each patient's particular needs. As these needs change, so should the therapy.

Successful treatment of the elderly often requires a high degree of cooperation between the practitioner, patient, and other supporting caregivers. Modified self-care routines may be necessary, such as use of a toothpick instead of floss, a toothbrush with a modified handle such as a tennis ball, and the frequent use of antimicrobial agents (such as fluorides or chlorhexidine) along with mechanical plaque control. Automated oral hygiene devices may facilitate more effective plaque control.

Summary

Research supports the majority of procedures routinely performed by the dental hygienist to prevent or arrest the progression of the common periodontal maladies. Science, combined with a century of clinical experience and inferential skills, has produced the periodontal parameters of care for today. As time passes, continued scientific testing of new and old therapeutic tactics along with clinical experience will continue to underpin future parameters for periodontal care.

At the beginning of the twenty-first century, periodontal treatment planning remains complicated. For now, ongoing periodontal care should be modulated based on the response of the patient to self-care and treatment rendered previously. If a desired and optimal response is not achieved, some other reasonable approach must be used and assessed. Critical analyses of outcomes will sometimes suggest that referral to a specialist is in the best interest of the patient.

Quality assessment has been defined as "a measure of care provided in a particular setting" (Burt & Eklund, 1992). Quality assurance is a broader concept that encompasses assessment of care along with the "implementation of any necessary changes to either maintain or improve the quality of care rendered" (Burt & Eklund, 1992).

Dental hygienists have the professional responsibility to promote the oral health of the public in the most effective ways possible. As excerpted from the American Dental Hygienists Association's (1998) Code of Ethics, "We acknowledge the following responsibilities to patients or clients:

- Provide oral health care utilizing high levels of professional knowledge, judgment, and skill.
- Serve as an advocate for the welfare of clients.
- Provide clients with the information necessary to make informed decisions about their oral health and encourage their full participation in treatment decisions and goals.
- Refer clients to other healthcare providers when their needs are beyond our ability or scope of practice.
- Educate clients about high-quality oral health care."

Key Points

- Evidence-based periodontal treatment based on dental literature focuses on the recognition of risk, prognosis, and treatment factors.
- The evidence-based approach is a good model for evaluating the results of periodontal therapy.
- Problem-based learning identifies patient's dental problems.

- The ideal goal of periodontal therapy is to restore the periodontium destroyed by disease to a comfortable and functional state of health.
- Periodontal treatment involves ongoing care and demands continued reassessments.

Web Sites

www.perio.org

www.ada.org

Self-Quiz

1. Which one of the following factors improves the treatment decisions made by dental/medical practitioners? (p. 310)

   a. clinical experience of the practitioner and use of scientific literature

   b. following the advice of fellow dental practitioners

   c. following the advice of fellow medical practitioners

   d. consulting with the dental companies

2. Which one of the following statements is the ideal goal of periodontal therapy? (p. 315)

   a. Control or eliminate and prevent the initiation, progression, or recurrence of periodontal diseases.

   b. Promote tissue healing by regeneration or replacement of the lost tissue with new bone, cementum, and periodontal ligament.

   c. Restore the periodontium to an attractive, comfortable, and functional state of health for the balance of the patient's life.

   d. Allow the attachment apparatus to relax.

   e. Remove all microbial plaque every day.

3. Which one of the following steps should be first in developing a plan to treat a patient? (p. 315)

   a. Teach proper use of oral hygiene aids.

   b. Determine the treatment goals.

   c. Discuss the case with the patient.

   d. Decide on the proper maintenance interval.

   e. Obtain informed consent for periodontal maintenance.

4. All the following are phases of treatment except one. Which one is the exception? (pp. 317–325)

   a. Phase I: disease control

   b. Phase II: surgical correction

   c. Phase III: restorative/prosthetic care

   d. Phase IV: maintenance care

   e. Phase V: implant care

5. In which one of the following phases of treatment is reevaluation of initial therapy completed? (p. 317)

   a. I

   b. II

   c. III

   d. IV

   e. V

6. Which one of the following treatment steps is most appropriate in controlling pregnancy-associated gingivitis? (p. 328)

   a. surgical intervention

   b. oral irrigation with chlorhexidine

   c. plaque control with toothbrushing and flossing

   d. systemic antibiotics

   e. estrogen supplements

7. Which one of the following treatments is most appropriate for patients with localized aggressive periodontitis? (pp. 328–329)

   a. periodontal debridement, systemic antibiotics, and surgery

   b. periodontal debridement and surgery

   c. oral rinsing and periodontal debridement

   d. oral irrigation and periodontal debridement

   e. improved oral hygiene and watchful waiting

8. Which one of the following sequences is the best initial treatment for a patient with gingival enlargement caused by phenytoin? (p. 327)

   a. oral hygiene instructions, periodontal debridement, systemic antibiotics, and surgery

   b. oral hygiene instructions and periodontal debridement

   c. periodontal debridement and systemic antibiotics

   d. periodontal debridement and surgery

   e. discontinuation of phenytoin

9. Which one of the following definitions best describes the term prognosis? (p. 330)

   a. prediction of the future course of a condition with or without treatment

   b. prediction of the future course of a condition without treatment

   c. identification and naming of the type of condition present

   d. patient's healing capacity

10. Which one of the following is the most important consideration when treating geriatric patients? (p. 330)

    a. Therapy may be complicated by multiple medical conditions.

    b. The ability to properly understand oral hygiene instructions may be impaired.

    c. Anxiety level is higher in this age group.

    d. Severe frailty inhibits normal maneuvering in the dental office.

    e. Physical impairments are possible.

References

American Academy of Periodontology. 1996. *Annals of periodontology: 1996 World Workshop in Periodontics*. Chicago: Author.

American Academy of Periodontology. 2000 Parameters of Care. *J. Periodontol 71* (Suppl.):847–883.

American Dental Hygienists Association. 1998. *1998–1999 Bylaws and code of ethics*. Chicago: Author.

Axelsson, P., and J. Lindhe. 1981. The significance of maintenance care in the treatment of periodontal disease. *J. Clin. Periodontol.* 8:281–294.

Burt, B., and S. Eklund. 1992. *Dentistry, dental practice and the community*. Philadelphia: W. B. Saunders.

Brangan, P. 1994. Dental hygiene care for the older adult. In eds. M. L. Darby and M. Walsh, *Dental hygiene theory and practice,* 873–912. Philadelphia: W. B. Saunders.

Grbic, J., and I. Lamster. 1992. Risk indicators for future periodontal attachment loss in adult periodontitis: Tooth and site variables. *J. Periodontol.* 63:262–269.

Grossi, S. G., R. J. Genco, E. E. Machtei, A. W. Ho, G. Koch, et al. 1995. Assessment of risk for periodontal disease: II. Risk indicators for alveolar bone loss. *J. Periodontol.* 66:23–29.

Grossi, S. G., J. J. Zambon, A. W. Ho, G. Koch, R. G. Dunford, et al. 1994. Assessment of risk for periodontal disease: I. Risk indicators for attachment loss. *J. Periodontol.* 65:260–267.

Haffajee, A. D., S. S. Socransky, J. Lindhe, R. L. Kent, H. Okamoto, and T. Yoneyama 1991. Clinical risk indicators for periodontal attachment loss. *J. Clin. Periodontol.* 18:117–125.

Hancock, E. B. 1996. Prevention. *Ann. Periodontol.* 1:223–249.

Ismail, A. I., E. C. Morrison, B. A. Burt, R. G. Caffesse, and M. T. Kavanagh. 1990. Natural history of periodontal disease in adults: Findings from the Tecumseh Periodontal Disease Study, 1959–1987. *J. Dent. Res.* 69:430–435.

Lang, K., R. Adler, A. Joss, and S. Nyman. 1990. Absence of bleeding on probing: An indicator of periodontal stability. *J. Clin. Periodontol.* 17:714–721.

Lindhe, J., E. Westfelt, S. Nyman, S.S. Socransky, I.L. Heij, G. Bratthall. 1984. Long-term effect of surgical/nonsurgical treatment of periodontal disease. *J. Clin. Periodontol.* 11:448–458.

Loesche, W. 1976. Chemotherapy of dental plaque infections. *Oral Sci. Rev.* 9:65–107.

McGuire, K. M., and M. E. Nunn. 1996. Prognosis versus actual outcome: II. The effectiveness of clinical parameters in developing an accurate prognosis. *J. Periodontol.* 67:658–665.

Newman, M. 1998. Improved clinical decision making using the evidence-based approach. *J. Am. Dent. Assoc.* 129:4S–8S.

Novak, M. J. 1999. Necrotizing ulcerative periodontitis. *Ann. Periodontol.* 4:74–77.

Pihlstrom, B., R. McHugh, T. Oliphant, and C. Ortiz-Campos. 1983. Comparison of surgical and nonsurgical treatment of periodontal disease: A review of current studies and additional results after 6 1/2 years. *J. Clin. Periodontol.* 10:524–541.

Ramfjord, S.P., R. G. Caffesse, E. C. Morrison, R. W. Hill, G. J. Kerry, et al. 1987. Four modalities of periodontal treatment compared over 5 years. *J. Clin. Periodontol.* 14:445–452.

Rowland, R. W. 1999. Necrotizing ulcerative gingivitis. *Ann. Periodontol.* 4:65–73.

Stambaugh, R. V., M. Dragoo, D. M. Smith, and L. Carasali. 1981. The limits of subgingival scaling. Int. *J. Periodont. Restor. Dent.* 1(5):31–41.

Tonetti, M. S., and A. Mombelli. 1999. Early-onset periodontitis. *Ann. Periodontol.* 4:39–52.

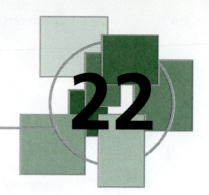

Oral Hygiene Self-Care

Diana L. Mercado Galvis, D.D.S., R.D.H., M.S.
Judith Kreismann, R.D.H., B.S., M.A.
Khalid Almas, B.D.S., M.Sc.

Outline

Goal

To provide information about the fundamentals of counseling periodontal patients on oral hygiene self-care.

Educational Objectives

Upon completion of this chapter, the reader should be able to:

Describe measures taken to prevent and control the progression of periodontal diseases.

Discuss preventive care as it relates to private practice.

Discuss the various toothbrushing methods used to maintain gingival health.

Compare the effectiveness of a powered toothbrush versus a manual toothbrush.

KEY WORDS
- oral biofilms
- halitosis
- oral hygiene self-care
- patient education
- primary prevention
- secondary prevention
- patient motivation
- oral rinses
- dentifrices

Discuss the importance of interdental cleaning in maintaining periodontal health.

Discuss the significance of halitosis.

Describe an effective plaque-control regimen following periodontal and implant surgery.

There is no alternative to well-performed oral hygiene self-care as a preventive measure. The willingness and ability of patients to keep dental plaque below the threshold for disease is essential. Preventive measures are important for a healthy periodontium as well as to achieve a successful outcome of periodontal therapy. Preventive measures in periodontics depend on the removal of supra- and subgingival dental plaque biofilms. The most common preventive methods involve both personal and professional mechanical plaque control. Preventive measures should address the control or elimination of etiologic factors as well as identified risk factors for inflammatory periodontal diseases (Hancock, 1996). The control of supragingival plaque in conjunction with professional tooth cleaning subgingivally forms the basis for the management of progressive periodontal diseases (Corbet & Davies, 1993). Supragingival plaque control contributes to preventing or moderating subgingival microbial recolonization, which can control progressive periodontal diseases. This chapter focuses on fundamental information related to oral hygiene self-care for the periodontal patient.

Definition of Oral Hygiene Self-Care

Oral hygiene self-care, also known as oral physiotherapy or oral home care, is defined as physical therapy for the mouth or oral cavity. It refers to daily oral health-care practices employed by the patient to prevent dental and gingival diseases and maintain optimal oral health. The rationale for oral hygiene self-care as well as professional periodontal debridement is the elimination or suppression of harmful microorganisms found in supragingival biofilms. Consequently, plaque control prevents the potential detrimental effects of pathogenic microorganisms on the teeth and periodontium. The primary method of oral hygiene self-care is the use of such mechanical oral hygiene measures as a toothbrush and interdental cleaning devices. Since not all bacteria in biofilms are pathogenic (disease-producing), the objective of treatment is not total elimination of all bacteria but rather control of the bacteria.

Periodontal Health: Motivation and Behavior

Since dental and periodontal health is taking on increasing importance for both patients and family members, evaluation of a patient's motivation and behavior in terms of oral self-care is important in the overall treatment plan.

In the process of evaluating a patient's oral hygiene, it is necessary to assess the clinical aspects of oral hygiene as well as relate the patient's attitude toward oral hygiene and his or her commitment to oral hygiene practices.

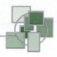

Periodontal Disease Control

There is overwhelming evidence that the accumulation of supragingival dental plaque on tooth surfaces near the free gingival margin is associated with the development of gingivitis. Thus removal of dental plaque from tooth surfaces is a basic step in the prevention and treatment of gingivitis. The subgingival plaque bacteria play an important role in the progression of periodontal diseases. The subgingival bacteria are derived from the supragingival dental plaque. If supragingival plaque is not removed, subgingival plaque develops. Therefore, meticulous mechanical supragingival plaque control can reduce the risk for the development of periodontitis or for disease recurrence after periodontal therapy or prevent further loss of attachment if periodontitis is already present (Addy & Adriaens, 1998; Westfelt, 1996). Clinical trials have shown that professionally delivered and frequently repeated supragingival tooth cleaning, combined with optimal self-performed plaque control, has a marked effect in controlling subgingival microbiota in moderate to deep periodontal pockets (Hellström, Romberg, Krok, & Lindhe, 1996).

Self-Cleansing Mechanism

The oral cavity possesses a "self-cleansing mechanism" that acts as a natural method for removing oral debris. The teeth, their alignment, occlusion, gingiva, tongue, cheeks, and saliva work together to remove oral debris. This self-cleansing mechanism is limited, however, and does not prevent dental caries and periodontal diseases. Therefore, mechanical plaque control is the most widely accepted method of preventing dental caries and periodontal diseases.

Patient Education

Educating the periodontal patient about oral hygiene self-care is one of the most important roles of the dental hygienist. Patient education provides the patient with the necessary information and skills for the prevention of dental caries and periodontal diseases. A thorough knowledge of oral hygiene self-care is essential for dental hygienists to help plan successful preventive strategies related to a patient's individual plaque-control needs.

One way to educate the patient on the importance of dental plaque is using disclosing agents. The purpose of using disclosing tablets or liquid is for supragingival plaque detection. The most commonly used disclosing agent is erythrosin, which is FD & C Red No. 28. Erythrosin stains newly formed dental plaque making it visible to the naked eye.

Studies have shown that the method used to educate patients about oral hygiene self-care techniques is not critical (Glavid, Christensen, Pedersen, Rosendahl, & Attström, 1985). Therefore, instructions can be given personally by the hygienist, or the patient may be provided with a self-instruction manual, pamphlet, or videotape.

Preventive Measures

The primary goal of prevention is to achieve the lowest plaque level possible. Total elimination of bacteria is neither possible nor desirable, because a number of beneficial bacteria exist in the oral cavity that are necessary for a balanced oral environment.

Preventive measures are classified into two main groups depending on when mechanical plaque control is instituted during the disease process. Primary prevention describes preventive measures taken to prevent disease from occurring. It aims at reducing plaque in all individuals regardless of their susceptibility to disease. On the other hand, if periodontal disease is already present in an individual, the goal of treatment changes from preventing the occurrence of disease to preventing the disease from progressing further or preventing the recurrence of the disease after treatment. This is secondary prevention (Garmyn, van Steenberghe, & Quirynen, 1998).

Halitosis

Halitosis is the general term used to describe unpleasant breath, regardless of its sources, oral or nonoral (e.g., expired air). Oral malodor is the term especially used to describe the odor from the oral cavity.

Oral malodor, bad breath, or halitosis is a common complaint encountered by dental practitioners. It may be due to poor oral hygiene, local factors, or systemic involvement. Oral malodor affects a large proportion of population and may cause a significant social or psychological handicap to those suffering from it. Dental hygienists should formulate informed choices while treating oral malodor patients to improve their quality of life through enhancing their social acceptance.

It has been estimated that 10 to 30% of the U.S. population suffers from bad breath on a regular basis (Meskin, 1996). In other studies, 20 to 60% of the population suffers from chronic oral malodor, and in approximately half of these individuals, the problem becomes serious enough to create personal discomfort and social embarrassment (Bosy, 1997; Brunete, Porskin, & Nelson, 1998). There is potential impact of oral malodor on personal life, so sufferers often make desperate attempts to mask their oral malodor with mints and chewing gum, compulsive brushing, and repeated use of mouthrinses.

In most cases, the problem of oral malodor has been shown to originate in the oral cavity, where conditions that favor the retention of anaerobic, mainly Gram–negative bacteria, lead to the development of bad breath (Ratcliff & Johnson, 1999). In addition to the periodontal pockets, the most important retention site is the dorsum of the tongue with its numerous papillae (Delanghe et al., 1999; Scully, 1997). There are various compounds that produce unpleasant smells in the human oral environment, such as hydrogen sulfide, methanethiol, dimethylsulfide, n-dodecanol, n-tetradecanol, phenol, indole, diphenylamine, pyridine, and others (Kostelc, Preti, Zelson, Stoller, & Tonzetich, 1980). Especially violatile sulfur compounds (VSC; hydrogen sulfide, methylmercaptan, and dimethyl sulfide), that arise from bacterial metabolism of amino acids, mainly contribute to oral malodor. It has been demonstrated that the intensity of clinical bad breath is significantly associated with amount of intraoral VSC level (Replogle & Beebe, 1996). The periodontal pocket is an ideal environment for VSC production with respect to the bacterial profile and sulfur source. In addition, VSC also accelerate periodontal tissue destruction. This may explain why patients with periodontal diseases often complain of oral malodor (Morita & Wang, 2001). Many people still believe that bad breath originates in the stomach. Halitosis is rarely a gastrointestinal condition (Page, 1997). Research reports now agree that, in the vast majority of cases, halitosis (80 to 90%) originates within the oral cavity, where anaerobic bacteria degrade sulfur-containing amino acids to the foul-smelling volatile sulfur compounds (Rosenberg,

Table 22–1	Oral Conditions that May Cause Bad Breath

- Periodontal pockets
- Xerostomia (dryness of mouth)
- Carious lesions
- Bacterial biofilms
- Interdental areas debris
- Papillae of the tongue
- Poor restorations
- Calculus
- Erupting wisdom teeth (Pericoronitis)
- Remaining roots
- Gangrenous pulps (necrosed pulp tissue)
- NUG (necrotizing ulcerative gingivitis)

1996; Tonzetich, 1997). The oral and systemic factors predisposing toward bad breath are given in Tables 22–1■ and 22–2■.

Classification of Halitosis Patients

Although halitosis involves oral, systemic, and psychological pathologies, a clear classification has not been established and mismanagement of psychological or systemic cases of halitosis can occur. The classification system reported by Miyazaki and colleagues (1999) has three categories: genuine halitosis, pseudo-halitosis, and halitophobia. Genuine halitosis is subclassified as physiologic halitosis and pathologic halitosis. Pathologic halitosis is categorized as oral pathologic halitosis and extraoral pathologic halitosis (Table 22–3■).

Table 22–2	Factors to Consider in a Patient with Halitosis

Non-pathologic causes
Oral: morning breath, xerostomia (mouth breathing, medications)
Aging
Hunger
Tobacco
Foods: onion, garlic, pastrami, other meats
Alcohol

Pathologic causes
Oral
Periodontal disease, xerostomia (underlying illness), gingivitis, stomatitis, glossitis, cancer, candidiasis, parotitis

Gastrointestinal disorders
Gastroesophageal reflux, hiatal hernia, cancer

Nasal
Rhinitis, sinusitis, tumors, foreign bodies

Pulmonary
Bronchitis, pneumonia, tuberculosis, cancer

Systemic
Diabetes, uremia, hepatic disease, blood dyscrasias, rheumatologic disease, dehydration, fever

Psychiatric
Delusions

Table 22–3   Classification of Halitosis with Corresponding Treatment Needs (TN) (Miyazaki et al., 1999)

Classification	Subdivision and Treatment Needs	Description
I. Genuine Halitosis A. Physiologic Halitosis	TN − 1	• Obvious malodor intensity beyond socially acceptable level. • Malodor arises through putrefactive process within the oral cavity. • Neither specific disease nor pathologic condition that could cause halitosis is found. • Origin is mainly the dorsoposterior region of the tongue. (Temporary halitosis as a result of dietary factors [e.g., garlic bread] should be excluded)
B. Pathologic Halitosis	1. Oral Pathologic TN-1 and TN-2	• Halitosis caused by disease, pathologic condition, or malfunction of oral tissues. • Halitosis derived from tongue coating modified by pathological condition (e.g. periodontal disease, xerostomia, etc) is included in this subdivision.
	2. Extraoral Pathologic TN-1 and TN-3	• Malodor originates from nasal, paranasal, and laryngeal regions. • Malodor originates from pulmonary tracts. • Malodor originates from upper digestive tracts. • Malodor originates from disorders anywhere in the body whereby the odor is blood-borne and emitted via lungs (Diabetes mellitus, hepatic cirrhosis, uremia, internal bleeding, etc).
II. Pseudo-Halitosis	TN-1 and TN-4	• Obvious malodor is not perceived by others, although a patient stubbornly complains of the existence of his/her halitosis. • Improvement of this condition is highly promising by explanation of examination results, counseling, and simple treatment measures.
III. Halitophobia	TN-1 and TN-5	• After treatment for genuine halitosis or pseudo-halitosis, a patient persists in believing that he or she has halitosis, although no physical or social evidence exists.

Pseudo-halitosis and halitophobia both involve a psychosomatic condition. Patients complain of the presence of bad breath, but offensive malodor is not perceived by others. Improvement of the condition of pseudo-halitosis is expected by the explanation of examination results, counseling, and simple treatment measures, such as tongue cleaning. Thus, pseudo-halitosis is treatable by dental practitioners. In contrast, halitophobic patients believed that there are definite physical or social factors that contribute to their belief in having halitosis. They cannot be convinced that they do not have malodor. Because of the difficulty in treating halitophobia, it is not considered within the realm of dentistry (Yaegaki & Coil, 2000b). Treatment needs for breath odor are described in detail in Table 22–4■.

Diagnosis and Assessment of Oral Malodor

There are many methods available for examination, diagnosis, and assessment of oral malodor.

Table 22–4	Treatment Needs (TN) for Breath Odor
Category	**Description**
TN-1*	Explanation of halitosis and instruction for oral hygiene. Support and reinforcement of the patient's self-care for further improvement of their oral hygiene.
TN-2	Oral prophylaxis, professional cleaning, and treatment for oral diseases, especially periodontal diseases.
TN-3	Referral to a physician or medical specialist.
TN-4	Explanation of examination data, further professional instruction, education, and reassurance for improvement.
TN-5	Referral to a clinical psychologist, psychiatrist, or other psychological specialist.

*TN-1 is applicable to all cases requiring TN-2 through TN-5.

1. Self Assessment

Patients have been found to be incapable of scoring their own malodor in an objective fashion. Inability to smell one's own oral malodor has been attributed to adaptation or dulling of sensation resulting from continued exposure. Patients should follow the instructions before receiving a breath examination (Table 22–5■).

2. Gas Chromatography

A few halitosis clinics use a gas chromatography (GC) equipped with a flame photometric detector for diagnosing halitosis (Yaegaki & Coil, 2000a). GC is the gold standard for oral malodor measurement (Miyazaki et al., 1999; Yaegaki & Coil, 2000a). It is an objective means to obtain exact values for the various odorous volatiles. It is a very sensitive method. A flame photometer detector is usually employed for the detection of VSC. Gas chromatography may also be combined with mass spectrometry, enlarging the scope of the method (Preti et al., 1992).

3. Halimeter®

The Halimeter (Interscan, CA), using an electrochemical gas sensor cell, has become the primary tool in chronic halitosis research and diagnosis. The Halimeter is approximately twice as sensitive to hydrogen sulfides as it is to methylmercaptan. Halimeter measurements are significantly influenced by other oral gases such as from chewing gum, strong mouth rinse odors, alcohol, shampoo, body lotion, smoking, and even water vapor.

Table 22–5	Instructions to Patients before Receiving Examination (Miyazaki et al., 1999)

Before the day of assessment, patients are instructed to abstain from:

1. Taking antibiotics for 3 weeks before the assessment.
2. Garlic, onions, and spicy foods for 48 hours before assessment.
3. Scented cosmetics for 24 hours before assessment.

On the day of the assessment, patients are instructed to abstain from:

1. Food and drink.
2. Oral hygiene practices.
3. Use of oral rinse or breath fresheners.
4. Smoking for 12 hours before assessment.

4. Organoleptic Measurement

Organoleptic scoring (Miyazaki et al., 1999), which is suitable for practitioners, is shown in Table 22–6■. When the recognition threshold (score 2 or over) is identified in a halitosis patient, a diagnosis of genuine halitosis is made.

The oral malodor judge is required to refrain from drinking coffee, tea, juice, smoking, and using scented cosmetics before the assessment. The judge must have a normal sense of smell and be examined by a specialist to evaluate the sense of smell. However, VSC standard gases for evaluating a judge's sense of smell are not available for clinicians. The judge can regularly check his or her specific sense of smell by sniffing VSC from a freshly boiled egg or Nori (seaweed that can be purchased in an Oriental food store) (Yaegaki, 2000).

5. Simple Determination of Oral Malodor

When a simple determination of oral malodor is required, the spoon test is preferred. In the spoon test, the posterior area of the dorsal surface of the tongue is assessed by thorough scraping, using a disposable plastic spoon. Afterwards, the spoon can be smelled; it has a very repulsive odor in patients with severe oral malodor (Yaegaki & Coil, 2000a).

6. Psychological Assessment

Halitophobia patients and many pseudo-halitosis patients have a psychosomatic condition (Miyazaki et al., 1999; Yaegaki, 2000). Because halitophobia is easily diagnosed using the halitosis classification of Miyazaki and colleagues (1999), corresponding patient management is improved. Psychological assessment is facilitated by specified, tested, and established questionnaires used to inquire medical history as a routine practice. Some patients may be diagnosed as psychological because of contradictions in their answer on the questionnaire (Yaegaki & Coil, 2000b).

7. Tongue Sulfide Probe

Recently a tongue sulfide probe for detecting oral malodor has been developed (Morita, Musinski, & Wang, 2001). The tongue sulfide level on the tongue dorsum (VSC level) is determined by using the tongue sulfide probe (Diamond General Development Corporation, Ann Arbor, MI). The probe is applied on the anterior, the middle, or the posterior part of the tongue along the median groove of the tongue dorsum with a light pressure for 30s. The probe is composed of an active sulfide–sensing element and a stable reference element. The sulfide-sensing element generates an electrochemical voltage proportional to the concentration of sulfide ions present. This voltage is measured relative to the operating point of the reference element.

Table 22–6	Organoleptic Scoring Scale (Miyazaki et al., 1999)	
0	*Absence of Odor*	Detectable odor is completely absent.
1	*Questionable*	Odor is detectable, although a judge could not recognize it as a malodor. This is defined as the detection threshold.
2	*Slight Malodor*	Odor is deemed to exceed the threshold of malodor recognition. This is defined as the recognition threshold.
3	*Moderate Malodor*	Malodor is definitely detected.
4	*Strong Malodor*	Strong malodor, but examiner can tolerate.
5	*Severe Malodor*	Overwhelming malodor. Examiner cannot tolerate malodor at this level (the examiner instinctively averts the nose).

Treatment of Oral Malodor

The first step in treating oral malodor is to assess all oral diseases and conditions that may contribute to oral malodor. The following methods have proven their effectiveness to a variable level.

1. **Tongue Cleaning**

Treatment needs (TN) corresponding to the classification of halitosis in dental practice has been categorized into five levels (see Table 22-4) (Miyazaki et al., 1999). Practical management of physiologic halitosis requires TN-1 with cleaning the tongue being more essential than mouth rinsing, because the origin of physiological halitosis is mainly the dorso-posterior region of the tongue. Tongue coating is comprised of desquamated epithelial cells, blood cells, and bacteria. Cleaning the tongue reduces VSC. Tongue brushing is preferred over tongue scraping (Yaegaki & Coil, 2000a). It is postulated that brush bristles sweep between papillae and remove microorganisms (Kleinberg & Codipilly, 2000). Tongue cleaning should be carried out before tooth brushing, because mint flavor in toothpaste sensitizes the oropharyx to an elevated gag reflex (Yaegaki & Coil, 2000b). The middle and posterior parts of the tongue dorsum should be focused for a cleaning as high proportional sulfide (pS) levels are found there (Morita, et al., 2001).

2. **Oral Hygiene and Mouthrinses**

Mechanical reduction of microorganisms through improved oral hygiene procedures has been associated with reductions in oral malodor.

Additional treatments in TN-1 include routine oral hygiene procedures and mouthrinsing. Some clinical trials of mouthrinses claim to reduce VSC determined by gas chromatography or Halimeter (Yaegaki & Coil, 2000a). Mouthrinses containing cetylpyridinium chloride (CPC), chlorhexidine, or hydrogen peroxide have very limited role in controlling VSC. Currently it has been recommended that patients use a zinc-containing mouthwash (Yaegaki & Coil, 2000b), because zinc strongly inhibits bacterial cysteine proteinase and inhibits the destruction of shed epithelial cells and blood cells (Yaegaki & Suetaka, 1989). Chemical methods of oral malodor control suffer from diversity of opinion to a large extent at the present time.

3. **Toothpastes**

Toothpastes containing triclosan and a copolymer or sodium bicarbonate were reported to reduce certain amounts of VSC, and these toothpastes also may be recommended (Niles et al., 1999).

4. **Chewing Gums**

When people are concerned with oral malodor, approximately 70% use chewing gum (Yaegaki et al. 1995). Chewing gum containing sugar was shown to reduce VSC in mouthair through an active pH change in the oral cavity (Kleinberg & Westbay, 1992). However, sugarless gum only masks halitosis with its flavors, producing a short-term effect (Reingewirtz, Girault, Reingewirtz, Senger, & Tenenbaum, 1999).

5. **Periodontal and Restorative Dental Treatment**

Periodontal treatment is frequently required as TN-2 because periodontal conditions contribute to oral pathologic halitosis. Also, because the reduction of salivary secretion may cause oral pathologic halitosis, the treatment of xerostomia may reduce oral malodor. Increased salivary flow may contribute to decreased oral malodor. Although dental caries may not be a significant cause of oral malodor, caries treatment may be recommend (Yaegaki & Coil, 2000b).

Management of Pseudo-Halitosis (Extraoral/Halitophobic Patients)

Because extraoral pathologic halitosis treatments are out of the realm of dental clinicians, those patients should be referred to medical practitioners (TN-3) (Yaegaki & Coil, 2000b). Pseudo-halitosis patients are able to accept the clinician's diagnosis that oral malodor does not exist after receiving literature support, education, and explanation of examination results (TN-4). If a patient is not able to accept the diagnosis of psuedo-halitosis or if a genuine halitosis patient still believes that halitosis exists after the halitosis was treated, the patient should be diagnosed as halitophobic. Such patients should be referred to a psychological specialist (TN-5) (Yaegaki & Coil, 2000b).

Over-the-Counter (OTC) Products

Over-the-counter oral health products are numerous in the market. Supermarkets are flooded with unsolicited oral hygiene and health products. They range from different tongue brushes, tongue scrapers, mouth rinses, chewing gums, chewable aromatic tablets, mouth fresheners, oral sprays, gels, and so on. Such OTC products may be genuinely effective as a result of actually reducing the number of bacteria, while others may mask the odors, though their masking effect may only last for a brief period (Loesche & Kazor, 2002).

Summary

1. The primary reference standard for detection of oral malodor is the human nose (organoleptic assessment), because it provides an overall evaluation of the existing malodor condition. For the treatment of bad breath, improved oral hygiene, especially tongue cleaning, has been shown to reduce VSC significantly. The value of some oral care products in reducing bad breath is less certain.

2. The incorporation of diagnosis and management of oral malodor should be considered seriously in comprehensive dental care. Although most oral malodor have a simple cause, no single therapy is always effective. A team approach to diagnosis and treatment involves the dentist, periodontist, an ear, nose, and throat specialist, dietition, pharmacist, internal medicine specialist, and psychologist.

3. It is hoped that dental hygienists will get help from the review to have better management of their patients with oral malodor. The effective treatment of oral malodor will boost self-esteem among their patients due to enhanced social acceptance and psychological well-being. It is highly recommended that physicians and dental practitioners should highlight the importance of oral malodor to their patients while examining them and offer their help to control the social and psychological handicap of oral malodor.

Mechanical Plaque Control

Plaque control involves the regular removal of dental plaque from the teeth and adjacent oral tissues and the prevention of its accumulation (Darby & Walsh, 1994). Removal of dental plaque and other deposits on the surface of the teeth can be accomplished by the self-cleansing mechanism or mechanical methods. Since dental plaque is not always visible to the naked eye, patients may be unaware of it until it is disclosed. For this reason, a disclosing agent is recommended for patient education and prior to the patient's daily oral hygiene self-care regimen.

Evaluation

Disclosing solutions show only gross changes and the quantity of stainable plaque. They do not differentiate between food and plaque, nor do they reveal the presence of microorganisms, but the disclosing dye in the form of a solution or tablet absorbs into the dental plaque. The red solution does not contain FD&C red #3 or saccharin. Nevertheless, exposure of plaque is a necessary first step in evaluation and can be accomplished with either disclosing tablets or liquid. The patient chews the tablet and passes the fragments along the teeth with the tongue. The liquid form is swabbed along the teeth and gingival margin with a cotton-tip applicator. With either method, once the disclosing solution has been placed on the teeth, the patient rinses lightly once with water. The dental plaque will appear the color of the dye in the disclosing agent. The dental hygienist can use this visual resource to demonstrate the appropriate techniques of oral hygiene self-care to the patient. It is important to show the patient areas where plaque accumulates in proximity to the gingiva. Patients can self-disclose dental plaque periodically to determine the effectiveness of their oral hygiene self-care techniques. However, merely teaching patients about the use of disclosing agents in their dental health education instruction frequently is not sufficient to motivate them to clean their teeth more effectively. Visual feedback may play an important part in health education, but it is just as important to show patients the results of their efforts by written methods or photography.

Oral Hygiene Self-Care Methods

Proper oral hygiene self-care accomplishes plaque control, improves appearance, refreshes the breath, and provides a sense of oral cleanliness. The oral hygiene plan designed for the patient should be based on the patient's specific oral hygiene needs. Numerous mechanical cleansing devices, including toothbrushes and interdental aids, are available commercially in today's highly competitive product market. The dental hygienist should be familiar with the particular characteristics of each product in order to make the most appropriate selection for each patient.

Toothbrushes

Manual Toothbrushes: Design

Clinical evaluation of the efficiency of toothbrushes and other oral hygiene devices is constrained by such factors as the time devoted to the method, the patient's hand pressure and dexterity, patient motivation, and the criteria used for measuring plaque (Yankell & Saxer, 1999). Therefore, toothbrush recommendations should be based on the toothbrushing method prescribed, the patient's intraoral characteristics, patient motivation, the patient's manual dexterity, and product cost.

The standard manual toothbrush consists of a handle and head with bristles and/or filaments. Toothbrush designs vary greatly depending on the desired characteristics. The handle may be straight (conventional) or angled, have a double angulation of the neck, come with or without thumb rests, and/or have a wavelike contour. The shank may be conventional (straight), offset, twisted, or curved. The head may have any of the following features: diamond shaped, squared, rounded, and of variable sizes for infants, children, young adults, and adults. The bristles/filaments (bristles are made of individual filaments) are most often made from nylon. Compared with natural bristles, nylon bristles have shown certain superior qualities, such as bristle durability, cleanliness, and resistance to the accumulation of bacteria and fungi. Bristle stiffness is classified as soft, medium, and hard. Soft bristles are the most highly recommended. Hard bristles have been shown to cause gingival recession and excessive tooth wear, resulting in cervical abrasion (Fig. 22–1■). Toothbrush bristle planes vary greatly. The flat (conventional), dome, bilevel, rippled, and tuft profiles are unique to each toothbrush. Frandsen (1986) reported that daily brushing with a conventional flat-bristle brush removes only 50% of plaque from tooth surfaces, with removal of plaque from interproximal surfaces especially lacking. Newer brushes using more tapered and narrow bristles have been designed to more effectively reach interproximal areas, but more research and data evaluation must be done. Research on toothbrush bristles has focused much attention on end rounding of the bristles. End-rounded bristles aid in reducing damage to the gingival tissue. Despite manufacturers' attempts to fabricate toothbrushes with a high percentage of acceptable end-rounded bristles, studies have shown that poorly rounded, sharp and pointed, or flat bristle tips may be present in significant numbers even among brushes making claims of superior end rounding (Dellerman, Hughes, & Burkett, 1994).

Alternatives to conventional toothbrushes have been studied. One example is a disposable polyester foam sponge on a stick impregnated with a nonfoaming dentifrice. These spongelike brushes have been used frequently in hospitals and nursing homes and are shown to possess plaque-preventive capabilities. The spongelike brush was found to be effective in retarding accumulation of plaque from a plaque-free baseline on both facial and lingual tooth surfaces (Lefkoff, Beck, & Horton, 1995). It is especially useful after periodontal surgery.

Figure 22–1 Improper use of a toothbrush caused gingival recession and tooth abrasion, identified by a notching in the cervical area of the maxillary lateral incisors and canines.

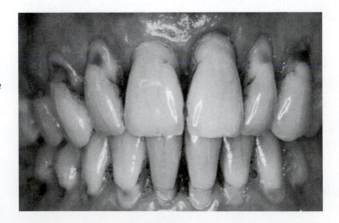

Care of Toothbrushes

The basic care of toothbrushes includes cleaning the brush after each use with a strong stream of warm water to force particles, toothpaste, and bacteria from the bristles. The toothbrush is then tapped against the edge of the sink to release excess particles and water. It is recommended that the brush be air dried in an upright position and have no contact with other toothbrushes. Portable toothbrush containers need to have air vents to prevent bacterial growth. The life of a toothbrush varies and is affected by the length of time in use, forcefulness of the toothbrushing stroke, amount of pressure exerted on the bristles as they are flexed, and bristle quality and design. Worn bristles are less effective in plaque removal than new ones. As a rule, once the bristles have lost their original shape (e.g., splayed or frayed), it is time to replace the toothbrush with a new one. The taper of the bristle tips may become worn as well and lose effectiveness. One manufacturer provides an indicator color strip within the toothbrush bristles. Once the color wears, the brush should be replaced.

Toothbrushing Methods

Numerous toothbrushing methods have been described in the dental literature. These methods are classified according to the direction of toothbrush movement: (1) horizontal—scrub method; (2) circular—Fones method; (3) roll—Rolling stroke technique; and (4) vibratory—Bass, Stillman, and Charters methods. Earlier studies on toothbrushing methods could not confirm clinically significant differences among various brushing methods, and no further research in this area has been done in recent years. Thus it can be concluded that improvement in oral hygiene may not depend on the type of toothbrushing method used (Jepsen, 1998). The correct method of brushing for an individual is that which best removes the plaque and does not cause damage to tooth or gingiva.

Horizontal Scrub Method   The horizontal scrub technique is probably the most commonly used method. The toothbrush bristles are placed perpendicular (90° angle) to the tooth, and the brush is moved back and forth in horizontal motions. For the anterior lingual and palatal tooth surfaces, the brush is held in a vertical position with the heel against the gingival margin, and the scrub stroke is performed in a vertical direction. This technique may be adequate for children with primary teeth, but long-term use in adults may result in gingival recession and cervical abrasion.

Fones Method   The Fones or circular toothbrushing method is performed by positioning the bristles perpendicular to the tooth and using a circular scrubbing stroke. Buccal surfaces are cleaned while the molars are in occlusion, and for cleaning the anterior facial surfaces, the teeth are placed edge to edge. The lingual and palatal tooth surfaces are brushed with an in-and-out stroke. This method is recommended as an easy-to-learn first technique for young children.

Rolling Stroke Technique   In the Rolling stroke technique, emphasis is placed on cleaning the facial and lingual tooth surfaces rather than the sulcular area. The bristles are placed at a 45° angle on the gingiva in an apical direction. The brush stroke is then activated by sweeping the bristles toward the occlusal or incisal surface in a rolling fashion. This stroke is repeated slowly three to four times for each facial and lingual area. The technique requires good manual dexterity and concentration.

Bass Method   Currently, the Bass method is the most widely used toothbrushing technique for adults presenting with or without periodontal diseases. It is also recommended for patients with dental implants. Other interchangeable names are sulcular or intrasulcular brushing. The Bass method is based on the use of a soft, multitufted toothbrush with rounded-end bristles guided at a 45° angle to the gingival margin (Fig. 22–2a,b■). The sides of the bristles are against the tooth surface. A vibratory action of the bristles using 10 strokes for each area disrupts the dental plaque at the gingival margin. With proper technique, plaque approximately 1 mm subgingivally also will be removed. The lingual and palatal surfaces of the anterior teeth are cleansed with the brush head placed vertically to the long axis of the tooth (Fig. 22–2c■), and the occlusal surfaces are brushed with a back-and-forth motion. Cleansing of the interdental areas is limited. The modified Bass method also uses the Rolling stroke toward the incisal or occlusal surface.

Stillman Method   The Stillman method was used originally for gingival stimulation and maintenance of normal gingival contour. The toothbrush is placed at a 45°

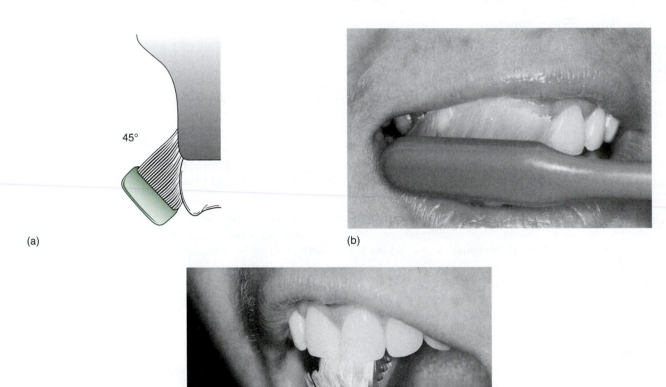

(a)

(b)

(c)

Figure 22–2   (a) Diagram of toothbrush placement in the Bass method. (Copyright © 1997. Rylander H. and Lindhe J. Cause-related periodontal therapy. Munksgaard, Copenhagen. Eds. Lindhe J., Karring T., and Lang N. P. *Clinical periodontology and implant dentistry.*) (b) Clinically: bristles are placed at a 45° angle to the gingival margin and placed into the interdental areas and gingival sulci without excessive force. With the brush in this position, small vibratory movements or rotary movements can effectively remove plaque. (c) Placement of toothbrush for the palatal surface of anterior teeth.

angle facing toward the gingival margin. The bristles are positioned partly on the gingival margin, causing the gingiva to blanch, and partly on the tooth and then shimmied (vibratory movement) approximately 1 mm in a mesiodistal direction to the count of 10 (Fig. 22–3■). The brush is repositioned by rotating the wrist with care not to force the bristles over the gingival margin. In the anterior lingual regions, the brush is held in a vertical direction. In the modified Stillman technique, as the brush is shimmied, the bristles roll down toward and over the occlusal or incisal third of each tooth. This is an attempt to enhance brushing of the entire facial and lingual tooth surfaces. The anterior lingual and palatal tooth surfaces are cleansed using the brush in the vertical position.

Charters Method   The Charters method is best indicated when the interdental papillae are missing, thus leaving interdental areas open. The original use of this method was for gingival stimulation or massage, but currently, there is no rationale for this purpose. The bristles are placed at a 45° angle toward the incisal or occlusal surface, with the sides of the bristles placed against the gingiva (Fig. 22–4■). The brush is then shimmied downward until the bristles engage the gingiva and interproximal area. The vibratory action extends the bristles into the proximal space. This is repeated four to six times in the same area. Occlusal surfaces are cleansed with a circular or rotary motion. This method should not be used when the contour of the interdental papillae is normal. The modified Charters method uses a Rolling stroke toward the occlusal or incisal surface.

Frequency of Toothbrushing

Toothbrushing must be carried out on a regular basis. It is difficult to determine the number of times a day an individual must brush, since the frequency of brushing is tailored to meet individual needs. An individual should brush as many times a day as it takes to effectively remove dental plaque. Factors that affect the recommendations for frequency of toothbrushing include rate of dental plaque formation,

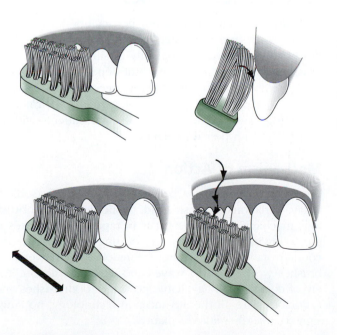

Figure 22–3   Modified Stillman method. The sides of the bristles are placed partly on the teeth and gingiva. The brush is shimmied in a lateral direction as the brush is moved coronally.

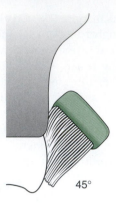

45°

Figure 22–4   Diagram showing the Charters method. The brush with the bristles is placed parallel to the long axis of the tooth pointing incisally. (Copyright © 1997. Rylander H. and Lindhe J. Cause-related periodontal therapy. Munksgaard, Copenhagen. Eds. Lindhe J., Jarring T., and Lang N.P. *Clinical peridontology and implant dentistry.*)

plaque visibility, state and susceptibility of oral disease, diet, and presence of contributory factors. Low-risk patients should be directed to brush at least twice a day. High-risk patients should brush more frequently, especially after meals. The use of disclosing agents is highly recommended because it allows meticulous removal of visible plaque from the teeth. The patient should individualize his or her own brushing technique to optimize plaque control. Current data on toothbrushing time suggests that people think they brush longer than they actually do. The average time spent brushing is between 24 and 60 seconds, but the recommended brushing time actually is about 3 minutes (Cancro & Fischman, 1995).

Powered Toothbrushes

Alternatives to manual toothbrushes include powered toothbrushes. A new generation of sonic and ultrasonic toothbrushes has become available. Powered toothbrushes were designed originally to simulate the action produced using a manual brush. However, effectiveness still depends on brush and bristle placement. Powered toothbrushes originally were recommended for patients lacking fine motor skills or patients with physical or mental impairments, but recent innovations in technology have increased their use for patients with periodontal disease, as well as patients with dental implants.

Mechanism of Action

There are many types of powered sonic and ultrasonic toothbrushes on the market today. Variations in brush head, bristle design, and brush movement exist. The various mechanical motions occur in rapid, short strokes in one or a combination of the following directions: reciprocating (in and out or up and down), rotational, counterrotational, oscillating (vibrational). A newer generation of powered toothbrushes work by sonic waves and ultrasonic action. Table 22–7■ describes a variety of commercially available powered toothbrushes and their respective modes of action. Despite all the advances in technology, no single powered toothbrush design completely removes plaque.

Table 22–7	Commercially Available Powered Toothbrushes
Product	**Features and Mode of Action**
Rotadent™ (Pro-Dentec, Batesville, AR)	This is the first of the new-generation powered toothbrushes that was designed differently from the conventional electric brush (rotary motion, no timer). This brush has three interchangeable brush heads that rotate similar to a prophy angle. One is shaped like a cut, with short bristles in the center, and is used on facial and lingual surfaces. The second is a single tuft of pointed bristles for the interproximal area. The third is a longer tuft of bristles for open embrasures.
Interplak® (Conair Corp., East Hanover, NJ)	Introduced into the market in the mid-1980s. Rectangular brushhead with six to eight bristle tufts that individually counterrotate; timer is available. Children's model is available. It consists of ten tufts of rotating bristles in a removable head. Each tuft rotates a turn and a half in one direction before changing direction to rotate a turn in a half in the opposite direction. The twisting action of the bristles accounts for facial, lingual, and interproximal effectiveness.
Braun Oral-B® 3D Plaque Remover (Braun, Oral-B, Belmont, CA)	Combines two distinct brushing motions: in-and-out high-frequency pulsations and side-to-side oscillations. Cup-shaped brushhead with FlexiSoft bristles that give with pressure. If the brush is pressed with too much force on the tooth, the brushing motion will stop. Interdental tips clean interproximal areas. The 3D neck is angled 3°, providing better maneuverability for posterior teeth. The brush is equipped with a memory timer that memorizes lapsed brushing time for when the brush may be briefly switched off.
Plaque Remover® Braun Oral-B (Belmont, CA)	Introduced into the market in 1996. Small round head oscillates 2800 times per minute. Movements are similar to a prophy angle, and the head rotates back and forth (oscillates). The small head allows the brush to be adapted to each tooth individually, reaching interproximally and subgingivally. Small head size necessitates longer than 2-minute brushing time for a complete dentition.
Sonicare® Plus with grip (Philips Oral Healthcare, Inc., Snoqualmie, WA)	Introduced in 1993. The brushhead is rectangular in shape. Moving at 31,000 strokes per minute, Sonicare's high-speed back-and-forth motion creates sonic (sound) waves that travel through toothpaste into difficult-to-clean areas. Attached plaque is removed by the effect of the vibrations carried through the dentifrice bubbles. The Smartimer® has a 2-minute automatic shutoff timer and the Quadpacer® quadrant timer beeps at 30-second intervals.
Plaque Control 3000™ Plaque Removal Instrument (Teledyne Water Pik, Fort Collins, CO)	2100 elliptical (circular) strokes per minute; no timer. This brush has a soft, compact, contoured brush head that moves in an elliptical motion similar to the motion of the manual Bass toothbrushing method. Ergonomically designed handle for comfort, control, and ease of use.
SenSonic® Plaque Removal Instrument (Teledyne Water Pik, Fort Collins, CO)	Sonic brushing with 30,000 brush strokes per minute and a soft, contoured, compact bristle design to remove plaque and reduce stains. The built-in electronic feedback system automatically adjusts speed for optimal performance, and the ergonomic handle is designed for comfort and brushing control. The SenSonic Advanced Plaque Removal Instrument has a timer, an automatic shutoff, and a battery indicator light.
Ultra Sonex® (Brewster, NY)	A manual toothbrush with a piezoelectric transducer embedded in the brushhead. Operates at 1.6 million cycles per second. A dentifrice is used to conduct the ultrasonic waves to the teeth and soft tissues.

Effectiveness

Various studies with conflicting results have examined the effectiveness of powered toothbrushes compared with conventional brushes in plaque removal. Since most studies in the 1960s and 1970s failed to show that powered toothbrushes remove plaque better than manual toothbrushes, they were not so popular. In the 1996 World Workshop in Periodontics it was concluded that limited evidence supports the fact that powered toothbrushes offer additional benefits compared with manual toothbrushes (Hancock, 1996).

A few powered toothbrushes may be superior in removing plaque from interproximal areas than conventional manual toothbrushes (Bader, 1992; Saxer & Yankell, 1997). One study suggests that the sonic toothbrush (Sonicare®, Optiva Corp., Bellevue, WA) is more beneficial in resolving inflammation and reducing pocket depths in patients with moderate periodontal disease (O'Beirne, Johnson, Rutger Persson, & Spektor, 1996). However, other randomized, controlled clinical studies have not proven conclusively any differences in the efficacy of plaque removal between manual and powered toothbrushes (Preber, Ylipaa, Bergström, & Ryden, 1991; Van der Weijden, Danser, Nijboer, Timmerman, & Vander Velden, 1993). A recent clinical study using 62 adult patients with significant amounts of plaque, calculus, and inflammation demonstrated that brushing with either a manual or ultrasonic toothbrush significantly reduced bleeding and gingival inflammation. Neither toothbrush showed superiority over the other in removing plaque (Forgas-Brockmann, Carter-Hanson, & Killoy, 1998). The novelty of using a new device may in part increase self-care efforts, thus improving oral hygiene.

Powered toothbrushes have been found to be superior in removing tooth stains (Grossman, Cronin, Dembling, & Proskin, 1996). The Braun Oral-B® Plaque Remover (Braun, Oral-B, Belmont, CA) and Sonicare® have been shown to be superior to a manual toothbrush in removal of chlorhexidine stains (Moran & Addy, 1995).

Recommending a Powered Toothbrush

Factors to consider when recommending a powered toothbrush include the toothbrush design, brushing motion, patient's interest and motivation, and the costs and benefits. Placement of bristles and the head of the toothbrush are important to avoid tissue trauma. The powered toothbrush should be moved slowly in sequence around the mouth using less pressure than with a manual toothbrush, thus producing less cervical abrasion and tissue trauma. Evaluation of a patient's ability to improve his or her plaque and gingival indices over time is the best method for determining the success of a specific powered toothbrush. Use of powered toothbrushes is safe on titanium dental implants.

The use of powered toothbrushes by patients with poor self-care compliance has shown some advantages (Hellstadius, Asman, & Gustafsson, 1993). Use of a powered toothbrush (counterrotational) in periodontal patients in a periodontal maintenance program has proved to be helpful in reducing plaque levels and enhancing gingival conditions (Yukna & Shaklee, 1993). Other patients that may benefit from the use of powered toothbrushes include those with limited manual dexterity, orthodontic patients, and children (parental brushing of children's teeth).

Interdental Care

Interdental cleaning is a primary area of neglect. A major factor in disease initiation and control is the anatomy of the interdental area. Cleansing of these interproximal areas depends on tooth alignment and tissue configuration. Supplemental aids are necessary because, despite new toothbrush designs, brushing alone is ineffective in the removal of interproximal plaque.

Various considerations are appropriate when recommending interdental cleaning devices. These factors are as follows:

1. The presence or absence of interdental papillae
2. Alignment of teeth
3. Shape of teeth
4. Tissue contour
5. Condition of restorations
6. Tightness of contact area
7. Presence of bridges, dental implants, and orthodontic appliances
8. Patient motivation and interest in interproximal cleaning
9. Effectiveness of patient's self-care
10. Size of gingival embrasure

Types of Gingival Embrasures

There are three types of gingival embrasures (Fig. 22–5■): Type I, in which the embrasure is completely filled with gingiva; Type II, in which there is slight to moderate recession of the interdental papillae; and Type III, in which there is extensive or complete loss of interdental papillae (Darby & Walsh, 1994).

Available interdental cleaning devices include dental floss, dental tape, interdental brushes, interdental stimulators, and oral irrigators (Table 22–8■). Determination of which interdental aid is to be used depends on the type of gingival embrasure.

Dental Floss and Dental Tape   Numerous types of nylon dental floss are available: waxed, unwaxed, flat, round, colored, flavored, shred resistant, and impregnated with substances such as fluoride, baking soda, and tetrasodium pyrophospate. Floss is indicated for use in Type I gingival embrasures, where the embrasures are completely filled with interdental papillae. It is also effective around implants. Dental floss is 80% effective in removing interproximal dental plaque. Waxed dental floss may be more resistant to tearing or shredding but may be too bulky for tight contacts. Teflon-coated floss is made of polytetrafluoroethylene and is inserted easily into difficult access areas and resists fraying (Ciancio, Shilby, & Farber, 1992). Unwaxed floss is thin and easily manipulated through tight contact areas. Even though patients prefer to use waxed floss rather than unwaxed floss (Beaumont, 1990), there is actually no difference between the two flosses in efficacy in removing interproximal plaque (Hill, Levi, & Glickman, 1973). Floss may fray and tear where teeth are crowded or in areas where restorations are defective. Dental tape is broad and flat and should be used in open interdental spaces or between teeth without tight contacts and for polishing proximal tooth surfaces. The major advantage of colored floss is patient appeal and the patient's ability to see what is removed by flossing. This factor may help motivate the patient to floss regularly.

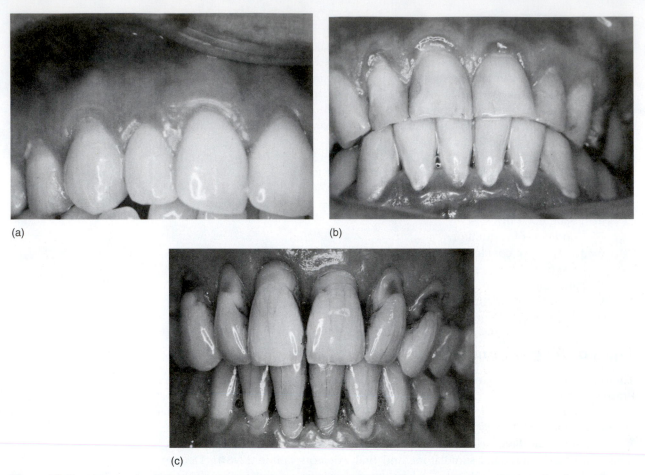

(a)

(b)

(c)

Figure 22–5   Three types of gingival embrasures. Interdental cleaning devices are specific for each type of embrasure. (a) Type I embrasure is completely filled with interdental gingiva. (b) Type II embrasure has partial loss of interdental gingiva (mandibular anterior teeth). (c) Type III embrasure has complete loss of interdental gingiva.

A floss modification called tufted dental floss, made by many manufacturers, has a stiff straight end with a section of unwaxed floss and an area of thicker nylon meshwork. The stiff end allows the floss to be passed easily under bridges, around implant abutments, through exposed furcations, or between orthodontic appliances.

The floss holder is a yoke-like device with a space between the two prongs of the yoke. The floss is secured tightly between the two prongs designed to facilitate movement of the floss interproximally, as shown in Figure 22–6■. It is recommended for patients with limited manual dexterity.

The floss threader is a needle-like device (Fig. 22–7■) to facilitate floss use under pontics and splinted crowns, between orthodontic appliances, through a gingival embrasure, or between teeth with tight contacts. It is used by threading approximately 12 inches of floss through the loop and then drawing it through the interproximal space. The floss is then engaged against the tooth surface.

Caution is necessary in flossing to avoid injury to the gingiva. The floss may cut the gingiva if it is pulled too quickly past the contact and/or if it is positioned too forcefully beneath the gingiva. Damage to the junctional epithelium may occur,

Table 22–8	Clinical Features of Interdental Cleaning Devices	
Type of Dental Device	**Use**	**Limitations**
Dental floss	Type I gingival embrasures.	Use caution not to cause tissue trauma. Not recommended for diastemas and Types II and III gingival embrasures.
Dental tape	Broad and flat for wider spaces and assists in polishing proximal surfaces.	Difficult to use for tight contact areas and Types II and III embrasures.
Dental floss threader	Floss is threaded through a plastic needle-like device. Best to use under pontics, around orthodontic wires, and where teeth are splinted or soldered.	Use caution not to injure the gingiva with the point of the threader.
Dental floss holder	Patients with limited manual dexterity or who do not want to place fingers in the mouth. For Type I embrasures.	Sometimes it is difficult to get the floss through the contact area; floss must be taut. Do not use in Types II or III embrasures.
Tufted floss	To clean beneath pontics, around orthodontic wires, and between splinted teeth. The yarn portion of the floss is used for actual cleaning where space permits.	Not intended for Type I gingival embrasures. Use caution with the tip of the floss.
Rubber-tip stimulator	Used for the removal of dental plaque along the gingival margin. Also can be used in an open embrasure.	To avoid tissue trauma, do not place tip subgingivally.
Wooden wedge	Use in Type II and III embrasures with shallow pockets.	Use caution not to cause tissue trauma. Difficult to adapt lingually.
Interdental brushes	Use in Type II and III embrasures and furcation involvement areas.	Do not use in Type I embrasures.
Implant floss	Use around implant posts or abutments.	Avoid forcing floss into the gingiva.
Electric interdental cleaner	Good for patients with limited manual dexterity. Good for all types of embrasures, including around bridges and implants. Available with a filament and FlexiTip stimulator.	Follow manufacturer's instructions.

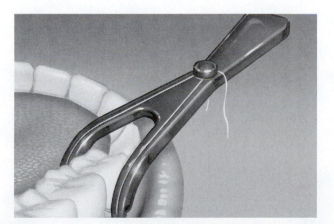

Figure 22–6   Floss holder. The floss is held tightly between two prongs. (Courtesy of John O. Butler Company, Chicago)

Figure 22–7 The floss threader is a needle-like device. Floss is placed through the loop for access underneath pontics, exposed furcations, orthodontic appliances, and splinted crowns. (Courtesy of John O. Butler Company, Chicago)

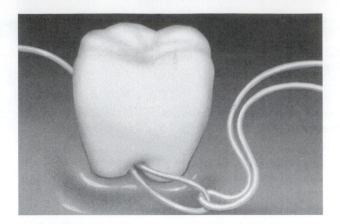

especially in healthy gingiva. The patient should be instructed to perform flossing procedures in a systematic fashion (hence all mandibular and maxillary teeth are included). Mastering the flossing technique requires time and patience. Patients are discouraged and less motivated to incorporate the flossing regimen into their oral hygiene program when they have difficulties with manual dexterity or when they do not have the patience to do the job well.

Floss also has been designed specifically for cleaning implants. The denture is removed before cleaning the abutments. The floss is looped from facial to lingual around the abutment and gently placed subgingivally until resistance is met. It is then crisscrossed and used in a sliding back-and-forth, up-and-down motion. Implant floss is made of braided nylon filaments and can be washed off after each use.

Interdental and Single-Tuft Brushes Exposed furcations, root concavities (e.g., mesial concavity on the maxillary first premolar), and Type II and III gingival embrasures usually are best cleaned with an interdental or single-tuft brush (also called end-tuft brush) (Fig. 22–8■). Other uses for such brushes include the distal surface of the terminal molar, around pontics and maligned teeth, and around orthodontic appliances or dental implant abutments. The premoistened brush is inserted interproximally and used in an in-and-out direction. However, such brushes should not be forced to fit into gingival embrasures.

Figure 22–8 Floss is not as effective as an interdental brush in removing interdental plaque from tooth concavities. (Courtesy of John O. Butler Company, Chicago)

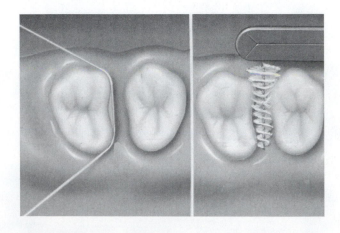

Interdental brushes consist of nylon filaments twisted onto a metal wire or a nylon-coated plastic wire that does not scratch or cause tissue trauma. Interchangeable bristles come in a variety of sizes, such as cylindrical, tapered, and large cylindrical (Fig. 22–9■). A unique wireless soft foam insert is available for postoperative periodontal care, implant maintenance, and medicament applications.

The single-tuft brush, also called an end-tuft brush, consists of a group of small bristles or tufts that are flat or tapered on a straight or angled handle (Fig. 22–10■).

Rubber-Tip Stimulator   The rubber-tip stimulator consists of a flexible rubber tip attached to a handle or at the end of a toothbrush. It is not recommended for healthy gingiva that completely fills the gingival embrasure, but it can be useful in Type II or Type III embrasures. Generally, it is used for removing plaque at the gingival margin, exposed furcation areas, concave surfaces, and open interdental areas. The tip is inserted gently into the interdental area and inclined approximately 45° toward the occlusal surface following the contour of the gingiva. It also can be placed interproximally at a 90° angle. A back-and-forth or rolling motion is used. It was thought originally that use of the rubber tip increased keratinization

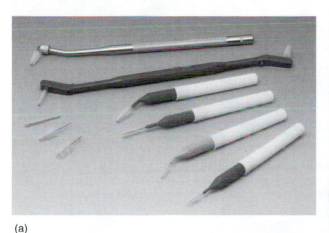

(a)

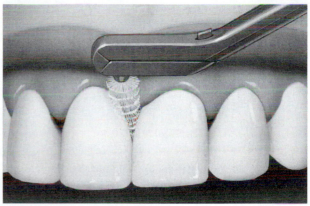

(b)

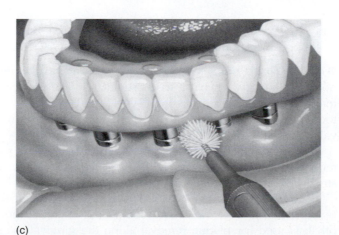

(c)

Figure 22–9   (a) Variations in types of interdental brushes. Uses of an interdental brush (b) in a Type II embrasure and (c) around implant abutments. (Courtesy of John O. Butler Company, Chicago)

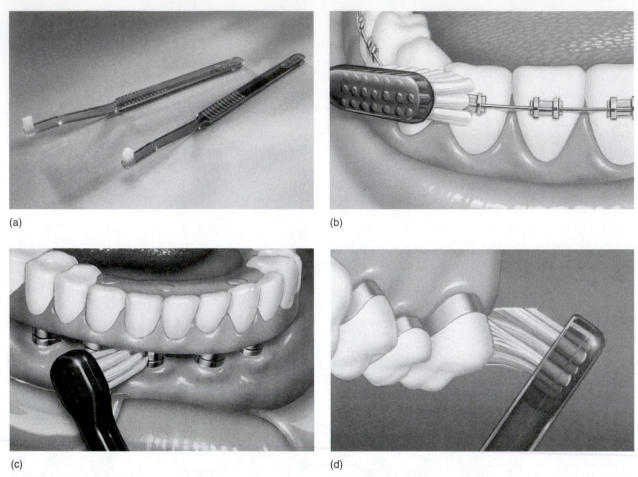

(a)

(b)

(c)

(d)

Figure 22–10 (a) Variations in single-tufted brushes (tapered and nontapered). (Courtesy of Oral-B Labs, Belmont, CA) Use of a single-tufted brush (b) around orthodontic appliances, (c) dental implants, and (d) the distal surface of the terminal tooth. (Courtesy of John O. Butler Company, Chicago)

and vascular function through gingival stimulation, but there is no clinical evidence to support this (Rounds & Tilliss, 1999).

Wooden Toothpicks Wooden toothpicks are available as either a toothpick-in-holder or a triangular balsa wood stimulator. These devices should be used where interdental papillae are missing (Type II and Type III embrasures). Since wooden toothpicks are difficult to use on lingual surfaces and they do not reach subgingivally, they are not as effective as dental floss.

The triangular stimulator should be moistened with saliva and then inserted interproximally, flat side toward the papilla, moving in an in-and-out burnishing stroke. Discard the wedge if it becomes splayed.

The toothpick-in-holder is a plastic-handled instrument with a tapered, conical opening at one end where the toothpick is inserted; the excess portion is broken off. It is used for plaque removal along the gingival margin, within the sulcus, in root concavities, in furcation areas, and around orthodontic appliances; it also can be used for the application of medicaments (e.g., fluoride or a desensitizing agent).

The blunt point and sides of the toothpick are placed in the sulcus to engage, debride, and dislodge adherent plaque.

Electric Interdental Cleaning Devices   One of the more recent advances in interdental cleaning is the Braun Oral-B Interclean® (Redwood City, CA), an electric interdental cleaning device that consists of a thin, flexible cleaning filament (Fig. 22–11■). The filament is placed into the interdental space and disrupts and sweeps away plaque by an elliptical movement using over 100 cleaning strokes per second. Individuals who are unable to floss or those who will not floss may find automated interproximal cleansing easier. This device has been shown to reduce plaque, gingivitis, and bleeding equal to or better than floss (Gordon, Frascella, & Reardon, 1996). Other automated interdental cleaners are available and include sonic devices, filament tips, brush tips, and flossers.

Tongue Cleansing

A number of tongue cleansing devices are available. These are used in a pull or forward motion. A soft-bristle toothbrush also may be used for tongue cleansing. When using a toothbrush, a brushing stroke starting on the posterior-most aspect of the dorsum of the tongue is performed with a roll to the tip of the tongue. Tongue brushing will improve tongue appearance and halitosis by removing coatings associated with bacteria, food, and smoking.

Dentifrices

A dentifrice is a toothpowder, toothpaste, or gel used in conjunction with a toothbrush to help remove plaque, materia alba, and stain from teeth. The word is derived from the Latin words dens ("teeth") and fricare ("to rub"). Although the

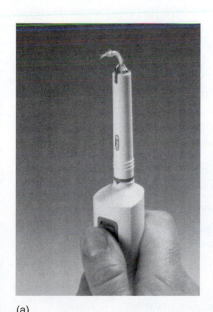
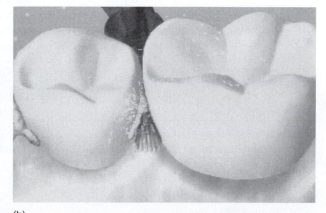

(a)   (b)

Figure 22–11   (a) Braun Oral-B Interclean®. (b) Interproximal use of the device. (Courtesy of Oral-B Labs, Belmont, CA)

Table 22–9	Dentifrices with Therapeutic Benefits (ADA Seal of Acceptance)
Product Name	**Active Ingredients**
Anticavity/antiplaque/antigingivitis	
Colgate® Total™ Toothpaste (Colgate-Palmolive Co., New York, NY)	0.30% triclosan 0.24% sodium fluoride
Prevention of calculus	
Colgate® Tarter Control Gel/Toothpaste (Colgate-Palmolive Co., New York, NY)	Tetrasodium pyrophosphate, 0.15% sodium fluoride
Aquafresh® Tartar Control Toothpaste (SmithKline Beecham Consumer Brands, Pittsburgh, PA)	Tetrapotassium pyrophosphate, tetrasodium pyrophosphate, 0.221% sodium fluoride
Crest® Tartar Protection Fluoride Gel/Toothpaste (Procter & Gamble, Cincinnati, OH)	Tetrapotassium pyrophosphate, disodium pyrophosphate, tetrasodium pyrophosphate, 0.15% sodium fluoride

Source: Adapted from Mariotti, A. J. Mouthrinses and dentifrices. In *ADA Guide to Dental Therapeutics,* 1st ed., 210–212. Chicago: ADA Publishing Co.

mechanical action of brushing and flossing is the primary means of plaque removal, a dentifrice facilitates the oral hygiene process.

Currently, dentifrices are considered to be either cosmetic or therapeutic. Cosmetically, they function in cleaning and polishing teeth, removing extrinsic stains, and freshening the oral cavity. There is a continuing effort to obtain additional dental benefits from dentifrices through the inclusion of agents designed to have a therapeutic action. This includes caries reduction; control of gingivitis, plaque, and calculus formation; and reduction of dentinal hypersensitivity (Tables 22–9■ and 22–10■).

The main limitation of dentifrices as a therapeutic agent is the issue of patient compliance. Dental hygienists cannot control the frequency of use or amount or type of dentifrice used by a patient. Dentifrice selection is based most often on cosmetic qualities such as flavor, texture, appearance, and dispensability rather than on its therapeutic value. The public looks to dental professionals for specific recommendations. The dental hygienist must be up to date with product information and be able to recommend a dentifrice that will provide oral health benefits yet appeal to the patient for continued use. Dentifrices should be chemically stable, effective, and nontoxic. Products with the ADA seal of acceptance have sustained scrutiny and testing and can be safely recommended by dental hygienists.

Table 22–10	Patient-Applied Dentifrices for the Treatment of Dentinal Hypersensitivity (ADA Seal of Acceptance)
Product Name	**Active Ingredient**
Crest Sensitivity Protection® (Procter & Gamble, Cincinnati, OH); Protect Sensitive Teeth Gel® (John O. Butler Co., Chicago, IL)	5% potassium nitrate, 0.15% sodium fluoride
Fresh Mint Sensodyne® Toothpaste (Block Drug, Jersey City, NJ)	5% potassium nitrate sodium monoflurophosphate
Gel-Kam® Gel (Colgate Oral Pharmaceuticals, Canton, MA)	0.4% stannous fluoride

Dentifrice Components

Dentifrices contain basic components along with an active ingredient for its intended use. The active agent provides the therapeutic benefit and can include fluoride for anticaries effect, potassium nitrate or strontium chloride for desensitization (reducing or eliminating dentin sensitivity), sodium pyrophosphate for calculus inhibition, or triclosan for plaque and gingivitis control. Recent formulations have incorporated a combination of these active ingredients for maximal patient benefits.

A typical dentifrice contains, besides water (15 to 50%), an abrasive (20 to 60%). Abrasives clean or polish tooth surfaces, allowing them to resist bacterial reaccumulation. The powders and pastes contain abrasives such as silicon oxides, chalk, hydrated aluminum oxide, and sodium bicarbonate. Generally speaking, commercial dentifrice powders are more abrasive than pastes. Abrasives usually do not damage the enamel, but they may dull tooth luster. Therefore, a polishing agent is incorporated into most dentifrices, forming an abrasive system (Fischman & Yankell, 1999). Although abrasives can result in tooth wear, other factors such as brushing habits, including technique, pressure, direction, and frequency of brushing, and toothbrush bristle stiffness can influence the incidence of tooth abrasion. The more abrasive the dentifrice, the more likely it is to cause tooth wear in the cervical area. This area is more prone to abrasion because enamel is approximately 20 times harder than dentin or cementum (Fischman & Yankell, 1999). There is no valid reason to use a dentifrice with a greater abrasiveness or polishing effect than necessary to prevent deposits, including stains on the teeth.

Humectants (20 to 40%) are a vehicle into which agents are incorporated to prevent hardening of the dentifrice when exposed to air. Common humectants are glycerin, sorbitol, mannitol, and polyethylene glycol. Surfactants (1 to 2%) act as detergents by contributing to the foaming action, lowering surface tension, and loosening deposits from the teeth. Sodium lauryl sulfate is the most commonly used detergent. Binders (1 to 2%; cellulose products, gums, alginates) prevent the separation of the solids and liquids in the dentifrice, maintain firmness and thickness, and ensure stability. Gels contain more binders to give the product a thicker quality. Flavoring and sweetening agents mask the poor-tasting ingredients and provide a pleasant flavor to the dentifrice. These include essential oils (peppermint, cinnamon, and wintergreen) and sodium saccharin. Colorants (1%) are dyes added to the dentifrice to enhance its attractiveness without staining or discoloring teeth or oral tissues or causing harm on ingestion.

Fluoride Dentifrices

Dentifrices are the most widely used form of self-applied fluoride. Recommended for both children and adults, fluoride dentifrices can reduce caries by 20 to 30% when used twice daily on a regular basis. First introduced in the 1950s, fluoride dentifrices contained stannous fluoride as the anticaries agent. Current fluoride dentifrices contain sodium fluoride (0.24%) or sodium monofluorophosphate (0.76%). The anticaries efficacy of these two fluoride agents continues to be evaluated (Proskin & Volpe, 1995). Although some analyses indicate that there is no statistically or clinically significant difference between the two fluoride agents (Volpe, Pretrone, Davies, & Proskin, 1995), it has been shown that the therapeutic benefit of fluoride depends on a dose-response relationship (Stephen, 1994). Sodium fluoride dentifrices appear to be retained longer, however, when compared with dentifrices containing sodium monofluorophosphate (Shellis & Duckworth, 1994) and thus may be more effective clinically (Duckworth, Jones, Nicholson, Jacobson, & Chestnutt, 1994).

Indications for fluoride gels include rampant caries, patients susceptible to caries, root caries, orthodontic appliances, dentinal hypersensitivity, and patients undergoing radiation therapy. Since over 95% of dentifrices contain fluoride and the benefits have been shown clinically for decades, issues of safety are of minor concern. Numerous studies have evaluated fluoride therapies for their impact on dental fluorosis (Stookey, 1994). Dentifrices have been identified as a causative factor in the increased prevalence of mild enamel fluorosis. For this reason, young children must be monitored for inadvertent dentifrice ingestion.

The mechanism of fluoride's anticaries effect in root caries is not well understood. Fluoride gels may have a beneficial effect in the prevention of caries on exposed root surfaces. An example of a home-applied gel prescription product is 1.1% sodium fluoride (Prevident® 5000 Plus Gel, Colgate Oral Pharmaceuticals, Canton, MA; Neutracare®, Oral-B, Belmont, CA). These gels should be applied daily after home-care procedures. The gel is applied either by brushing it on the root surface for 1 minute or using a custom-made or disposable tray for 4 minutes.

Clinical studies report that the daily use of a fluoride paste reduces root surface caries by more than 65% (Jensen & Kohout, 1988). More research is needed to truly confirm fluoride's role in the prevention of root caries. Therefore, fluoride dentifrices are recommended primarily for dental caries prevention.

Stannous Fluoride Dentifrices

Initially, before the introduction of sodium fluoride and sodium monofluorophosphate, stannous fluoride was incorporated into dentifrices. Stannous fluoride, in concentrations of greater than 0.3%, has been the most widely studied fluoride in controlling plaque and gingivitis. Clinical studies show mixed results, and stannous fluoride does not have the ADA seal of acceptance.

When compared with a sodium fluoride dentifrice, stannous fluoride did not demonstrate significant effects on supragingival plaque (Beiswanger, Doyle, & Jackson, 1995).

Commonly reported adverse side effects include extrinsic tooth staining caused by the tin molecule and a metallic, bitter taste. Recent dentifrice formulations contain flavoring agents that mask the taste. Removal of stains caused by stannous fluoride is no more difficult than stain removal resulting from other product use (Beiswanger et al., 1995). Stannous fluoride is available as a brush-on gel, a mouthrinse, and a dentifrice.

Triclosan-Containing Dentifrices

Triclosan is another type of therapeutic dentifrice. Triclosan is a phenolic compound with antiplaque/antigingivitis properties. It is a broad-spectrum antibacterial agent effective against Gram-positive and Gram-negative bacteria. Used as an antibacterial agent in soaps, deodorants, and cosmetics, triclosan recently has become available in the United States in a dentifrice formulation (Total™, Colgate Oral Pharmaceuticals, Canton, MA).

This product contains 0.3% triclosan and 2.0% polyvinylmethylether maleic acid (PVM/MA), which enhances its retention (substantivity) onto hard and soft oral surfaces and adds anticalculus properties (Ciancio, 1997). Triclosan binds to plaque, resulting in a sustained impact on bacteria for over 12 hours after brushing (Volpe, Petrone, DeVizio, & Davies, 1996). Triclosan affects the quality of existing plaque (Lindhe, Rosling, Socransky, & Volpe, 1993) and plaque regrowth (Binney, Addy, McKeowns, & Everatt, 1996). When compared with other dentifrices, triclosan is as effective as stannous fluoride (Binney, Addy, Owens, & Faulkner, 1997) and sodium fluoride dentifrices (Binney, Addy, McKeowns, & Everatt, 1995) in inhibiting plaque. In addition, this product is also claimed to prevent caries. No adverse side effects have been reported, and it is safe for oral use. Anionic agents, which are also present in most dentifrices, do not alter their antibacterial effectiveness. Triclosan has the ADA seal of acceptance.

Sodium Bicarbonate/Hydrogen Peroxide Dentifrices

Sodium bicarbonate (baking soda) has been used as a cleansing agent for many years and has been the primary abrasive agent in dentifrices. The therapeutic benefit of sodium bicarbonate dentifrices results from reduction of plaque and gingivitis and stain removal (Koertge, 1996; Zambon, Mather, & Gonzales, 1996). The mechanism of action is disruption of the bacterial cell membrane (Drake, Vargas, Cardenzana, & Srikantha, 1995). Even though baking soda disintegrates quickly during brushing (so that its abrasive action is not sustained), it still removes stains (Koertge, 1996). An additional benefit of baking soda dentifrices is their control of oral malodor (Brunette, 1996).

Hydrogen peroxide is added to dentifrices for its antigingivitis properties. Some manufacturers claim that hydrogen peroxide–containing dentifrices were developed to whiten teeth by decolorizing stains. Others claim that hydrogen peroxide freshens the mouth because of its bubbling action. Consumers often view these agents as more "natural." The concept of combining sodium bicarbonate with hydrogen peroxide is based on the regimen supported by the Keyes technique. Most dentifrices contain a low level of hydrogen peroxide (<1%) that causes no harm to tissues (Marshall, Cancro, & Fischman, 1995).

The Keyes technique has received much attention in the lay press for the treatment of periodontal disease without surgical intervention. The Keyes technique, originally developed by Dr. Paul Keyes in the late 1970s, is based on monitoring of the disease with phase-contrast microscopy and treatment. The first phase of treatment involves mechanical therapy, and this is followed by local antimicrobial therapy, in which the patient uses a toothpaste composed of 3% hydrogen peroxide, salt, and sodium bicarbonate. Oral irrigation at home and in the office is also done. In the last phase of treatment, patients are administered systemic antibiotics such as tetracycline. This type of treatment was found not to be any more effective than conventional periodontal therapy (Pihlstrom et al., 1987). In addition, oral ulcerations have been reported to result from short-term use of 3% hydrogen peroxide in combination with a salt solution (Levine, 1987).

Research findings on the efficacy of these dentifrices are mixed. A 52% reduction in bleeding sites was found after a 3-month test (Fischman, Kugel, Truelove, Nelson, & Cancro, 1992). Dentifrices containing hydrogen peroxide may decrease plaque and gingivitis, but mechanical access to submarginal sites is required for them to deliver a therapeutic effect (Marshall et al., 1995). When applied with a sulcular brush and an interproximal toothpick, sodium bicarbonate/hydrogen peroxide had no benefit in reducing the microbial biota in 4- to 7-mm pockets (Cerra & Killoy, 1982). No antimicrobial benefits were exhibited when compared with conventional dentifrices (sodium fluoride, stannous fluoride) and mouth rinses (essential oils) (Bacca et al., 1997).

Given these mixed findings, dental hygienists should educate their patients about the limited benefits of these dentifrices. These products have the ADA seal of acceptance on the basis of their anticaries benefit, not antiplaque/antigingivitis claims.

Most home bleaching products contain as the active ingredient 0.75 to 10% hydrogen peroxide or 10 to 15% carbamide peroxide. Carbamide peroxide breaks down into hydrogen peroxide. Another component is urea, which helps in plaque removal. High levels (35%) of peroxide can penetrate the dentin and cause toxicity to the pulp. Broken down, leaky restorations near the cementoenamel junction are major routes of entrance of peroxide (Marshall et al., 1995).

Tartar-Control Dentifrices

Calculus, although not a primary causative factor for periodontal disease, does play a role in dental plaque retention. Any attempt by patients to reduce calculus by home-care practices and preventive product use aids in improved oral health and cosmetic appearance. The introduction of soluble pyrophosphates into dentifrices provides a chemical means of reducing supragingival calculus formation. Calcium and phosphorous from saliva are prevented from incorporating into the plaque matrix to form calculus.

Pyrophosphates act as crystal growth inhibitors, especially large, organized crystals. This may delay mineralization of the plaque and make it more susceptible to mechanical removal. Once calculus has formed into an organized matrix, pyrophosphates are ineffective. Their effectiveness is limited to new supragingival calculus. For this reason, recommendations for use are appropriate after prophylaxis or scaling/root planing.

Many studies have evaluated the effectiveness of pyrophosphates on calculus formation (Addy & Koltai, 1994; Gaengler, Kurbad, & Weinert, 1993). Not only is there a reduction in new calculus formation, but also the number of sites in the mouth that are calculus-free is increased (Lobene, 1989). Results after 3 and 6 months indicated significant reductions in supragingival deposits (Schiff, 1987) by 35.5 and 45.9%, respectively. Calculus inhibitors cause the newly formed deposits to be softer and easier for the clinician to remove. The amount of force and number of strokes by the dental hygienist are reduced (White et al., 1996). The addition of a copolymer (methoxyethylene and maleic acid) to a pyrophosphate dentifrice enhances the anticalculus effect (Singh, Petrone, Volpe, Rustogi, & Norfleet, 1990).

Besides the effect on hard deposits, anticalculus dentifrices also may exhibit antimicrobial activity by killing or inhibiting bacterial growth (Drake, Grigsby, & Drotz-Dieleman, 1994). Pyrophosphates have been found to reduce chlorhexidine-induced extrinsic stain (Bollmer, Sturzenberger, Vick, & Grossman, 1995).

True allergic reactions and mucosal (tissue) irritation are rare and most likely due to flavoring agents rather than the pyrophosphates. Tissue irritation has been reported in the form of tissue sloughing (peeling) and tooth surface sensitivity. Pyrophosphates in dentifrices also have been thought to interact with the fluoride compounds and interfere with the remineralization process. Fluoride uptake is not altered by pyrophosphates, however. The anticaries benefits are similar for regular-formula and tartar-control dentifrices. The ADA seal of acceptance has been given to tartar control dentifrices based on their anticaries properties. Because calculus inhibition is of cosmetic rather than therapeutic value, pyrophosphate dentifrices are not evaluated on the basis of their primary mode of action.

Zinc Citrate–Containing Dentrifices

Viadent™ Advanced Care (Colgate Oral Pharmaceuticals, Canton, MA) has as its active ingredients 2% zinc citrate trihydrate, which is an antibacterial agent, and 0.8% sodium monofluorophosphate, which has anticaries properties. This formulation is also available as an oral rinse. Sanguinarine is not in this new formulation.

Other Dentifrice Categories

Herbal-based and "natural" dentifrices are attractive alternatives to some patients interested in maintaining oral hygiene. Although these products have been documented to perhaps be as effective as conventional dentifrices in their ability to control plaque and gingivitis (Mullaby, James, Coulter, & Linden, 1995), their efficacy remains questionable. As long as these "natural" toothpastes contain fluoride, patients receive anticaries benefit. Patients must be educated on the limitations of their choice of dentifrice. The primary benefit of some of these alternatives is motivational, in that patients may be encouraged to brush more regularly with their chosen dentifrice.

A relatively new toothpaste containing essential oils in its formulation relies on support of data from studies evaluating the antiseptic mouthrinse (Listerine®, Warner-Lambert, Morris Plains, NJ). Product acceptance is based on fluoride content, not on plaque and gingivitis benefits.

Dentifrices containing a lactoperoxidase system (Biotene®, Laclede Professional Products, Rancho Dominguez, CA) may be beneficial for special patient groups. Patients with xerostomia were relieved of their symptoms after a 4-week daily use of a lactoperoxidase dentifrice and mouthrinse (Kirstila, Lenander-Lumikari, Soderling, & Tenovuo, 1996).

Home Care for Periodontal Patients

Post-Periodontal Surgical Home Care

The important role of oral hygiene in controlling dental plaque growth and recolonization immediately after periodontal surgery cannot be overestimated (Sanz & Herrera, 1998). The degree of oral hygiene maintained by the patient also influences the healing response after periodontal surgery (Flores-de-Jacoby & Mengel, 1995; Palcanis, 1996). Presently, it is unknown if the healing response results from the improvement in and maintenance of low plaque levels by the patient (Westfelt, 1996) or is related to the increased frequency of periodontal maintenance visits after surgery (Ramfjord, 1987).

Following periodontal surgery, patients should be cautious around the periodontal dressing. It is likely that they will be inclined to avoid brushing the area, but they should be instructed to lightly brush the exposed tooth surfaces and all other areas of the dentition with a soft or ultrasoft toothbrush. The Bass method should be avoided; other methods that do not place the bristles directly into the gingival crevice are recommended to prevent trauma to the healing tissue.

Periodontal patients frequently have localized or generalized blunted papillae due to the disease process or as a consequence of periodontal surgery. Because of the open interdental spaces, the use of interdental brushes and single-tuft brushes is recommended.

Implant Home Care

Diligent home care around tissue-integrated prostheses is imperative for long-term success. Plaque-control procedures must start immediately after uncovering the implants. It is important that the dental hygienist customize a home-care regimen based on the patient's awareness and ability and the type of prosthesis present (Orton, Steele, & Wolinsky, 1987).

There are two specific areas of focus for home-care procedures around implants. The first is the portion of the titanium abutment exposed above the soft tissues in the oral cavity, as well as the small portion just below the gingiva. The second area requiring plaque control is the prosthetic component, consisting of the rigid cast framework and tooth replacement materials.

A multitude of home-care devices exist to assist in mechanical oral hygiene regimes. These devices include various manual (Fig. 22–12■) or powered toothbrushes (Fig. 22–13■) and specific interdental aids (Balshi, 1986). Soft or ultrasoft manual toothbrushes are the traditional means of plaque removal. However, brush heads come in many different shapes and sizes, and brushes should be prescribed individually depending on the implant type and the patient's abilities. An excellent area-specific soft nylon brush is the single-tufted brush. This brush is for use on individual implants, one implant at a time, and the shaft can be bent for better access.

Various interdental devices are available, including interdental brushes, rubber-tip stimulators, wooden cleaners, and numerous types of dental floss. The brush attachment for interdental brushes is available as a plastic or nylon-coated wire rather than a metal wire to prevent scratching of implant surfaces. Interdental brushes are used only if sufficient interdental embrasure exists. Various floss types, such as tufted floss or floss cords (PostCare™, J. O. Butler, Chicago), along with folded gauze or traditional floss, are effective and safe interproximal plaque-removal aids (Fig. 22–14■).

Clinical use of antimicrobials (chemotherapeutic agents) can adjunctively help to inhibit plaque and gingivitis around implants. These agents may be delivered by rinsing or applied topically (via toothbrush, floss, or cotton-tipped applicator). Irrigation can be used if pathologic changes are present (Meffert, Langer, & Frutz, 1992). A study conducted by Felo, Shibly, Ciancio, Lauciello, and Ho (1997) investigated the effects of subgingival irrigation with chlorhexidine gluconate diluted with water on peri-implant gingival health compared with rinsing with chlorhexidine when used as an adjunct to routine peri-implant maintenance. Results suggested that powered subgingival irrigation with chlorhexidine may be better than rinsing in implant maintenance. However, even though the results of this study were fa-

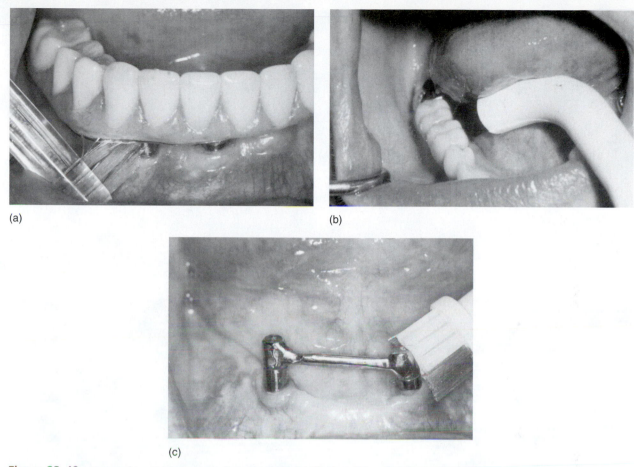

(a)

(b)

(c)

Figure 22–12   Types of toothbrushes used on implants. (a) Single-tuft brush (also referred to as an end-tuft brush). (b) Powered brush used with fixed partial denture superstructure. (c) Powered brush used with overdenture abutments and retention bar.

vorable toward the use of irrigation at home, patients should not irrigate routinely until more controlled clinical studies can support its use.

The use of chlorhexidine gluconate (Peridex®, Zila Pharmaceuticals, Cincinnati, OH; or PerioGard®, Colgate Oral Pharmaceuticals, Canton, MA) and Listerine® (Warner-Lambert, Morris Plains, NJ) has been shown to be advantageous in the inhibition of bacterial plaque in implant patients (Ciancio et al., 1995).

Some practitioners may recommend home irrigation devices, but patients should be advised to use gentle pressure, ensuring that the irrigant is not forced into the sulcus. Excessive fluid pressure with the tip positioned apically could damage the perimucosal seal. Using either a sideport blunt-tipped canula or a rubber-tip irrigating device is less likely to violate this seal.

While rinsing with antimicrobials has been proven to be beneficial, some rinses do have unwanted side effects, such as staining, altered taste, and increased calculus formation. Awareness of potential side effects may indicate alternative delivery by applying the solution in a site-specific fashion so as to avoid undesirable effects.

Figure 22–13 Various types of powered brush heads. Many clinicians recommend powered brushes for use around dental implants.

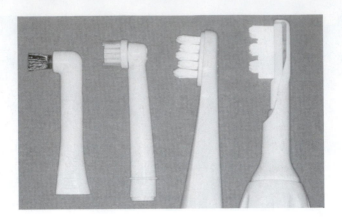

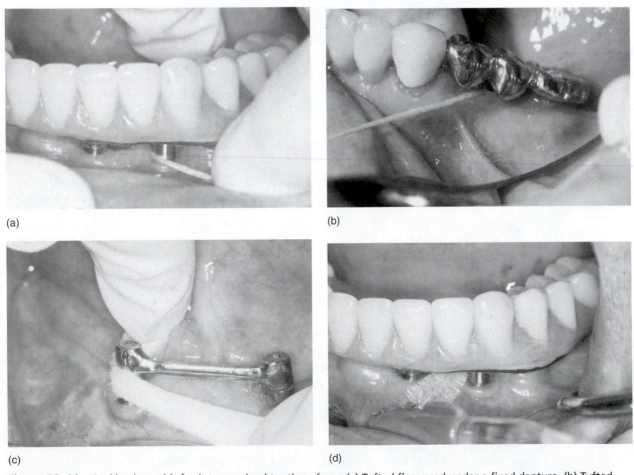

(a)

(b)

(c)

(d)

Figure 22–14 Oral hygiene aids for interproximal tooth surfaces. (a) Tufted floss used under a fixed denture. (b) Tufted floss used under a fixed bridge. (c) Folded gauze strip can be efficient when access is good. (d) Interdental brush used under a fixed partial denture.

Orthodontic Home Care

Orthodontic appliances tend to increase the accumulation of supragingival plaque on the teeth leading to the development of gingival inflammation and bleeding. Meticulous oral hygiene is important to control the development of gingival inflammation. During orthodontic treatment, the patient should be evaluated regularly. A soft-bristled toothbrush designed specifically for orthodontic appliances should be recommended to the patient, including an oral rinse if needed to supplement brushing. The Charters method of brushing is used to clean the brackets of cervical areas of the teeth. For interdental home care, use of a floss threader with floss or Super Floss is recommended.

Advice to the Patient

Noncompliance with oral hygiene self-care is a major factor in the recurrence of periodontal diseases. One role of the dental hygienist is to determine the patient's enthusiasm and manual dexterity in performing plaque control (Baker, 1995). This entails having good professional communications skills and patience, since it is not easy for patients to change their habits. Besides lack of motivation, other reasons for plaque control failure include poor technique, lack of knowledge, and inconsistent performance (Van Dyke, Offenbacher, Pihlstrom, Putt, & Trummel, 1999).

Flossing can be done either before or after toothbrushing, but most patients floss before brushing. Patients often find flossing to be a difficult experience. Therefore, the dental hygienist must introduce flossing from an educational perspective and then gradually instruct the patient about technique. It is best not to have the patient start with too many plaque-control devices at one time. Rather, it may be advantageous to introduce effective toothbrushing at the first appointment and then reinforce it at subsequent visits. The patient's toothbrushing method should only be changed or modified if it is ineffective in removing plaque or causing trauma. Flossing or other methods of interdental cleaning can be introduced at a later time. By gradually having the patient master each technique separately, he or she will not be overwhelmed.

Oral hygiene self-care programs are based on a patient's individual needs. Keeping the program simple will increase patient compliance. Try to adapt the oral hygiene program to the patient's lifestyle. Establishing good oral hygiene habits involves having patients clean their teeth in a systematic pattern (e.g., starting on the maxillary right and ending on the mandibular right). However, strict adherence to one approach may not always be in the best interests of thorough plaque removal and improved gingival health.

Oral physiotherapeutic products have limitations. Brushing and flossing are effective in the mechanical removal of most supragingival plaque but are limited in removing subgingival plaque due to the design of the devices and the contour of the gingiva. A periodontal patient may be able to access the subgingiva only slightly. The techniques described in this chapter can be modified to permit cleansing of all accessible areas of the dentition. A different regimen is applied after periodontal surgery, and the patient must be familiar with the various cleaning aids needed. The dental hygienist must introduce these new aids to the patient.

The iatrogenic effects of dentistry need to be eliminated prior to setting expectations for plaque removal. For example, unpolished amalgam restorations retain more plaque than polished ones. Composite materials may accumulate plaque greater than amalgam. Ill-fitting margins, overhangs, and rough surfaces on restorations should be evaluated for replacement or finishing because of plaque-retentive possibilities.

Patients with gingival enlargement (drug-induced or hormonal) must be especially compliant with frequent maintenance visits and good oral hygiene self-care. Keeping plaque levels to a minimum has been shown to reduce the development of gingival enlargement in some patients. Since the gingiva is overgrown and pseudopockets result, it is difficult for such patients to practice optimal toothbrushing and flossing.

Effects of Improper Use of Oral Hygiene Devices

Once the importance of oral hygiene is explained to the patient and he or she begins to use numerous oral hygiene devices, the next step is to ensure that the patient is using each device correctly.

Toothbrushing

Factors that can cause acute or chronic tissue problems include incorrect bristle angulation or placement, heavy or long brushing strokes, a toothbrush with hard bristles, extremely abrasive toothpaste, and loss of concentration. Acute soft tissue lesions appear as small ulcers, red areas, or denuded gingiva. Chronic, long-standing gingival lesions present as gingival recession, rolled marginal gingiva, or gingival clefting (Fig. 22–15■). Gingival recession was found to occur mostly on the buccal surfaces of maxillary first molars, premolars, and canines (Björn, Andersson, & Olsson, 1981). Hard tissue lesions present as toothbrush abrasions occurring at the cervical area of teeth (see Fig. 22–1). Tooth abrasion in most cases is due to the combined effect of toothbrushing and the use of dentifrices containing abrasives (Sangnes, 1976). Cervical abrasion may occur once the root surface has been exposed by gingival recession. Thus, in order for cervical abrasions to occur, they must be preceded by gingival recession.

Figure 22–15   Soft tissue trauma caused by improper toothbrushing. Note rolled free gingival margins.

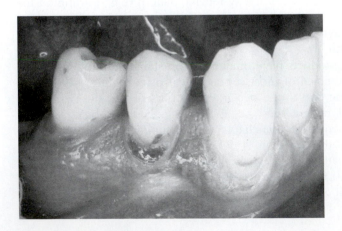

The Bass method is one of the more technique-sensitive toothbrushing methods. This method requires the patient to have good manual dexterity and concentration when applying the bristles to each area along both dental arches to minimize damage to soft tissue. The soft tissue needs to be evaluated at each maintenance visit for signs of improper brushing. If used correctly, powered toothbrushes do not cause soft or hard tissue damage.

Interdental Devices

Dental floss, interdental brushes, and single-tufted brushes can cause injury to the gingiva if improper techniques are used. Each device is indicated in different types of gingival embrasures. Gingival ulcers, cuts, and clefts can result from improper technique.

Floss should not be forced too deeply into the gingival crevices. When floss is used as part of the daily plaque-control routine, the junctional epithelial cells adhering to the enamel are in a continuous state of disruption and healing (Waerhaug, 1981). Interdental brushes and single-tufted brushes should not be forced into a gingival embrasure that has an intact papilla.

Interdental cleaning is easy to master if the dental hygienist provides proper teaching and supervision to the patient.

Dentinal Hypersensitivity

Maintaining plaque control is of utmost importance in reducing the sensitivity of exposed root surfaces. Often patients have difficulty complying with oral hygiene procedures because of the discomfort experienced during toothbrushing. Thus these areas are not cleaned and become more sensitive. Identification of a lesion is difficult, and frequently, toothbrushing is a major factor in localizing the sensitivity. Accordingly, root surfaces must be desensitized and an adequate oral hygiene self-care program maintained. In patients with good oral hygiene but with dentinal hypersensitivity, use of a desensitizing agent is recommended.

Gingival recession as a result of disease processes (inflammation and attachment loss), tooth malposition, faulty toothbrushing, or periodontal surgery can result in exposed dentin. This can result in hypersensitivity near the cervical area of the tooth. Usually, movement of fluid within the dentinal tubules causes discomfort in the exposed areas.

Desensitization

A number of treatments are available for sensitive teeth. The type of treatment depends on the severity of the problem and the history of prior intervention. The following steps are recommended for desensitization:

1. Use the air syringe to assess whether there is sensitivity. Write on the tooth being evaluated a "+" if the tooth has a positive response to the stimulus.
2. Recommend use of a desensitizing dentifrice for about 4 to 6 weeks. The patient is instructed to brush two times a day for 1 minute.
3. Instruct the patient on proper brushing so that the situation does not get worse. The patient's brushing technique must be corrected if treatment is to be successful.

4. Discuss the role of diet with the patient. Acidic and citrus foods should be limited in the patient's diet. If the patient frequently consumes acidic foods or juices, he or she should be instructed to rinse the mouth with sodium bicarbonate to help neutralize the acidity.

5. At the next examination, do the air syringe test again, and if the sensitivity is gone, the patient can go back to his or her regular dentifrice. If the sensitivity reappears later, the patient can use the desensitizing dentifrice again. If the sensitivity is still present, an in-office treatment should be tried.

Treatment

Treatment of dentin hypersensitivity focuses on blocking the opened dentinal tubules to prevent transmission of the noxious external stimuli and decreasing the intradental nerve excitability. Therapeutic products can be applied either professionally or by the patient. Most of the patient-applied over-the-counter (OTC) products must be used for a prolonged period of time for greatest effect. Since it takes many weeks for efficacy, manufacturers have added fluoride to the formula for its anticaries effect. It must be stressed to patients that optimal plaque control also will help to reduce the sensitivity.

Table 22–10 lists the more commonly used dentifrices for dentinal hypersensitivity. Potassium nitrate is effective in reducing cold and tactile sensitivity as compared with regular toothpaste (Silverman et al., 1996). Potassium nitrate acts quickly and directly on the pulpal nerves.

Other agents in dentifrices include dibasic sodium citrate and 0.4% stannous fluoride. Stinging and extrinsic staining may contribute to patient noncompliance with stannous fluoride. These dentifrices are ADA approved for the relief of dentin sensitivity. Since these products are dentifrices (pastes and gels), application is by means of a soft-bristle toothbrush, brushing for at least 1 minute and making sure that all surfaces are brushed and then expectorated.

Strontium chloride is no longer used in dentifrices because fluoride could not be incorporated into the formulation. It used to be marketed as Sensodyne-SC® (Block Drug, Jersey City, NJ).

Minimal research has been done to evaluate the duration of the sensitivity decrease following cessation of use of desensitizing dentifrices. Some sensitivity may return within 6 to 12 weeks following use of such a dentifrice for 6 to 8 weeks.

Patient-Applied Treatment

Basically, potassium nitrate and stannous fluoride products are available for patient-applied treatments (Table 22–11■).

Dentifrices

Patient-applied medicaments are available as dentifrices, gels, and rinses. Dentifrices are helpful when many tooth surfaces are sensitive. For patients with mild sensitivity without loss of substantial tooth structure, a densensitizing dentifrice is recommended. Because it can take several weeks to see results, fluoride has been added to most dentifrices. It appears that a potassium nitrate–containing dentifrice works the fastest.

The longer the dentifrice is in contact with the dentin surface, the greater is its success. Thus more frequent applications are advised. Instead of using a dentifrice

Table 22–11	Patient-Applied Desensitizing Agents (other than dentifrices)	
Product	**Active Ingredient**	**Method of Use**
Gel-Kam® gel (Colgate Oral Pharm., Canton, MA)	0.4% stannous fluoride	Apply to toothbrush and brush teeth. This product is available over-the-counter without a prescription. Available in 4.3-oz tubes or a pack with 2-to 3.5-oz tubes.
Gel-Kam® Oral Care Rinse (Colgate Oral Pharm., Canton, MA)	0.63% stannous fluoride	Patient places 1/8 fluid oz of concentrate in marked mixing vial (included in box) and adds water as directed to prepare a 0.1% stannous fluoride rinse. Rinse over a 3-week period.
STANIMAX™ Perio Rinse (SDI Labs, Glenview, IL)	0.63% stannous fluoride	1/8 fluid oz is diluted with warm water to make 1 oz of the rinse in a measuring cup that is provided.
STANIMAX™ Brush-on Gel (SDI Labs, Glenview, IL)	0.4% stannous fluoride	Apply gel to a toothbrush.

in the usual manner, it may be more effective if the undiluted dentifrice is applied with a cotton applicator directly on the tooth surface.

Fluorides

Of all the fluorides, stannous fluoride shows the most promise for topical application in periodontal therapy as an antibacterial and desensitizing agent. Application of stannous fluoride (0.4%) on a daily basis, after some time, can be therapeutic in reducing dentinal hypersensitivity. However, it often stings the gingiva, and patients may not comply with treatment. In addition, stannous fluoride will stain dentin more than enamel because of its porous nature, making it unaesthetic. Because it is nonabrasive, extrinsic stains will build up if it is used instead of toothpaste. Stannous fluoride is also available in a 0.63% oral rinse that dilutes to a 0.1% solution.

In-Office Treatment

If therapeutic dentifrices are not successful, in-office application of medicaments is recommended. Several products are available, including ferric oxalate, fluoride (with or without iontophoresis), bonding agents, varnishes, and glass ionomers (Table 22–12■).

Oxalate Salts

Most oxalates (ferric oxalate and potassium oxalate) are available as acidic solutions. Oxalates are capable of blocking the dentinal tubules when they are placed on an area of exposed dentin. Often the patient brushes the oxalate off. Thus the patient must be instructed not to brush too vigorously so that the dentin will not be removed. It is best to evaluate the patient's brushing technique in the office.

Table 22–12	Chairside Desensitizing Products	
Product	**Active Ingredient**	**Method of Use**
Dentinbloc® (Colgate Oral Pharm., Canton, MA)	1.09% sodium fluoride, 0.40% stannous fluoride, 0.14% hydrogen fluoride	Saturate a cotton pellet and apply to dry exposed dentin. Do not burnish; use light pressure.
Sensodyne® Sealant (Block Drug Corp., Jersey City, NJ)	6% ferric oxalate	Saturate a cotton pellet and apply to dry exposed dentin. Do not burnish; use light pressure.
Protect® Drops (John O. Butler Co., Chicago, IL, available in a dropper bottle or unit dose ampule)	2.7% potassium oxalate	Saturate a cotton pellet and apply to dry exposed dentin. Do not burnish; use light pressure.
Dentin conditioners	Aluminum oxalate	Saturate a cotton pellet and apply to dry exposed dentin. Use light pressure; do not burnish.
STANIMAX-PRO™ (SDI Labs, Glenview, IL)	3.28% stannous fluoride	Can be used as a gel or diluted one-to-one with water to form a 1.64% stannous fluoride rinse.
Duraflor® (Pharmascience Inc., Montréal, Canada)	50 mg sodium fluoride varnish	Apply to affected area with a cotton pellet.
Duraphat® (Colgate Oral Pharm., Canton, MA)	5% sodium fluoride varnish	Apply to affected area with a brush that comes with kit or with a cotton pellet.

Fluorides

Most dental practitioners use fluoride for management of hypersensitivity. Stannous fluoride is applied topically on the exposed dentin, forming a sort of granular layer over the dentin surface that does not come off with simple washing, so it seals or decreases dentin permeability.

Sodium fluoride is available as a paste (33% sodium fluoride, 33% kaolin, 33% glycerin). Sodium fluoride works best for about 7 to 14 days, and then its effects dissipate.

Various sodium fluoride solutions have been tried with limited success. When iontophoresis is used to allow the fluoride ion to penetrate into the dentinal tubules, longer-lasting effects, up to 3 to 4 months, are seen. A second application usually is necessary.

Restorative Materials

Bonding agents are improving rapidly, but they are not used very much at this time. Use of such agents is a technique-sensitive procedure. Often the restoration is finished with a diamond bur, which may open up new tubules below the restoration, recreating sensitive dentin. Since the restoration is located at the cervical third of the tooth, overhangs or rough surfaces may create more problems.

If the sensitivity can be narrowed down to just one or two teeth, a glass ionomer can be used as a last resort.

Summary

Supragingival and subgingival dental plaque biofilms play a major role in the initiation of periodontal diseases. Since the subgingival microbiota is derived originally from supragingival plaque, it is necessary to disrupt both groups of bacteria. This is accomplished through mechanical supragingival plaque removal by the patient using toothbrushes and interdental devices and by the dental hygienist by removaling subgingival plaque.

It would seem that gingivitis should be treated easily with plaque removal. Unfortunately, many obstacles prevent the timely removal of plaque. Besides lack of motivation to learn and perform toothbrushing and flossing skills, many patients also perform inconsistently, lack knowledge, and employ poor technique.

Fluorides have successfully decreased the rate of dental caries. Thereafter, few advances in chemical plaque control (dentifrices) have been achieved in recent years, except for the introduction of triclosan. Tartar-control dentifrices offer a cosmetic benefit. Desensitizing toothpastes may aid in the alleviation of dentinal hypersensitivity. Baking soda/hydrogen peroxide dentifrices have not been shown to consistently elicit antiplaque/antigingivitis effects. Triclosan is the first chemical agent used in dentifrices that can claim benefits to periodontal health.

Key Points

- Plaque removal prevents gingivitis.
- The removal of plaque through daily plaque-control practices and professional cleanings is important in controlling subgingival plaque formation.
- There are numerous periodontal and medical causes of bad breath that need to be explored to effectively treat halitosis.
- The removal of supragingival plaque is important in controlling the development of subgingival plaque and periodontitis.
- The main goal of prevention is to achieve the lowest plaque level possible.
- Plaque-control measures by the patient and professional maintenance appointments are both important in maintaining gingival health and are essential parts of primary and secondary prevention of periodontitis.
- Dental floss is indicated for interproximal plaque removal in Type I gingival embrasures.
- There is no difference in efficacy of plaque removal with waxed or unwaxed dental floss.

Web Sites

www.perio.org

www.adha.org

www.dentalcare.com

www.colgate.com

Self-Quiz

1. Which one of the following statements describes the rationale for periodontal oral hygiene self-care? (p. 338)
   a. reduction in the risk for development of dental caries
   b. augmentation of the immune reaction to a bacterial insult
   c. elimination or suppression of harmful microorganisms found in supragingival plaque biofilms
   d. disruption of the number of subgingival microbial biota with a delay in the repopulation of pathogens

2. Which one of the following oral hygiene regimens is best for a patient after periodontal surgery? (p. 367)
   a. Resume regular brushing and flossing regimens.
   b. Use a soft-bristle toothbrush and an antimicrobial mouthrinse.
   c. Use powered toothbrush and floss.
   d. Use oral irrigation with chlorhexidine.

3. A patient says that he is doing the best he can with his home care, but he still has moderate to heavy supragingival deposits. Which of the following recommendations should the dental hygienist give to this patient? (pp. 338–339)
   a. Don't worry because everyone gets some accumulations.
   b. Use an antimicrobial mouthrinse.
   c. Improve or change method of home care.
   d. Refer to a specialist.

4. Waxed dental floss has proven to be more effective in interdental cleaning than unwaxed dental floss because it is easier for the patient to handle. (p. 335)
   a. Both the statement and the reason are correct and related.
   b. Both the statement and the reason are correct but not related.
   c. The statement is correct, but the reason is not.
   d. The statement is not correct, but the reason is correct.
   e. Neither the statement nor the reason is correct.

5. Various toothbrushing methods are described in the literature because some methods are superior in removing plaque than others. (p. 349)
   a. Both the statement and the reason are correct and related.
   b. Both the statement and the reason are correct but not related.
   c. The statement is correct, but the reason is not.
   d. The statement is not correct, but the reason is correct.
   e. Neither the statement nor the reason is correct.

6. All the following factors need to be considered when recommending interdental cleansing devices except one. Which one is the exception? (p. 355)
   a. amount of plaque
   b. manual dexterity
   c. presence of a bridge
   d. type of gingival embrasure

7. Which one of the following methods best evaluates for effectiveness of a patient's oral hygiene? (p. 339)
   a. show and tell
   b. feedback
   c. disclosing agents
   d. self-documentation

8. Which one of the following oral hygiene aids is best to remove dental plaque on the proximal surface of a tooth that has a Type I gingival embrasure? (p. 357)
   a. toothbrush
   b. interdental brush
   c. rubber-tip stimulator
   d. wooden wedge
   e. dental floss

9. Which one of the following steps should be done first when treating a patient for dentinal hypersensitivity? (p. 373)

   a. Recommend a desensitizing dentifrice for 4 to 6 weeks.

   b. Instruct the patient on the proper tooth-brushing method.

   c. Identify the tooth that is painful.

   d. Apply sodium fluoride.

10. Which of the following oral hygiene aids is best used for interdental removal of plaque from implants? (p. 368)

    a. toothbrush

    b. powered toothbrush

    c. interproximal brush with plastic core

    d. interproximal brush with metal core

References

Addy, M., and P. Adriaens. 1998. Epidemiology and etiology of periodontal diseases and the role of plaque control in dental caries: Consensus report of group A. In eds. N. P. Lang, R. Attström, and H. Löe, *Proceedings of the European Workshop on Mechanical Plaque Control*, 99–101. Chicago: Quintessence.

Addy, M., and R. Koltai. 1994. Control of supragingival calculus. Scaling and polishing and anticalculus toothpastes: An opinion. *J. Clin. Periodontol.* 21:342–346.

Bacca, L. A., M. Leusch, A. C. Lanzalaco, D. Macksood, and O. J. Bouwsma, et al. 1997. A comparison of intraoral antimicrobial effects of stabilized fluoride dentifrice, baking soda/hydrogen peroxide dentifrice, conventional NaF dentifrice and essential oil mouthrinse. *J. Clin. Dent.* 8:54–61.

Bader, H. J. 1992. Review of currently available battery operated toothbrushes. *Compend. Contin. Educ. Dent.* 13:1163–1169.

Baker, K. 1995. The role of dental professionals and the patient in plaque control. *Periodontology 2000* 8:108–113.

Balshi, T. J. 1986. Hygiene maintenance procedures for patients treated with the tissue integrated prosthesis (osseointegration). *Quintessence Int.* 17:95–102.

Beaumont, R. H. 1990. Patient preference for waxed or unwaxed dental floss. *J. Periodontol.* 61:123–125.

Beiswanger, B. B., P. M. Doyle, and R. D. Jackson. 1995. The clinical effect of dentifrices containing stabilized stannous fluoride on plaque formation and gingivitis: A six-month study with ad libitum brushing. *J. Clin. Dent.* 6:46–53.

Binney, A., M. Addy, S. McKeowns, and L. Everatt. 1995. The effect of commercially available triclosan-containing toothpaste compared to a sodium-fluoride containing toothpaste and a chlorhexidine rinse on 4-day plaque regrowth. *J. Clin. Periodontol.* 22(1):830–834.

Binney, A., M. Addy, S. McKeowns, and L. Everatt. 1996. The choice of controls in toothpaste studies: The effect of a number of commercially available toothpastes compared to water on a 4-day plaque regrowth. *J. Clin. Periodontol.* 23(5):456–459.

Binney, A., M. Addy, J. Owens, and J. Faulkner. 1997. A comparison of triclosan and stannous fluoride toothpastes for inhibition of plaque regrowth: A crossover study designed to assess carryover. *J. Clin. Periodontol.* 24(3):166–170.

Björn, A. L., U. Andersson, and A. Olsson. 1981. Gingival recession in 15-year-old pupils. *Swed. Dent. J.* 5:141–146.

Bollmer, B. L. V., O. P. Sturzenberger, V. Vick, and E. Grossman. 1995. Reduction of calculus and Peridex stain with Tarter Control Crest. *J. Clin. Dent.* 6(4):185–187.

Borden, L.C., E.S. Chaves, J.P. Bowman, B. M. Faith, and G. L. Hollar. 2002. The effect of four mouthrinses on oral malodor. *Compendium* 23:531–546.

Bosy, A. 1997. Oral malodor: philosophical and practical aspects. *J. Can. Dent. Assoc.* 63:196–201.

Brunette, D. M. 1996. Effects of baking soda–containing dentifrices on oral malodor. *Compend. Contin. Educ. Dent.* 17 (Suppl. 19):22–31.

Brunette D.M., H.M. Proskin, and B.J. Nelson. 1998. The effects of dentifrice systems on oral malodor. *J. Clin. Dent.* 9:76–82.

Cancro, L. P., and S. L. Fischman. 1995. The expected effect on oral health of dental plaque control through mechanical removal. *Periodontology 2000.* 8:60–74.

Cerra, M. B., and W. J. Killoy. 1982. The effect of sodium bicarbonate and hydrogen peroxide on the microbial flora of periodontal pockets: A preliminary report. *J. Periodontol.* 53:599–603.

Ciancio, S. G. 1997. Triclosan: A new antigingivitis agent. *Biol. Ther. Dent.* 13:23–26.

Ciancio, S. G., O. Shilby, and G. A. Farber. 1992. Clinical evaluation of the effect of two types of dental floss on plaque and gingival health. *Clin. Prevent. Dent.* 14:14–18.

Corbet, E. F., and W. I. R. Davies. 1993. The flow of supragingival plaque in the control of progressive periodontal disease: A review. *J. Clin. Peridontol.* 20:307–313.

Darby, M., and M. Walsh. 1994. *Dental hygiene theory and practice*. Philadelphia: W. B. Saunders.

Delanghe, G., J. Ghyselen, C. Bollen, D. van Steenberghe, B. Vanderkerckhove, and L. Feenstra. 1999. An inventory of patients response to treatment at a multidisciplinary breath odor clinic. *Quintessence Int.* 30:307–310.

Dellerman, P. A., T. J. Hughes, and T. A. Burkett. 1994. A comparative evaluation of the percent acceptable end-round bristles in the Crest Complete, the Improved Crest Complete and the Oral-B Advantage toothbrushes. *J. Clin. Dent.* 5:74–81.

Drake, D. R., B. Grigsby, and D. Drotz-Dieleman. 1994. Growth-inhibitory effect of pyrophosphate on oral bacteria. *Oral Micro. Immunol.* 9(1):25–28.

Drake, D., K. Vargas, A. Cardenzana, and R. Srikantha. 1995. Enhanced bacterial activity of Arm and Hammer Dental Care. *Am. J. Dent.* 8(6):308–312.

Duckworth, R. M., Y. Jones, J. Nicholson, A. P. Jacobson, and I. G. Chestnutt. 1994. Studies on plaque fluoride after use of F-containing dentifrices. *Adv. Dent. Res.* 8(2):202–207.

Felo, A., O. Shibly, S. G. Ciancio, F. R. Lauciello, and A. Ho. 1997. Effects of subgingival chlorhexidine irrigation of peri-implant maintenance. *Am. J. Dent.* 10:107–110.

Fischman, S. L., G. Kugel, R. B. Truelove, B. J. Nelson, and L. P. Cancro. 1992. Motivational benefits of a dentifrice containing baking soda and hydrogen peroxide. *J. Clin. Dent.* 3:88–94.

Fishman, S. L., and S. Yankell. 1999. Dentifrices, mouth rinses, and tooth whiteners. In eds. N. O. Harris and F. García-Godoy, *Primary preventive dentistry,* 5th ed., 103–125. Stamford, CT: Appleton and Lange.

Flores-de-Jacoby, L., and R. Mengel. 1995. Conventional surgical procedures. *Periodontology 2000.* 9:38–54.

Forgas-Brockmann, L. B., C. Carter-Hanson, and W. J. Killoy. 1998. The effects of an ultrasonic toothbrush on plaque accumulation and gingival inflammation. *J. Clin. Periodontol.* 25:375–379.

Frandsen, A. 1986. Mechanical oral hygiene practices. In eds. H. Löe and D. V. Kleinman, *Dental plaque control measures and oral hygiene practices,* 93–116. Oxford: IRL Press.

Gaengler, P., A. Kurbad, and W. Weinert. 1993. Evaluation of anti-calculus efficacy: An SEM method of evaluating the effectiveness of pyrophosphate dentifrice on calculus formation. *J. Clin. Periodontol.* 20:144–146.

Garmyn, P., D. van Steenberghe, and M. Quirynen. 1998. Efficacy of plaque control in the maintenance of gingival health: Plaque control in primary and secondary prevention. In eds. N. P. Lang, R. Attström, and H. Löe, *Proceedings of the European Workshop on Mechanical Plaque Control,* 107–120. Chicago: Quintessence.

Glavid, L., H. Christensen, E. Pedersen, H. Rosendahl, and R. Attström. 1985. Oral hygiene instruction in general dental practice by means of self-teaching manuals. *J. Clin. Periodontol.* 12:27–34.

Gordon, J. M., J. A. Frascella, and R. C. Reardon. 1996. A clinical study of the safety and efficacy of a novel electric interdental cleaning device. *J. Clin. Dent.* 7:70–73.

Grossman, E., M. Cronin, W. Dembling, and H. Proskin. 1996. A comparative study of extrinsic tooth stain removal with two electric toothbrushes and a manual brush. *Am. J. Dent.* 9:25–29.

Hancock, E. B. 1996. Prevention. *Ann. Periodontol.* 1:223–249.

Hellstadius, K., B. Asman, and A. Gustafsson. 1993. Improved maintenance of plaque control by electric tooth brushing in periodontitis patients with low compliance. *J. Clin. Periodontol.* 20:235–237.

Hellström, M. K., P. Ramberg, L. Krok, and J. Lindhe. 1996. The effect of supragingival plaque control on the microflora in human periodontitis. *J. Clin. Periodontol.* 23:934–940.

Hill, H. C., P. A. Levi, and I. Glickman. 1973. The effects of waxed and unwaxed dental floss on interdental plaque accumulation and interdental gingival health. *J. Periodontol.* 53:411–414.

Jensen, M. E., and F. J. Kohout. 1988. The effect of a fluoridated dentifrice on root and coronal caries in an older adult population. *J. Am. Dent. Assoc.* 117:829–832.

Jepsen, S. 1998. The role of manual toothbrushes in effective plaque control: Advantages and limitations. In eds. N. P. Lang, R. Attström, and H. Löe, *Proceedings of the European Workshop on Mechanical Plaque Control,* 121–137. Chicago: Quintessence.

Kirstila, V., M. Lenander-Lumikari, E. Soderling, and J. Tenovuo. 1996. Effects of oral hygiene products containing lactoperoxidase, lysozyme, and lactoferrin on the composition of whole saliva and on subjective oral symptoms in patients with xerostomia. *Acta Odontol. Scand.* 54:391–397.

Kleinberg, I., and M. Codipilly. 2001. Cysteine challenge testing as a method of determining the effectiveness of oral hygiene procedures for reducing oral malodor. *J. Dent. Rest.* 79 (special issue):425.

Kleinberg, I., and G. Westbay. 1992. Salivary and metabolic factors involved in oral malodor formation. *J Periodontol.* 63:768–775.

Koertge, T. E. 1996. Management of dental staining: Can low-abrasive dentifrices play a role? *Compend. Contin. Educ. Dent.* 17(Suppl 19):33–38.

Kostelc, J. G., G. Preti, P. R. Zelson, et al. 1980. Salivary volatiles as indicators of periodontitis. *J Periodont Res.* 1980;15:185–192.

Lefkoff, M. H., F. M. Beck, and J. E. Horton. 1995. The effectiveness of a disposable tooth cleansing device on plaque. *J. Periodontol.* 66:218–221.

Levine, R. A. 1987. The Keyes technique as a cofactor in self-inflicted gingival lesions: A case report. *Compend. Contin. Educ. Dent.* 8:266–269.

Lindhe, J., B. Rosling, S. S. Socransky, and A.R. Volpe. 1993. The effect of a triclosan containing dentifrice on established plaque and gingivitis. *J. Clin. Periodontol.* 20:327–334.

Lobene, R. R. 1989. A study to compare the effects of two dentifrices on adult dental calculus formation. *Clin. Dent.* 1:67–69.

Loesche, W. J. and C. Kazor. 2002. Microbiology and treatment of halitosis. *J. Periodontol.* 28:256–79.

Mariotti, A. J. 1998. Mouthrinses and dentifrices. In *ADA Guide to Dental Therapeutics,* 1st ed. 210–212. Chicago: ADA Publishing Co.

Marshall, M. V., L. P. O. Cancro, and S.F. Fischman. 1995. Hydrogen peroxide: A review of its use in dentistry. *J. Periodontol.* 66:786–796.

Meffert, R., B. Langer, and M. Frutz. 1992. Dental implants: A review. *J. Periodontol.* 63:859–870.

Meskin, L. H. 1996. A breath of fresh air. *J. Am. Dent. Assoc.*127:1282–86.

Miyazaki, H., M. Arao, K. Okamura, K. Yaegaki, and T. Matsuo. 1999. Tentative classification of halitosis and its treatment needs. *Niigata Dent. J.* 32:7–11.

Moran, J. M., and M. Addy. 1995. A comparative study of stain removal with two electric toothbrushes and a manual brush. *J. Clin. Dent.* 6:188–193.

Morita M., D.L. Musinski, and H.L. Wang. 2001. Assessment of newly developed tongue sulfide probe for detecting oral malodor. *J. Clin. Periodontol.* 28:494–496.

Morita, M., and H.L. Wang. 2001. Association between oral malodor and adult periodontitis: a review. *J. Clin. Periodontol.* 28:813–819.

Mullaby, B. H., J. A. James, W. A. Coulter, and G. H. Linden. 1995. The efficacy of a herbal-based toothpaste on the control of plaque and gingivitis. *J. Clin. Periodontol.* 22:686–689.

Niles H.P., K. Rustogi, M. Pestrone, et al. 1999. Long lasting breath freshening effects of a trichlosan/coplymer/NaF toothpaste pp. 13. *Proceedings of the 4th International Conference on Breath Odor,* Los Angeles, CA.

O'Beirne, G. O., R. H. Johnson, G. Rutger Persson, and M. D. Spektor. 1996. Efficacy of a sonic toothbrush on inflammation and probing depth in adult periodontitis. *J. Periodontol.* 67:900–908.

Page, R. C. 1997. Causes of halitosis. *Oral Care Rep.* 7(4):7–8.

Palcanis, K. G. 1996. Surgical pocket therapy. *Ann. Periodontol.* 1:589–617.

Pihlstrom, B. L., L. F. Wolff, M. B. Bakdash, E. M. Schaffer, J. R. Jensen, et al. 1987. Salt and peroxide compared with conventional oral hygiene: I. Clinical results. *J. Periodontol.* 58:291–300.

Preber, H., V. Ylipaa, J. Bergström, and H. Ryden. 1991. A comparative study of plaque removing efficiency using rotary electric and manual toothbrushes. *Swed. Dent. J.* 15:229–234.

Preti G., Clark L., B.J. Cowart, R.S. Feldman, L.D. Lowry, et al. 1992. Non-oral etiologies of oral malodor and altered chemosensation. *J. Periodontol.* 63:790–796.

Proskin, H.M., and A.R. Volpe. 1995. Comparison of the anticaries efficacy of dentifrices containing fluoride as sodium fluoride or sodium monofluorophosphate. *Am. J. Dent.* 8:51–58.

Ramfjord, S. P. 1987. Maintenance care for treated patients. *J. Clin. Periodontol.* 14:433–437.

Ratcliff P.A., and P.W. Johnson. 1999. The relationship between oral malodor, gingivitis, and periodontists. A review. *J. Periodontol.* 70:485–489.

Reingewirtz Y., O. Girault, N. Reingewirtz, B. Senger, and H. Tenenbaum. 1999. Mechanical effects and volatile sulfur compounds reducing effects of chewing gums and a control group. *Quintessence Int.* 30:319–323.

Replogle, W.H., and D.E. Beebe. 1996. Halitosis. *American Family Physician.* 53:1215–1223.

Rosenberg M.J. 1996. Clinical assessment of bad breath: Current Concepts. *J. Am. Dent. Assoc.* 127:475–482.

Rounds, M. C., and T. S. I. Tilliss. 1999. Personal oral hygiene: Auxiliary measures to complement toothbrushing. In eds. N. O. Harris, and F. Garcia-Godoy,

Primary preventive dentistry, 125–154. Norwalk, CT: Appleton & Lange.

Sangnes, G. 1976. Traumatization of teeth and gingiva related to habitual tooth cleaning procedures. *J. Clin. Periodontol.* 3:94–103.

Sanz, M., and D. Herrera. 1998. Role of oral hygiene during the healing phase of periodontal therapy. In eds. N. P. Lang, R. Attström, and H. Löe, *Proceedings of the European Workshop on Mechanical Plaque Control,* 248–267. Chicago: Quintessence.

Saxer, U. P., and S. L. Yankell. 1997. Impact of improved toothbrushes on dental diseases: II. *Quintessence Int.* 28:573–593.

Schiff, T. G. 1987. The effect of a dentifrice containing soluble pyrophosphate and sodium fluoride on calculus deposits. *Clin. Prev. Dent.* 9:13–16.

Scully C., M. El-Maaytah, S. R. Porter, and J. Greenman. 1997. Breath odor: etiopathogenesis, assessment and management. *Eur. J. Oral Sci.* 105:287–293.

Shellis, R. P., and R. M. Duckworth. 1994. Studies on the cariostatic mechanisms of fluoride. *Int. Dent. J.* 44(3 Suppl. 1):263–273.

Silverman, G., E. Berman, C. B. Hanna, A. Salvato, P. Fratarcangelo, et al. 1996. Assessing the efficacy of three dentifrices in the treatment of dentinal hypersensitivity. *J. Am. Dent. Assoc.* 127:191–201.

Singh, S. M., M. E. Petrone, A. R. Volpe, K. N. Rustogi, and J. Norfleet. 1990. Comparison of the anticalculus effect of two soluble pyrophosphate dentifrices with and without a copolymer. *J. Clin. Dent.* 2:53–55.

Stephen, K. W. 1994. Fluoride toothpastes, rinses and tablets. *Adv. Dent. Res.* 8:185–189.

Stookey, O. K. 1994. Review of fluorosis risk of self-applied topical fluorides, dentifrices, mouthrinses and gels. *Comm. Dent. Oral Epidemiol.* 22(3):181–186.

Tonzetich, J. 1997. Production and origin of oral malodor: a review of mechanisms and methods of analysis. *J. Periodontal.* 48:13–20.

Van der Weijden, G. A., M. M. Danser, A. Nijboer, M. F. Timmerman, and U. Van der Velden. 1993. The plaque-removing efficacy of an oscillating/rotation toothbrush: A short-term study. *J. Clin. Periodontol.* 20:273–278.

Van Dyke, T., S. Offenbacher, B. Pihlstrom, M. Putt, and C. Trummel. 1999. What is gingivitis? Current understanding of prevention, treatment, measurement, pathogenesis and relation to periodontitis. *J. Int. Acad. Periodontol.* 1:3–10.

Volpe, A. R., M. E. Petrone, R. Davies, and H. M. Proskin. 1995. Clinical anticaries efficacy of NaF and SMFP dentifrices: Overview and resolution of the scientific controversy. *J. Clin. Dent.* 6:1–28.

Volpe, A. R., M. E. Petrone, W. DeVizio, and R. M. Davies. 1996. A review of plaque, gingivitis, calculus and caries clinical efficacy studies with a fluoride dentifrice containing triclosan and PVM/MA copolymer *J. Clin. Dent.* 7(Suppl):1–14.

Waerhaug, J. 1981. Healing of the dentoepithelial junction following the use of dental floss. *J. Clin. Periodontol.* 8:144–150.

Westfelt, E. 1996. Rationale of mechanical plaque control. *J. Clin. Periodontol.* 23:263–267.

White, D. J., B. W. Bollmer, R. A. Baker, E. R. Cox, M. A. Perlich, et al. 1996. Quanticale assessment of the clinical scaling benefits provided by phyrophosphate dentifrices with and without triclosan. *J. Clin. Dent.* 7(special issue):46–49.

Yaegaki K. 2000. Organoleptic measurement of oral malodor. In ed. K. Yaegaki, *Clinical guideline for halitosis,* 35–44. Tokyo: Quintessence.

Yaegaki, K., and J.M. Coil. 2000b. Genuine Halitosis, Pseudo-Halitosis, and Halitophobia: classification, diagnosis and treatment. *Compendium.* 21:880–890.

Yaegaki, K., and J.M. Coil. 2000a. Examination, classification, and treatment of halitosis, clinical perspectives. *J. Can. Dent. Assoc.* 66:257–261.

Yaegaki, K., and T. Suetaka, 1989. The effect of zinc chloride mouthwash on the production of oral malodor, the degradation of salivary cellular elements and proteins. *J. Dent. Health.* 9:377–386.

Yankell, S. L., and U. P. Saxer. 1999. Toothbrushing and toothbrushing techniques. In eds. N. O. Harris and F. Garcia-Godoy, *Primary preventive dentistry,* 77–102. Norwalk, CT: Appleton and Lange.

Yukna, R. A., and R. L. Shaklee. 1993. Evaluation of a counterrotational powered brush in patients in supportive periodontal therapy. *J. Periodontol.* 64:859–864.

Zambon, J. J., M. L. Mather, and Y. Gonzales. 1996. A microbiological and clinical study of the safety and efficacy of baking-soda dentifrices. *Compend. Contin. Educ. Dent. Suppl.* 17:39–44.

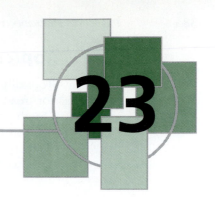

23

Topical Drug Delivery Systems: Oral Rinses and Irrigation

Mea A. Weinberg, D.M.D., M.S.D., R.Ph.

Outline

Goal

To provide an understanding of the fundamentals of counseling periodontal patients on the adjunctive use of chemotherapeutic agents for supragingival plaque control.

Educational Objectives

Upon completion of this chapter, the reader should be able to:

Describe measures, using chemical agents, taken to prevent and control the progression of periodontal diseases.

List the different oral rinses available for the periodontal patient.

KEY WORDS

- chemotherapeutic agents
- topical delivery
- periodontal pathogens
- topical drug devices
- oral biofilms
- substantivity

Topical Delivery Systems

Topically applied chemotherapeutic agents have been developed based on a need for treatment of gingival bleeding and inflammation in association with gingivitis. Mouth rinsing and oral irrigation are two approaches used for supragingival application of antiseptic solutions. Oral rinses are the most common form of topical delivery. Oral rinses are ideal vehicles for the delivery of topical antimicrobials because of their relative simplicity of formulation and ease of use for patients.

Oral Rinses

Mouth rinses generally are divided into two classifications: therapeutic rinses, used to treat diseases such as gingival diseases, and cosmetic rinses, used to freshen the breath. Indications for using oral rinses are as follows:

1. as an addition to home care regimens that have failed to achieve plaque-control goals by other means;
2. as an addition to periodontal instrumentation;
3. where oral hygiene may be inadequate or difficult to accomplish for many people, as in the physically or mentally compromised;
4. following surgical procedures, when brushing and flossing are generally not practical;
5. as a preprocedural rinse, to reduce aerosolized bacteria in the dental office (when masked, the clinician is protected; however, after the mask is removed, aerosols remain in the dental operatory);
6. for maintenance of dental implants.

Topical antimicrobial agents delivered by a rinse are effective only against supragingival bacteria. No antimicrobial rinse has been shown to be effective against periodontitis because oral rinses do not reach the subgingival area. Mouth rinses may be discontinued if oral health conditions can be maintained without their use.

Antiplaque/Antigingivitis Agents

Antimicrobial agents ideally should inhibit microbial colonization on tooth surfaces and prevent the subsequent formation of plaque. They also should eliminate or suppress the pathogenicity of existing plaque. Antiseptics have a greater potential to prevent the formation of plaque than to resolve established plaque and gingivitis.

An antimicrobial agent relies on two factors for efficacy. Success depends on the amount of time the agent stays in contact with the target site and how well the agent gains access to the target site. A major requirement for the success of antimicrobial therapy is substantivity, which is the ability of the drug to adsorb or bind to intraoral surfaces such as teeth and soft tissues with subsequent release of the drug in its active form (Stabholz et al., 1993). Substantivity involves the ability of the drug to stay at the target site for longer periods of time, thus maintaining therapeutic levels. It is ideal to have a drug with high substantivity that will be bound in the oral cavity and released over a period of hours in order to prolong the effects. Lack of substantivity can be overcome by more frequent use of the agent, but this would likely result in noncompliance and undesirable side effects.

Classification of Oral Rinses

Topical antimicrobial oral rinses can be classified as either first- or second-generation agents. First-generation agents have antibacterial properties with low substantivity and limited therapeutic value in reducing plaque and gingivitis. Examples include phenolic compounds, quaternary ammonium compounds, peroxide, and sanguinarine. Second-generation agents have antibacterial properties in addition to substantivity. Chlorhexidine gluconate is an example of a second-generation agent and is currently the only second-generation agent proven to prevent and control gingivitis. It is available in the United States only by prescription. All first-generation mouth rinses are available over the counter (OTC) without a prescription.

In 1986, the American Dental Association (ADA) established guidelines for evaluation of the therapeutic effectiveness of products against gingivitis. For example, studies should be conducted over a minimum of 6 months, two studies with independent investigators should be conducted, and the active product should be used as part of a normal regimen and compared with a placebo or control product.

Most mouth rinses contain alcohol as a flavor enhancer and as a vehicle for the active ingredients. There has been some concern about the association of alcohol in mouth rinses with oral cancer. Various studies have shown inconsistent findings. Some studies document that there is no reason for patients to refrain from use of alcohol-containing mouth rinses (Ciancio, 1993), while research from the National Cancer Institute has drawn an association between alcoholic mouth rinses to mouth and throat cancers (Winn et al., 1991). Additionally, a vitro (laboratory) studied the effect of acetaldehyde, a toxic compound produced by alcohol metabolism (breakdown) in the body. It was reported that acetaldehyde caused changes in gingival fibroblasts (cells involved in oral connective tissue maintenance) (Poggi, Rodriguez y Baena, Rizzo, & Rota, 2003).

Bisbiguanides

Description and Mechanism of Action   Chlorhexidine gluconate (Peridex®, Zila Pharmaceuticals, Cincinnati, OH; PerioGard®, Colgate Oral Pharmaceuticals, Canton, MA) is a cationic (positively charged) molecule. Originally, chlorhexidine was used in medicine as an antiseptic cream for wounds, as a preoperative skin cleanser, and as a surgical scrub. In 1970, the first study on the ability of chlorhexidine to inhibit the formation of plaque and maintain soft tissue health was released (Löe & Schiott, 1970). It was not until 1986 that chlorhexidine became available in the United States by prescription at a 0.12% concentration with an alcohol concentration of 11.6%. It has the ADA seal of acceptance for the treatment of gingivitis.

After rinsing, chlorhexidine (positively charged) is attracted to and attaches onto the negatively charged bacterial cell walls, causing lysis or breakage of the cell wall and the contents of the cells leak out. Chlorhexidine enters the cell through the opening, resulting in death of the bacteria. By binding to the pellicle on the tooth surface, chlorhexidine inhibits plaque attachment. Chlorhexidine exhibits substantivity, with approximately 30% of the drug binding to oral tissues and the plaque on the teeth (Rölla, Löe, & Schiott, 1971) and showing antimicrobial activity for 8 to 12 hours afterwards (Addy & Wright, 1978; Schiott et al., 1970).

Indications   Rinsing with chlorhexidine is indicated before, during, and after periodontal debridement to reduce plaque levels and gingival inflammation. Chlorhexidine rinses can improve wound healing and provide better plaque control after periodontal surgery when brushing and flossing is not feasible (Sanz, Newman, Anderson, & Motaska, 1987). In the office, before using dental devices that produce an aerosol, such as power-assisted instruments or air polishing, it has been shown that a preoperative rinse with chlorhexidine markedly reduces contamination of the dental office (Warrall, Knibbs, & Glenwright, 1987). Rinsing with chlorhexidine has been shown to decrease the severity of mucositis in patients receiving chemotherapy. Since peri-implantitis is similar to gingivitis, rinsing with chlorhexidine may be effective in implant plaque control.

Usage   It is recommended to rinse twice a day for 30 seconds. The positive charge of chlorhexidine causes it to bind to the negatively charged molecules in toothpastes such as fluorides and sodium lauryl sulfate (a detergent) and thus inactivates them. Therefore, it is best to rinse either 30 minutes before or after toothbrushing or rinse very well with water after toothbrushing. Because of this inactivation by anionic compounds, chlorhexidine is not available in toothpaste form. Chlorhexidine can be used as an irrigant, but it is usually diluted with water to reduce the incidence of staining.

Adverse Side Effects   Chlorhexidine is a relatively safe drug because it is poorly absorbed from the oral membranes and systemic circulation if swallowed. The most common adverse side effect is a yellow, brownish extrinsic staining of the teeth, tongue, and restorations within the first few days of use. Staining is more frequent with chlorhexidine than with other agents because of its affinity for oral surfaces. The staining may be associated with food dyes found within certain foods and beverages. This staining is not permanent and can be removed mechanically during professional prophylaxis. If the patient is compliant with oral home care, the staining is more likely on proximal tooth surfaces than facial or lingual surfaces. Other adverse side effects include a temporarily impaired taste perception and increased supragingival calculus formation.

Phenolic Compounds

Listerine® (Warner-Lambert, Morris Plains, NJ) is a combination of phenolic compounds or essential oils, including thymol, eucalyptol, menthol, and methyl salicylate, in an alcohol vehicle. The mechanism of action is cell wall disruption, resulting in leakage of intracellular components and lysis of the cell. The original-formula Listerine contains 26.9% alcohol, whereas Cool Mint and Fresh Burst Listerine contain 21.6% alcohol. The newest product, Natural Citrus, also contains 21.6% alcohol.

Because of low substantivity, effectiveness is strongly related to the duration of tooth contact. Clinical studies have shown it to significantly reduce plaque development in patients with minimal plaque levels (Gordon, Lamster, & Sieger, 1985). A 6-month study comparing Listerine with a control product found that Listerine reduced plaque and gingivitis from 20 to 34%. The subjects had preexisting plaque and gingivitis, and no prophylaxis was performed at the beginning of the study

(Lamster, Alfano, Seiger, & Gordon, 1983). In-office preprocedure rinsing with Listerine reduced the level of bacteria in the aerosol generated during ultrasonic scaling (Fine et al., 1992).

Recommendations are to rinse for 30 seconds with 2/3 oz once in the morning and once at night. Possible adverse side effects include a burning sensation and bitter taste.

Quaternary Ammonium Compounds

Quaternary ammonium compounds are positively charged (cationic) compounds similar to chlorhexidine, except that after rinsing they readily bind to oral surfaces and are released more rapidly or lose their activity upon binding to the surface (Moran & Addy, 1984). Substantivity is only approximately 3 hours (Roberts & Addy, 1981). An increase in bacterial cell wall permeability leads to cell lysis and decreased attachment of bacteria to tooth surfaces. Cetylpyridinium chloride is the active ingredient in Scope® Original (Procter & Gamble, Cincinnati, OH), Cepacol® (J. B. Williams, Glen Rock, NJ), and Viadent™ Advanced Care (Colgate Oral Pharmaceuticals, Canton, MA). The alcohol concentration is 14% for Cepacol, 18.9% for Scope Original, and 5.5% for Viadent™ Advanced Care.

Clinical data on plaque reduction and gingivitis control have been relatively inconclusive because of the variability in results between studies. Following an initial professional prophylaxis and suspension of all oral hygiene, chlorhexidine was found to be superior to cetylpyridinium in the reduction of plaque (Renton-Harper, Addy, Moran, Doherty, & Newcombe, 1996). Cetylpyridinium chloride may have some antiplaque action but less effect on gingivitis when used as an adjunct to conventional oral home care. Lack of substantivity limits clinical efficacy. As with chlorhexidine, to obtain the maximum effect, the patient should rinse very well or wait 30 minutes after brushing with a dentifrice before using the rinse. Adverse side effects are similar to those of chlorhexidine, including some staining, calculus formation, and mucosal ulceration.

Oxygenating Agents

Oxygenating agents such as peroxides and perborates have been used in mouth rinse formulations primarily for acute necrotizing ulcerative gingivitis and pericoronitis. Since hydrogen peroxide liberates gaseous oxygen, it provides a cleansing action and gentle effervescence for oral wounds. Its antimicrobial effect is directed at anaerobic microorganisms that cannot live in the presence of oxygen, and it has a physical effect on plaque through the bubbling of oxygen as it is released from the peroxide (Marshall, Cancro, & Fischman, 1995). The Food and Drug Administration has approved its use as a temporary debriding agent in the oral cavity. However, antiplaque/antigingivitis claims are not well supported.

The safety of hydrogen peroxide has been disputed. Long-term use of 3% hydrogen peroxide has resulted in gingival irritation (Marshall et al., 1995; Rees & Orth, 1986) and delayed tissue healing, and it may serve as a cocarcinogen in animals (Weitzman, Weitberg, Stossel, Schwartz, & Shklar, 1986). A cocarcinogen is a compound that when administered with a low dose of a known carcinogen results in increased incidence of tumors. On the other hand, other studies found that adverse effects from exposure to 3% or less hydrogen peroxide were rare. It was concluded that exposure to less than 3% hydrogen peroxide was safe (Marshall et al., 1995).

Long-term studies do not demonstrate any additional benefit over regular home care, however. Since many patients use hydrogen peroxide on a regular basis, the dental hygienist should question patients about their oral home-care practices.

Povidone-Iodine

Povidone-iodine is antibacterial and antiseptic. Its primary use is in the prevention and treatment of surface infections. Often povidone-iodine is combined with hydrogen peroxide as a subgingival irrigant for the reduction of gram-negative microorganisms. Most studies confirm that iodine may be a beneficial adjunctive treatment for the prevention and control of gingivitis when used with optimal oral hygiene self-care procedures (Clark, Magnusson, Walker, & Marks, 1989). Iodine can stain teeth, clothing, skin, and restorations, however.

Fluorides

Fluorides have been used in dentistry primarily for dental caries prevention by reducing demineralization and enhancing remineralization. Fluoride rinses have not been proven clinically to prevent root caries (Paine, Slots, & Rich, 1998). Its role as an antiplaque/antigingivitis agent is less well documented and shows controversial results.

Stannous fluoride (SnF_2) has been documented to exhibit antimicrobial properties in the control of gingival inflammation and bacterial repopulation. The tin molecule supposedly prevents bacterial adhesion to the tooth surface. Another indication for stannous fluoride is for dentinal hypersensitivity. Stannous fluoride is available as a dentifrice, a gel, and a concentrated oral rinse that is diluted with water. For home rinsing, available products include Gel-Kam® (available over-the-counter; Colgate Oral Pharmaceuticals, Canton, MA) and Stanimax (0.63% SnF_2). Extrinsic tooth staining occurs with extended use. Sodium fluoride is indicated for caries prevention and has not been documented to have any antiplaque/antigingivitis action.

Prebrushing Rinses

A prebrushing rinse (Plax®, Pfizer, New York) that contains surfactants such as sodium lauryl sulfate (which functions as a detergent to help loosen and remove plaque), sodium benzoate (a preservative), and tetrasodium pyrophosphate (an anticalculus agent) is intended to be used before brushing. Studies have shown limited beneficial effects of this agent over rinsing with water alone (Grossman, 1988).

Alcohol-Free Mouth Rinses

Most mouth rinses contain alcohol as a vehicle to carry other ingredients and as a flavor enhancer. The form of alcohol in the rinse is either ethanol (ethyl alcohol) or a specially denatured (SD) alcohol that is made synthetically. Alcohol can cause drying of the oral mucosal tissues, especially when the agent is used for extended periods of time. Indications for a nonalcoholic mouth rinse include pregnant women, former alcoholics, patients who are taking medications that would additionally dry the mouth, patients taking metronidazole (an antibiotic), and patients who prefer to avoid alcohol. Table 23–1■ lists some nonalcoholic antimicrobial mouthrinses.

Table 23–1	Alcohol-Free Antimicrobial Mouth Rinses

Rembrandt® (DenMat, Santa Maria, CA)
Oral B® Plaque Rinse (Redwood City, CA)
Listermint® (Warner-Lambert, Morris Plains, NJ)
BreathRX® (Discus Dental, Culver City, CA)

Oral Irrigation

Oral irrigation emerged in the late 1960s as an adjunct to brushing and flossing. Early studies indicated that mechanical water-pressure devices did not remove significant amounts of supragingival plaque but only loosened food debris and less adherent materials (Lobene, 1969). However, regardless of the plaque index, reductions in gingivitis and calculus formation were evident as early as 1969 (Lobene, 1969; Lobene & Soparkar, 1970). Today, there is a preponderance of clinical studies that address the use of oral irrigation on gingivitis and periodontitis maintenance patients and show significant reductions in clinical parameters (e.g., bleeding on probing and gingival inflammation).

Home Oral Irrigation

The primary use of oral irrigation is to nonspecifically reduce bacteria and their by-products that lead to the initiation or progression of periodontal diseases (Drisko, 1996). The target area of irrigation is unattached or loosely attached microorganisms at the subgingival level, regardless of where the tip of the device is placed. It is a misconception that if the tip is placed at the gingival margin, it is only effective on supragingival plaque; it is effective against both supragingival and subgingival bacteria. Cobb, Rodgers, and Killoy (1988) found that supragingival irrigation had an effect on subgingival microorganisms at probing depths of up to 6 mm. Irrigation attempts to reduce the potential of developing gingivitis or decreases existing gingivitis and directly reduces pocket microbiota in an attempt to control or prevent the initiation of periodontitis.

With our current understanding of the pathogenesis of periodontal infections and the role endotoxins play in the immune response, irrigation may have a more significant place in self-care routines, especially since the highest concentrations of endotoxins have been found within the loosely adherent subgingival plaque. Supragingival irrigation dilutes (Ciancio, 1990) and flushes away bacteria coronal to the gingiva, which helps to prevent or treat gingivitis (Drisko, 1996) and also reduces subgingival bacteria. Subgingival irrigation attempts to directly reduce the pocket microbiota in an effort to prevent initiation of periodontitis or to help its reduction (American Academy of Periodontology, 1995). However, irrigation does not remove adherent dental plaque, calculus, or stains.

Home irrigation has been proven to reach farther into the pocket than rinsing (Braun & Ciancio, 1992; Eakle, Ford, & Boyd, 1986; Flotra, Gjermo, Rölla, & Waerhaug, 1972; Mashimo, Umemoto, Slots, Genco, & Ellison, 1980). The addition of an antimicrobial agent has reduced clinical parameters in some studies. Flemming and colleagues (1990) demonstrated an enhanced effect on reducing gingivitis when a 0.06% solution of chlorhexidine was used as the irrigant compared with rinsing and water irrigation. Conversely, the addition of Listerine® (Warner-Lambert, Morris

Plains, NJ) as an irrigant was as effective as placebo in reducing gingivitis and improving gingival health (Ciancio, Mather, Zambon, & Reynolds, 1989). However, the addition of Listerine® resulted in greater reductions in plaque and gingival bleeding and a moderate decrease in total bacteria counts, although it was not statistically significant. Subgingival irrigation with chlorhexidine has been shown to decrease subgingival microbiota and inflammation around implants (Lavigne, Drust-Bay, Williams, Killoy, & Theisen, 1994).

Devices

Oral irrigation devices generally are power-driven pulsating devices that deliver water or a medicament to the site. The pulsations create two zones of hydrokinetic activity. The impact zone is the area where the irrigant comes in contact with the tooth surface, and the flushing zone is the deflection of the irrigant subgingivally (Cobb et al., 1988). A pulsating stream of water provides better flushing than a continuous stream because it incorporates a compression and decompression phase, which allows debris and bacteria to be displaced more efficiently. Products are available that are nonpulsating and non-power-driven, but to date, there is no evidence that they are clinically effective.

A Water Pik (Teledyne Water Pik, Fort Collins, CO; Fig. 23–1a■) is one such home irrigation device (Table 23–2■). Water or a medicament is delivered to the gingival margin with a standard jet tip (Fig. 23–1b■) placed at a 90° angle to the long axis of the tooth. The jet tip is positioned directly interproximally so that the stream of water or medicament reaches the target slightly subgingivally. The tip is passed along the gingival margin to the next proximal area and held in place for 5 to 6 seconds. The procedure is usually performed over a bathroom sink beginning with a low-pressure setting. Pressure may be increased as needed or according to patient comfort and gingival health. Eakle and colleagues (1986) found that

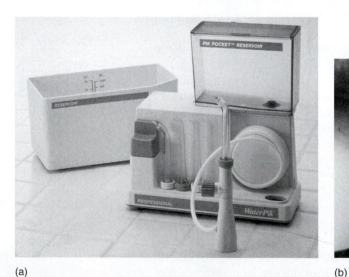

(a)

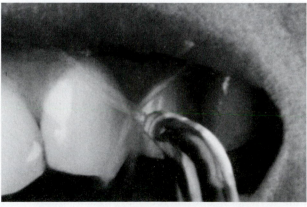

(b)

Figure 23–1   (a) Water Pik® dental systems. (b) Placement of standard jet tip. (Courtesy of Teledyne Water Pik, Fort Collins, CO)

Table 23–2	Home Oral Irrigators
Product	**Description**
Water Pik™ dental systems (various) (Teledyne Water Pik, Fort Collins, CO)	Two tips are available; standard jet tip for supragingival irrigation and the Pik Pocket™ tip for subgingival irrigation.
Braun Oral-B™ Oxy Jet (Oral-B, Belmont, CA)	Mixes air and water, then pressurizes it to form micro-bubbles that attack bacteria. Use in conjunction with toothbrush.
Viajet™ (Oratec Corporation, Herndon, VA)	Two standard tips for supragingival irrigation and two sulcus tips for marginal application are available. For office use: A cannula (stainless steel tube) adapter for subgingival application is also available.
Braun Oral-B™ Plaque Removal System (Oral-B, Belmont, CA)	This device is only available with the powered brush (sold as one unit). Plastic tips are available for supragingival use only, and the tips cannot be removed.

a standard jet tip delivered an irrigant 44 to 71% into the depth of pockets. In addition, use of a standard jet tip with a Water Pik® oral irrigator placed on medium pressure was found to have a positive effect on subgingival microorganisms at probing depths of up to 6 mm (Cobb et al., 1988). Some home irrigation devices have accessory delivery tips designed for targeted direct subgingival delivery. A Water Pik® oral irrigator using a Pik Pocket® subgingival irrigation tip (Fig. 23–2■) delivers an irrigant to approximately 90% of the depth of pockets ranging from 0 to 6 mm (Braun & Ciancio, 1992). The Pik Pocket® tip is designed for controlled, targeted low-pressure delivery of a medicament or water. Waterpik® dental water jets come in many models including a cordless unit.

In-Office Irrigation

Efficacy   An alternate route of topical drug delivery is through patient or professionally applied oral irrigation. An antimicrobial agent also can be applied professionally in-office. This can be accomplished by using an air- or powered-driven device (e.g., Perio Pik Subgingival Irrigation Handpiece, Teledyne Water Pik®, Fort

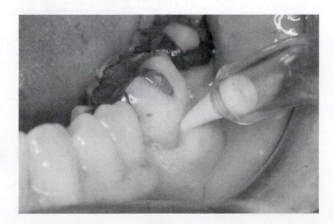

Figure 23–2   Pik Pocket® subgingival delivery tip placement in furcation of mandibular first molar. (Courtesy of Teledyne Water Pik, Fort Collins, CO)

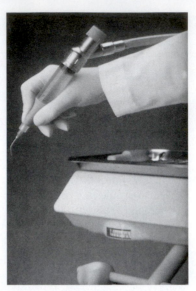

Figure 23–3   Perio Pik™ subgingival irrigation handpiece for in-office subgingival irrigation fits into a standard handpiece holder. (Courtesy of Teledyne Water Pik®, Fort Collins, CO)

Collins, CO; Fig. 23–3■), ultrasonic unit (piezoelectric) scaler (Piezon Master 400, EMS, Richardson, TX; Fig. 23–4■), or handheld syringe. Caution must be taken when using a handheld syringe because the delivery pressure cannot be controlled and may exceed a safe pressure for delivery into a periodontal pocket. Control is also compromised because of the inability to fulcrum and may affect the delivery to the apical aspect of the pocket. Penetration of an irrigant with an ultrasonic unit may be limited due to little lateral dispersion of agents and inaccessibility of the tip to certain areas (Nosel, Scheidt, O'Neal, & Van Dyke, 1991).

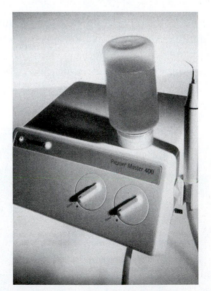

Figure 23–4   Ultrasonic scaler (Piezon Master 400, EMS, Richardson, TX) for professional in-office subgingival irrigation of solutions during ultrasonic scaling. There is a built-in reservoir for the irrigant.

At present, a single episode of in-office irrigation has been shown only to have limited or no beneficial effects by itself, but it may be of some advantage if patients perform subgingival irrigation at home between continuing-care appointments (Jolkovsky et al., 1990). Repeated irrigations over a period of time or longer exposure to an antibiotic has shown efficacy in some patients (Christersson, Norderyd, & Puchalsky, 1993; Clark et al., 1989). The use of 2% chlorhexidine alone over a 15-week period was nearly as effective in reducing clinical parameters as periodontal debridement alone (Southard, Drisko, Killoy, Cobb, & Tira, 1989).

Many different chemical agents have been used as irrigants (Table 23–3■). Owing to differences in protocol, type of agent used, concentrations, and levels of disease, oral irrigation is inconclusive in terms of efficacy, and research is ongoing.

Studies repeatedly show statistically significant reductions in gingivitis, bleeding on probing, probing depth, and periodontal pathogens in gingivitis and periodontal maintenance patients with the use of oral irrigation over normal oral hygiene (Cobb et al., 1988; Flemming et al., 1990; Newman et al., 1994). Subgingival calculus must be removed before irrigation because it interferes with penetration of the agent (Pitcher, Newman, & Strahan, 1980).

It appears that using a standard jet tip or a specialized delivery tip is effective with specific home irrigation devices. Caution must be taken when evaluating the research because not all products have been studied in clinical trials. Therefore, established efficacy with one product may not be true for another. It is always advisable to contact the manufacturer and request copies of the clinical trials that support product claims.

Indications

Adjunctive oral irrigation may not be necessary for all patients. However, Chaves and colleagues (1994) found an added benefit for patients with good oral hygiene. Oral irrigation is an ideal adjunct when supragingival mechanical aids (e.g., toothbrushes, floss, and interproximal brushes and devices) are not sufficient to keep the bacterial load below the threshold of disease. It is also ideal for delivering antimicrobial agents deeper into pockets. Patients with physical challenges, orthodontic appliances, or prosthodontic replacements such as implants and crowns or those who need an adjunctive method to reduce repopulation of bacteria between periodontal maintenance appointments are also ideal candidates for supplemental home oral irrigation. Subgingival irrigation may be better than rinsing in the maintenance of gingival health around dental implants (Felo, Shibly, Ciancio, Lauciello, & Ho, 1997).

Patients with plaque-induced gingivitis can benefit most from oral irrigation because the disease is in its early stage. Patients with slight and moderate chronic periodontitis also may benefit from oral irrigation. However, patients with severe

Table 23–3	Chemical Agents Used as Irrigants

- Water
- Chlorhexidine
- Povidone-iodine
- Essential oils
- Hydrogen peroxide
- Fluoride
- Tetracycline

chronic periodontitis and refractory periodontitis require more aggressive treatment and referral to a periodontist.

Cautions

Controlled powered-driven home irrigation devices are safe for patients to use on a daily basis. Thorough patient evaluation is always necessary prior to recommending any device or aid to a patient. It is important to match the correct product with the patient's specific needs. Also, take the time to instruct patients on the proper use of their device.

Oral irrigation should not be used when a periodontal abscess or ulcerations are present. Once the problem has been resolved, it then may be appropriate to recommend irrigation therapy. Since the American Heart Association (AHA) has not established guidelines for patients requiring antibiotic prophylaxis and use of home oral irrigation, it is recommended that these patients do not use oral irrigation (Drisko, 1996).

Irrigation versus Toothbrushing

Controversy exists over whether irrigation provides an additional benefit over toothbrushing and flossing. Irrigation is not a substitute for toothbrushing or flossing. Toothbrushing plus irrigation may be better than toothbrushing alone in patients with poor oral home care (Flemming et al., 1990). Supragingival irrigation is adequate as an adjunctive therapy to decrease inflammation (e.g., redness and bleeding), but there is no significant reduction in probing depth or gain in clinical attachment. Irrigation distributes antimicrobial agents into interproximal areas better than rinsing. There may be no difference between irrigating with a medicament (chemical agent) or with water, however. In patients with good oral hygiene, daily brushing and flossing remain the most efficient methods for controlling gingivitis.

Summary

Antiseptics deserve continued evaluation, and their importance should not be underestimated. Currently, the most valuable application of antiplaque/antigingivitis agents is as an adjunct to conventional mechanical debridement and oral home care for short- to medium-term usage.

An important factor in the efficacy of any antiplaque/antigingivitis agent is an adequate contact time with the target site. Accordingly, the well-proven success of chlorhexidine is related to its substantivity more than to any unique action on the microbiota (bacteria). It is the function of the dental hygienist to advise patients on the role of oral rinses and dentifrices in the hygienic phase of treatment. The hygienist should use his or her knowledge of clinical studies to decide on the appropriate product for each patient.

Key Points

- Oral rinses and irrigation are types of topical delivery systems.
- Oral rinses are only effective supragingivally and do not have any effect on subgingival plaque.
- Oral irrigation may be useful between maintenance appointments to reduce bacterial reinfection (repopulation).

Web Sites

www.ada.org

www.perio.org

www.collagenex.com

www.adha.org

www.cdc.gov/oralhealth/infectioncontrol.htm

Self-Quiz

1. Which one of the following procedures most effectively removes supra/subgingival oral biofilms? (p. 384)

   a. oral rinsing

   b. oral irrigation

   c. systemic antibiotics

   d. periodontal debridement

   e. controlled-release drugs

2. All the following are indications for the use of mouth rinses in periodontics except one. Which one is the exception? (p. 384)

   a. limited manual dexterity

   b. gingivitis

   c. periodontitis

   d. peri-implantitis

3. Which one of the following antimicrobial agents possesses high substantivity to the oral soft tissues? (p. 385)

   a. cetylpyrimidium

   b. alcohol

   c. chlorhexidine

   d. erythromycin

   e. tetracycline

4. Which one of the following instructions should be given to a patient rinsing with chlorhexidine? (p. 385)

   a. Rinse immediately after brushing.

   b. Rinse immediately before brushing.

   c. Wait about 30 minutes after brushing.

   d. Wait about 1 hour after brushing.

5. Which one of the following antimicrobial mouth rinses contains the highest concentration of alcohol? (pp. 385–388)

   a. Listerine®

   b. PerioGard®

   c. Scope®

   d. Viadent™ Advanced Care

References

Addy, M., and R. Wright. 1978. Comparison of the in vivo and in vitro antibacterial properties of povidone-iodine and chlorhexidine gluconate mouth rinses. *J. Clin. Periodontol.* 5:198–205.

Braun, R., and S. Ciancio. 1992. Subgingival delivery by an oral irrigation device. *J. Periodontol.* 63:469–472.

Christersson, L. A., O. M. Norderyd, and C. S. Puchalsky, 1993. Topical application of tetracycline HCl in human periodontitis. *J. Clin. Periodontol.* 20:80–95.

Ciancio, S. G. 1990. Powered oral irrigation and control of gingivitis. *Biol. Ther. Dent.* 5:21–24.

Ciancio, S. G. 1993. Alcohol in mouth rinse: Lack of association with cancer. *Biol. Ther. Dent.* 9(1):2–3.

Ciancio, S. G., C. Lauciello, O. Shibly, M. Vitello, and M. Mather. 1995. The effect of an antiseptic mouth rinse on implant maintenance: Plaque and peri-implant gingival tissues. *J. Peridontol.* 66:962–965.

Ciancio, S. G., M. L. Mather, J. J. Zambon, and H. S. Reynolds. 1989. Effect of a chemotherapeutic agent delivered by an oral irrigation device on plaque, gingivitis, and subgingival microflora. *J. Periodontol.* 60:310–315.

Clark, W. B., I. Magnusson, C. B. Walker, and R. G. Marks. 1989. Efficacy of Perimed antibacterial system on established gingivitis I. Clinical results. *J. Clin. Periodontol.* 16:630–635.

Cobb, C. M., R. L. Rodgers, and W. J. Killoy. 1988. Ultrastructural examination of human periodontal pockets following the use of an oral irrigation device in vivo. *J. Periodontol.* 59:155–163.

Drisko, C. H. 1996. Non-surgical pocket therapy: Pharmacotherapeutics. *Ann. Periodontol.* 1:491–566.

Eakle, W. S., C. Ford, and R. L. Boyd. 1986. Depth of penetration in periodontal pockets with oral irrigation. *J. Clin. Periodontol.* 13:39–44.

Elworthy, A., J. Greenman, F. M. Doherty, R. G. Newcombe, and M. Addy. 1996. The substantivity of a number of oral hygiene products determined by the duration of effects on salivary bacteria. *J. Periodontol.* 67:572–576.

Felo, A., O. Shibly, S. G. Ciancio, F. R. Lauciello, and A. Ho. 1997. Effects of subgingival chlorhexidine irrigation on peri-implant maintenance. *Am. J. Dent.* 10:107–110.

Fine, D. H., C. Mendieta, M. L. Barnett, D. Furgang, R. Meyers, et al. 1992. Efficacy of preprocedural rinsing with an antiseptic in reducing viable bacteria in dental aerosols. *J. Periodontol.* 63:821–824.

Flemming, T. F., M. G. Newman, F. M. Doherty, E. Grossman, A. H. Mechkel, and M. B. Bakdash. 1990. Supragingival irrigation with 0.06% chlorhexidine in naturally occurring gingivitis: I. Six-month clinical observations. *J. Periodontol.* 61:112–117.

Flotra, L., P. Gjermo, G. Rölla, and J. Waerhaug. 1972. A 4-month study on the effect of chlorhexidine mouth rinses on 50 soldiers. *Can. J. Dent. Res.* 80:10–16.

Gordon, J. M., I. B. Lamster, and M. C. Sieger. 1985. Efficacy of Listerine antiseptic in inhibiting the development of plaque and gingivitis. *J. Clin. Periodontol.* 12:697–704.

Grossman, E. 1988. Effectiveness of a prebrushing mouthrinse under single-trial and home-use conditions. *Clin. Prev. Dent.* 10:3–9.

Jolkovsky, D. L., M. Y. Waki, M. G. Newman, et al. 1990. Clinical and microbiological effects of subgingival and gingival marginal irrigation with chlorhexidine gluconate. *J. Periodontol.* 61:663–669.

Lamster, I. B., M. C. Alfano, M. C. Seiger, J. M. Gordon. 1983. The effect of Listerine antiseptic on existing plaque and gingivitis. *J. Clin. Prev. Dent.* 5:12–16.

Lavigne, S. E., K. S. Drust-Bay, K. B. Williams, W. J. Killoy, and F. Theisen. 1994. Effects of chlorhexidine on

the periodontal status of patients with HA-coated integral dental implants. *Int. J. Oral Maxillofax. Implants.* 9:156–162.

Lobene, R. R. 1969. The effect of a pulsed water pressure cleansing device on oral health. *J. Periodontol.* 40:51–54.

Lobene, R. R., and P. M. Soparkar. 1970, March. The effect of a pulsating water pressure device on gingivitis, plaque and calculus. In *Program and Abstracts of the 48th General Meeting International Association for Dental Research.*

Löe, H., and C. R. Schiott. 1970. The effect of mouthrinses and topical application of chlorhexidine on the development of dental plaque and gingivitis in man. *J. Periodont. Res.* 5:79–83.

Marshall, M. V., L. P. O. Cancro, and S. F. Fischman. 1995. Hydrogen peroxide: A review of its use in dentistry. *J. Periodontol.* 66:786–796.

Mashimo, P. A., T. Umemoto, J. Slots, R. J. Genco, and S. A. Ellison. 1980. Pathogenicity testing of Macaca arctoides subgingival plaque following chlorhexidine treatment. *J. Periodontol.* 51:190–199.

Meffert, R., B. Langer, and M. Frutz. 1992. Dental implants: A review. *J. Periodontol.* 63:859–870.

Moran, J., and M. Addy. 1984. The effect of surface adsorption and staining reactions on the antimicrobial properties of some cationic antiseptic mouth rinse. *J. Periodontol.* 55:278–282.

Newman, M., M. Cattabriga, D. Etienne, T. Flemmig, M. Sanz, et al. 1994. Effectiveness of adjunctive irrigation in early periodontitis: Multicenter evaluation. *J. Periodontol.* 65:224–229.

Nosel, G., M. Scheidt, R. O'Neal, and T. Van Dyke. 1991. The penetration of lavage solution into the periodontal pocket during ultrasonic instrumentation. *J. Periodontol.* 62:554–557.

Paine, M., J. Slots, and S. Rich. 1998. Fluoride use in periodontal therapy: A review of the literature. *J. Am. Dent. Assoc.* 129:69–77.

Pitcher, G. R., H. N. Newman, and J. D. Strahan. 1980. Access to subgingival plaque by disclosing agents using mouth rinsing and direct irrigation. *J. Clin. Periodontol.* 7:300–308.

Poggi P, R. Rodriguez y Baena, S. Rizzo, and M. T. Rota. Mouth rinses with alcohol: cytotoxic effects on human gingival fibroblasts in vitro. *J. Periodontol.* 74: 623–629.

Rees, T. D., and C. E. Orth. 1986. Oral ulcerations with use of hydrogen peroxide. *J. Periodontol.* 57:689–692.

Renton-Harper, P., M. Addy, J. Moran, R. M. Doherty, and R. G. Newcombe. 1996. A comparison of chlorhexidine, cetylpyridium chloride, triclosan, and C3LG mouth rinse products for plaque inhibition. *J. Periodontol.* 67:486–489.

Roberts, W. R., and M. Addy. 1981. Comparison of in vitro and in vivo antibacterial properties of antiseptic mouth rinses containing chlorhexidine, alexidine, CPC and hexetidine: Relevance to mode of action. *J. Clin. Periodontol.* 8:295–310.

Rölla, G., H. Löe, and R. C. Schiott. 1971. Retention of chlorhexidine in the human oral cavity. *Arch. Oral Biol.* 16:1109–1116.

Sanz, M., M. G. Newman, L. Anderson, and W. Motaska. 1987. A comparison of the effect of a 0.12 percent chlorhexidine gluconate mouth rinse and placebo on postperiodontal surgical therapy. *J. Dent. Res.* 66:280 (Abstract).

Schiott, C. R., H. Löe, S. B. Jensen, M. Kilian, R. M. Davies, and L. Glavid. 1970. The effect of chlorhexidine mouth rinses on the human oral flora. *J. Periodont. Res.* 5:84–89.

Southard, S. R., C. L. Drisko, W. J. Killoy, C. M. Cobb, and D. E. Tira. 1989. The effect of 2 percent chlorhexidine digluconate irrigation on clinical parameters and the level of Bacteroides gingivalis in periodontal pockets. *J. Periodontol.* 60:302–309.

Stabholz, A., J. Kettering, R. Aprecio, G. Zimmerman, P. J. Baker, and U. M. E. Wikesjo. 1993. Antimicrobial properties of human dentin impregnated with tetracycline HCl or chlorhexidine: An in vitro study. *J. Clin. Periodontol.* 20:557–562.

Warrall, S. F., P. J. Knibbs, and H. D. Glenwright. 1987. Methods of reducing contamination of the atmosphere from use of an air polisher. *Br. Dent. J.* 163:118–119.

Weitzman, S. A., A. B. Weitberg, T. P. Stossel, J. Schwartz, and G. Shklar. 1986. Effects of hydrogen peroxide on oral carcinogenesis in hamsters. *J. Periodontol.* 57:685–688.

Winn, D. M., W. J., Blot, J. K. McLaughlin, D. F. Austin, R. S. Greenberg, S. Preston-Martin. 1991. Mouthwash use and oral conditions in the risk of oral and pharyngeal cancer. *Cancer Res.* 51:3044–3047.

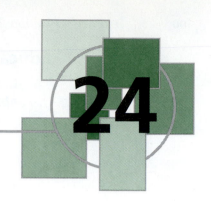

24

Systemic and Local Drug Delivery Systems: Systemic Antibiotics, Local Drug Devices, and Enzyme Suppression Therapy

Mea A. Weinberg, D.M.D., M.S.D., R.Ph.

Outline

KEY WORDS

- chemotherapeutic agents
- periodontal pathogens
- antibiotic resistance
- topical drug devices
- controlled-release drug devices
- systemic drug delivery
- biofilm
- substantivity

Goal

To provide an understanding of current concepts about the adjunctive use of chemical agents in the prevention and treatment of the inflammatory periodontal diseases.

Educational Objectives

Upon completion of this chapter, the reader should be able to:

Discuss the rationale for the use of antimicrobials in the treatment of the inflammatory periodontal diseases.

List and discuss the various types of drug delivery systems.

Describe the newest types of controlled-release devices.

Discuss enzyme suppression therapy.

Periodontal therapy can be divided into three types of treatment:

- *Mechanical therapy.* This deals with the removal of plaque through mechanical (periodontal) debridement and toothbrushing and flossing.
- *Chemical therapy.* This is the administration of chemical agents to aid in the removal/suppression of the bacterial load.
- *Enzyme suppression therapy.* The newest approach to the treatment of inflammatory periodontal diseases, this deals with inhibiting the enzyme collagenase, which causes destruction of collagen, rather than focusing on bacterial reduction.

Selected Drug Information Resources

It is important for the dental hygienist to be aware of the generic names and trade names of drugs. The generic name is the official name of the drug as determined by the United States Adopted Names Council. The trade name of a drug is the registered property of a specific manufacturer and is protected for 17 years so that the manufacturer has the exclusive rights for that specific drug.

Numerous drug reference books are available. Selected resources include the following:

- *The Physicians' Desk Reference* (PDR®) (Medical Economics Company, Inc., Montvale, NJ). This is published once a year and is essentially a conglomerate of the patient package inserts that the manufacturers supply for each drug.
- *Delmar's Dental Drug Reference* (Delmar Thompson™ Learning, Albany, NY).
- *Mosby's Dental Drug Reference* (Mosby-Year Book, Inc., St. Louis, MO).
- *Drug Information Handbook for Dentistry* (Lexi-Comp, Inc., Hudson, OH).
- *ADA Guide to Dental Therapeutics* (ADA, Chicago).

Rationale for Use of Antibiotics

Although periodontal debridement and periodontal surgery are currently and will always be the foundation for controlling inflammatory periodontal diseases, several factors can substantiate the adjunctive use of chemical or chemotherapeutic agents (e.g., antiseptic mouthrinses and antibiotics). An antiseptic is a substance that prevents or inhibits the growth of microorganisms or kills microbes on contact. An antibiotic is a substance that is synthesized by microorgansims that prevents or inhibits the growth of bacteria by either stopping multiplication or killing the bacteria.

Instrumentation often leaves behind significant numbers of periodontal pathogens (Waerhaug, 1978). Repopulation of these pathogens can occur within 60 days of periodontal debridement (Sbordone et al. 1990). In addition, certain periodontal pathogens such as *Actinobacillus actinomycetemcomitans* and *Porphyromonas gingivalis* invade the gingival epithelium and connective tissue and elude removal by periodontal debridement (de Graaf, van Winkelhoff, & Goené, 1989; Renvert, Wikström, Dablén, Slots, & Egelberg, 1990). Other periodontal pathogens, such as *Bacteroides forsythus* (renamed *Tannerella forsythensis*), *Prevotella intermedia,* and *Peptostreptococcus micros,* live in nonperiodontal sites such as the tongue, tonsils, saliva, and buccal mucosa (Asikainen, Alaluusua, & Saxén, 1991). These sites are a source for reinfection and must be considered in the overall treatment process. Other factors influencing the use of chemical plaque-control agents include the manual dexterity of the patient.

A number of chemical agents have been studied clinically and shown to be successful in the further suppression of dental plaque in certain types of periodontal diseases when used in conjunction with periodontal debridement and surgery. The role of antimicrobial agents as part of the periodontal treatment plan in certain patients has gained significant importance in recent years since the acknowledgment that periodontal diseases are infectious diseases with specific bacteria as the cause (Loesche, 1976). Based on the specific plaque hypothesis, treatment is geared toward the elimination or reduction of specific bacteria (e.g., *A. actinomycetemcomitans, P. gingivalis, P. intermedia,* and spirochetes). Thus antimicrobial agents can be instituted as a supplement, not a replacement, during nonsurgical and surgical therapy. Since there are also beneficial bacteria living in the mouth, it is not desirable nor a goal to eliminate all intraoral bacteria. Unfortunately, systemic antibiotics used indiscriminately can result in antibiotic resistance, in which an antibiotic is ineffective against certain bacteria. This is becoming a worldwide problem.

Delivery Systems

Currently, two systems are available for the delivery of chemotherapeutic agents: local and systemic systems. Topical and controlled (sustained)-release drug devices are local delivery systems. Each delivery system has advantages and limitations (Table 24–1■).

Topical application delivers the agent or drug to an exposed surface such as the teeth and gingiva. The most common route for the supragingival topical delivery of antimicrobial agents is by a mouthrinse, a dentifrice, or an oral irrigator. Subgingival topical delivery of antimicrobial agents is by oral irrigation or the use of controlled-release devices.

Controlled-release delivery devices are placed directly into the periodontal pocket and are designed to release a drug slowly over 24 hours for prolonged drug action. Antimicrobials are delivered into the periodontal pocket by fibers, gels, chips, powder, ointments, acrylic strips, or collagen films.

Table 24–1 Main Features of Drug Delivery Systems

Delivery System	Target Site	Adequate Concentration at Target Site	Stays at Target Site Long Enough	Reaches the GCF	Advantages
Systemic: tablets, capsules	Periodontal pocket; epithelium and connective tissue; nonperiodontal sites (e.g., saliva, tongue, buccal mucosa, tonsils)	Fair concentrations reached due to some dilution by the time it reaches pocket area; frequent dosing is necessary to maintain therapeutic levels	No	Yes	Reaches all intraoral sites where bacterial reservoirs are found
Topical: oral rinses	Supragingival	Adequate concentrations, but therapeutic level dramatically declines by being washed out by saliva	No	No	No systemic adverse side effects; no antibiotic resistance develops
Topical: dentifrices	Supragingival	Adequate concentrations, but therapeutic level dramatically declines by being washed out by saliva	No	No	No systemic adverse effects; high patient compliance
Topical: subgingival irrigation	Periodontal pocket	Adequate concentrations, but therapeutic level dramatically declines by being washed out by GCF	No	No	No systemic adverse side effects
Controlled-release: powder, gel, chip	Periodontal pocket	Adequate concentrations; therapeutic levels are relatively constant for several days	Yes	Yes	Maintains therapeutic levels in the GCF for several days; no systemic adverse side effects; concentrates in pocket without dilution through entire body; possible development of bacterial resistance to the antibiotic (more studies needed)

Systemic drug delivery involves taking a tablet or a capsule orally with subsequent distribution of the agent through the circulation to the subgingival pocket area.

Choice of the delivery system is based on the target site. For instance, if gingivitis were being treated, oral rinses or irrigation would be chosen for supragingival plaque control. If, on the other hand, a certain type of periodontitis is being treated, the target site is the base of the periodontal pocket. Since oral rinses do not reach subgingivally, the delivery system of choice would be either oral irrigation or systemic or controlled-release delivery.

Dental Plaque as a Biofilm

As mentioned earlier, dental plaque exists as a biofilm. A plaque or oral biofilm is defined as "matrix-enclosed bacterial populations adherent to each other and/or to surfaces or interfaces" (Costerton et al., 1994). Plaque biofilms are of varying thicknesses, and in order to penetrate the biofilm, antibiotic concentrations must be several times greater than that needed to kill bacteria in a test tube (laboratory conditions) (Kleinfelder, Müller, & Lange, 1999). Subgingival biofilms cannot be removed by toothbrushing, flossing, or the use of antimicrobial agents. It is necessary to physically remove the biofilm by instrumentation, and then the antimicrobial agent can be administered. For this reason, administration of antimicrobial agents should never be the sole treatment and always should be as an adjunct to periodontal debridement and/or periodontal surgery. The biofilm structure also may account for the rapid rebound or repopulation of the pathogenic bacteria, which occurs frequently after the use of antimicrobial agents (Page, Offenbacher, Schroeder, Seymour, & Kornman, 1997).

Drug Actions

When considering the use of chemotherapeutic agents, the dental hygienist should be aware of the pharmacokinetics and pharmacodynamics of the drug. Pharmacokinetics involves knowledge of the drug's absorption, distribution, metabolism, and excretion. Pharmacodynamics relates to the drug's mechanism of action. In addition, any adverse side effects and drug–food interactions should be noted, and the patient should be informed.

Systemic Drug Delivery

Indications

Systemic drug delivery through oral administration has several advantages and disadvantages (see Table 24–1). Antibiotics generally are unnecessary and inappropriate for reducing plaque levels and treating gingivitis, with the exception of necrotizing periodontal diseases. Bacterial invasion (spirochetes) of periodontal tissues seen in NUG eludes mechanical removal with instruments.

Systemic antibiotics are useful as adjuncts in periodontal treatment for patients with aggressive periodontitis, all types of refractory periodontitis, and immunodeficiency diseases. Patients with refractory periodontal diseases usually harbor persistent subgingival pathogens that are likely to be resistant to conventional treatment. In localized aggressive periodontitis patients, *A. actinomycetemcomitans* invades the gingival connective tissue and thus evades removal by mechanical instrumentation. Antibiotics will benefit patients with a periodontal abscess when there is accompanied systemic signs such as fever or lymphadenopathy.

Selection

Adjunctive systemic antibiotics may be used during initial and/or surgical therapy. It may be advantageous to perform microbiologic testing to determine the presence of specific bacteria to reduce the possibility of antibiotic resistance. Reevaluation with microbiologic testing 1 to 3 months after antimicrobial therapy may be done to verify elimination or suppression of the pathogens. However, the expense of this procedure may preclude its generalized use. Long-term use (1 to 2 months or longer) of systemic antibiotics is considered to be without foundation.

Proper selection and dosing of the appropriate antibiotic are necessary to avoid untoward reactions and antibiotic resistance. Many categories of antibiotics are available, and several are indicated in periodontal infections (Table 24–2■). The dental hygienist must be familiar with both the generic and brand or trade names of each drug. If the generic name of the drug is not listed in the PDR®, use another drug reference book. Not all drug names are found in the PDR. For example, Sumycin is a trade name for tetracycline HCl and is manufactured by a specific company.

Good oral hygiene is still mandatory and will favor a positive clinical response when patients are prescribed systemic antibiotics. As mentioned earlier, periodontal debridement must be performed before the administration of any antimicrobial agent. This will remove the biofilm that protects subgingival microorganisms, except in cases where the bacteria have invaded the soft tissue. Systemic antibiotics are given in certain situations and are always used as a supplement or adjunct to

Table 24–2   Classification of Systemic Antibiotics Used in Periodontics
Tetracyclines
Tetracycline HCl
Doxycycline hyclate
Minocycline HCl
Beta-lactam
Penicillin VK
Amoxicillin trihydrate
Amoxicillin
+ clavulanic acid
Nitroimadazoles
Metronidazole
Azalides (derivative of erythromycin)
Azithromycin dihydrate
Lincomycins
Clindamycin HCl
Fluoroquinolones
Ciprofloxacin HCl

conventional periodontal debridement and oral hygiene self-care. Antibiotics should never be given as the only treatment regimen. Antibiotics are classified as being either bacteriostatic, which means they suppress the multiplication of the bacteria, or bactericidal, which means they kill the bacteria.

Adverse Drug Events

Heightened public interest in adverse drug events has motivated the government to require pharmaceutical companies to provide adverse drug reaction (ADR) information (Smith, 1999). The requirement is to provide information on the percentage of adverse drug reactions caused by antibiotics in both hospital and nonhospital settings.

ADRs can range from mild reactions that disappear when the antibiotic is discontinued to severe reactions that are life-threatening, disabling, or result in hospitalization (Smith, 1999). Table 24–3■ lists common adverse effects associated with antimicrobial agents.

Systemic Antibiotics

Tetracyclines

Tetracyclines as a group are bacteriostatic, inhibiting bacterial growth and multiplication by inhibiting protein synthesis. Two semisynthetic analogues of tetracycline, doxycycline hyclate and minocycline HCl, are broad-spectrum antibiotics, affecting both gram-positive and gram-negative microorganisms. Doxycycline and minocycline have been used in the treatment of *A. actinomycetemcomitans* infections in

Table 24–3	Classification of Adverse Effects of Systemic Antimicrobial Agents
Adverse Effect	**Features**
Hypersensitivity reactions	Involves allergic reactions to the antibiotic (e.g., rashes).
Gastrointestinal disturbances	Very common; includes nausea, vomiting, and diarrhea. Pseudomembranous colitis is the most severe gastrointestinal complication that requires immediate discontinuation of the antibiotic. Although initially believed to be a complication associated primarily with clindamycin, most oral and injectable antibiotics may produce this side effect.
Hepatotoxicity	Liver disease can occur with commonly administered antibiotics such as erythromycin, amoxicillin-clavulanic acid, and quinolones.
Photosensitivity reactions	Occurs with fluoroquinolones and tetracyclines (less with minocycline). Seen as an exaggerated sunburn. Patients should not be exposed to sun when taking these antibiotics.
Fungal infection	Fungal infections can occur especially with use of broad-spectrum antibiotics, which destroy bacteria, allowing fungi (*Candida albicans*) to overgrow, which may produce gastrointestinal irritation, stomatitis, and vaginal infection. Acidophilus (available in a soft gel tablet) or yogurt taken in conjunction with the antibiotic (except tetracycline) will replace some of the bacteria, thereby possibly preventing a fungal infection.

localized aggressive periodontitis (formerly known as localized juvenile periodontitis) and refractory periodontitis. Mandell, Tripodi, Savitt, Goodson, and Socransky (1986) reported that while surgery and treatment with tetracycline were superior in localized aggressive periodontitis patients, it appeared that there was a possibility of reinfection with or incomplete elimination of *A. actinomycetemcomitans*.

Anticollagenase Feature   Tetracyclines have both antibacterial and nonantibacterial properties. Besides affecting bacterial growth, they also affect the host response by inhibiting the production and secretion of collagenase by cells in the body such as polymorphonuclear leukocytes (PMNs) (Golub, Ramanurthy, McNamara, Greenwald, & Rifkin, 1984). Collagenase is an enzyme responsible for the destruction of collagen, which makes up the connective tissue of the periodontium. Tetracyclines also were found to inhibit bone resorption by affecting osteoclast function (Rifkin, Vernillo, & Golub, 1993). This anticollagenase property does not depend on the drug's antibacterial actions.

Concentration in Gingival Crevicular Fluid   Another property of tetracyclines is their ability to concentrate in the gingival crevicular fluid (GCF) at two to four times blood levels following multiple doses (Gordon, Walker, Murphy, Goodson, & Socransky, 1981). Doxycycline (Pascale et al., 1986) and minocycline also concentrate in higher levels in the GCF than in serum. Tetracyclines exhibit higher substantivity than other antibiotics (Baker, Evans, Coburn, & Genco, 1983; Stabholz et al., 1993), which allows binding to root surfaces with a slow release into the GCF. The binding of tetracyclines to calcium ions in the GCF enhances their substantivity. These properties allow the drug to maintain high therapeutic levels in the GCF. It is advantageous for a drug to concentrate in high levels in the GCF because the GCF bathes the subgingival pocket area where the periodontal pathogens live.

Adverse Side Effects and Drug–Drug and Drug–Food Interactions
Common adverse side effects of tetracyclines include nausea, vomiting, and diarrhea. Gastrointestinal (stomach) upset is much less with the semisynthetic drugs because they are more highly absorbed from the gastrointestinal tract. Tetracyclines stain newly formed teeth during enamel deposition and should not be used during the last half of pregnancy or in children up to 8 years of age. A complex is formed with calcium orthophosphate that produces a yellow-gray fluorescent discoloration. Photosensitivity is another adverse side effect, resulting in exaggerated sunburn when patients are exposed to the sun.

Tetracyclines, except doxycycline and minocycline, should not be taken concomitantly with dairy products because tetracycline binds to calcium, inhibiting its absorption. Tetracycline should be taken on an empty stomach (1 hour before or 2 hours after meals) because food delays its absorption. Doxycycline and minocycline can be taken without regard to meals. Absorption of all tetracyclines into the bloodstream is delayed with antacids. Tetracyclines, as well as other antibiotics, interfere with the metabolism of oral contraceptives. Estrogens, a component in oral contraceptives, must be metabolized (broken down) to its active form in the stomach by bacteria. Most antibiotics kill or stop the growth of these bacteria, inhibiting estrogen breakdown. Patients must use other forms of birth control if they are taking antibiotics concomitantly. Tetracyclines or any other bacteriostatic drug should not be given together with bactericidal antibiotics such as penicillin, metronidazole, or ciprofloxacin that would interfere with the bactericidal action of that drug. In order for a bactericidal drug to work, the bacteria need to be multiplying.

How Supplied   Tetracycline HCl (Sumycin): 100- and 250-mg capsules. Doxy-cycline hyclate (Vibramycin®, Pfizer, New York, NY, Vibra-Tabs®, Pfizer, New York, NY, Doryx®, Warner Chilcott Prof. Prod., Rockaway, NJ): 100-mg tablets and 50- and 100-mg capsules.

Penicillins (Beta-lactams)

Penicillins as a group are bactericidal, and their mechanism of action is to inhibit bacterial cell wall synthesis. Penicillin VK has limited activity against gram-negative periodontal pathogens. It is indicated primarily in certain acute periodontal infections such as abscesses. Amoxicillin, a broad-spectrum penicillin, is used frequently in periodontics. Some bacteria produce enzymes called beta-lactamases that inactivate the penicillin molecule. To overcome this vulnerability, a beta-lactamase inhibitor such as clavulanic acid is combined with amoxicillin (Augmentin®, SmithKline Beecham, Philadelphia).

Adverse Side Effects and Drug–Drug and Drug–Food Interactions
Approximately 5 to 10% of individuals are allergic to penicillin. It is best to take Augmentin® with food to decrease gastrointestinal upset. Severe gastrointestinal upset (e.g., nausea, vomiting, and diarrhea) occurs as a result of the acid component. Food does not interfere with absorption of amoxicillin into the bloodstream. Penicillins should not be taken together with bacteriostatic antibiotics because for a bactericidal antibiotic to work, the bacteria need to be multiplying, and this would be inhibited if a bacteriostatic antibiotic were administered concomitantly with penicillin.

How Supplied   Penicillin VK (Pen-Vee K, Penicillin VK): 250- and 500-mg tablets. Amoxicillin trihydrate (Polymox, Trimox, Amoxil): 250-mg capsules and 125-mg chewable tablets. Augmentin®, SmithKline Beecham, Philadelphia: A "250" tablet contains: 250 mg amoxicillin and 125 mg potassium clavulanate; a "500" tablet contains 500 mg amoxicillin and 125 mg potassium clavulanate.

Cephalosporins

Cephalosporins are not considered to be the drug of choice for most types of dental infections, including periodontal diseases. These antibiotics do not provide an advantage over amoxicillin or penicillin.

Nitroimadazoles

Mechanism of Action and Indications   Metronidazole is specifically effective against obligate or strict anaerobic (live in a pure nonoxygen environment) microorganisms. Metronidazole penetrates well into the GCF, but not as high as the tetracyclines. Metronidazole is bactericidal, and its mechanism of action is to inhibit bacterial DNA synthesis.

Metronidazole is indicated in the treatment of acute nectrotizing gingivitis (ANUG). Metronidazole is also indicated when barrier membranes are used during guided tissue regeneration surgery. *P. gingivalis,* a strict anaerobe, is the primary bacteria that colonize on porous membrane material. It has been reported in both professional journals and in the lay press that periodontal debridement in conjunction with metronidazole may reduce the need for periodontal surgery (Loesche, Giordano, Soehren, & Kaciroti, 1996), but this remains controversial. Metronidazole in combination with amoxicillin or Augmentin may be effective against refactory and aggressive forms of periodontitis associated with *A. actinomycetemcomitans* and *P. gingivalis* infection. However, a recent study of 21 patients with moderate, untreated periodontal diseases evaluated the benefits of amoxicillin and Augmentin® after initial therapy. Patients received periodontal debridement twice during the study. After the second debridement, patients were assigned randomly to either the group that received the drug combination or the placebo group. Results indicated no added benefit when amoxicillin and Augmentin were taken after initial therapy (Winkel et al., 1999).

Adverse Side Effects and Drug–Drug Interactions Antibiotic resistance to metronidazole is rare, but there are numerous adverse side effects. Gastrointestinal upset is seen frequently, especially nausea. A metallic taste in the mouth has been reported, as well as darkened urine. Consumption of alcohol beverages, including use of alcohol-containing mouthrinses, while taking metronidazole results in a disulfiram-like reaction. Disulfiram is a drug given to wean alcoholics off alcohol by acting to deter further ingestion of alcohol. It works by inhibition of the enzyme aldehyde dehydrogenase, causing a buildup of acetaldehyde, a toxic by-product of ethanol metabolism (Garey & Rodvold, 1999). Within 5 to 10 minutes after metronidazole is taken with alcohol, serious non-life-threatening adverse side effects occur including headache, flushing, nausea, vomiting, and cramps. The reaction usually lasts for up to 1 hour; however, it may continue for a few days after discontinuation of the medication (Walker, 1996). Alcohol should not be consumed during metronidazole therapy and for at least 3 days after discontinuing the drug. Metronidazole is contraindicated in patients taking anticoagulants (e.g., warfarin), lithium (a drug used for manic depression), and cimetadine (an antiulcer drug).

How Supplied Metronidazole (Flagyl®, Searle, Chicago): 375-mg capsules and 250- and 500-mg tablets.

Macrolides

Erythromycin, a macrolide antibiotic, is not used in the treatment of periodontal diseases because it is primarily effective against Gram-positive microorganisms and does not penetrate gram-negative bacterial cells. Erythromycin also does not penetrate the GCF to effective levels. Erythromycins are bacteriostatic and inhibit bacterial protein synthesis. Adverse side effects include severe gastrointestinal disturbances, including nausea, vomiting, and diarrhea.

Second-Generation Drugs: Azalides The newer second-generation erythromycins, referred to as azilides, have a broader spectrum of action with fewer adverse side effects. Azithromycin dihydrate shows promising results in periodontics. Azithromycin has several unique features. Azithromycin concentrates in phagocytes such as PMNs and macrophages, which contribute to its distribution into inflamed periodontal tissues (gingival connective tissue) in greater amounts than in plasma (Malizia, Tejada, Ghelardi, Senesi, & Gabriele, 1997). In addition, a post-antibiotic effect is seen, whereby high antibiotic levels remain after the drug is discontinued (Malizia et al., 1997).

Adverse Side Effects and Drug–Drug and Drug–Food Interactions All erythromycins, except for azithromycin, should not be taken with nonsedating antihistamines such as astemizole (Hismanal®, Janssen Pharmaceuticals, Titusville, NJ).

Erythromycin inhibits the metabolism or breakdown of these drugs, causing high blood levels, which can lead to cardiotoxicity. There are no contraindications to the use of fexofenadine (Allegra®, Hoescht Marion Roussel, Kansas City, MO) or loratadine (Claritin®, Schering Corporation, Kenilworth, NJ). Concurrent use of erythromycins and theophylline (an antiasthma drug) increases blood levels of theophylline. Capsules of azithromycin should be taken on an empty stomach, but tablets can be taken with food.

How Supplied   Azithromycin (Zithromax®, Pfizer, New York, NY): 250-mg capsules and 600-mg tablets.

Lincomycins

Clindamycin HCl penetrates well into the GCF and is active against most periodontal pathogens except *A. actinomycetemcomitans* and *Eikenella corrodens* and is especially useful in treating refractory periodontitis. Clindamycin HCl inhibits bacterial protein synthesis and is bacteriostatic. Although the development of pseudomembranous colitis has been associated with the use of clindamycin, it can occur with any antibiotic; however, its occurrence is usually hospital based. Suppression of normal intestinal bacteria allows the overgrowth of *Clostridium difficile,* which produces a toxin that causes severe watery diarrhea and fever. The antibiotic should be discontinued as soon as such signs appear. Clindamycin can be taken with food.

How Supplied   Clindamycin HCl (Cleocin®, Pharmacia & Upjohn, Bridgewater, NJ): 75-, 150-, and 300-mg capsules.

Quinolones (fluoroquinolone)

Fluoroquinolones are bactericidal because they inhibit bacterial DNA replication. Quinolones are not actually an antibiotic, however, because they are totally synthetic. Nevertheless, they are frequently referred to as broad-spectrum antimicrobials with good activity against facultative gram-negative anaerobes. Adverse side effects include dizziness, convulsions, headache, hallucinations, and joint and cartilage damage (do not give to athletes). Ciprofloxacin should not be given to children younger than 18 years of age because of its effect on cell growth. Ciprofloxacin should not be administered with theophylline or caffeine because it inhibits their metabolism, resulting in increased blood levels. Dairy products and antacids delay absorption. Food does not slow absorption.

How Supplied   Ciprofloxacin HCl (Cipro®, Bayer, New Haven, CT): 100-, 250-, 500-, and 750-mg tablets.

Controlled (Sustained)-Release Drug Delivery

The development of site-specific, controlled (sustained)-release delivery systems has provided a further option for antimicrobial therapy by allowing therapeutic levels of a drug to be maintained in the periodontal pocket for prolonged periods of time. If the drug is released from the device past 24 hours it is called a controlled-release device and if the drug is released within 24 hours it is called a sustained-release device. Many devices are available in the United States and Europe that incorporate an antimicrobial agent into a specific material (a polymer) that is placed into the periodontal pocket. The active ingredient is then released from the material, which subsequently exerts its antibacterial activity on subgingival bacteria over several days. Then the material is absorbed (dissolves). The concentration of antimicrobials administered in a controlled (sustained)-release device does not enter the bloodstream and thus does not trigger adverse side effects. Types of materials used to incorporate antimicrobial drugs include fibers, gels, chips, collagen film, and acrylic strips. Controlled (sustained)-release drug therapy is used as an adjunct to periodontal debridement and should not replace conventional mechanical therapy. In fact, the American Academy of Periodontology reported in the 2003 Annals that it "would be premature to conclude that insertion of sustained-release antimicrobial systems is as effective as scaling and root planing in all populations of patients" (Hanes & Purvis, 2003). They are indicated for use in recurrent pockets of 5 mm or greater that continue to bleed on probing. The intended results with these devices are gains in clinical attachment levels and reductions in probing depths and bleeding on probing.

Currently in the United States, PerioChip®, Atridox®, and Arestin™ are available commercially. Other controlled-release systems are available in Europe that have not been approved for use in the United States.

Nonresorbable Controlled-Release Devices

Tetracycline HCl Fibers

The first controlled-release device approved in the United States in the early 1990s was Actisite®. Actisite® is an ethylene vinyl acetate flexible fiber impregnated with 12.7 mg of tetracycline HCl. It is placed subgingivally into the periodontal pocket, where the tetracycline is released slowly over 7 to 10 days. Disadvantages in using tetracycline fibers include difficulty in placing and keeping the fiber in the pocket, bacterial resistance to tetracycline, and the inaccessibility of the drug to the adjacent gingival connective tissue and nondental sites such as the tongue, tonsils, and buccal mucosa, where bacteria also live. Currently, newer, more user-friendly and efficacious products have precluded the use of Actisite.

Resorbable Controlled (Sustained)-Release Devices

Chlorhexidine Gluconate Chip

The PerioChip® (DEXCEL Pharma, Israel; OMNII Oral Pharmaceuticals) is a gelatin maxtrix (bovine origin) containing 2.5 mg of chlorhexidine gluconate. This product received Food and Drug Administration approval in June 1998. PerioChip® is indicated for use as an adjunct to instrumentation in maintenance patients with pockets 5 mm or larger that bleed recurrently on probing (Jeffcoat et al., 1998). A recent clinical study comparing the efficacy of periodontal debridement alone with that of periodontal debridement plus PerioChip® revealed statistically significant reduc-

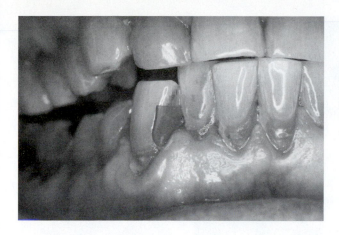

Figure 24–1 PerioChip® is a film or chip containing the antimicrobial chlorhexidine gluconate. After a periodontal maintenance visit, PerioChip® is placed subgingivally in pockets 5 mm or greater in depth and bleed on probing.

tions in probing depth and gains in clinical attachment in the periodontal debridement plus PerioChip® group. However, the magnitude of these changes was small (0.3 mm), so the results are not clinically significant (Jeffcoat et al., 1998). In this study, mechanical debridement was limited to only 1 hour in patients with moderately advanced peridontitis (5- to 8-mm pockets), which does not seem realistic.

After periodontal debridement, the chip is placed into the periodontal pocket (Fig. 24–1■). In contact with subgingival fluids it becomes sticky and binds to the epithelium lining the pocket, so no periodontal dressing is indicated. Its antibacterial action occurs when chlorhexidine is released over 7 to 10 days, after which it resorbs and does not have to be removed. Up to eight chips can be inserted into pockets in one visit. Another round of treatment can be done at 3 months.

Doxycycline Hyclate Gel

Atridox® is composed of 10% (42.5 mg) doxycycline hyclate in a gel formulation that is biodegradable and subsequently will resorb. The ingredients are available in two syringes (powder and liquid) that are mixed together (Fig. 24–2■) and injected into the pocket around the entire tooth (Fig. 24–3■). The gel form

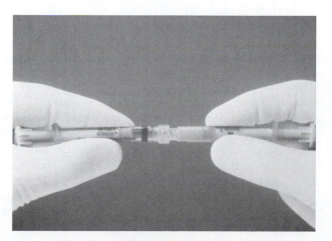

Figure 24–2 Atridox® is prepared by joining/interlocking the two syringes. (Courtesy of CollaGenex Pharm., Newton, PA [formerly Block Drug Corp., Jersey City, NJ])

Figure 24–3 After pumping the materials between the two joined syringes, a cannula is connected to the syringe to apply into the pocket. (Courtesy of CollaGenex Pharm., Newton, PA [formerly Block Drug Corp., Jersey City, NJ])

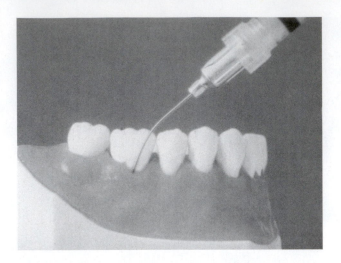

allows for ease of flow, readily adapting to subgingival root morphology. When the gel comes in contact with gingival fluid in the pocket, it solidifies to a wax-like substance.

Atridox® is indicated as an adjunct to scaling and root planing procedures in patients with chronic periodontitis. Local anesthesia is not required. Results of therapy are to promote attachment level gain, to reduce pocket depths, and to reduce bleeding on probing. Atridox® may also be used in patients who refuse to have periodontal debridement or periodontal surgery, and who are medically, physically, or emotionally compromised.

A randomized, controlled clinical study (Garrett, Johnson, & Stoller, 1998) comparing Atridox® alone (all patients had a history of periodontal debridement at least 2 months before the study) and periodontal debridement alone reported that Atridox® produced clinical results comparable with periodontal debridement alone. Both groups showed a statistically significant reduction in pocket depths (an average of 1.3 mm) and gains in attachment levels (average of 0.8 mm).

Levels of doxycycline in the pocket (GCF) peaked at 2 hours after placement into the pocket, and effective drug levels were maintained at 28 days (Stoller, Johnson, Trapnell, Harrold, & Garrett, 1998). Although, within a few days levels of doxycycline has peaked.

Minocycline Hydrocholoride Microspheres

The most recently FDA-approved sustained-release device is Arestin™ (OraPharm, Warminster, PA). Arestin microspheres is a sustained-release product containing the antibiotic minocycline hydrochloride. Minocycline is a type of tetracycline but it is longer acting and has a broader spectrum of antibiotic activity. Each cartridge of Arestin contains 1 mg of minocycline (Fig. 24–4■). Arestin is indicated as an adjunct to scaling and root planing procedures for the reduction of pocket depth in patients with chronic localized periodontitis. Studies have shown that scaling and root planing followed by the application of Arestin resulted in a greater percentage reduction in pocket depths (≥2mm) at 9 months compared to scaling and root planing alone.

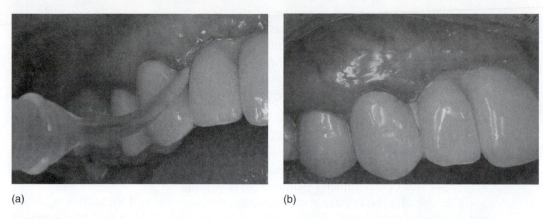

(a)   (b)

Figure 24–4   Arestin™ being administered into a pocket. Arestin is a powder containing minocycline. (Courtesy of Dr. Stuart J. Froum, New York, New York)

Many periodontal pathogens including *Porphyromonas gingivalis, Prevotella intermedia, Fusobacterium nucleatum, Eikenella corrodens,* and *Actinobacillus actinomycetemcomitans* are susceptible to minocycline.

Other Products

Some controlled-release products are available in other countries. Elyzol® (Dumex, Copenhagen, Denmark) is a 25% metronidazole gel that is injected into the pocket. Periocline® (Sunstar Corp., Osaka, Japan) and Dentomycin® (Cyanamid International, Wayne, NJ) are a 2% minocycline gel.

Precautions

Antibiotic Resistance

Bacterial resistance to antibiotics raises serious questions for health care providers. The danger is that an antibiotic will not be effective if administered later on for a truly life-threatening bacterial infection because the bacteria have become resistant to that antibiotic. Thus antibiotic resistance can lead to an increase in the incidence of disease. Patterns of antibiotic use in the United States also contribute significantly to the global problem. Patients often stop their antibiotic treatment prematurely, believing that if they feel better, it is not necessary to take the full course. Patients also self-medicate with leftover antibiotics from a previous infection. Patients may request antibiotics or other medications because they believe they will be beneficial. Many practitioners comply with such patient requests without evaluating the situation clinically, and many practitioners simply overprescribe antibiotics.

Therefore, it is extremely important to use antibiotics and antimicrobials conservatively, only when indicated, and with the narrowest possible spectrum of activity. Prolonged or repetitive courses of antibiotic treatment should be avoided. Antibiotics are an adjunct to treatment.

Other Precautions/Contraindications

Subgingival placement of devices containing antibiotics or antimicrobials is not recommended in an acutely abscessed periodontal pocket. Any antibiotic product should be used with caution in patients having a history of predisposition to oral candidasis because antibiotics suppress the growth of or kill bacteria, which allows for the growth of other microorganisms such as fungi.

The use of tetraycycline and its analogs, doxycycline and minocycline, should not be used during tooth development, which includes the last half of pregnancy, infancy, and childhood up to the age of 8 years.

Enzyme-Suppression Therapy

Although bacteria are the culprits in initiating inflammatory periodontal diseases, the inflammatory mediators, including cytokines and prostaglandins produced by the host (body) cells in response to the bacteria, are partly responsible for periodontal tissue breakdown. When produced in excess, inflammatory mediators induce destruction of healthy periodontal tissues. For example, prostaglandins facilitate bone resorption by stimulating the activity of osteoclasts.

Matrix Metalloproteinases

Host cells, including PMNs and fibroblasts, also respond to bacterial products by synthesizing and secreting matrix metalloproteinases (MMPs) in the host connective tissue. The MMPs are a family of enzymes that work together to break down connective tissue proteins, including collagen. MMPs that cause the breakdown of the periodontium include collagenase and gelatinase.

In healthy oral tissues, as part of the normal turnover of connective tissue, fibroblasts synthesize and secrete collagenase, which removes "old" collagen while new collagen is laid down. However, in the presence of disease (bacterial infection), PMNs produce collagenase in excessive amounts, which destroys periodontal tissues (collagen). Thus the third approach to therapy is to inhibit the collagenase synthesized and released by PMNs. Antibiotics are aimed at reducing or eliminating the periodontal pathogens but do not target the enzyme-producing PMNs.

Subantimicrobial-Dose Doxycycline

Golub and colleagues (1984) found that tetracyclines, especially doxycycline, have anticollagenase properties and inhibit collagenase activity. This group of investigators discovered that by using only 20-mg tablets of doxycycline, instead of the customary 50- or 100-mg tablets, collagenase would be inhibited. At these subantimicrobial doses, doxycycline only has anticollagenase activity and no antibacterial action. This subantimicrobial or low-dose doxycycline (SDD) formulation is avail-

able under the trade name Periostat® (CollaGenex, Newton, PA; www
.collagenex.com). Periostat® is indicated as an adjunct to periodontal debridement
to promote attachment level gain and to reduce pocket depths in patients with
chronic periodontitis. It is intended to improve the clinical outcome of periodontal
debridement. Periostat is also used in the treatment of certain medical conditions
including dermatologic and ophthalmologic lesions. Periostat® tablets are taken
twice daily. Efficacy beyond 9 months of continuous dosing and safety beyond 12
months of continuous dosing have not been established.

In a large-scale clinical study, patients received debridement and either Perio-
stat® or a placebo twice a day for 9 months. The results of the study showed that
after 3 months of daily use, reductions in probing depth and improvements in attachment levels were statistically greater with SDD and debridement than with
placebo and debridement (Ciancio & Ashley, 1998). Reductions in probing depth
from baseline were up to 38% greater with SDD in tooth sites with mild to moderate periodontitis (probing depths of 4 to 6 mm) and severe periodontitis (probing
depths of 7 mm or more). Improvements in attachment from baseline were up to
54% greater with the SDD than with placebo in severely diseased sites. Although
treatment differences in the per-patient mean change in probing depth and clinical
attachment level were statistically significant, these differences were relatively
small. However, the frequency of probing depth reduction of 2 mm or more was
greater in the Periostat group than in the placebo group.

Summary

The multifaceted approach to treating periodontal diseases uses mechanical instrumentation, which reduces the bacterial load, and locally and systemically administered antibiotics and host-modulating pharmacotherapies as treatment adjuncts.

Treatment of patients with gingivitis or chronic periodontitis is related to reducing the number of bacteria to a level conducive to health (Loesche, 1976). This
involves periodontal debridement, periodontal surgery, and, if needed, oral rinses
and oral irrigation. Frequently, these patients are overtreated using systemic antibiotics, which can lead to the development of bacteria that become resistant to
antibiotics. Systemic antibiotics are contraindicated in these patients.

In a small percentage (around 20%) of patients with periodontitis (Loesche,
1976), specific bacteria (e.g., *A. actinomycetemcomitans, P. gingivalis, P. intermedia,* and spirochetes) can be implicated in the diseases (Loesche, 1976; Slots,
1986). Since these bacteria invade the soft tissues, treatment may include systemic
antibiotics to eliminate the bacteria in the tissues. It is more difficult to recognize
these types of patients. Examples include patients with localized aggressive periodontitis, necrotizing periodontal diseases, and refractory forms of periodontal diseases. In addition, patients with a compromised immune system, such as AIDS
patients, can benefit from the use of antimicrobial agents.

The controlled (sustained) drug devices may be useful in the adjunctive treatment of chronic periodontitis. The clinician's decision to use local antimicrobial
agents remains the matter of individual clinical judgement. Even though scaling
and root planing disrupts the subgingival biofilms that cause periodontitis, the
placement of sustained-release antimicrobial devices subgingivally may help in
slowing the rapid return of the biofilm and thus may slow the progression of
disease.

Antibiotic resistance of bacteria has enormous clinical and societal implications. In essence, when bacteria become resistant to an antibiotic, that antibiotic becomes ineffective. Although the prudent use of antibiotics will continue to be a valuable treatment option for certain forms of periodontal disease, the abuse and misuse of antibiotics must be addressed and monitored to prevent antibiotic resistance.

As advances are made in the development of new antimicrobial and antibiotic agents, the oral health care team will continue to play an integral part in ensuring that these agents are used appropriately. No data are available to support the long-term effectiveness of the newly approved controlled-release devices. Although many studies on site-specific drug therapy and submicrobial-dose doxycycline report statistically significant reductions in probing depths and improvements in attachment levels, the clinical benefit may not be significant. Further clinical studies are needed to determine clinical significance.

Key Points

- Systemic antibiotics are indicated in certain inflammatory periodontal diseases such as localized or generalized aggressive periodontitis, and refractory forms of periodontal diseases.
- Controlled-release drug devices that slowly release antimicrobial agents are used in site-specific (recurrent) areas in chronic periodontitis.
- Enzyme-suppression therapy involves the inhibition of collagenase that is synthesized and released by neutrophils.
- Dental practitioners should contribute to limiting antibiotic resistance.

Web Sites

www.rxlist.com

www.collagenex.com

www.pdr.net

www.gsm.com

www.drugs.com

www.nchi.nlm.nih.gov

Self-Quiz

1. All the following results are possible after site-specific chemotherapy except one. Which one is the exception? (pp. 410–413)
   a. reduction in probing depth
   b. gain in clinical attachment
   c. reduction in bleeding
   d. formation of alveolar bone

2. Which one of the following procedures most effectively removes supra/subgingival plaque biofilms? (p. 403)
   a. oral irrigation
   b. systemic antibiotics
   c. periodontal debridement
   d. controlled-release drugs

3. Which of the following controlled-release devices is in a gel form? (p. 411)

   a. Arestin

   b. Atridox

   c. Actisite

   d. PerioChip

4. Which of the following agents is the active ingredient in Arestin? (p. 412)

   a. tetracycline HCl

   b. minocycline HCl

   c. doxycycline hyclate

   d. chlorhexidine gluconate

5. Which one of the following antimicrobial agents possesses high substantivity to the root surface? (p. 406)

   a. cetylpyrimidium

   b. sanguinarine

   c. tetracycline

   d. erythromycin

   e. chlorhexidine

6. All the following are ways a dental practitioner can contribute to limiting antibiotic resistance except one. Which one is the exception? (p. 413)

   a. Prescribe drug at the first sign of purulent exudate.

   b. Avoid prolonged course of the medication.

   c. Instruct the patient on proper use.

   d. Prescribe an antibiotic with the narrowest possible spectrum of activity.

7. All the following properties of tetracyclines favor its use in periodontics except one. Which one is the exception? (p. 406)

   a. substantivity

   b. antifungal

   c. antibacterial

   d. anticollagenase

8. Which one of the following indications is for site-specific drug delivery? (p. 409)

   a. probing depths of less than 4 mm

   b. pockets with suppuration and bleeding

   c. nonresponding bleeding sites with probing depths of 5 mm or more

   d. sites with bone loss, suppuration, bleeding, and probing depths of less than 5 mm

9. Which of the following is an adverse side effect that may occur when taking antibiotics? (p. 413)

   a. bacterial resistance

   b. mucosa inflammation

   c. bone degeneration

   d. tissue mucositis

10. Which of the following drugs is used in chronic periodontitis to suppress the production and secretion of host cell collagenase? (p. 414)

    a. Arestin

    b. Periostat

    c. Vibramycin

    d. Tetracycline

    e. Atridox

References

Asikainen, S., S. Alaluusua, and L. Saxén. 1991. Recovery of A. actinomycetemcomitans from teeth, tongue, and saliva. *J. Periodontol*. 62:203–206.

Baker, P., T. Evans, R. Coburn, and R. Genco. 1983. Tetracycline and its derivatives strongly bind to and are released from the tooth surface in active form. *J. Periodontol*. 54:580–585.

Ciancio, S. G., and R. Ashley. 1998. Safety and efficacy of subantimicrobial-dose doxycycline therapy in patients with adult periodontitis. *Adv. Dent. Res*. 12:27–31.

Costerton, J. W., Z. Lewandowski, D. DeBeer, D. Caldwell, D. Korber, and G. James. 1994. Biofilms, the customized microniche. *J. Bacteriol*. 176:2137–2142.

Cummins, D. 1997. Vehicles: How to deliver the goods. *Periodontology 2000* 15:84–99.

De Graaf, J., A. J. van Winkelhoff, and R. J. Goené. 1989. The role of *Actinobacillus actinomycetemcomitans* in periodontal disease. *Infection* 17:269–271.

Garey, K. W., and K. A. Rodvold. 1999. Disulfiram reactions and anti-infective agents. *Infect Med*. 16(11): 741–744.

Garrett, S., L. Johnson, and N. Stoller. 1998. The influence of subgingival calculus levels on outcomes following treatment of periodontitis with subgingivally delivered doxycycline or periodontal debridement. *J. Dent. Res*. 77:923 (Abstract 2336).

Golub, L. M., N. S. Ramamurthy, T. F. McNamara, R. A. Greenwald, and B. R. Rifkin. 1984. Tetracyclines inhibit tissue collagenase activity: A new mechanism in the treatment of periodontal diseases. *J. Periodont. Res.* 19:651–655.

Gordon, J. M., C. B. Walker, J. C. Murphy, J. M. Goodson, and S. S. Socransky. 1981. Tetracycline: Levels achievable in gingival crevice fluid and in vitro effect on subgingival organisms: 1. Concentrations in crevicular fluid after repeated doses. *J. Periodontol.* 52:609–612.

Hanes, P.J., and J.P. Purvis. 2003. Local anti-infecctive therapy: Pharacological agents. A systematic review. *Ann Periodontol,* 8:79–98.

Jeffcoat, M. K., K. S. Bray, S. G. Ciancio, A. R. Dentino, D. H. Fine, et al. 1998. Adjunctive use of a subgingival controlled-release chlorhexidine chip reduces probing depth and improves attachment level compared with periodontal debridement alone. *J. Periodontol.* 69:989–997.

Kleinfelder, J., R. Müller, and D. Lange. 1999. Antibiotic susceptibility of putative periodontal pathogens in advanced periodontitis patients. *J. Clin. Periodontol.* 26:347–352.

Loesche, W. 1976. Chemotherapy of dental plaque infections. *Oral Sci. Rev.* 9:65–107.

Loesche, W. J., J. Giordano, S. Soehren, and N. Kaciroti. 1996. The nonsurgical treatment of patients with periodontal disease. *Oral Surg. Oral Med. Oral Pathol.* 81:533–543.

Malizia, T., M. R. Tejada, E. Ghelardi, S. Senesi, M. Gabriele, et al. 1997. Periodontal tissue disposition of azithromycin. *J. Periodontol.* 68:1206–1209.

Mandell, R. L., L. S. Tripodi, E. Savitt, J. M. Goodson, and S. S. Socransky. 1986. The effect of treatment on *Aa* in local juvenile periodontitis. *J. Periodontol.* 57:94–97.

Page, R. C., S. Offenbacher, H. E. Schroeder, G. J. Seymour, and K. S. Kornman. 1997. Advances in the pathogenesis of periodontitis: Summary of developments, clinical implications and future directions. *Periodontology 2000* 14:216–248.

Pascale, D., J. Gordon, I. Lamster, P. Mann, M. Seiger, and W. Arndt. 1986. Concentration of doxycycline in human gingival fluid. *J. Clin. Periodontol.* 13:841–844.

Renvert, S., M. Wikström, G. Dahlén, J. Slots, and J. Egelberg. 1990. On the inability of root debridement and periodontal surgery to eliminate *Actinobacillus actinomycemtemcomitans* from periodontal pockets. *J. Clin. Periodontol.* 17:351–355.

Rifkin, B. R., A. T. Vernillo, and L. M. Golub. 1993. Blocking periodontal disease progression by inhibiting tissue destructive enzymes: A potential therapeutic role of tetracyclines and their chemically modified analogs. *J. Periodontol.* 64:819–827.

Smith, C. 1999. Adverse effects of antibiotics. *U.S. Pharmacist* (May):46–60.

Slots, J. 1986. Bacterial specificity in adult periodontitis: A summary of recent work. *J. Clin. Periodontol.* 13:912–917.

Stabholz, A., J. Kettering, R. Aprecio, G. Zimmerman, P. J. Baker, and U. M. E. Wikesjo. 1993. Antimicrobial properties of human dentin impregnated with tetracycline HCl or chlorhexidine: An in vitro study. *J. Clin. Periodontol.* 20:557–562.

Stoller, N., L. Johnson, S. Trapnell, C. Harrold, and S. Garrett. 1998. The pharmacokinetic profile of a biodegradable controlled-release delivery system containing doxycycline compared to systemically delivered doxycycline in gingival crevicular fluid, saliva, and serum. *J. Periodontol.* 69:1085–1091.

Waerhaug, J. 1978. Healing of the dentoepithelial junction following subgingival plaque control: II. As observed on extracted teeth. *J. Periodontol.* 49:119–134.

Walker, C. B. 1996. Selected antimicrobial agents: Mechanism of action, side effects and drug interactions. *Periodontology 2000* 10:12–28.

Winkel, E., A. van Winkelhoff, D. Barendregt, G. van der Weijden, M. Timmerman, and U. van der Velden. 1999. Clinical and microbiological effects of initial periodontal therapy in conjunction with amoxicillin and clavulanic acid in patient with adult periodontitis. *J. Clin. Periodontol.* 26:461–468.

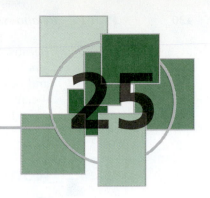

Healing after Nonsurgical Periodontal Therapy

Mea A. Weinberg, D.M.D., M.S.D., R.Ph.
Cynthia Fong, R.D.H., M.S.

Outline

Goal

To provide an understanding of tissue healing after non-surgical therapy.

Educational Objectives

Upon completion of this chapter, the reader should be able to:

Discuss the rationale for periodontal debridement.

Explain the clinical outcomes of periodontal debridement.

Discuss the effects of nonsurgical treatment on the subgingival microbiota.

Describe the effects of combined oral hygiene self-care with subgingival periodontal debridement on clinical attachment loss.

Describe the healing response in gingivitis and periodontitis after periodontal debridement.

KEY WORDS

- periodontal therapy
- periodontal debridement
- supragingival debridement
- subgingival debridement
- deplaquing
- prophylaxis
- inflammatory periodontal diseases
- soft tissue healing
- gain in clinical attachment

Because periodontal disease activity is site-specific within the same mouth and differs between individuals, choice of treatment is determined on a site-to-site basis and/or on a patient-to-patient basis. The critical factor in the success of periodontal therapy is not only the thoroughness of the professional debridement but rather the achievement of a high standard of oral hygiene self-care.

Nonsurgical Periodontal Therapy

The traditional emphasis of the initial phase of periodontal therapy or nonsurgical therapy is control of the supragingival microbial plaque and disruption or removal of subgingival gram-negative microbiota, thus delaying the repopulation of pathogenic microorganisms (Magnusson, Lindhe, Yoneyama, & Liljenberg, 1984). Subgingival plaque originates either from an apical extension of growing supragingival plaque (Waerhaug, 1978) and/or from incomplete subgingival instrumentation. In either case, it is essential to control the supragingival microbial activity through oral hygiene self-care and subgingival plaque removal by professional mechanical instrumentation (Cobb, 1996; Dahlen, Lindhe, Sato, Hanamura, & Okamoto, 1992; Katsanoulas, Renee, & Attström, 1992; Sbordone, Ramaglia, Gulletta, & Iacono, 1990). Subgingival debridement decreases the number of periodontal pathogens such as *Porphyromonas gingivalis* and *Prevotella intermedia* in subgingival plaque and shifts the plaque composition to a predominately Gram-positive aerobic species associated with periodontal health.

Thus nonsurgical therapy is based on returning the gingival tissue to a healthy, noninflamed state that can be maintained easily by the patient and the practitioner.

Terminology

The traditional therapy for removing supragingival and subgingival plaque, its by-products and toxins, and calculus has been scaling and root planing. Scaling is defined as the mechanical removal of supragingival and subgingival dental plaque, calculus, and stains (tooth-accumulated materials) from the crown and root surfaces. Thus scaling is performed both supragingivally and subgingivally. Subgingival scaling removes the adherent plaque and calculus attached to the root surface. Subgingival calculus is mineralized plaque that often adheres tenaciously to root surfaces and thus is very difficult to remove. Root planing is defined as a "definitive treatment procedure designed to remove cementum or surface dentin that is rough, impregnated with calculus, or contaminated with toxins or microorganisms" (Ciancio, 1989). The rationale for root planing is to smooth the root surface so as to decrease the surface area to which calculus and plaque attach. Another aim is to obtain a smooth root surface by removing cementum (including some dentin) that is impregnated with bacterial toxins.

Over the past few years, the term periodontal debridement has emerged in the literature, and it is defined as the removal of any foreign material, including dental plaque, its by-products and toxins, calculus, and diseased or dead tissue, from the coronal tooth surfaces, root surfaces, sulcus or pocket, and periodontium (e.g., supporting bone). Thus the difference between periodontal debridement and scaling and root planing is that it encompasses more than just the root surfaces. It includes the pocket space, the pocket wall, and the underlying tissues (O'Hehir, 1999). Rather than total removal of cementum and the attainment of smooth root surfaces, conservation of cementum and the achievement of a good tissue healing response through control of bacterial infection are the objectives of periodontal debridement (O'Hehir, 1999). Supragingival debridement is the mechanical removal of dental plaque and calculus from tooth surfaces above the gingival margin. Subgingival debridement is the mechanical removal of dental plaque and calculus from tooth surfaces below the gingival margin. Even though periodontal debridement encompasses many procedures and currently is the newest terminology for instrumentation, the terms scaling and root planing should not be completely eliminated from the periodontal vocabulary.

Deplaquing describes the mechanical disruption of nonattached, free-floating subgingival plaque and its by-products from the sulcus or pocket. Deplaquing is recommended at reevaluation and maintenance appointments.

There are numerous definitions of oral prophylaxis in the literature. The American Dental Hygienist's Association (ADHA) reversed a change made to the prophylaxis definition published in the Current Dental Terminology (CDT)-4, which stated that prophylaxis was a scaling and/or polishing procedure to remove coronal plaque, calculus, and stains. The change to this definition involved removal of the term "/or", thereby restoring the 1992 ADA Current Dental Terminology definition, which reads scaling and polishing. The American Academy of Periodontology provides the most comprehensive definition of oral prophylaxis. An oral prophylaxis is the removal of plaque, calculus, and stains from the exposed and unexposed surfaces of the teeth by scaling and polishing as a preventive measure for the control of local irritants (American Academy of Periodontology, 2003).

Polishing is performed to remove stains from the teeth and has not been shown to have any therapeutic benefits. For this reason, the American Dental Hygienist's Association's position on polishing is that it is a procedure that should be performed selectively when teeth have extrinsic stains (American Dental Hygienist's Association, 1995).

In some states, dental hygienists are permitted to perform closed gingival curettage or soft tissue curettage. According to the American Academy of Periodontology, curettage is not an accepted procedure in periodontics. Curettage involves removal of the diseased lining of the soft tissue pocket wall (soft tissue debridement), including the junctional epithelium and the underlying inflamed connective tissue. The goal of gingival curettage is to reduce or eliminate periodontal inflammation. Indications for performing curettage include the presence of inflamed gingival tissues and shallow suprabony pockets. However, the benefits of soft tissue curettage are questionable, and as a separate procedure, it has no justifiable application during active therapy for chronic periodontitis (Ciancio, 1989). Kalkwarf (1989) demonstrated that the healing effects of curettage were not any better than scaling and root planing alone. It is noteworthy, however, that some inadvertent gingival curettage does occur as a result of scaling and root planing procedures.

Periodontal Debridement

Treatment of inflammatory periodontal diseases has evolved significantly during the past decades. It was once thought that a primary goal of traditional scaling and root planing was the achievement of smooth root surfaces that were free of deposits. This intent was based on the assumption that bacteria would attach to rough surfaces (e.g., calculus and irregular root topography) and interfere with soft tissue healing. It is now known that bacteria adhere to any surface, rough or smooth. Therefore, evaluation of successful periodontal debridement depends primarily on the soft tissue response. The clinical significance of root surface roughness or smoothness is still undetermined (Jacobson, Blomlöf, & Lindskog, 1994), but the dental hygienist nevertheless should strive to remove as much subgingival calculus as possible and to achieve root smoothness because they may affect plaque accumulation. Oberholzer and Rateitschak (1996) concluded that striving for total root smoothness during periodontal surgery seems to be unnecessary; however, the value of a cleaned tooth surface cannot be minimized in periodontal tissue healing response.

Mechanical nonsurgical therapy consisting of oral hygiene self-care and periodontal instrumentation is intended to prevent, arrest, control, or eliminate periodontal diseases in order to ultimately maintain the teeth in a functional state of health (Cobb, 1996). Periodontal debridement remains the current basis of nonsurgical periodontal therapy.

Combined Personal and Professional Debridement

Periodontal instrumentation is performed during the initial or preliminary phase of periodontal therapy. The beneficial effects of periodontal debridement combined with oral hygiene self-care in the treatment and prevention of periodontal diseases have been well documented. These include reduction of clinical inflammation, establishment of more beneficial microorganisms and less pathogenic microorganisms, reduction in probing depths, and a gain in attachment (American Academy of Periodontology, 1997; Kaldahl et al., 1996).

One clinical study reported that in the presence of supragingival plaque, a subgingival microbiota containing greater than 5% spirochetes and motile rods was reestablished in 4 to 8 weeks after mechanical instrumentation. Sites devoid of supragingival plaque following supervised oral hygiene and mechanical instrumentation had less than 5% gram-negative bacteria (Magnusson et al., 1984). A more recent investigation studied the effects of supragingival plaque control alone and plaque control combined with subgingival debridement on clinical attachment loss over a 3-year period (Westfelt, Rylander, Dahlen, & Lindhe, 1998). Results showed a reduction in bleeding scores following the combined treatment of plaque control and subgingival debridement. Plaque scores were reduced in both groups. Increased attachment loss of 2 mm or more was low in the combined treatment group. This study demonstrated that supragingival plaque control is not enough to prevent further attachment loss in periodontitis patients.

Rationale and Indications for Periodontal Debridement

The purpose of periodontal debridement is to treat and resolve inflammation in the periodontal soft tissues by removing the irritants, which are the supragingival and subgingival plaque and calculus. In conjunction with oral hygiene self-care, which also decreases supragingival plaque accumulation, repopulation of subgingival pathogenic microbiota is delayed and shifts the composition of pocket material from a pathogenic gram-negative microbiota to gram-positive species, which are more conducive to periodontal health.

Periodontal debridement is indicated at sites showing (1) signs of gingival inflammation, (2) elevated levels of bacterial pathogens, and (3) progressive attachment or alveolar bone loss (Cobb, 1996). Various forms of instrumentation are used, including hand-activated instrumentation and powered-driven instrumentation (e.g., sonic and ultrasonic instrumentation).

Outcomes of Periodontal Debridement

The ultimate long-term outcome or end point for mechanical nonsurgical therapy is preservation of the form and function of the dentition (Cobb, 1996). Determining the effects of nonsurgical periodontal treatment requires the use of measurable clinical end points. Most clinical studies, as well as private practices, measure the probing depths, gain or loss of clinical attachment (measuring the clinical attachment levels), and alveolar bone height and document bleeding on probing, visual signs of gingival inflammation, and changes in subgingingival microbiota (Cobb, 1996).

Reduction of the fluid and cellular components of an inflammatory lesion in the lamina propria should result in an increased proportion of collagen fibers, which when combined with reattachment of the junctional epithelium or the formation of a long junctional epithelium will produce increased resistance to passage of the probe tip. This results in a gain in clinical attachment.

Probing Depths/Clinical Attachment Level

Subgingival root debridement is contraindicated in sites that do not have periodontal pockets. A landmark clinical study showed that subgingival root debridement of teeth with initially shallow probing depths of less than 3 mm slightly decreased or did not alter probing depths, but loss of clinical attachment did occur (Lindhe, Socransky, Nyman, & Haffajee, 1982). Taking into consideration a number of clinical studies over the past years, Cobb (1996) determined that thorough debridement of moderately deep pockets (4 to 6 mm) usually results in a mean reduction in probing depth of 1.29 mm and a mean gain in clinical attachment of 0.55 mm, whereas sites with deeper probing depth (7 mm or more) showed a mean reduction in probing depth of 2.16 mm and a gain in clinical attachment of 1.29 mm. Care in selecting sites that will benefit from subgingival debridement is essential in the prevention of clinical attachment loss.

Subgingival Microbiota

Periodontal debridement of pockets causes profound shifts in the composition of the subgingival microbiota. After subgingival debridement, the number of gram-negative microorganisms decreases, especially spirochetes, and the number of gram-positive rods and cocci increases. However, this therapy may be ineffective in eliminating *Actinobacillus actinomycetemcomitans* from affected subgingival sites (Cobb, 1996) because it invades soft tissue (Renvert, Wikström, Dahlen, Slots, & Egelberg, 1990).

Unfortunately, shifts in microbiotal composition are transient, and usually the pocket area becomes repopulated with subgingival microorganisms within days to months. Since the subgingival microbiota originate in supragingival areas (Waerhaug, 1978), regular and effective plaque control and professional subgingival therapy are absolutely critical for long-term control of inflammatory periodontal diseases (Cobb, 1996).

Bleeding on Probing

Periodontal debridement has predictably reduced the levels of inflammation. A vast number of clinical studies conducted over recent years have shown that periodontal debridement has reduced bleeding in approximately 57% of sites (Cobb, 1996).

Treatment Sequence

The treatment sequence for periodontal debridement varies depending on clinical findings and diagnosis. The first step, after the disease is classified and a treatment plan is developed, is oral hygiene self-care instructions specifically designed for the patient's needs. Instrumentation procedures should be performed in a logical and orderly manner and usually are done to completion by quadrant.

Some patients with severe inflammation due to heavy plaque and calculus deposits may require initial debridement followed by a waiting period of a few weeks to allow the inflammation in the lamina propria to subside. The tissues will then be more resistant to penetration by instruments, and more definitive treatment can then be given.

Most patients undergoing subgingival debridement require topical and/or local anesthesia (Palmer & Floyd, 1995). However, the patient must not have any allergy or sensitivity to the agent used. Two types of topical anesthetics are available: amide types, such as 5 or 10% lidocaine, and ester types, such as benzocaine (varied concentrations are available, but usually it is 20%). The possibility of allergic reactions is greater with lidocaine because it shows greater absorption into the systemic circulation than benzocaine. When a topical anesthetic is used, best results are obtained when a small amount is applied on a cotton-tip applicator, the tissues are dried prior to application of the agent, and the applicator is held in contact with the mucous membranes for 1 to 2 minutes. Alternatives include the use of an anesthetic patch, an anesthetic rinse, or electronic anesthesia. Topical anesthetic sprays should not be used because high doses of the agent can be absorbed into the circulatory system.

Local anesthesia is best applied by quadrant. It is recommended to treat one or two quadrants during a single visit depending on the number of teeth present as well as the degree of difficulty of the intervention. When two quadrants are treated during the same appointment, usual practice is to treat the upper and lower quadrants on either the right or the left side of the face. Both mandibular quadrants should not be treated during the same appointment so as to avoid patient discomfort and to prevent an inability on the part of the patient to control his or her mandible with both sides anesthetized.

Posttreatment care focuses on the prevention of dental plaque formation. A long-term plaque-free dentition is an unrealistic goal, and for this reason, periodic periodontal maintenance visits are required to monitor and identify disease recurrence (Westfelt, 1996).

Periodontal Debridement Procedures

Before debridement procedures are started, it is necessary to obtain a written informed consent from the patient. The procedure and its expected outcomes are explained to the patient. It is important for the patient to understand that the decreased probing depths primarily due to gingival shrinkage may cause gingival recession and "longer looking" teeth and that teeth may respond with hypersensitivity to cold, toothbrushing, or sweets. Such hypersensitivity is usually not permanent, but it may cause pain and discomfort that lasts for a few weeks to months.

Subgingival Debridement

Calculus Removal As periodontal debridement is started on a patient, the primary goal is to remove gross deposits from supragingival and subgingival tooth surfaces. The ultimate goal of subgingival debridement is to render a root surface free of plaque, calculus, and endotoxins to enable soft tissue healing. Complete calculus removal is essentially not attainable (Kepic, O'Leary, & Kafrawy, 1990), and total root smoothness is not necessary for adequate tissue healing. Clinical studies have shown that practitioners who spent an average of 12 to 15 minutes to complete the debridement of each tooth with hand and ultrasonic instruments fail to remove calculus from all surfaces. After debridement, about 47% of all nonfurcated surfaces and 63% of 6 mm or larger pockets showed residual calculus. Surgical access reduced the frequency of residual calculus to 20 and 38%, respectively. Teeth with furcations had a higher frequency of residual calculus, and surgical access did not provide any additional benefit (Buchanan & Robertson, 1987; Caffesse, Sweeney, & Smith, 1986; Fleischer, Mellonig, Brayer, Gray, & Barnett, 1989).

While total elimination of causative factors is an appropriate treatment goal, reduction of dental plaque and calculus below threshold levels appears to control the disease process and improve clinical signs of inflammation (Robertson, 1990), producing significant reductions in gingivitis, tooth loss, attachment loss, severity of disease, and probing depths (American Academy of Periodontology, 1997). Thus, if periodontal debridement can achieve elimination of inflammation and disease progression, then no further treatment is necessary. If periodontal debridement fails to achieve these objectives, then periodontal surgery may be necessary.

Root Surface Characteristics With the development of a gram-negative bacterial flora in the gingival crevice, events occur that eventually cause breakdown of the attachment apparatus. If elimination or disruption of the subgingival bacteria is not accomplished, rapid growth and maturation occur. During growth and after the death of subgingival gram-negative microorganisms, endotoxins or lipooligosaccharides are released from their cell walls. Endotoxins are highly toxic compounds that are capable of penetrating the junctional epithelium and entering the connective tissue, resulting in destruction of periodontal tissues. This causes loss of connective tissue attachment from the root surface, apical migration of the junctional epithelium, and bone loss. A periodontal pocket forms, and the root surface (cementum) becomes contaminated when exposed to this new subgingival pocket environment. The cementum is sufficiently porous to allow binding of endotoxins and colonization of dental plaque and calculus onto the altered root surfaces. Cementum that is rough and impregnated with calculus or contaminated with toxins or microorganisms and dentin is referred to as contaminated, altered, or necrotic cementum.

Cementum Removal The periodontal literature offers no firm conclusions about either the feasibility of or the need for removal of all contaminated cementum. In the past it was thought that the presence of cementum-bound endotoxins inhibited tissue healing after periodontal debridement. Much investigation has been directed toward the elimination of this contaminated or necrotic cementum. It is the consensus that endotoxins found on diseased root surfaces are weakly and superficially bound and that 99% may be removed by brushing (Moore, Wilson, & Kieser, 1986; Nakib, Bissada, Simmelnik, & Goldstine, 1982). The primary reason for removing the superficial layer of cementum by subgingival debridement is to remove plaque and calculus from the irregularities on the root surface. Extensive subgingival debridement for a prolonged amount of time is unnecessary (Cheetham, Wilson, & Kieser, 1988), and total removal of cementum is not the goal because the attachment of new soft tissue to the root surface is enhanced by the presence of cementum (Somerman, Archer, Shteyer, & Foster, 1987). O'Leary and Kafrawy (1983) concluded that total removal of cementum under routine clinical conditions is not a realistic objective of therapy. Smart, Wilson, Davies, and Kieser (1990), using ultrasonic instrumentation, showed that contaminated root surfaces could be rendered comparable to healthy teeth. Therefore, the key to periodontal therapy is the removal of plaque and calculus in order to reduce the number of oral bacteria below the threshold level capable of initiating inflammation (American Academy of Periodontology, 1997). Precisely how much cementum is removed as a result of root planing is uncertain.

Therefore, it is important to attain relatively smooth root surfaces only for the purpose of reducing plaque retention without excessive and unnecessary removal of cementum and dentin. The therapeutic goal of debridement therapy is to control bacterial infection as opposed to simply removing deposits from root surfaces.

Adverse Effects of Periodontal Debridement

Subgingival debridement may cause soft tissue recession, making the teeth look longer and exposing the root surface to the oral environment. This may result in dentinal hypersensitivity as a result of removal of the thin outer layer of cementum and exposure of the underlying dentin. Usually, teeth are not sensitive immediately after the periodontal debridement; hypersensitivity may take about 3 to 4 days to appear. Treatment of dentinal hypersensitivity is discussed in Chapter 22.

Limitations of Periodontal Debridement

Pocket Depth

The effectiveness of periodontal debridement depends on the effectiveness of the mechanical removal of dental plaque and calculus. Root debridement does not always remove all plaque and calculus from subgingival tooth surfaces. Studies have shown that considerable amounts (54 to 57%) of calculus remain on the root surfaces of teeth with moderate or advanced pockets and that more residual calculus is found on tooth surfaces with increasing probing depths (Wylam, Mealey, Mills, Waldrop, & Moskowicz, 1993). There was no significant difference whether an anterior or a posterior tooth was debrided (Sherman et al., 1990).

Current conclusions about the effectiveness of periodontal debridement in deeper pockets are conflicting, and there is as yet no agreement on whether non-surgical instrumentation is effective in advanced periodontal lesions (Forabosco, Galetti, Spinato, Colao, & Casolari, 1996). The most frequently lost teeth in patients receiving comprehensive periodontal treatment are the molars. Explanations for this relate to the difficulty in achieving adequate daily plaque removal and the difficulty in properly debriding molars. Stambaugh, Dragoo, Smith, and Carasali (1981) found that the average probing depth for "efficient" removal of plaque, calculus, and necrotic cementum was 3.73 mm. Rateitschak, Schwarz, Guggenheim, Duggelin, and Rateitschak (1992) found that surfaces where curets could reach usually were free of plaque and calculus, but in deep pockets the curet did not reach the base of the pocket. Consequently, modified curets with longer shanks were developed to increase treatment effectiveness in deeper pockets.

Furcations and Root Anatomy

Access for adequate instrumentation in the furcation area is often difficult, if not impossible, given the special anatomic characteristics of multirooted teeth (Fleischer et al., 1989; Greene, 1995). Pathogenic microbiota frequently persists in furcation lesions (Loos, Claffey, & Egelberg, 1988). Narrow furcation openings make periodontal debridement a challenge. Fifty-eight percent of molars have furcation entrance diameters that are smaller than the smallest diameter of a relatively new curet, which is 0.75 mm (Bower, 1979a; Parashis, Anagnon-Vareltzides, & Demetriou, 1990).

Knowledge about the morphology of the furcation area and the variations in root form and structure is important for effective instrumentation. Root concavities, which are depressions found on the proximal root surfaces, are plaque and calculus traps, making instrumentation extremely difficult. For instance, a deep mesial concavity is found on the maxillary first premolar. On the maxillary first molars, the mesiobuccal root has the greatest incidence of concavities, whereas both the mesio- and distobuccal roots of the mandibular first molars have concavities (Bower, 1979b; Fig. 25–1■). Moreover, any other root also may have root concavities.

Time Spent and Clinician Skill

Controversy exists over how much time should be spent on subgingival debridement. Subgingival debridement is sensitive to both technique and operator skill. Since endotoxins are just weakly bound to the root surface (Moore, Wilson, & Kieser, 1986), it is not necessary to spend a great deal of time debriding. However, a considerable amount of time still should be spent in effectively removing subgingival plaque, calculus, and necrotic cementum. If this procedure is done incorrectly, root gouging may occur, resulting in the production of grooves and pits in the root surface.

A clinical study (Anderson, Palmer, Bye, Smith, & Caffesse, 1996) evaluating single versus multiple episodes of subgingival instrumentation to determine effectiveness concluded that there was no significant difference between the two treatments. It was suggested that calculus remaining after one thorough episode of instrumenta-

Figure 25–1 Root morphology. Root concavities in the maxillary molar decrease the effectiveness of debridement.

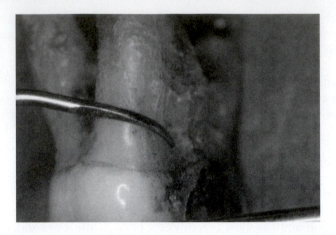

tion is not likely to be removed by repeated instrumentation. How much time is enough? Most researchers suggest that periodontal debridement should take at least 10 minutes per tooth (Lowenguth & Greenstein, 1995). Coldiron, Yukna, Weir, and Caudill (1990) found that cementum removal was generally achieved on periodontally healthy roots with 20 strokes of a curet, but residual calculus remained.

The results of a clinical study assessing periodontal debridement forces in periodontally involved molars show a broad range of forces being applied by the practitioner (Zappa, Röthlisberger, Simona, & Case, 1993). Additionally, the quality of periodontal debridement done on a molar may be primarily determined by the attitude of the practitioner, who subjectively treats the tooth according to his or her habits, rather than according to the characteristics of the root surfaces being treated (Zappa et al., 1993).

Most studies confirm that the more experienced the clinician, the more calculus-free the root surfaces were in deeper pockets and in hard-to-reach areas such as furcations (Brayer, Mellonig, Dunlap, Marinak, & Carson, 1989).

Healing Response and the Outcome of Therapy

Diseased Periodontal Unit

When a periodontal probe is inserted into the pocket of a diseased and inflamed pocket, the probe penetrates the tissue apical to the junctional (pocket) epithelium. This occurs because the connective tissue contains less collagen and more inflammatory cells. Once the periodontium is treated the thin junctional epithelium is closely adapted to the tooth or root surface and collagen replaces the inflammatory cells in the connective tissue. This is responsible for the increased resistance to probing force so that the probe tip stops at a more coronal level of the junctional epithelium than when inflammation was present.

Healing Periodontal Unit

An expected outcome of debridement is tissue healing. Healing results in tissue repair, shrinkage of gingival tissue, and the renewal of epithelial cells in contact with tooth surfaces (Caffesse, Mota, & Morrison, 1995; Caton, Nyman, & Zander, 1980).

Generally, the same healing features of periodontal tissues are seen following debridement of any chronically inflamed site. Initially, following debridement, there is an acute inflammatory reaction due to the traumatic nature of the therapy. This inflammation subsides within 24 to 48 hours. Over the next week, there is a gradual reduction of inflammatory cells, epithelial tissue healing, and finally, connective tissue maturation with collagen deposition.

Gingivitis: Healing after Periodontal Debridement

Histologically, in gingivitis, once dental plaque and calculus are removed, the pocket epithelium will reform into junctional epithelium and reattach to the adjacent tooth surface as it was in health. The inflammatory cells in the gingival connective tissue are replaced by collagen; this improvement results in an apparent "gain in clinical attachment."

Clinically, there is a reduction in or elimination of inflammation (e.g., bleeding) and the elimination of edema, both of which result in tissue shrinkage and occasionally gingival recession. Gingiva that is fibrotic will not shrink, as does edematous tissue. The gingiva often returns to its salmon pink color. The greatest reduction in probing depths occurs after 4 to 6 weeks and is primarily due to (1) tissue shrinkage, which may result in gingival recession, and (2) reformation of collagen, which results in greater resistance to probing (Fig. 25–2a■). The reductions obtained in probing depths as a result of nonsurgical therapy are in the range of 1 to 2 mm.

Periodontitis: Healing after Periodontal Debridement

Histologically, in periodontitis, after the removal of dental plaque, calculus, and necrotic cementum, some healing will occur. In most patients, healing occurs by repair rather than regeneration (e.g., formation of new bone, cementum, and periodontal ligament). Histologically, repair of the root epithelial interface has been described as a long junctional epithelial attachment that prevents the formation of a new connective tissue attachment (Cobb, 1996). Research has shown, however, that the presence of a long junctional epithelium does not represent an area of less resistance to infection (Beaumont, O'Leary, & Kafrawy, 1983; Caffesse et al., 1986). However, patients who are erratic in their compliance with oral hygiene self-care do not do as well with a long junctional epithelium as patients with complete compliance (Wilson, Schoen, & Fallon, 1989).

The pocket epithelium transforms back into junctional epithelium, which begins to reattach along the root surface between the gingival connective tissue and the root (Fig. 25–2b■). The formation of a long junctional epithelium results in closure of the pocket. This reestablishment of the junctional epithelium most likely occurs within 1 (Caton & Zander, 1979) or 2 (Waerhaug, 1978) weeks. The inflammatory cells in the gingival connective tissue are replaced by collagen, but a long junctional epithelium prevents the formation of a gingival connective tissue attachment (gingival fibers). The greatest reduction in probing depths and gain in clinical attachment level can be measured after 4 to 6 weeks (Barrington, 1981), although true gains in clinical attachment are seen primarily after periodontal surgery, if at all. Gains in clinical attachment level after treatment do not necessarily mean that

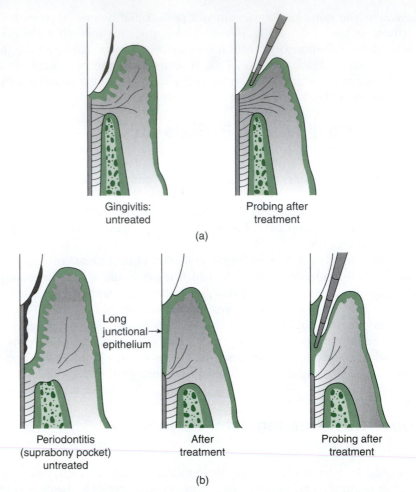

Figure 25–2   Healing of the gingival tissues after subgingival debridement. (a) In gingivitis, the tissues will heal, with approximation of the junctional epithelium to the tooth surface. (b) In periodontitis, after root planing, the tissues heal by formation of a long junctional epithelial attachment to the root surface.

new gingival connective tissue attachment has been achieved (Armitage, 1996). It may simply indicate that the probe is more resistant to penetration once the gingival collagen has reformed and that the probe tip when placed into the gingival crevice stops at a more *coronal* location of the junctional epithelium. This gives the appearance of a gain in clinical attachment when it actually may not be. It is the distance between the base of the periodontal pocket (before treatment) and the tip of the periodontal probe when placed into the crevice (after treatment). A true gain in clinical attachment after periodontal treatment indicates that a new connective tissue attachment (collagen fibers inserting) to the root has occurred.

Residual or undetected calculus that instrumentation has failed to remove is often present. Despite incomplete calculus removal, Sherman and colleagues (1990) showed that sites still could respond favorably. Haffajee and colleagues (1997) found that periodontal debridement demonstrated clinical improvement in subjects with chronic periodontitis even though only modest changes in subgingival microbiota were seen. This suggests potential targets for therapy and indicates that radical alterations in subgingival microbiota may not be necessary.

Reevaluation of Initial Therapy: Tissue Response

After appropriate initial therapy, a planned reevaluation should assess the current state of health or disease. The treatment sequence for the reevaluation appointment consists of a medical history update, a soft tissue examination, a plaque index, determination of the presence of bleeding, an oral hygiene self-care evaluation, and periodontal probing. Pretreatment findings are compared with the current status of the patient. It is important to evaluate and emphasize the patient's oral hygiene self-care techniques. Controversy exists regarding the recommended time interval between the initial therapy and the reevaluation appointment. Recommendations range from a minimum of 2 weeks to a maximum of 6 weeks after periodontal debridement to allow for tissue healing, although waiting longer than 6 weeks may augment the healing response. A shorter time period may be indicated if the patient has been classified as a potential surgical patient. If results of initial therapy show improvement, but with some residual 5-mm probing depths, the patient should be placed on periodontal maintenance and reevaluated in a few months. Reevaluation at regular intervals is essential to alert the dental hygienist to areas where plaque control has failed and inflammation has returned. Unstable sites should be retreated or monitored closely for signs of attachment loss. At the reevaluation appointment, a decision is made regarding whether the patient qualifies for surgical intervention, continues with initial therapy, or is placed on a periodontal maintenance schedule. Factors that may influence this decision include the overall treatment plan, including restorative procedures, as well as the desires of the patient.

Reevaluation includes an examination of the gingival tissues. If inflammation persists, which is apparent clinically as bleeding on probing and redness, the cause needs to be determined. Persistent inflammation may result from incomplete debridement, patient noncompliance with home care, or a systemic disease. The desired microbial response is a change in the composition of the bacteria found within the pocket from a pathogenic Gram-negative species (e.g., spirochetes, *P. gingivalis, P. intermedia*) to a more beneficial Gram-positive species such as cocci or nonmotile bacteria (Mousques, Listgarten, & Phillips, 1980).

Ultrasonic versus Hand-Activated Instrumentation

Studies comparing hand- and power-driven scalers are difficult to assess because of the wide variety of study designs. With the advent of modified periodontal inserts, subgingival root debridement became possible. Most studies have had comparable results with hand- and power-driven scalers when considering residual plaque and calculus. The ultimate determinant of treatment success with power-driven scalers (e.g., ultrasonics and sonics) is observation of the response of the tissues. Posttreatment evaluation consists of monitoring the soft tissue response and determining the critical levels of periodontal pathogenic organisms present within the gingival crevice. Thus, the outcome of scaling and root planing is similar for hand-activated instrumentation and power-driven scalers.

It has been documented that ultrasonic scalers with modified tips produced smoother roots with less damage, better access to the base of the pocket, and superior plaque and calculus removal than hand-activated instruments and also required less time (Dragoo, 1992; Kocher & Plagmann, 1997).

Comparing manual and ultrasonic instrumentation of deep pockets (6–9 mm), it was found that both methods were equal in reducing total microbial counts and colony-forming units (Oosterwal, Matee, Mikx, van't Hof, & Renggli, 1987). However, Leon and Vogel (1987) found that ultrasonic instrumentation was more effective at reducing spirochetes and motile rods when treating advanced bone loss in furcations. Thus, the tissue healing response is similar with manual and ultrasonic instrumentation.

Summary

The philosophy of periodontal therapy has changed over the past decade as a result of further understanding of the disease process. Therapy is based on up-to-date clinical and microbial studies. The decision to perform periodontal debridement as a definitive treatment should depend on the severity of periodontal disease, the inflammatory status of the gingiva, the treatment objectives of the dental hygienist, treatment time, and the skill of the operator (Lowenguth & Greenstein, 1995).

Selection of the proper instrument involves considering the following factors: the amount of calculus, the type of tissue tone (e.g., firm, edematous, or hard and fibrotic), probing depths (or type of disease present), root morphology, and location of the calculus. Root smoothness is no longer the main criterion for periodontal instrumentation, although all detectable deposits should be removed so as to achieve a successful soft tissue response. The primary goal of periodontal debridement is to make the root and the soft tissue biologically compatible (Wilson et al., 1989). In most cases, periodontal debridement improves clinical parameters, decreasing both gingival inflammation (evidenced by less bleeding) and probing depths. Improvements in microbial parameters are transient, and the microbiota soon return to pretreatment levels. Therefore, the patient requires continuous maintenance or plaque control. Both periodontal debridement and daily plaque removal by the patient are equally important for the maintenance of periodontal health and will continue to be the standard of periodontal therapy. Healing after nonsurgical therapy (scaling/root planing) is clinical/histologically complete at about 3 to 6 months after final instrumentation. Clinically, there should be less number of bleeding sites, more soft tissue recession, and a gain of clinical attachment as seen by an increased resistance of the probe.

Key Points

- Successful periodontal treatment, maintenance of periodontal health, and the regeneration of periodontal tissues depend on the removal of supra- and subgingival deposits.
- Oral hygiene self-care and mechanical subgingival instrumentation are indicated in the treatment of inflammatory periodontal diseases to reduce inflammation and microbial levels. The clinical end point to periodontal debridement is a good tissue healing response.
- Periodontal debridement has been shown to disrupt or alter the subgingival microbiota, thus slowing down repopulation.
- Although meticulous debridement may remove some cementum, the intentional, aggressive removal of diseased cementum does not seem to be nec-

essary; endotoxins are loosely attached to the root surface and can be removed easily.

- The type of healing occurring after subgingival debridement is a long junctional epithelium attachment to the root surface, which is considered to be a type of repair.

Self-Quiz

1. Which one of the following healing responses is seen in gingivitis after periodontal debridement? (p. 429)

    a. formation of new bone, cementum, and periodontal ligament

    b. formation of new cementum and periodontal ligament

    c. reattachment of the junctional epithelium

    d. reattachment of the alveolar mucosa

2. Which one of the following healing responses is seen in periodontitis after periodontal debridement? (p. 429)

    a. reattachment of the sulcular epithelium

    b. reattachment of the desmosomes

    c. formation of new bone, cementum, and periodontal ligament

    d. formation of a long junctional epithelium

3. Which one of the following definitions describes a gain in clinical attachment after periodontal debridement? (p. 430)

    a. bone fill and formation of new cementum

    b. improved gingival tone and reattachment of the junctional epithelium

    c. improved gingival tone and increased mature collagen fibers

    d. gingival recession, bone fill, and establishment of a new periodontal ligament attachment

4. After periodontal debridement, on which one of the following does clinical success depend? (p. 431)

    a. amount of time spent on the procedure

    b. number of quadrants completed

    c. total removal of calculus

    d. tissue response

5. Which one of the following benefits is seen after subgingival debridement? (p. 422)

    a. disruption of the Gram-negative microbial flora

    b. repopulation of Gram-negative anaerobic flora

    c. removal of Gram-positive facultative flora

    d. interference with attachment of Gram-positive anaerobic flora to root surfaces

References

American Academy of Periodontology. 1997. Treatment of gingivitis and periodontitis. *J. Periodontol.* 68:1246–1253.

American Academy of Periodontology. 2003. *Glossary of periodontal terms,* 4th ed. Chicago: Author.

American Dental Hygienist's Association. 1995. *A position paper on selective tooth polishing.* Chicago: Author.

Anderson, G. B., J. Palmer, F. Bye, B. Smith, and R. Caffesse. 1996. Effectiveness of subgingival scaling and root planing: Single versus multiple episodes of instrumentation. *J. Periodontol.* 67:367–373.

Armitage, G. C. 1996. Periodontal diseases: Diagnosis. *Ann. Periodontol.* 1:37–215.

Barrington, E. P. 1981. An overview of periodontal surgical procedures. *J. Periodontol.* 52:697–702.

Beaumont, R., T. O'Leary, and A. Kafrawy. 1984. Relative resistance of long junctional epithelial adhesions and connective tissue attachments to plaque-induced inflammation. *J. Periodontol.* 55:213–223.

Bower, R. C. 1979a. Furcation morphology relative to periodontal treatment: Furcation entrance architecture. *J. Periodontol.* 50:23–27.

Bower, R. C. 1979b. Furcation morphology relative to periodontal treatment: Furcation root surface anatomy. *J. Periodontol.* 50:366–374.

Brayer, W. K., J. T. Mellonig, R. M. Dunlap, K. W. Marinak, and R. E. Carson. 1989. Scaling and root planing effectiveness: The effect of root surface access and operator experience. *J. Periodontol.* 60:67–72.

Buchanan, S. A., and P. S. Robertson. 1987. Calculus removal by scaling and root planing with and without surgical access. *J. Periodontol.* 58:159–163.

Caffesse, R. G., L. F. Mota, and E. D. Morrison. 1995. The rationale for periodontal therapy. *Periodontology 2000.* 9:7–13.

Caffesse, R. G., P. L. Sweeney, and B. A. Smith. 1986. Scaling and root planing with and without periodontal flap surgery. *J. Clin. Periodontol.* 13:205–210.

Caton, J., S. Nyman, and H. Zander. 1980. Histometric evaluation of periodontal surgery: II. Connective tissue attachment after four regenerative procedures. *J. Clin. Periodontol.* 7:224–231.

Caton, J., and H. Zander. 1979. The attachment between tooth and gingival tissues after periodontic root planing and soft tissue curettage. *J. Periodontol.* 50:462–466.

Cheetham, W. A., M. Wilson, and J. B. Kieser. 1988. Root surface debridement: An in vitro assessment. *J. Clin. Periodontol.* 15:288–292.

Ciancio, S. G. 1989. Non-surgical periodontal treatment. In eds. M. Nevins, W. Becker, and K. Kornman, *Proceedings of the World Workshop in Clinical Periodontics,* Vol. 2, 1–22. Chicago: American Academy of Periodontology.

Cobb, C. M. 1996. Non-surgical pocket therapy: Mechanical. *Ann. Periodontol.* 1:443–490.

Coldiron, N. B., R. A. Yukna, J. Weir, and R. F. Caudill. 1990. A quantitative study of cementum removal with hand curettes. *J. Periodontol.* 61:293–299.

Dahlen, G., J. Lindhe, K. Sato, H. Hanamura, and H. Okamoto. 1992. The effect of supragingival plaque control on the subgingival microbiota in subjects with periodontal disease. *J. Clin. Periodontol.* 19:802–809.

Dragoo, M. R. 1992. A clinical evaluation of hand and ultrasonic instruments on subgingival debridement: I. With unmodified and modified ultrasonic scalers. *Int. J. Periodont. Rest. Dent.* 12:310–323.

Fleischer, H. C., J. T. Mellonig, W. K. Brayer, J. L. Gray, and J. D. Barnett. 1989. Scaling and root planing efficacy in multirooted teeth. *J. Periodontol.* 60:402–409.

Forabosco, A., R. Galetti, S. Spinato, P. Colao, and C. Casolari. 1996. A comparative study of a surgical method and scaling and root planing using Odontoson. *J. Clin. Periodontol.* 23:611–614.

Greene, P. R. 1995. Non-surgical periodontal therapy: Essential and adjunctive methods. *Br. Dent. J.* 179:28–34.

Haffajee, A. D., M. A. Cugini, S. Dibart, C. Smith, L. R. Kent, Jr., and S. S. Socransky. 1997. The effect of scaling and root planing on the clinical and microbiological parameters of periodontal diseases. *J. Clin. Periodontol.* 24:324–334.

Jacobson, L., J. Blomlöf, and S. Lindskog. 1994. Root surface texture after different scaling modalities. *Scand. J. Dent. Res.* 102:156–160.

Kaldahl, W. B., K. L. Kalkwarf, D. Kashinath, D. Patil, M. P. Molvar, and J. K. Dyer. 1996. Long-term evaluation of periodontal therapy: I. Response to four therapeutic modalities. *J. Periodontol.* 67:93–102.

Kalkwarf, K. L. 1989. Tissue attachment. In eds. M. Nevins, W. Becker, and K. Kornman, *Proceedings of the World Workshop in Clinical Periodontics,* Vol. 5, 1–21. Chicago: American Academy of Periodontology.

Katsanoulas, T., I. Renee, and R. Attström. 1992. The effect of supragingival plaque control on the composition of the subgingival flora in periodontal pockets. *J. Clin. Periodontol.* 19:760–765.

Kepic, T. J., T. J. O'Leary, and A. H. Kafrawy. 1990. Total calculus removal: An attainable objective? *J. Periodontol.* 61:16–20.

Kocher, T., and H. C. Plagmann. 1997. The diamond-coated sonic scaler tip: Part II: Loss of substance and alteration of root surface texture after different scaling modalities. *Int. J. Periodontics Restorative Dent.* 17(5):484–493.

Leon, L. E., and R.I. Vogel. 1987. A comparison of the effectiveness of hand scaling and ultrasonic debridement in furcations as evaluated by differential dark-field microscopy. *J Periodontol.* 58:86–94.

Lindhe, J., S. S. Socransky, S. Nyman, and A. Haffajee. 1982. Critical probing depth. *J. Clin. Periodontol.* 9:323–336.

Loos, B., N. Claffey, and J. Egelberg. 1988. Clinical and microbiological effects of subgingival debridement in periodontal furcation pockets. *J. Clin. Periodontol.* 15:453–463.

Lowenguth, R. A., and G. Greenstein. 1995. Clinical and microbiological response to nonsurgical mechanical periodontal therapy. *Periodontology 2000.* 9:14–22.

Magnusson, I., J. Lindhe, T. Yoneyama, and B. Liljenberg. 1984. Recolonization of a subgingival microbiota following scaling in deep pockets. *J. Clin. Periodontol.* 11:193–207.

Moore, J., M. Wilson, and J. B. Kieser. 1986. The distribution of bacterial lipopolysaccharide (endotoxins) in relation to periodontal involved root surfaces. *J. Clin. Periodontol.* 13:748–751.

Mousques, T., M. A. Listgarten, and R. W. Phillips. 1980. Effect of scaling and root planing on the composition of the human subgingival microbial flora. *J. Periodont. Res.* 15:144–151.

Nakib, N. M., N. F. Bissada, J. W. Simmelnik, and S. N. Goldstine. 1982. Endotoxin penetration into root cementum of periodontally healthy and diseased human teeth. *J. Periodontol.* 53:368–378.

Oberholzer, R., and K. H. Rateitschak. 1996. Root cleaning or root smoothing: An in vivo study. *J. Clin. Periodontol.* 23:326–330.

O'Hehir, T. E. 1999. Debridement 5 scaling and root planing plus. *RDH.* 14, 62.

O'Leary, T. J., and A. D. Kafrawy. 1983. Total cementum removal: A realistic objective. *J. Periodontol.* 54:221–226.

Oosterwaal, P. J., M. I. Matee, F. H. Mikx, M. A. van't Hof, and H. H. Renggli. 1987. The effect of subgingival debridement with hand and ultrasonic instruments on the subgingival microbflora. *J Clin Periodontol.* 14:528–533.

Palmer, R. M., and F. D. Floyd. 1995. Periodontology: A clinical approach: 3. Non-surgical treatment and maintenance. *Br. Dent. J.* 178:263–268.

Parashis, A. O., A. Anagnou-Vareltzides, and N. Demetriou. 1990. Calculus removal from multirooted teeth with and without surgical access: II. Comparison between external and furcation surfaces and effect of furcation entrance width. *J. Clin. Periodontol.* 20:294–298.

Rateitschak, P., J. Schwarz, R. Guggenheim, M. Duggelin, and K. Rateitschak. 1992. Nonsurgical periodontal treatment: Where are the limits? An SEM study. *J. Clin. Periodontol.* 19:240–244.

Renvert, S., M. Wikström, G. Dahlen, J. Slots, and J. Egelberg. 1990. Effect of subgingival debridement on the elimination of *Actinobacillus actinomycetemcomitans* and *Bacteroides gingivalis* from periodontal pockets. *J. Clin. Periodontol.* 17:345–350.

Robertson, P. B. 1990. The residual calculus paradox. *J. Periodontol.* 61:65–66.

Sbordone, L., L. Ramaglia, E. Gulletta, and V. Iacono. 1990. Recolonization of the subgingival microbiota after scaling and root planing in human periodontitis. *J. Periodontol.* 61:579–584.

Sherman, P. R., L. H. Hutchens, Jr., L. G. Jewson, J. M. Moriarty, G. W. Greco, and W. T. McFall, Jr. 1990. The effectiveness of subgingival scaling and root planing: I. Clinical detection of residual calculus. *J. Periodontol.* 61:3–8.

Smart, G. J., M. Wilson, E. H. Davies, and J. B. Kieser. 1990. The assessment of ultrasonic root surface debridement by determination of residual endotoxins levels. *J. Clin. Periodontol.* 17:174–178.

Somerman, M. J., S. Y. Archer, A. Shteyer, and R. A. Foster. 1987. Protein production by human gingival fibroblasts is enhanced by guanidine EDTA extracts of cementum. *J. Periodont. Res.* 22:75–77.

Stambaugh, R. V., M. Dragoo, D. M. Smith, and L. Carasali. 1981. The limits of subgingival scaling. *Int. J. Periodont. Restor. Dent.* 1(5):31–41.

Waerhaug, J. 1978. Healing of the dentoepithelial junction following subgingival plaque control: II. As observed on extracted teeth. *J. Periodontol.* 49:119–134.

Westfelt, E. 1996. Rationale of mechanical plaque control. *J. Clin. Periodontol.* 23:263–267.

Westfelt, E., H. Rylander, G. Dahlen, and J. Lindhe. 1998. The effect of supragingival plaque control on the progression of advanced periodontal disease. *J. Clin. Periodontol.* 25:536–541.

Wilson, T. G., Jr., J. Schoen, and P. Fallon. 1989. Removing tooth-borne dental deposits: Mechanical means by the professional. In ed. T. G. Wilson, Jr., Dental maintenance for patients with periodontal diseases, 67–96. Chicago: Quintessence.

Wylam, J. M., B. L. Mealey, M. P. Mills, T. C. Waldrop, and D. C. Moskowicz. 1993. The clinical effectiveness of open versus closed scaling and root planing on multirooted teeth. *J. Periodontol.* 64:1023–1028.

Zappa, U., J. P. Röthlisberger, C. Simona, and D. Case. 1993. In vivo scaling and root planing forces in molars. *J. Periodontol.* 64:349–354.

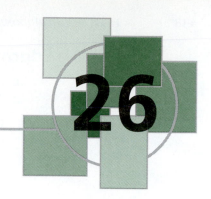

Principles of Periodontal Surgery: Gingivectomy, Osseous Resection, and Periodontal Plastic Surgery

Stuart J. Froum, D.D.S.

Outline

KEY WORDS

- periodontal surgery
- periodontal diseases
- healing
- gingivectomy
- flap surgery
- mucogingival surgery
- periodontal dressing
- postoperative care

Goal

To provide an understanding of the basic indications and principles of periodontal surgery and post-operative care.

Educational Objectives

Upon completion of this chapter, the reader should be able to:

Discuss the rationale for periodontal surgical therapy.

Describe the indications and contraindications for periodontal surgical therapy.

Compare and contrast the currently accepted surgical treatment modalities.

Demonstrate postoperative care following periodontal surgery.

Identify and explain the management of postoperative complications.

Discuss surgical wound healing and how soon after surgery a reevaluation can be performed.

The term "surgery" is a generic word to describe the branch of medical science concerned with the treatment of diseases or injuries by manual or operative means. Periodontal debridement (scaling and root planing) meets this definition, but it is not considered surgery. Periodontal surgery, as used in the dental literature, is applied only to surgical procedures used to treat periodontal diseases or to modify the morphology of soft tissues and bone.

Different surgical procedures have been proposed to treat gingivitis and periodontitis, as well as to gain access to the underlying root surface and supporting bone. The most common surgical procedures include the gingivectomy and the apically positioned flap with or without osseous (bone) resection.

Objectives, Indications, and Contraindications of Periodontal Surgery

Over the past several years, root instrumentation techniques and local and systemic antibiotic periodontal therapy have improved dramatically. Nevertheless, periodontal surgery remains a valid option for many patients. It is imperative for the dental hygienist to have a thorough knowledge of various basic periodontal surgical procedures as well as a clear understanding of the indications and contraindications of these procedures. This is particularly important upon consideration of the limitations of scaling and root planning. Egelberg (1995) reviewed these limitations, which include the fact that complete removal of subgingival calculus may not be predictably attainable after subgingival root planning. This was demonstrated in one study in which pockets with initial probing depths of ≥ 5 mm showed inadequately debrided root 65% of the time (Greenstein, 2000).

The primary objectives of periodontal surgery include the following (Palcanis, 1996):

1. Reduction in the pocket depth, which allows the patient and the dental practitioner access for plaque control.
2. The aim is not necessarily to eliminate the pocket (e.g., in patients with very deep pockets and bone loss) but to gain access to the root and underlying bone to achieve more effective removal of calculus and subgingi-

val bacterial biofilm so as to maintain periodontal attachment levels and perhaps even gain "new attachment." New attachment is defined as the union of connective tissue with a root surface that has been deprived previously of its original attachment apparatus (American Academy of Periodontology, 2001).

3. To regenerate periodontal tissues lost due to the disease.
4. To arrest disease progression.
5. To create an oral environment that is maintainable by both the patient and the dental team.

After the surgical procedures have been performed, the therapeutic end points of clinical success are measured by the attainment of stable or improved clinical attachment levels, minimal inflammation (bleeding on probing), and reduced and stable probing depths (Palcanis, 1996).

Indications for periodontal surgery include the following:

1. Pocket elimination/reduction on teeth with gingival/periodontal pockets;
2. Correction of mucogingival defects (e.g., for root coverage, increasing the zone of keratinized/attached gingiva, augmentation of alveolar ridges);
3. To improve aesthetics; that is esthetic crown lengthening
4. Creation of a favorable restorative environment such as lengthening of the clinical crown;
5. Placement of dental implants;
6. Incision and drainage of a gingival or periodontal abscess; and
7. Regeneration of the attachment apparatus that was destroyed as a result of periodontal disease.

Periodontal surgical therapy is contraindicated or at least delayed for the following reasons:

1. Systemic diseases that cannot be controlled by medications or otherwise, such as diabetes mellitus, cardiovascular conditions (e.g., hypertension), or in immunodeficiency diseases (e.g., HIV infection) (in these patients, a medical consultation with the patient's physician is warranted).
2. Systemic diseases that are associated with excessive bleeding, such as leukemia, hemophilia, and renal (kidney) dialysis (consult with the patient's physician).
3. Patients taking anticoagulation medication (Coumadin, heparin), which would result in extensive and difficult-to-control bleeding.
4. Patients who are mentally unable to undergo periodontal surgery.
5. Patients who are noncompliant with plaque control or periodontal maintenance appointments.
6. Concern for cosmetic outcome (i.e., postsurgical gingival shrinkage), especially in anterior areas.
7. Treating teeth that have hopeless prognoses.

Preoperative Preparation

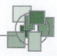

Preoperative management involving patient preparation for surgery includes removal of soft and hard deposits, reinforcement of oral hygiene self-care, selective occlusal adjustment, and selective adjunctive antimicrobial or antibiotic agents. It is important to complete initial therapy because this may eliminate the need for surgery or at least reduce or eliminate gingival inflammation, which will increase the manageability of the tissues during surgery and allow for better healing. Evaluation for surgery is done at a minimum of 4 to 6 weeks after completion of the initial phase of therapy. At this time, a soft tissue examination will determine the tissue healing or response to the initial therapy. An evaluation of the patient's oral hygiene status also is made. If there is residual calculus, additional sessions of periodontal debridement may be necessary. A complete periodontal charting is done, including identification and cause of bleeding sites and sites with clinical attachment loss (Carranza, 1996).

Requirements for Periodontal Surgery

Specific requirements must be met before surgery is performed. Any uncontrolled or poorly controlled systemic disease (i.e., diabetes) should be addressed by referring the patient to their physician prior to surgery. Elimination of plaque-retentive restorations should be performed before surgery (e.g., overhanging margins of restorations or overcontoured restorations) (Flores-de-Jacoby & Mengel, 1995). Any carious lesions should be repaired and hopeless teeth extracted. Necessary endodontic treatment should be performed prior to periodontal therapy. The hygienist and dentist should recommend a smoking cessation program to the patient prior to surgery. Risk factors such as smoking have been shown to delay wound healing after surgery (Boström, Linder, & Bergström, 1998; Preber & Bergström, 1990), and this may need to be addressed with the patient.

Types of Periodontal Surgery

There are many types of surgical procedures, and selection of the appropriate surgery depends on the pattern of bone loss (e.g., horizontal vs. vertical or a combination of both) and the presence of mucogingival involvement. Periodontal surgery usually is done in quadrants or sextants depending on the number of teeth involved and the decision of the surgeon. Most important, the practitioner and the patient should be aware of the limitations of periodontal surgery (Table 26–1■).

Lang and Löe (1993) proposed a convenient classification of periodontal surgical procedures. It includes five categories:

1. Procedures for pocket reduction or elimination (gingivectomy)
2. Procedures for gaining access to root surfaces for debridement (periodontal flap surgery)

Table 26–1	Limitations of Periodontal Surgery

- Periodontal surgery does not compensate for the patient's poor plaque control.
- Some adverse effects from surgery include gingival recession, which may compromise aesthetics to some degree.
- It will not routinely produce miraculous and complete regeneration of all lost periodontal tissues.

3. Procedures for treatment of osseous defects (flap surgery with osseous reduction)
4. Procedures for correcting mucogingival defects (periodontal plastic surgery)
5. Procedures for regeneration of lost periodontium (periodontal regeneration)

Healing Following Periodontal Surgery

There are four types of healing responses of periodontal tissues that can occur after periodontal treatment (Carranza, 1996). Repair is the healing of periodontal tissues with tissues that do not replicate the original lost periodontium. After periodontal surgery and periodontal debridement, instead of the gingival connective tissue attaching to the tooth, the junctional epithelium reforms on the root surface by migrating along the root surface, forming a long junctional epithelium attachment. Another example of repair is scar formation, in which the new tissue formed is considered epithelium and connective tissue but does not replicate the original tissue that was lost or damaged. Reattachment is the reunion of epithelial or connective tissue to a root surface that was not damaged by periodontal disease. This would occur after an incision, or injury, or where a surgical flap has to be extended to a tooth with a healthy periodontium for better access. New attachment is the union of connective tissue or epithelium with a root surface that was deprived of its original attachment apparatus. This new attachment can include new periodontal ligament, cementum, or bone, but only two of the three tissues. Regeneration is the reformation of the periodontal tissues that were destroyed by periodontal disease with the formation of new cementum, periodontal ligament, and bone. This is the ideal treatment result and is the goal of various surgical procedures. However, it is not always attained. Rather, a partial regeneration or new attachment is more often obtained. Epithelium is the first tissue to move or migrate into the wound area. Epithelium migrates up to 0.5 mm a day, which is faster than connective tissue or bone cells. This can interfere with the formation of a new attachment or regeneration.

Procedures for Pocket Reduction/Elimination

Gingivectomy/Gingivoplasty

Definition   Gingivectomy is the excision or removal of the soft tissue walls (gingiva) in order to eliminate a pocket. Gingivoplasty, on the other hand, refers to surgical reshaping or recontouring of the oral surface of the gingiva without removing any portion of the gingiva that is attached to the tooth.

Indications   The main objectives of gingivectomy/gingivoplasty procedures are to reduce or eliminate suprabony periodontal pockets that are associated with horizontal patterns of bone loss and to eliminate pseudopockets (gingival overgrowth) induced by certain medications, such as phenytoin, cyclosporine, valproic acid, and nifedipine. Enlarged gingiva and interdental papillae seen in mouth breathers also can be treated with these techniques. Oftentimes, localized or generalized gingival enlargement is seen during pregnancy, which may or may not resolve postpartum. Surgery in these cases, unless the gingival overgrowth becomes infected or interferes with chewing, is delayed until a reevaluation is made postpartum. Frequently, the gingival enlargement will recur, and gingivectomy procedures may have to be repeated. Less frequently, lengthening of the clinical crown can be achieved using gingivectomy.

Contraindications   Contraindications for gingivectomy include lack of attached gingiva and the presence of infrabony pockets associated with vertical bone loss.

Technique   After the patient receives local anesthesia, the gingivectomy is begun by marking the base of the pockets with a periodontal probe or other instrument. Incisions are made with a surgical blade angled at 45 degrees to the gingiva slightly coronal to the base of the pocket (Fig. 26–1■). Incisions are not made into the sulcus, but rather on the outer epithelium, with the blade directed in an occlusal or incisal direction rather than apically. Root debridement is performed followed by gingivoplasty to reestablish a physiologic gingiva. After hemostasis is obtained (bleeding is controlled), the area is dried, and a periodontal dressing is placed. The patient is given postoperative instructions. A sample of postoperative instructions to the patient for any surgical procedure is given in Table 26–2■. This includes care of the surgical wound, oral hygiene measures taken during initial healing, and reporting adverse signs and symptoms. The dental hygienist's role in postoperative care is reviewed in Table 26–3■. The patient then returns in 1 week for a postoperative visit.

Healing Epithelialization of the wound surface starts within a few days of surgery and usually takes 7–14 days depending on the size of the wound. Soft tissue healing is completed within 4 to 5 weeks, although clinically it may appear healed within 2 weeks. Clinically it is important to avoid probing the area until the connective tissue has healed.

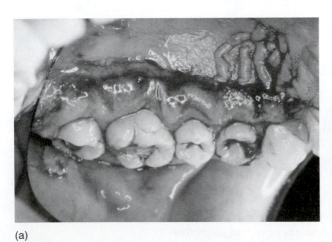
(a)

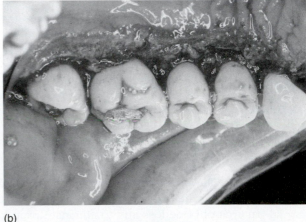
(b)

Figure 26–1   (a) Clinical picture of a gingivectomy procedure. A 38-year-old patient with pseudopockets (gingival enlargement) due to phenytoin therapy. The incision is made apical to the bleeding points, which demarcate the base of the pocket. (b) After the incision is made, the tissue is removed, exposing the underlying bleeding connective tissue.

Table 26–2	Postoperative Instructions
Discomfort	Usually minimal discomfort is expected, especially after the anesthesia wears off. If you have been given a prescription, fill it and take the medication as directed. Aspirin should not be used. If discomfort persists, call the office.
Swelling	If swelling occurs, it will peak 48 to 72 hours after the surgery. You may use an ice pack on the outside of your face, 15 minutes on and 15 minutes off, for the next 2 hours. If swelling occurs after the first day, a moistened heated towel may be used on the area. If excessive swelling occurs, call the office.
Bleeding	There may be occasional blood stains in the saliva for the first 4 or 5 hours. This is not unusual; do not be alarmed. If bleeding continues, do not rinse to stop bleeding. Apply firm pressure using a moistened gauze pad or fresh tea bag for 20 minutes, without interruption. Repeat as necessary. If the bleeding does not stop, call the office.
Physical activity	It is recommended that you rest and limit your activities for the rest of the day. Avoid excessive exertion (jogging, swimming, tennis, etc.) for the next week.
Eating	Limit your diet to soft foods on the day of the surgery. Do not drink hot liquids (tea, coffee, soup) for 24 hours following surgery. Do not chew on the area where the surgery was performed. Avoid alcoholic beverages for 1 week following the surgery.
Sutures	If sutures were used, avoid that area. They will be removed approximately 7 to 14 days following surgery.
Dressing	To help minimize irritation, a periodontal dressing may be placed around the surgical area. It will harden within about 2 hours and should not be removed. It is of no concern if a few pieces of the dressing break off. However, if the dressing seems to be loose or has come off, contact the office for instructions.
Smoking	Do not smoke. Smoking may negatively affect the healing process, which may result in a poor outcome.
Home care	The most important element required for good healing is meticulous oral hygiene. If a dressing is placed, avoid pressing down on it. Use a soft or ultrasoft toothbrush to carefully clean the occlusal surface and the surface of the dressing. If no dressing was placed, gently use a soft or ultrasoft toothbrush to cleanse the area. Do not floss the surgical site. Brush and floss the untreated areas as usual. Do not rinse on the day of the surgery. On the second day, use the prescribed mouth rinse as directed.
Medications	In some cases, medications will be prescribed. Use prescribed medications as directed.

Periodontal Flap Surgery

A flap is defined as that loosened portion of the gingiva, alveolar mucosa, and/or periosteum that is separated from the underlying structures except at its base, from which the flap receives its blood supply. Flaps are the most commonly used periodontal surgical procedure. Flap procedures are designed to gain access to the underlying bone and root surface for the purpose of debridement, bone recontouring, or regeneration. Generally, a flap is made by an incision with a surgical blade or knife into the pocket (intracrevicular) or slightly subgingival to the gingival margin

Table 26–3	Surgical Care Procedures	
Surgical Procedure	**Postoperative Care**	**Reevaluation Procedures**
Gingivectomy	1. Instruct patient not to brush the area where the periodontal dressing is located. 2. At postoperative visit, carefully remove the dressing, irrigate with sterile water or saline and wipe off the white film (this consists of dead epithelial cells). 3. Reapply dressing if needed. 4. Patient may start to brush surgical site gently with a roll technique. Bleeding will occur but will gradually lessen. The patient should continue to brush even if light bleeding is seen.	1. Periodontal probing should not be done until a minimum of 6 weeks after surgery. 2. Final prosthetic restorations should not be completed until 6 weeks or more after surgery. 3. Supragingival scaling can be done after 1 week, but subgingival periodontal debridement should not be performed until 6 weeks after surgery.
Flap surgery	1. Instruct patient not to brush the area where the periodontal dressing is located. 2. At postoperative visit, carefully remove the dressing, irrigate with sterile water or saline and wipe off the white film (this consists of dead epithelial cells). 3. Reapply dressing if needed; patient may start to brush surgical site gently with a roll technique. Bleeding will occur but will gradually lessen. The patient should continue to brush even if bleeding is seen. 4. Avoid smoking.	1. Periodontal probing should not be done until a minimum of 3 months after surgery. 2. Final prosthetic restorations should not be completed until a minimum of 3 months after surgery. 3. Supragingival scaling can be done after 1 week, but subgingival periodontal debridement should not be performed until 3 months after surgery.
Mucogingival surgery	1. Instruct patient not to brush the area where the periodontal dressing is located. 2. At postoperative visit, carefully remove the dressing, irrigate with sterile water or saline and wipe off the white film (this consists of dead epithelial cells). 3. Avoid smoking. 4. Reapply dressing if needed; patient may start to brush surgical site gently with a roll technique. Advise the patient not to hit the gums with the toothbrush. The patient discontinue brushing if bleeding is seen and only rinse the area with warm water.	1. Gingival grafts with root coverage would be reevaluated a minimum of 6 months after surgery. 2. Gingival grafts without root coverage can be reevaluated a minimum of 2 months after surgery.

(internal bevel incision). The amount of attached gingiva present and the depth of the pockets primarily determine the type of incision made. The flap is then reflected away from the tooth with an instrument called a periosteal elevator to expose the underlying tooth and root surface.

Flap Classification

Flaps are classified on the basis of tissue components included in the flap and the positioning of the flap at the end of the procedure. In a full-thickness or mucoperiosteal flap, the gingiva, alveolar mucosa, and periosteum are reflected from the root and the underlying bone surfaces (see Fig. 26–2a■). A partial- or split-thickness flap is a flap in which the periosteum and some connective tissue are left attached to the bone and is not included in the flap. Partial-thickness flaps are used when the bone is thin and exposure to the environment is not desirable, since this would increase the chances of bone resorption. Based on the final positioning of the flap at the end of the surgical procedure, flaps are classified as apically, coronally, and laterally positioned. The most frequently used periodontal flap procedures are the modified Widman flap and apically positioned flap.

Healing Following Flap Surgery

Following traditional flap surgery, the debrided root surface becomes repopulated with epithelial cells that form a long junctional epithelium along the root surface with no new connective tissue attachment (gingival fibers inserting into the cementum) (Fig. 26–2b■).

Modified Widman Flap

Ramfjord and Nissle (1974) described the modified Widman flap (MWF) as a flap for better visualization of the area.

Objective   The specific objective of the MWF is to gain access to root surfaces for improved periodontal debridement and a reduction in inflammation and pocket depths.

Indications   The procedure is indicated for deep pockets, infrabony pockets, and where aesthetics is important, such as in the anterior region. An advantage of this procedure is direct visualization with debridement of deep pockets. Widman flap procedures also allow complete removal of pocket epithelium, and since the flaps can be placed in close approximation, healing takes place by primary intention.

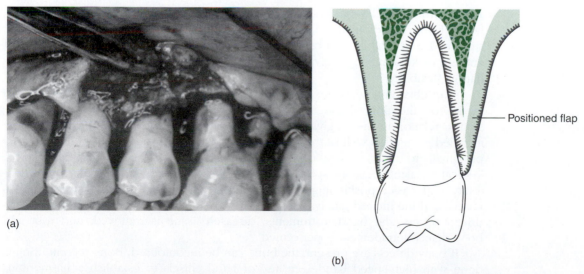

(a)

Positioned flap

(b)

Figure 26–2   (a) This flap was made to gain access to the underlying root and bone to modify defects in the bone and for root and defect debridement. Since connective tissue remains on the bone, it is called a split-thickness flap. (b) Replaced flap postoperative.

Contraindications   The MWF is contraindicated if there are bony defects that need to be recontoured or regenerated.

Technique   After adequate anesthesia is obtained, incisions are made through the crest of the gingiva approximately 1 mm from the margin. This is called an inverse bevel incision. This incision is scalloped and extended as far interproximally as possible to preserve the interdental papillae. Gingival tissues are then reflected only far enough to allow the surgeon direct vision of the root surfaces and the crest of bone. After complete debridement of plaque, calculus, and diseased tissue from the root surfaces and bony defects, the flap is readapted to cover the crest of bone. In some cases, bone recontouring is required for better flap adaptation. Interrupted interproximal sutures are then placed, and the surgical area is covered with a periodontal dressing. The patient receives postoperative instructions. The dressing and sutures are removed after 1 week, and the patient is placed on a chlorhexidine mouth rinse.

Apically Positioned Flap

An apically positioned flap is a full-thickness flap made with an internal bevel incision that following suturing is apically positioned at or near the level of the alveolar crest.

Objective   The main objective is to surgically reduce or eliminate deep pockets by apically positioning the gingival complex while retaining the entire width of gingiva.

Indications   This procedure is used to (1) eliminate moderate or deep pockets by positioning the gingival tissue apically, (2) lengthen the clinical crown for restorative/prosthetic procedures, and (3) increase the zone of attached gingiva.

Contraindications   The apically positioned flap is contraindicated where aesthetics is a concern, such as in the anterior region, where root exposure would be unaesthetic. This type of surgery is also contraindicated in patients at high risk for root caries. It is also contraindicated in areas of advanced bone loss.

Technique   (Fig. 26–3■) The apically positioned flap can be used on buccal surfaces of both mandibular and maxillary arches as well as on the mandibular lingual surface. The palatal gingiva cannot be displaced or moved because it is composed entirely of keratinized gingiva without alveolar mucosa, which is what gives the flap its flexibility.

After obtaining adequate local anesthesia, a reverse (internal) bevel incision is made from the gingival margin to the crest of bone. The location of the initial incision in relation to the gingival margin depends on the width and thickness of the attached gingiva, as well as the depth of the pocket. The incision is scalloped interproximally to obtain optimal coverage of alveolar bone when the flaps are sutured. Vertical releasing incisions at the ends of the initial incision may be placed for flexibility and easier positioning of the flap apically. Next, a full-thickness flap is raised, and the incised gingival tissue collar is removed with a curet. Using power-driven scalers and hand instruments, diseased tissue is removed, and root and bony defect debridement is performed.

If bony defects are present, the bone can be recontoured. Bone recontouring is done with high-speed handpiece and/or hand chisels to establish a harmonious

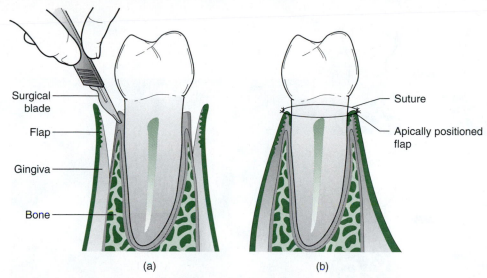

Surgical blade
Flap
Gingiva
Bone
(a)

Suture
Apically positioned flap
(b)

Figure 26–3   The apically positioned flap procedure. (a) An inverse bevel incision is made slightly apical to the free gingival margin and the flap is reflected from the alveolar process. (b) The flap is positioned apically and it is sutured. This procedure attempts to help eliminate or reduce the soft tissue pocket depth.

relationship between the gingiva and the bone. The flap is then positioned apically to cover the bone and is sutured. A periodontal dressing can be applied.

Healing   The attachment or closure of the soft tissue to the root surface in the apically positioned flap is by a long junctional epithelium, with no new connective tissue attachment. Complete healing occurs within 30 to 35 days. Postoperative care procedures are reviewed in Table 26–3.

Procedures for Treating Osseous Defects

Periodontal Flap Surgery with Osseous Resection

Periodontitis is a disease that involves loss of connective tissue attachment and loss of alveolar bone. This loss creates osseous defects and deformities leading to an uneven gingival architecture, which makes it difficult for the patient and the dental hygienist to maintain a healthy dentition. Osseous surgery is periodontal surgery involving modification of the bone supporting the teeth in order to eliminate pockets and obtain optimal physiologic gingival contours. The elimination or modification of bone defects can be either by resection or recontouring, which is removing bone, or by adding bone, which is termed periodontal regeneration (Fig. 26–4■). Periodontal regeneration is discussed in Chapter 27.

Ostectomy and Osteoplasty

Ostectomy and osteoplasty are the two types of osseous recontouring during osseous surgery (Fig. 26–5■). Ostectomy is the removal of supporting bone or bone that is in contact with the root, and osteoplasty is the reshaping or recontouring of

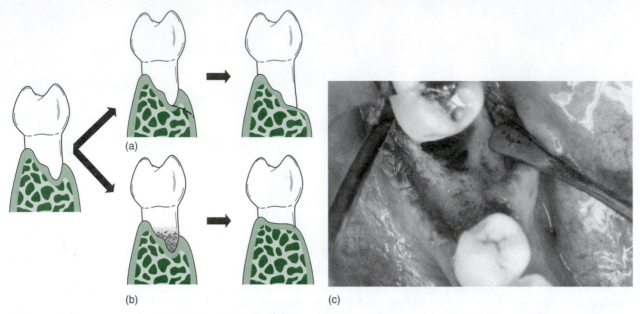

Figure 26–4   A periodontal bony defect is treated either by (a) reshaping or recontouring the bone (top diagram) or (b) filling in the defect (bottom diagram) with bone or a bone substitute (regeneration). (c) This three-wall bony defect on the mesial surface of the molar (the buccal, lingual, and mesial walls remain) is best treated with a regenerative procedure.

nonsupporting bone or bone that is not in contact with the root (e.g., bony ledges) to achieve physiologic contours.

Classification of Osseous Defects

The surgical approach (e.g., resection or regeneration) depends on the pattern of bone loss. The base of a suprabony pocket is coronal to the alveolar crest. The pattern of bone destruction is horizontal, where the bone height is reduced evenly between two adjacent teeth, creating flat interproximal bone. On the other hand, in infrabony pockets, the base of the osseous defect is apical to the crest of the alveolar bone. The pattern of bone destruction is vertical (angular), where the bone is "scooped out" along the side of the root. Intraosseous or infrabony defects are classified according to the number of remaining osseous walls and by their predominant morphology: one-, two-, and three-wall defects. Most infrabony defects are a combination of 1–2- or 2–3-walled morphology. Most infrabony defects are interproximal, but they can be located on the direct facial or lingual surface. A crater is a specific type of two-wall defect in which the remaining osseous walls are the fa-

Figure 26–5
(a) Ostectomy removes bone attached to the tooth, which is called supporting bone.
(b) Osteoplasty is the reshaping of the nonsupporting bone.

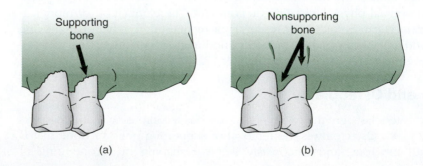

cial and lingual walls. A hemiseptal defect is a type of one-wall defect in which the remaining wall is usually the facial or lingual. A circumferential defect is a three-wall defect that wraps around the line angle of the tooth to involve the lingual or facial surface. Only by probing through the soft tissue pocket (bone sounding), but more precisely by surgical entry, can a determination of the type of infrabony defect be made.

Objectives   The objectives of osseous resective surgery are to create optimal physiologic contours that reduce bony ledges or irregular contours in order to permit primary flap closure and to eliminate infrabony pockets by eliminating the bony walls of the defect.

Indications   Indications for osseous resective surgery include the following: (1) to permit optimal flap adaptation by removing bony ledges or exostosis, (2) to eliminate shallow infrabony pockets (1 to 2 mm deep), (3) to open furcations for easier maintenance, and (4) to lengthen crowns for restorative procedures (e.g., crowns).

Contraindications   Osseous resective surgery is contraindicated in the following situations: (1) patients with advanced periodontitis (teeth in these patients already have compromised bone support; additional resection of tooth-supporting structures would be contraindicated), (2) aesthetics (removal of bone in aesthetic areas, especially the anterior maxillary area, will result in an aesthetically unacceptable appearance), (3) isolated deep vertical defects (attempts to reduce or eliminate such defects would result in removing too much supporting bone from the adjacent tooth), and (4) the existence of local anatomic factors, such as the external oblique ridge, maxillary sinus, and flat palate limits achieving the intended results from osseous resection.

Technique   (Fig. 26–6■) The patient receives local anesthesia. The flap is reflected from the root and bone. When the flaps are elevated, the alveolar crest and marginal bone are inspected. If the marginal bone is thick with ledges, osteoplasty is performed with burs on a high-speed handpiece with copious irrigation. If infrabony defects are present, ostectomy is performed with burs and hand instruments to flatten the interproximal bone. A question arises to how much bone should be removed. The answer is enough bone is removed to eliminate or significantly reduce the depth of the defect but not enough to compromise the tooth or adjacent teeth. These procedures will create a harmonious environment for the alveolar process and the overlying gingiva. The apically positioned flap is the technique of choice when pocket elimination is anticipated. If desired, periodontal dressing may be placed over the surgical area. Postoperative instructions are given.

Healing   The soft tissue attachment to the root surface is by a long junctional epithelium. Healing also results in gingival recession with root exposure. Healing is complete by 2 to 3 months.

Crown Lengthening Procedures

Crown lengthening or crown extension is a surgical procedure designed to expose more tooth structure for restorative purposes (e.g., placement of a crown or other restoration). Indications for crown lengthening are as follows: (1) a tooth that is

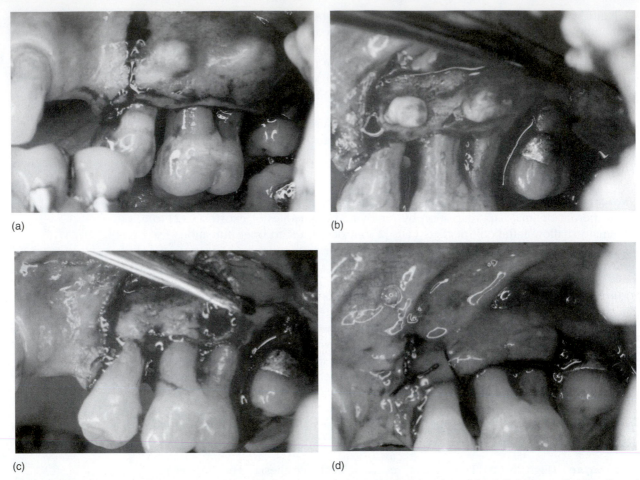

(a)

(b)

(c)

(d)

Figure 26–6   (a) A horizontal and vertical releasing incision is made on the facial surface. (b) A full-thickness flap is reflected away from the bone. There is a furcation involvement on the first molar. Note the two bony protuberances called exostoses (singular: exostosis) on the facial surface. A two-wall bony crater exists between the premolar and molar. (c) Osteoplasty removed the exostoses, resulting in a thin, smooth, bony surface. Ostectomy removed the bony crater. (d) An apically positioned flap. The flap is moved in an apical position to the crest of bone to eliminate the depth of the pocket.

fractured close to the gingival margin and/or alveolar crest and (2) subgingival caries.

Before surgery is performed, the concept of the biologic width must be considered. Biologic width is the soft tissue dimension that is occupied by the junctional epithelium and the gingival connective tissue attachment (gingival fibers). The average length of the junctional epithelium is 0.97 mm, and the average length of the gingival fibers is 1.07 mm, making the dimension of the biologic width approximately 2.04 mm. Thus the biologic width is the soft tissue attachment from the base of the sulcus to the crest of alveolar bone. There must be enough length of root surface to allow for these two attachments. This distance is necessary for gingival health. The margin of a crown or other restoration should not be placed within this space. When a margin is placed less than 2 mm from the alveolar crest it causes gingival inflammation and damage to the attachment apparatus. Bone resorption will then take place to reestablish this biologic width. Thus, if a tooth is fractured, a radiograph will indicate how close the most coronal part of the remaining tooth structure is to the alveolar bone. Osseous resective surgery may be indicated to create more exposed tooth structure and allow for reestablishment of soft tissue attachments and proper placement of restorative margins (Fig. 26–7■).

Root Resection

In patients with substantial furcation involvements (class III or IV) with extensive bone loss around the roots of molar teeth and defective, decayed, or resorbed roots, root resection or hemisection may be indicated. Root resection or amputation is defined as the removal of a root while leaving the crown on a multirooted tooth (Fig. 26–8■). Root resection is usually done on maxillary molars. Hemisection is the surgical sectioning and removal of one root and the crown portion and is usually done on mandibular molars that have a furcation involvement with severe bone loss around the root. If a molar is adequately stable with sufficient bony support but displays a class III or IV furcation involvement, a bisection or bicuspidization procedure can be done. This involves the sectioning or cutting of the molar in

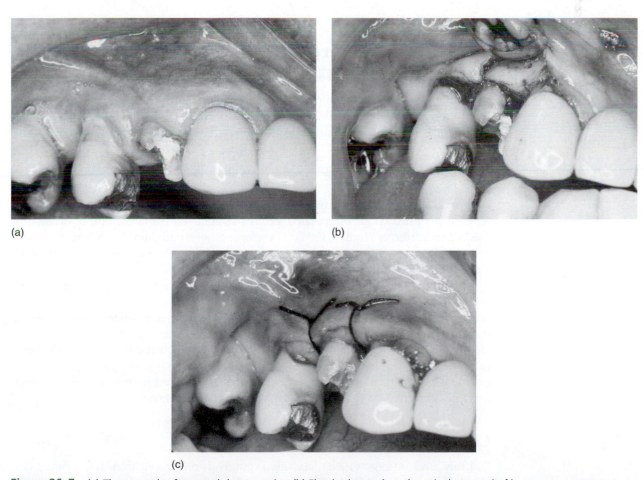

(a)

(b)

(c)

Figure 26–7   (a) The premolar fractured due to caries. (b) Flap is elevated, and surgical removal of bone was necessary to lengthen the crown so a crown could be placed without impinging on the biologic width. (c) The flap was positioned apically and sutured.

Figure 26–8 Root amputation: surgical blade used to reflect the flap; buccal furcation involvement with bone loss of the mesiobuccal root of the mandibular first molar allows for the surgical amputation of the mesiobuccal root.

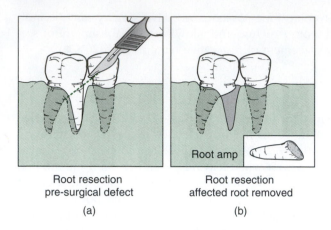

Root resection
pre-surgical defect

(a)

Root amp

Root resection
affected root removed

(b)

half, creating two separate teeth. Endodontics (root canal therapy) must be done before any of these procedures.

Mucogingival Surgical Procedures (Periodontal Plastic Surgery)

The mucogingival relationship is important in sustaining the health of the gingival attachment. Mucogingival surgery is a periodontal surgical procedure used to correct defects in the morphology, position, and/or amount of gingiva.

Indications Historically, the use of mucogingival surgical procedures was limited to treatment of gingival recession. A certain amount of attached gingiva was considered necessary to maintain gingival health and prevent further recession. However, several studies have shown that periodontal health can be maintained regardless of the width of attached gingiva (Salkin, Freedman, Stein, & Bassiouny, 1987; Wennström & Lindhe, 1983). Therefore, gingival augmentation is used in sites with inadequate width and thickness of attached gingiva that exhibit persistent inflammation (bleeding) or progressive recession and sites with inadequate dimensions of gingiva that have subgingival restorations or orthodontics. In sites where crown margins are to be placed subgingivally, recession with exposure of the crown margins may occur when there is inadequate gingival dimensions. Other indications for mucogingival procedures include (1) elimination of frenum and muscle pull at or near the gingival margin, (2) areas in which the base of a periodontal pocket extends to or beyond the mucogingival junction, (3) deepening of the buccal vestibule, (4) aesthetic reasons (e.g., to cover exposed roots), and (5) modifications of edentulous ridges prior to prosthetic reconstruction.

Classification of Gingival Recession

Sullivan and Atkins (1968) classified gingival recession into four categories: (1) shallow-narrow, (2) shallow-wide, (3) deep-narrow, and (4) deep-wide. Miller (1985) expanded this classification (Fig. 26–9■). Miller's classification includes gingival recession not extending to the mucogingival junction and gingival recession extending to the mucogingival junction with bone or soft tissue loss in the interdental area.

Types of Soft Tissue Grafts

Mucogingival defects are corrected using different types of soft tissue grafts. In addition, guided tissue regeneration procedures also may be used for this purpose.

Pedicle Graft or Laterally Positioned Flap

The pedicle graft, as the name implies, is used to move gingiva from an adjacent tooth or edentulous area to a prepared recipient site on another tooth with an inadequate amount of attached gingiva. The pedicle graft is "freed" on three aspects but retains its attachment (blood supply) from its base. This procedure requires sufficient width and thickness of gingiva to be present in the donor site. There should be no underlying bone dehiscence or fenestration. The pedicle graft is best used for single-site recession for root coverage and augmentation (increasing the amount) of attached gingiva.

Technique   (Fig. 26–10■) A V-shaped incision is made around the recipient site. Incised tissue is removed, and root planing of the root surface is performed. A full- or split-thickness flap is elevated on the tooth away from the defect and rotated to cover the defect. The flap is sutured, and pressure is applied (this is done with all soft tissue grafts) for about 4 to 5 minutes, ensuring that no blood clot has formed under the graft. A periodontal dressing to protect the flap can be placed. If a periodontal dressing is not used, the patient should not brush the area. Postoperative instructions are given to the patient (see Table 26–3), and the patient returns 1–2

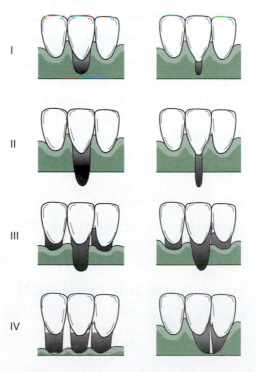

Figure 26–9 P. D. Miller's classification of gingival recession. (Adapted from Miller, P.D., A classification of marginal tissue recession. *Int. J. Periodont. Rest. Dent.*, 1985.)

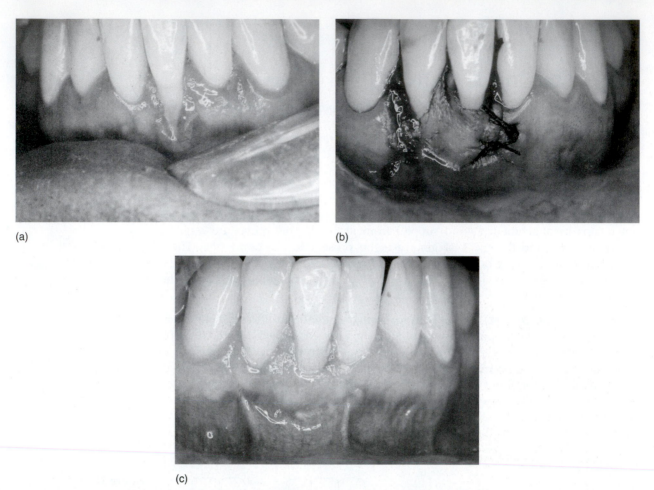

(a)

(b)

(c)

Figure 26–10 (a) Lateral incisor with severe gingival recession with root exposure. (b) A laterally positioned flap was used to move gingiva from the right central incisor to the left central incisor. An anchor suture is around the lateral incisor. (c) Two months of healing shows good root coverage and increased width of attached gingiva.

weeks later. At the first postoperative visit, the sutures and the dressing are removed, and the area either may be left uncovered or may be redressed for an additional week.

Healing Usually clinical healing occurs in about 1 month. However, complete maturation can take up to 1 year.

Double Papillae Flap

The double papillae flap is a modification of the laterally positioned flap. The papillae from each side of the tooth with the defect are reflected and rotated over the midfacial aspect of the recipient tooth and sutured.

Free Gingival Soft Tissue Graft

Unlike a pedicle graft, a free gingival graft (FGG) has a donor site located away from the grafted site. Thus the blood supply is not attached to the graft but depends on the recipient bed. The most common site for donor tissue is the palate, but in many cases, edentulous areas also can be used. Free gingival grafts are more predictable for augmentation of attached gingiva than for root coverage because significant shrinkage of the graft occurs during healing. Thicker free gingival grafts can be used for root coverage because there is less tissue shrinkage.

Technique   (Fig. 26–11■) After local anesthesia is administered on the palate and the recipient area, split-thickness flaps are reflected at the recipient site. A piece of gingiva about 1.5 mm thick is obtained from an intraoral area. Although the most common donor site is the hard palate, edentulous areas also can be used. The donor tissue (graft) is placed on the recipient bed, and the graft is sutured in place, usually with absorbable sutures, making sure that it does not move, since this will interfere with the establishment of a blood supply from the recipient bed and the graft may fail. A periodontal dressing may be applied. Postoperative instructions are given, and the patient returns in 1 week (see Table 26–3). Smoking is strictly prohibited because soft tissue grafts are more likely to fail if the patient smokes. This was demonstrated by Miller (1987), where he found a 100% correlation between failure to obtain root coverage and heaving smoking. A major disadvantage

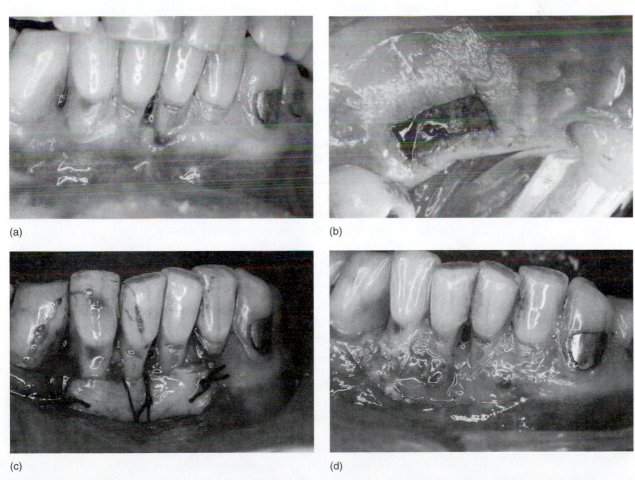

(a)

(b)

(c)

(d)

Figure 26–11   (a) Mandibular central and right lateral incisors have no attached gingiva. (b) A free gingival graft was harvested from the palate and (c) sutured into place at the recipient site. (d) Posttreatment view of the grafted site. Increased width of attached gingiva was achieved. Note that root coverage was not obtained using this type of grafting procedure.

of free gingival grafts is the poor color match between the graft and the existing gingiva.

Healing   The graft will swell initially, and then shrinkage occurs. The graft receives blood and nutrients from the underlying connective tissue. Complete healing with keratinization occurs in about 1 month.

Subepithelial Connective Tissue Graft

The subepithelial connective tissue graft is the procedure of choice for root coverage of single or multiple teeth. The subepithelial connective tissue graft was first described by Langer and Calagna (1982) as having several advantages over the other grafts: (1) there is no open wound on the palate as in a free gingival graft, (2) the graft has a better blood supply coming from both the underlying connective tissue and the overlaying flap, and (3) better aesthetics and tissue and color blend are seen.

Indications   The subepithelial connective tissue graft may be used for both single and multiple adjacent teeth with gingival recession and root exposure. It is limited by the amount of donor tissue able to be harvested.

Technique   (Fig. 26–12■) After local anesthesia is obtained, a split-thickness flap is raised at the recipient site using a surgical blade. A flap is raised at the donor site on the palate, and connective tissue is harvested while leaving the epithelium on the outside of the flap. This palatal flap is sutured into place. The connective tissue is placed on the recipient site and sutured in place with absorbable sutures. A periodontal dressing may be applied. Postoperative instructions are given to the patient, and the patient returns in 1 to 2 weeks (see Table 26–3). At 1–2 weeks, the dressing and sutures are removed, and the area is either left uncovered or redressed for another week.

Healing   Healing occurs through a double blood supply. Both the connective tissue from the recipient site and the overlying flap aid in healing of the soft tissue graft. Complete healing occurs in approximately 1 month.

Guided Tissue Regeneration for Root Coverage

Guided tissue regeneration (GTR) will be discussed further in Chapter 27. Essentially, GTR involves the use of a barrier membrane that is designed to prevent the gingival tissue from establishing contact with the root surface, creating a space for the formation of a new attachment and new bone rather than a long junctional epithelial attachment. This concept was intended originally for the treatment of class II buccal furcation defects and certain infrabony defects. A newer application is for the treatment of gingival recession and for root coverage (Pini Prato, et al. 1992).

Alloderm® (LifeCell Corporation, New Jersey) is a biomaterial that is processed from human tissue. The process removes all epidermal and dermal cells (acellular dermal matrix), while preserving the remaining biological dermal matrix. All cells are removed to remove the risk of rejection or inflammation. This material is indicated for recession defects and for periodontal sites that have little to no attached gingiva where the goal is to increase the amount of keratinized/attached gingiva and to obtain root coverage (Tal, Moses, Zohar, Meir, & Nemcovsky, 2002).

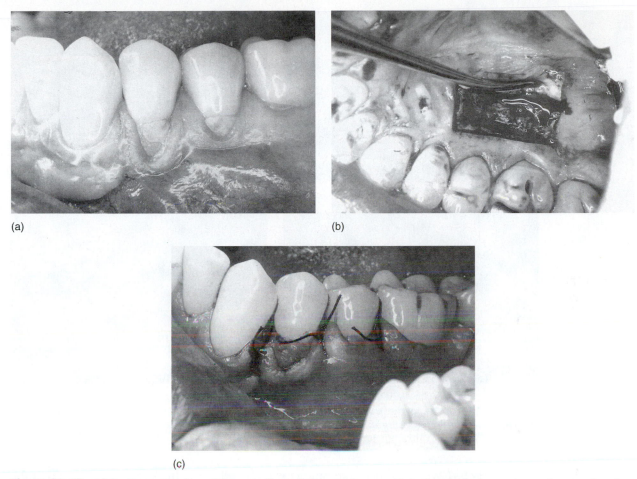

(a)   (b)

(c)

Figure 26–12 (a) Pretreatment view of the mandibular left premolar area. Note the gingival recession and exposed root surfaces. A connective tissue graft was selected to cover the root surfaces. (b) The subepithelial connective tissue graft was harvested from the palate. Incisions were made, and the epithelium was reflected. Note the vascular connective tissue underlying the epithelium. (c) The graft was sutured to the recipient site. Part of the connective tissue is visible on the premolars. (Courtesy of Dr. Stuart J. Froum, New York, New York)

Alloderm is used in a similar way that an autograft is used except there is no harvesting of donor tissue (e.g., palatal tissue) and thus less pain is involved. At the time of surgery, AlloDerm is rehydrated in sterile saline before it is sutured in place on the recipient bed. AlloDerm acts like a scaffold to support regeneration of the patient's own tissue. Six to eight months postsurgery, AlloDerm becomes integrated into the patient's own soft tissue. A surgical case using Alloderm is presented in Figure 26–13■.

When treatment planning a case involving Alloderm, it is important to coordinate periodontal and restorative therapies that will enhance the esthetics of the completed case.

A clinical study showed that treatment with a coronally positioned graft plus Alloderm significantly increased gingival thickness when compared with a coronally positioned flap alone. Coverage of a recession defect was significantly improved with the use Alloderm (Woodyard, Greenwell, Hill, Dirisko, Iasella et al., 2004).

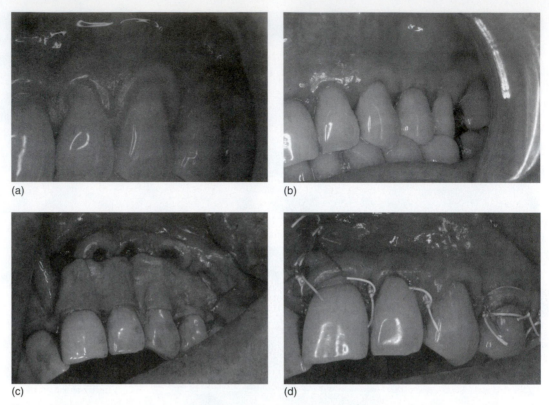

Figure 26–13   (a) Preoperative view of the maxillary left quadrant. Note the gingival recession. (b) Placement of Alloderm at recipient site. (c) Flap sutured in place, covering the Alloderm. (d) 3 weeks post-op. Note the root coverage obtainted. (Courtesy of Dr. Stuart J. Froum, New York, New York)

Technique   After local anesthesia is obtained, a full-thickness flap is raised at the recipient site. Root planing is completed on the root surface. A barrier membrane is placed over the recession and bone and sutured. The flap is repositioned coronally covering both the membrane and the enamel. If the membrane is resorbable, it is not removed and will resorb in about 6 to 8 weeks after surgery. The flap sutures are removed after 2 to 4 weeks. Patients should not brush the area for at least 6 weeks and are recommended to rinse with chlorhexidine gluconate.

Sutures

Sutures are used to co-apt or closely adapt a flap to a tooth surface until the wound has healed sufficiently to withstand normal functional stresses. Closure of the wound provides good hemostasis and covers exposed bone. Suture material is broadly classified as absorbable or nonabsorbable and synthetic or nonsynthetic. Absorbable sutures are absorbed by the healing tissues by the breakdown process of hydrolysis (process by which water gradually penetrates the suture filaments, causing the breakdown of the suture's polymer chain) or proteolysis (process by which the suture filaments are absorbed by protein [salivary] enzymes and then digested by body enzymes). Nonabsorbable sutures do not get absorbed and remain in the tissues until removed.

Absorbable Sutures

Surgical gut is a *natural* material from the intestines of sheep or cows and is absorbable. Surgical gut is not too strong and is hard to handle, getting knotted easily. Chromic gut is plain gut that has been treated with chromic salts, which make it more resistant to absorption. Through proteolysis, enzymes in saliva will absorb surgical gut sutures within 7 to 10 days and chromic gut in about 14 days. However, depending upon the patient's saliva, sutures may still be seen up to 2–4 weeks later.

The other type of absorbable suture is synthetic. Examples of *synthetic* absorbable sutures include polyglactin 910 (Vicryl™, Coated Vicryl™, Johnson & Johnson, Somerville, NJ), poliglecaprone 25 (Monocryl™, Johnson & Johnson), and PGA FA (Hu-Friedy, Chicago, IL). These sutures are easier to handle, the knot will not loosen easily, and they cause less tissue irritation and inflammation than surgical gut because of the more reliable, constant rate of absorption through hydrolysis. Resorption of sutures begins between 10 and 15 days and is usually completed in 28 to 70 days.

Nonabsorbable Sutures

Silk, a type of nonabsorbable natural suture, is the most frequently used suture material because of its ease in handling and superior visibility. Examples of nonabsorbable synthetic sutures include nylon (Ethilon™, Johnson & Johnson, Somerville, NJ), polyester (Ethibond™, Johnson & Johnson), and expanded polytetrafluoroethylene (e-PTFE, Gore-Tex®, W. L. Gore & Associates, Flagstaff, AZ). Silk sutures can elicit tissue inflammation, so they should be removed not later than 10 days after surgery. If sutures need to be left in place for several weeks, e-PTFE sutures are recommended.

Needle and suture material come in various sizes. Needles also are classified according to their shape and curvature. Needles are available in a 1/4-, 3/8-, 1/2-, and 5/8-inch circle, with 3/8- or 1/2-inch being employed most commonly in periodontal surgery. Suture size is classified numerically. An increase in the number of zeros indicates a decrease in the diameter of the suture. Thus 4-0 and 3-0 sutures are used most often in periodontal flap surgery. The 6-0 and 5-0 sutures are smaller and are used in more delicate mucogingival surgical procedures (Hutchens, 1995).

Suturing Techniques

Suturing technique varies among surgeons. Basically, there are different ways to tie the suture. The most common and simplest suture is the interrupted suture, which is tied with a square, or surgeon's, knot (Fig. 26–14■). After the needle engages the buccal and lingual gingiva, it should be tied on the buccal rather than the lingual so that it is easier to remove and the sutures are in a more protected area. When tying a suture, leave about a 2-mm end. Other types of sutures include continuous sutures, mattress sutures, and sling sutures (Fig. 26–15■).

The number of sutures placed should be documented in the chart. When the patient returns for the postoperative visit, count the number of sutures before removing them. This will verify that all sutures were removed.

Figure 26–14
An interrupted
circumferential (loop)
suture.

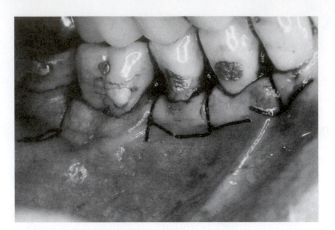

Periodontal Dressing

In today's clinical practice, periodontal dressings are of the noneugenol type that does not cause irritation or burning to the tissue or bone. The primary purpose of using a periodontal dressing over a surgical area is for patient comfort. Periodontal dressings also protect the wound area after surgery. Some practitioners prefer not to use a dressing because the dressing creates an anaerobic (nonoxygen) area under itself that favors the growth of pathogenic microorganisms. However, this theory has not been proven.

The most widely used noneugenol dressing is a COE-pak® (GC America, Inc., Alsip, IL). It is supplied in two tubes: the accelerator tube and the base tube. Equal amounts of dressing from each tube are mixed for 30 to 45 seconds. In the hard and fast set, the working time is about 5 to 8 minutes; in the regular set, it is 10 to 15 minutes. The material is then formed into a strip. Hemostasis should be achieved before the dressing is applied, and the area should be dried. The end of the facial strip is wrapped around the distal aspect of the last tooth and meets with the lingual strip. Finger pressure is applied interproximally to wedge the dressing into place. A dressing placed on a surgical site should not overextend onto the gingiva, vestibule, or occlusal surfaces (Fig. 26–16■). Any excess dressing should be trimmed with a curet.

Figure 26–15
Horizontal mattress
sutures using 4-0 silk.

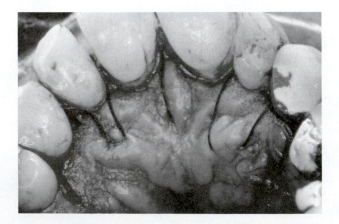

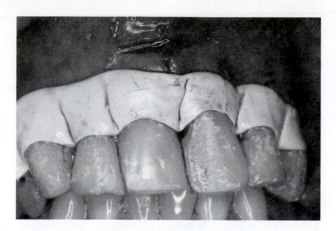

Figure 26–16
Placement of a
periodontal dressing. The
packing should not
interfere with occlusion
or impinge on the
gingiva.

A light-cured periodontal dressing is available (Barricaid™, Dentsply International, Inc., Milford, DE). It is transparent and is used frequently on anterior areas where aesthetics are a concern. The material is first applied to the area (which does not necessarily have to be completely dry) and then is light-cured.

Surgical and Postoperative Care

The dental hygienist plays an important role in the postoperative care of patients.

Surgical Complications

Syncope is defined as a temporary loss of consciousness caused by a loss of blood flow to the brain. Patients have been known to faint before, during, or after surgical procedures. If a patient faints, treatment should be stopped and the patient positioned with the head lower than the body. The patient's vital signs, including blood pressure, respiration, and pulse, should be monitored. Oxygen can be administered if necessary. Causes for patient syncope include fear or anxiety about the procedure, the site of blood, pain, or low blood sugar.

Immediately after the administration of a local anesthetic containing epinephrine, patients may complain of a fast heartbeat or begin to shake or shiver. This is caused by the inadvertent injection of the anesthetic solution into a vein rather than a nerve. Keep the patient calm by reassuring that this will pass very soon and in most cases the patient will be fine. To prevent this situation, it is essential to aspirate while injecting.

During periodontal surgery, bleeding will occur because blood vessels are severed and the diseased tissue is vascular. Small blood vessels will be severed or broken when making incisions. However, it is important not to severe certain arteries such as the greater palatine artery in the maxillary palatal area. Once the diseased tissue is removed and the flaps are raised, bleeding should diminish. Excessive bleeding is controlled by finding the source of the bleeding and applying pressure by administering a vasoconstrictor (e.g., lidocaine 2% with 1:50,000 epinephrine) or by tying the offending artery.

It is important to avoid unnecessary or excessive hemorrhaging or bleeding. The patient's medical history should be evaluated carefully and updated to help avoid these situations. For example, a patient may be taking aspirin every day or even several times a week as a preventive measure for stroke. Aspirin (acetylsalicylic acid) binds to platelets and inhibits the formation of prostaglandins, resulting in a prolonged bleeding time that lasts for approximately 7 days, until new platelets are formed. A similar situation occurs with nonsteroidal anti-inflammatory drugs such as ibuprofen. It is best to consult with such a patient's physician before performing surgery for patients taking these drugs and with the physician's consent suggesting halting these drugs several days prior to surgery.

Postoperative Complications

After periodontal surgery, the patient is given a number of written suggestions and instructions. These instructions must be reviewed carefully with the patient before he or she is allowed to leave the office. An example of postoperative patient instructions is given in Table 26–2. During the first postoperative week, the patient may experience swelling, pain, and sensitivity; these are usually mild and transient. Swelling generally can be controlled by the use of ice packs for the first 2 days. An ice pack should be applied extraorally 20 minutes on and 20 minutes off for the first day. If swelling continues, the patient should switch to warm packs. Swelling can be due to soft tissue inflammation from the surgical procedure or an infection. If swelling continues, advise the patient to return to the office. Pain is usually due to swelling. If there is severe pain, the patient should return to the office. The patient may be given systemic antibiotics and analgesics (pain medication). The dental hygienist should confirm that the patient is taking the appropriate medications as prescribed. The patient should be asked if he or she is taking any over-the-counter medications, vitamins, or herbal remedies.

The patient may complain of seeing blood in the mouth for a few hours after the surgery. Most of the time this is residual blood in the saliva probably remaining on the tongue after surgery. If there is frank bleeding coming from the surgical site, the patient should apply pressure to the site and return to the office as soon as possible. Rinsing should not be done because it will prevent a blood clot from forming.

Oral Hygiene Instructions

Maintenance of the surgical area is important, and the dental hygienist must instruct the client on proper care (see Tables 26–2 and 26–3). It has been demonstrated that regardless of the type of surgery performed (i.e., gingivectomy, MWF, or osseous recontouring), all will fail and probing depths recur if plaque control is not meticulously controlled following surgery (Nyman, Lindhe, & Rosling, 1977). Vigorous toothbrushing and flossing should not be done until healing is complete, yet it must be stressed to patients that removal of dental plaque is important for healing. The period of time the patient refrains from toothbrushing varies with each surgeon. While a periodontal dressing is in place, the patient should not brush that area. Rinsing with chlorhexidine gluconate is recommended. After the dressing and sutures are removed, patients are instructed to brush gently with a roll technique. Gradually, as healing occurs, regular brushing can be resumed. After surgery, the interdental papillae are usually absent or blunted, creating large gingival embrasures. Plaque removal in these areas is best accomplished with an interdental brush (single-tuft brush). Also, plaque removal on teeth with Class III/IV furcation involvement is best with a single-tuft brush. If no large interdental spaces develop after surgery, the patient can continue to use dental floss or a small interdental brush.

Postoperative Visit Management

The dental hygienist may be called on to attend to a patient at the first postoperative visit. Table 26–3 describes various reevaluation procedures that may be performed at this visit. At the 7- to 10-day postoperative visit, the dressing and sutures are removed. After the dressing is carefully removed, the number of sutures are counted and compared with the number of documented sutures placed at the time of the surgery. Frequently, parts of or all of the periodontal dressing may have come off during the week. When the dressing is removed, care must be taken not to pull the sutures. If the sutures are being pulled by the dressing, cut the interfering sutures before the dressing is further removed. Once the dressing is removed, a white layer can be seen on the tissue surface. This represents dead epithelial cells. A moistened (with water, saline, or chlorhexidine) cotton-tipped applicator is used to carefully cleanse the area. Following suture removal, the area is again thoroughly irrigated with water or saline. Only supragingival debridement should be performed; subgingival debridement should be postponed until complete healing has occurred. The decision to apply another dressing to the area depends on the amount of discomfort the patient is experiencing and the rate of healing.

Effects of Surgical Procedures

As a consequence of surgery, several problems may arise. Patients should be informed about these adverse side effects before surgery. All patients also should sign an informed consent form.

Tooth Mobility

Tooth mobility may increase immediately after surgery and may not return to preoperative levels for as long as 6 months. The patient should be told that this is a normal consequence of surgery. Increased tooth mobility is due to the extension of inflammation into the periodontal ligament and to the surgical manipulation. The occlusion should be checked to verify that there is no occlusal trauma. Any occlusal interferences should be eliminated. Check for fremitus to help determine occlusal interferences.

Gingival Recession: Dentinal Hypersensitivity and Root Caries

Gingival recession with longer clinical crowns may occur after surgery. With exposure of the root surface, the patient may experience dentinal hypersensitivity and can develop root caries due to demineralization.

Maintaining adequate plaque control can reduce both the sensitivity and risk for root caries. For immediate hypersensitivity relief, an in-office application of DentinBloc® (Colgate Oral Pharmaceuticals, Canton, MA) is done. Other in-office desensitizing products are available, including chemical agents (oxalates, fluorides), sealants, and bonding agents (see Chapter 22).

It is also helpful for the patient to use at home a dentifrice containing potassium nitrate (Fresh Mint Sensodyne®, Block Drug Corp., Jersey City, NJ; Protect®, John O. Butler Co., Chicago). Unfortunately, the use of dentifrices is controversial, and they may take several weeks to have a positive effect. Once the patient has relief from the hypersensitivity, he or she can start to use the regular dentifrice but should return to the desensitizing dentifrice if the sensitivity returns. An over-the-counter 0.4% stannous fluoride gel (Gel-Kam®, Colgate Oral Pharmaceuticals) that is applied to the toothbrush may reduce dentinal hypersensitivity and prevent demineralization of the exposed root surfaces. A 0.63% stannous fluoride oral rinse (Gel-Kam® Oral Care Rinse, Colgate Oral Pharmaceuticals) is available by prescription for patient use at home. Adverse side effects of stannous fluoride include staining of the dentin and stinging of the soft tissue.

Summary

The range of treatment alternatives for periodontitis is wide. The type of treatment depends on a number of factors, including the patient's level of plaque control, the type of gingival or periodontal pocket, and the type of periodontal defect. Careful assessment and planning of a case are important in the overall surgical treatment.

Key Points

- Periodontal flap surgery is indicated for increasing access to the underlying root and bone in deeper periodontal pockets.
- The patient must be able to maintain excellent plaque control before periodontal surgery is performed.
- The therapeutic clinical end point of success for surgical pocket therapy is an oral environment that is easily maintainable by the patient and the clinician; there should be minimal inflammation (bleeding) and minimal probing depths.
- Cigarette smoking adversely affects the outcome of surgery.

Web Sites

www.perio.org (videotape: Introduction to Periodontal Surgery for Dental Hygienists; Periodontal Plastic Surgery)

www.dentl.ucla.edu

Self-Quiz

1. Which one of the following prerequisites for periodontal surgery is of primary importance? (p. 438)
   a. meticulous plaque control
   b. placement of interim restorations
   c. low anxiety level
   d. desire to continue treatment

2. Which one of the following healing responses is usually seen after periodontal flap surgery? (p. 445)
   a. new bone, cementum, and periodontal ligament
   b. new bone and cementum
   c. long junctional epithelium
   d. connective tissue attachment

3. Which one of the following surgical procedures is indicated for gingival enlargement in a patient who is taking phenytoin? (p. 441)
   a. mucogingival
   b. gingivectomy
   c. periodontal flap
   d. excisional new attachment

4. When placing sutures, the knot is usually tied on the palatal surface because this is a protected area. (p. 459)
   a. Both the statement and the reason are correct and related.
   b. Both the statement and the reason are correct but not related.
   c. The statement is correct, but the reason is not.
   d. The statement is not correct, but the reason is correct.
   e. Neither the statement nor the reason is correct.

5. After periodontal surgery, which one of the following hygiene aids is best recommended to clean exposed furcations? (p. 462)
   a. dental floss
   b. manual toothbrush
   c. powered toothbrush
   d. single-tuft brush

6. Which one of the following surgical procedures is best recommended for augmenting the amount of attached gingiva and covering exposed root surfaces before a patient undergoes orthodontic treatment? (p. 456)
   a. gingivectomy
   b. connective tissue graft
   c. modified Widman flap
   d. crown lengthening

7. Which one of the following measures should be advised to a patient who calls the office 2 days after periodontal surgery and states that he or she has bleeding from the surgical site? (p. 462)
   a. rinse with warm salt water
   b. lie down on a couch
   c. remove the packing
   d. apply pressure

8. Which of the following is the primary objective of periodontal flap surgery? (p. 438)
   a. Gain access to the bone and root surface
   b. Augment the amount of free gingiva
   c. Provide easy-to-maintain areas
   d. Allow for healing by regeneration

9. A patient has experienced some root sensitivity in the area of flap surgery. Which one of the following recommendations can the dental hygienist make to alleviate the pain? (p. 463)
   a. Floss the area
   b. Rinse with a nonfluoride mouth rinse
   c. Rinse and brush with a baking soda solution
   d. Brush with a potassium nitrate dentifrice

10. All the following adverse effects the patient should be informed about before periodontal surgery is performed except one. Which one is the exception? (p. 463)
    a. dentinal hypersensitivity
    b. gingival recession
    c. tooth mobility
    d. root caries
    e. open bite

References

American Academy of Periodontology. 2001. *Glossary of periodontal terms,* 4th ed. Chicago: Author.

Boström, L., L. E. Linder, and J. Bergström. 1998. Influence of smoking on the outcome of periodontal surgery: A 5-year follow-up. *J. Clin. Periodontol.* 25: 194–201.

Carranza, F. A., Jr. 1996. The surgical phase of therapy. In eds. F. A. Carranza, Jr., and M. G. Newman, *Clinical periodontology,* 565–569, 584–587. Philadelphia: W. B. Saunders.

Egelberg J. 1995. Effectiveness of subgingival scaling and root planning. In Periodontics the scientic way. Synopses of human clinical studies, 2nd ed. 71–90. Malmo, Sweden: OdontosSience.

Flores-de-Jacoby, L., and R. Mengel. 1995. Conventional surgical procedures. *Periodontology 2000.* 9:38–54.

Greenstein G. 2000. Nonsurgical periodontal therapy in 2000; a literature review. *J. Am. Dent. Assoc.* 131: 1580–1592.

Hutchens, J. L., Jr. 1995. Periodontal suturing: A review of needles, material, and techniques. *Postgrad. Dent.* 2(4):3–14.

Lang, N. P., and H. Löe. 1993. Clinical management of periodontal diseases. *Periodontology 2000.* 2:128–139.

Langer, B., and L. Calagna. 1982. The subepithelial connective tissue graft: A new approach to the enhancement of anterior cosmetics. *Int. J. Periodont. Rest. Dent.* 2:22–23.

Miller, P. D. 1985. A classification of marginal tissue recession. *Int. J. Periodont. Rest. Dent.* 5:15–37.

Miller, P.D. 1987. Root coverage with free gingival grafts. Factors associated with incomplete coverage. *J. Periodontol.* 58:674–681.

Nyman S., J. Lindhe, and B. Rosling. 1977. Periodontal surgery in plaque infected dentitions. *J. Clin. Periodontol.* 4:240–249.

Palcanis, K. G. 1996. Surgical pocket therapy. *Ann. Periodontol.* 1:589–617.

Pini Prato, G., C. Clauser, P. Cortellini, C. Tinti, G. Vincenzi, and U. Pagliaro. 1992. Guided tissue regeneration versus mucogingival surgery in the treatment of human buccal gingival recession. *J. Periodontol.* 63:919–928.

Preber, H., and J. Berström. 1990. Effect of cigarette smoking on periodontal healing following surgical therapy. *J. Clin. Periodontol.* 17:324–328.

Ramfjord, S. P., and R. R. Nissle. 1974. The modified Widman flap. *J. Periodontol.* 45:601–607.

Salkin, L. M., A. L. Freedman, M. D. Stein, and N. A. Bassiouny. 1987. A longitudinal study of untreated mucogingival defects. *J. Periodontol.* 58:164–166.

Sullivan, H. C., and J. H. Atkins. 1968. Free autogenous gingival grafts: I. Principles of successful grafting. *Periodontics* l6:121–129.

Tal, H., O. Moses, R. Zohar, H. Meir, C. Nemcovsky. 2002. Root coverage of advanced gingival recession: A comparative study between acellular dermal matrix allograft and subepithelial connective tissue grafts. *J. Periodontol.* 73:1405–1411.

Wennström, J. L., and J. Lindhe. 1983. Role of attached gingiva for maintenance of periodontal health. *J. Clin. Periodontol.* 10:206–221.

Woodyard J. G., H. Greenwell, M. Hill, C. Drisdo, J. M. Iasella, J. Scheetz. 2004. The clinical effects of acellular dermal matrix on gingival thickness and root coverage compared to coronally positioned flap alone. *J. Periodontol.* 75:44–56.

Yukna, R. A., and J. L. Lawrence. 1980. Five-year evaluation of the excisional new attachment procedure. *J. Periodontol.* 51:382–385.

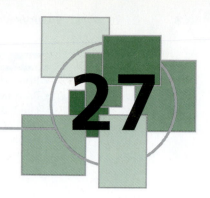

27

Principles of Periodontal Surgery: Periodontal Regeneration

Stuart J. Froum, D.D.S.

Outline

Goal

To provide an understanding of the basic principles of periodontal surgical regeneration.

Educational Objectives

Upon completion of this chapter, the dental hygiene student should be able to:

Describe the process of periodontal regeneration, including the type and origin of cells involved in the regenerative process.

Describe the different bone grafts and bone substitutes that are used in periodontal regeneration.

Discuss the role of enamel matrix protein derivatives and growth factors in regeneration of bony defects.

Compare and contrast the different clinical procedures used to attain periodontal regeneration.

KEY WORDS

- periodontal therapy
- periodontal regeneration
- bone grafts
- bone substitute materials
- guided tissue regeneration (GTR)
- barrier membranes
- growth factors

467

Table 27–1	Procedures Used to Enhance Periodontal Regeneration

- Bone and bone substitute grafting to fill the periodontal defect
- Prevention or retardation of junctional epithelial downgrowth:
  Guided tissue regeneration (GTR)
  Acid conditioning of the root surface
- Application of enamel matrix protein derivatives
- Growth factor application to promote specific cell proliferation

The goals of periodontal therapy have long included arresting the disease process, preventing disease recurrence, and providing for the regeneration of periodontium lost as a result of the disease. Over the past four decades, great strides have been made in the field of periodontal regeneration. Periodontal regeneration is defined as healing after periodontal surgery that results in the reconstruction of lost tissues, including supporting alveolar bone, cementum, and a functionally oriented periodontal ligament (American Academy of Periodontology, 2001). This chapter provides a review of the various regenerative therapies and materials currently in use today (Table 27–1■). Future directions in this ever-changing field also will be discussed. Techniques currently in use include open flap debridement, the use of bone grafts and bone substitutes, guided tissue regeneration, combination techniques, and root surface treatment, and the use of biomimetics and growth factors.

Periodontal Regenerative Surgery

Objectives

Once inflammation of the gingiva is resolved with initial therapy (e.g., periodontal debridement and oral hygiene self-care instruction), the periodontitis component still must be treated. Periodontitis is characterized by apical migration of the junctional epithelium resulting in periodontal pocket formation, loss of clinical attachment (connective tissue fibers attached to the tooth surface), and alveolar bone loss. Periodontal regenerative surgery using bone grafts, bone substitute materials, and/or barrier membranes and modulators of tissue healing is aimed at regenerating the periodontal attachment apparatus lost due to periodontitis (Froum, Gomez, & Breault, 2001).

The primary goal of regenerating lost attachment is the preservation of the natural tooth. Secondary goals of using such bone-replacement materials as bone grafts and bone substitutes in infrabony defects include the following: (1) a reduction in probing depths, (2) a gain in clinical attachment level (this refers to a reduction in probing depth caused by decreased penetration of the probe at the base of the pocket), (3) filling of the osseous defects with new bone, and (4) regeneration of new supporting alveolar bone, new cementum, and a functionally oriented periodontal ligament (Brunsvold & Mellonig, 1993; Schallhorn, 1977). The latter can only be determined by histologic examination of the healed periodontal tissues.

Regenerative surgery significantly differs from osseous resective procedures, in which the osseous (bony) walls are removed surgically to eliminate the intraosseous component of the defect. Often the morphology of the defect requires the removal of too much bone to obtain complete elimination of the defect (parabolic interdental bone), which would further compromise the affected tooth. Periodontal regenerative surgery involves "adding" bone (bone fill) into the intraosseous defect instead of its removal. Certain bony defects are more amenable to regeneration than others (Table 27–2■). The type of periodontal defects that respond best to the use of bone grafts include three-wall, two-wall, and combination-type intraosseous defects. This is because the remaining bony walls contain and hold the bone graft in the defect. The depth and width of these infrabony type defects influence the amount of bone and connective tissue attachment gain. For example, an infrabony defect that is deep and narrow will most likely achieve better regeneration than a defect that is deep and wide (Tonetti, Pini Prato, & Cortellini, 1993). Moreover, the additional surrounding bony walls provide more surface area upon which bone can form. Horizontal patterns of bone loss, loss of buccal or lingual plates of bone, and furcation defects cannot be treated predictably with bone graft and bone substitute materials. However, Class II buccal furcation defects on the mandibular molars are most predictable for periodontal regeneration.

The following are different types of regenerative techniques.

Open Flap Debridement

As a surgical technique, open flap debridement (OFD), in which a flap is reflected and the roots and pocket area are debrided without the addition of any bone or bone substitute material, has been used primarily as a control for comparison in assessing other treatment modalities (Laurell, Gottlow, Zybetz, & Persson, 1998). In most histologic studies, open flap debridement resulted in repair rather than regeneration of periodontal tissues. A greater recurrence of probing depth over time has been shown with open flap debridement alone (Smith, Ammons, & van Belle, 1980) when compared with traditional osseous resective procedures. A review of the literature shows that OFD results in an average clinical attachment level gain of 1.5 mm and average bone fill of 1.1 mm (Laurell et al., 1998).

Bone Grafts and Bone Substitutes

Bone-replacement materials are classified into four categories: autografts, allografts, alloplasts, and xenografts. Bone substitutes can be synthetic (manufactured, not naturally occurring) materials (alloplasts) or processed from the bone of other species (xenografts). Table 27–3■ describes the different types of bone graft materials.

Table 27–2	Bony Defects: Response to Regeneration
Defects healing best after regeneration	**Defects with a lesser chance for regeneration**
3-wall infrabony defect	1-wall infrabony defect
Class II buccal furcation involvement on mandibular molars	Class III furcation involvement
Deeper bony defects (deeper than 3 mm)	Shallower bony defects

Table 27–3	Types of Bone Grafts/Bone Replacement Materials
Name	**Features**
Autografts	Bone harvested from one part of the body and grafted to another part of the same patient's body. The bone can be obtained from an intraoral site such as the maxillary tuberosity area, edentulous area, healing extraction site, or mandibular torus during implant placement or an extraoral site (e.g., iliac crest of the pelvis).
Allografts	Bone material obtained from other individuals of the same species but genetically different. Donors include human cadavers. Allografts are processed under complete sterility and stored in bone banks. The main forms of bone allografts used in clinical practice are demineralized freeze-dried bone (DFDBA) and freeze-dried bone (FDBA).
Alloplasts	A synthetic type of bone substitute. Inert, biologically compatible substances. Synthetic alloplasts include hydroxyapatite, calcium phosphate, bioactive glass, and calcified polymers.
Xenografts	A type of natural bone substitute derived from a genetically different species (e.g., bovine).

Autografts (Autogenous Grafts)

Autogenous bone is living bone derived directly from the patient's own body and has shown the best potential of any of the bone fill material for periodontal regeneration and bone fill. This bone is often mixed with the patient's blood. However, when a sufficient amount of bone is not available intraorally, or if the patient does not want bone obtained from extraoral sites such as the hip, other materials must be considered. Autogenous bone has long been considered to be the gold standard of grafting materials in terms of stimulating new bone formation.

Allografts (Allogeneic Grafts)

Allografts such as demineralized freeze-dried bone (DFDBA) obtained from human cadavers have demonstrated bone-forming properties. Bone allografts are obtained from bone banks. The issue of safety (e.g., nontransmission of hepatitis, HIV, and other known diseases) when using allografts has been well established, thus minimizing this factor as a concern (Marx & Carlson, 1993; Mellonig, Preuett, & Moyer, 1992). Controlled clinical studies have shown greater bone fill in sites treated with DFDBA than in nongrafted controls, with DFDBA reporting a mean bone fill of 2.6 mm (65% defect fill) compared with 1.3 mm (30% defect fill) in nongrafted controls (Mellonig, 1984). A recent review of the literature concluded that both autogenous bone and DRDBA support the formation of a new attachment apparaturs (Reynolds, Aichelmann-Reidy, Branch-Mays, & Gunsolley, 2003).

Alloplasts (Alloplastic Grafts)

Alloplastic bone substitutes are manufactured synthetic materials. They are classified as implant material. Alloplasts (implants) are differentiated from grafts, which are defined as "any tissue or organ used for implantation or transplantation" (Hallmon, Carranza, Drisko, Rapley, & Robinson, 1996). Advantages of alloplasts include zero risk of disease transmission as compared with allografts and no additional surgical sites required in the mouth or body to harvest bone (as with autografts). However, alloplasts are not as effective in forming bone as are graft materials. Alloplasts are inert (nonliving) materials acting as a bone "filler" in the defect, and when effective, they act as a scaffold for bone to form around them.

A number of alloplastic materials have been introduced in an attempt to create a readily available material for bone fill of infrabony periodontal defects. Synthetic alloplasts may be divided into ceramic and nonceramic categories. These may be further divided into absorbable and nonabsorbable materials. Absorbable materials will absorb or dissolve (it may take years) and be replaced with new bone, whereas nonabsorbable grafts may never absorb. Ceramic alloplasts are materials that include calcium phosphate such as hydroxyapatite and tricalcium phosphate. The most commonly used ceramic materials are nonporous hydroxyapatite, porous hydroxyapatite, and tricalcium phosphate. Frequently, these materials result in a repair that evidences a long junctional epithelium to the root surface and/or adhesion of connective tissue fibers oriented parallel to the root (Yukna, 1993).

Bioactive glass is another type of alloplast. In a recent clinical study of the treatment of infrabony periodontal defects, a bioactive glass (Perioglas®, John O. Butler Co., Chicago) showed significant clinical superiority in gain of clinical attachment and defect fill compared with sites that were treated with open flap debridement alone (Froum, Weinberg, and Tarnow 1998). Bioactive glass particles contain silicon dioxide, sodium oxide, calcium oxide, and phosphorous pentoxide. Advantages of this material include the ability to bond to both hard and soft tissue (Hench, 1988), its cohesiveness (Hench & West, 1996), and its ability to inhibit the apical migration of junctional epithelium (Fetner, Martigan, & Low, 1994). One human histological study showed the clinical improvement to be a repair rather than a regenerative response (Nevins et al., 2000).

While many of these materials serve as scaffolds or fillers that allow bone from the surrounding area to grow over and into them, to date alloplasts have failed to demonstrate human histologic evidence of new cementum and a functionally oriented periodontal ligament. From a clinical standpoint, these materials appear to be biocompatible, nontoxic, nonallergenic, noncarciogenic, and noninflammatory.

Xenografts (Xenogeneic Grafts)

Heterografts or xenografts are taken from a donor of another species. Bio-Oss® (Osteohealth Co., Shirley, NY) and Osteograf®/N (CeraMed Dental, Lakewood, CO) are types of natural bone mineral obtained from the cow (bovine). This bone is anorganic and deproteinated. One histological study showed that Bio-Oss used in periodontal osseous defects has the potential to regenerate lost periodontal support (Camelo et al., 1998).

Objectives of Bone-Replacement Materials

Ideally, bone-replacement materials should be able to enhance the formation of new cementum, bone, and periodontal ligament. They should be osteogenic. That is, they should cause bone cells, osteoblasts, to migrate and proliferate into the healing surgical site. Bone graft materials (autogenous and allogeneic) may be osteoinductive (provide a stimulus for noncommitted stem cells to form bone). These osteoinductive materials induce the transformation of immature cells into bone-producing osteoblasts through growth factors that are found only in living bone

(Fox, 1997). Autogenous bone is the ideal grafting material because grafted autogenous bone stimulates bone growth by osteoconduction and osteoinduction during surgical healing.

This differs from alloplastic grafts, which when placed into a periodontal defect at best function as an osteoconductive material. In these situations, the bone-replacement material acts as a scaffold or framework to allow bone apposition against its surface, with cells originating from the surrounding existing bone. Such osteoconductive materials require the presence of existing bone, and the more bone there is (greater number of bony walls in an intraosseous defect), the greater is the chance of a successful bone fill (Fox, 1997). These materials are not osteoinductive and do not produce new bone. The size and shape of the bone-replacement particles influence their osteoconductive capacity. Eventually, the particles of material are either replaced by the bone growing over them or incorporated into the new forming bone.

Biologics and Devices

This is a rapidly developing field that has generated few clinical studies thus far. Wound healing is a complex, well-orchestrated sequence of events. In studying the dynamics of cell-to-cell and cell-to-tissue interaction, scientists discovered the presence of growth factors. Attempts have been made to use these factors to enhance wound healing (repair and regeneration).

Growth factors are naturally occurring proteins that mediate or regulate cellular events such as cell proliferation. Growth factors are found only in living tissue in cells such as bone, platelets, and macrophages. Bone morphogenic proteins (BMPs) are factors found in bone that help induce new bone formation (Wozney, 1995). Platelet-derived growth factors are proteins naturally released from platelets during the healing phase following injury.

There are several problems that have to be addressed before *growth factors* become part of the clinical periodontal armamentarium. The proper vehicle or delivery system for specific factors has not been identified. There are still questions about the concentration of growth factors when they are used by themselves or in combination with other factors. The variability of growth factor responses locally and systemically is still unknown. However, growth factors may have potential for clinical use in the near future. A recent review of growth factors concluded that there is insufficient data to draw definitive conclusions regarding their use in periodontal regenerative surgery at this time (Giannobile & Somerman, 2003).

Recent clinical trials have been performed utilizing a porcine (pig) enamel matrix protein derivative (Emdogain®, Straumann, Switzerland; Chicago), in periodontal regenerative techniques. These clinical studies have shown improved clinical results and gain in clinical attachment and bone fill in sites treated with Emdogain® versus open flap debridement (Froum, Weinberg, Rosenberg, & Tarnow, 2001). Multicenter studies have been performed with this material and verifies the safety of multiple uses in the same patient (no allergies or immunologic problems (Froum, Weinberg, Novak, Mailhot, Mellonig et al., 2004).

Slavkin and Boyde (1975) proposed that enamel-related proteins from Hertwig's epithelial root sheath (HERS), which is the apical extension of the dental organ, are involved in the formation of cementum. In human teeth these enamel proteins are present in areas where cementogenesis (formation of cementum) is initiated.

This gel-like material is available in a premixed, one-vial preparation that is syringed onto the root surface, and the flap is sutured (Fig. 27–1■).

Bone Grafts and Bone Substitutes: Surgical Procedure

Intracrevicular incisions are made, and a gingival flap is reflected. The root surface and osseous defect are debrided to remove all granulomatous (diseased) tissue. A combination of power-driven and hand instruments is commonly used to ensure that all calculus and plaque as well as altered cementum are removed from the root surface (Brunsvold & Mellonig, 1993). The defect is filled and packed with bone or a bone replacement material. The flap is replaced and sutured in an attempt to fully cover the material (Figs. 27–2■ and 27–3■). A periodontal dressing may be placed if desired. The patient returns 7 to 14 days later for suture removal, light debridement, and oral hygiene instruction during the first postoperative visit.

Guided Tissue Regeneration

Cells Involved in Regeneration

The periodontal unit can be divided into five tissue components: the gingival epithelium, the gingival connective tissue, the periodontal ligament (PDL), the supporting alveolar bone, and cementum. In 1976 it was theorized that the type of tissue that predominates in the healing wound after periodontal surgery determines

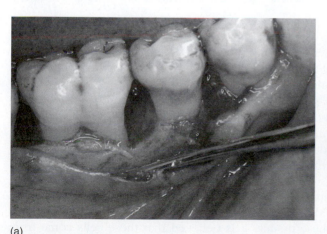

(a)

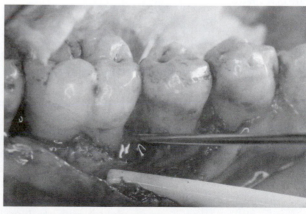

(b)

Figure 27–1   (a) An 8-mm two-wall intraosseous defect on the mandibular first molar. (b) After flaps are reflected and the roots and defect thoroughly debrided, Emdogain was syringed onto the root surface and the flap sutured to cover the material. (Courtesy of Dr. Stuart J. Froum, New York, New York)

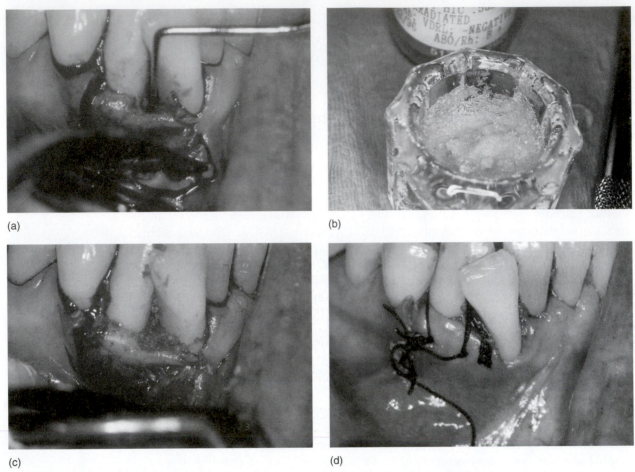

(a)

(b)

(c)

(d)

Figure 27–2 (a) A 9-mm intraosseous periodontal defect is present on the mesial aspect of the mandibular incisor. (b) Following reflection of a periodontal flap and defect and root debridement, a demineralized freeze-dried bone allograft (DFDBA) was reconstituted with sterile saline and (c) placed into the defect. (d) The flap is sutured with silk sutures to cover the graft material.

whether the response is either repair (e.g., long junctional epithelial attachment or connective tissue adherence) or regeneration (e.g., new bone, new cementum, and new periodontal ligament) (Melcher, 1976).

Epithelium is the fastest growing tissue, migrating at a rate of 0.5 to 1.0 mm per day. A periodontal wound in which unimpeded epithelial migration is allowed to occur results in repair with a long junctional epithelium. This type of healing occurs after open flap debridement and osseous resective surgical procedures. Regeneration does not occur when either gingival (junctional) epithelium or gingival connective tissues (e.g., tissue inside the flap) contact the root surface during healing. In order for regeneration to occur, cells capable of forming new cementum, PDL, and supporting alveolar bone must migrate into the periodontal osseous defect and produce these tissues. It is believed that these cells come from the PDL (osteoblasts, fiberblasts, and cementoblasts) and/or alveolar bone remaining around the tooth (Melcher, McCulloch, Cheong, Nemeth, & Shiga, 1987). In order for these cells to migrate into the periodontal defect, apical epithelial migra-

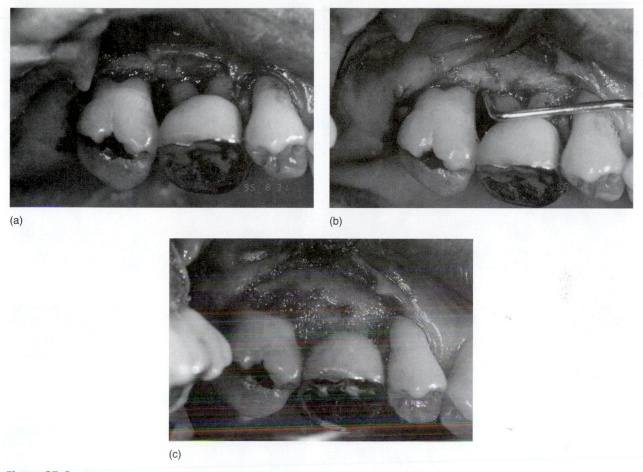

Figure 27–3 (a) A deep crater between the maxillary first and second molars. (b) Probing of the 10-mm-deep defect. (c) After thorough tooth and root debridement, Perioglas® was placed into the defects and furcation involvement of the first molar and the flaps were sutured with silk sutures to cover the graft material.

tion must be delayed, and the gingival connective tissue from the gingival flap must be excluded. If the flap makes contact with the tooth surface, a long junctional epithelium forms along the root and may prevent the necessary regenerative cells from gaining access to the periodontal defect. This concept led to the theory of selective cell repopulation or guided tissue regeneration (GTR) (Gottlow, Nyman, Karring, & Wennström, 1986; Nyman, Gottlow, Karring, & Lindhe, 1982).

This concept has been the basis for clinical techniques using barrier membranes inserted between the gingival flap and the root surface. The membrane maintains a "space" between the tooth and the flap. This procedure is designed to retard apical migration of the junctional epithelium and exclude the gingival connective tissue cells from making contact with the root surface and defect. This then allows cells originating from the PDL space and/or alveolar bone cells to migrate coronally into the defect to form new bone, cementum, and attachment (Fig. 27–4■).

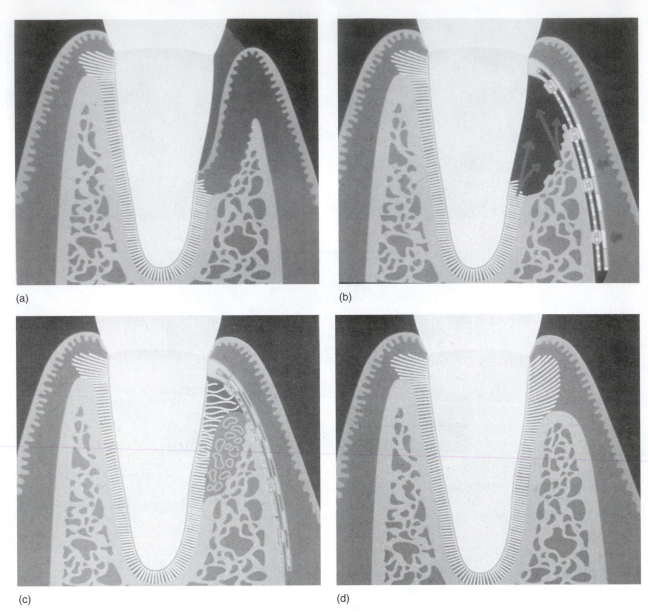

(a)

(b)

(c)

(d)

Figure 27–4   Schematic illustration of a guided tissue regeneration procedure. (a) The periodontal defect with the junctional epithelium on the root surface. (b) After a flap is raised and the defect debrided, a barrier membrane is placed over the defect to create a space for the defect to heal. The periodontal ligament and bone cells attempt to migrate coronally (arrows) into the defect to produce new cementum, periodontal ligament, and supporting alveolar bone. The flap is then sutured over the membrane covering it. (c) Healing by regeneration. (d) The result of therapy after healing.

Surgical Procedure

Barrier membranes have been used in the treatment of Grade II buccal furcation defects in both maxillary and mandibular molars and in two- and three-wall inter-proximal infrabony periodontal defects. Optimal results are obtained in patients that are healthy nonsmokers who demonstrate adequate oral home care.

Clinically, GTR techniques are performed by making intrasulcular incisions and full-thickness flap reflection. Following debridement of the periodontal defect and the root surface, a membrane barrier is placed on the tooth so as to cover the periodontal bony defect (Fig. 27–5■). The membrane is situated between the inner flap and the tooth and bone. The flap is sutured so that the membrane is fully covered and not exposed to the oral cavity. Frequently, a bone graft is first placed into the periodontal defect to prevent the membrane from collapsing into the defect and to aid in regeneration.

Types of Membranes

Nonabsorbable Membranes

Membranes are classified as nonabsorbable or absorbable. Nonabsorbable membranes were the first to be used and studied clinically. Since the body does not absorb (dissolve) a nonabsorbable membrane, it has to be removed. A second surgical procedure therefore is performed a minimum of 6 to 8 weeks later to remove the barrier. The most commonly used nonabsorbable barrier membrane is expanded polytetrafluoroethylene (e-PTFE). Examples of an e-PTFE membrane are Gore-Tex® and Gore-Tex® Regenerative Membrane Titanium Reinforced, in which the titanium enhances the shape ability of the membrane. (Gore Associates, Flagstaff, AZ). A similar nonresorbable barrier is TefGen-FD™ and TefGen-RE™ (Lifecore Biomedical, Chaska, MN). Which are less porous than Gore-Tex®, and thus may limit the amount of connective tissue ingrowth.

Most studies using nonabsorbable membranes in infrabony defects showed positive results. Over the past two decades, studies of infrabony defects in human beings treated with e-PTFE barriers showed definitive clinical gains in new attachment, with three-wall defects having the greatest improvement (Gottlow et al., 1986). A 12-month study of one-, two-, and three-wall infrabony defects treated with e-PTFE barriers showed a 93% fill of three-wall defects, an 82% fill of two-wall defects, and a 39% fill of one-wall defects (Cortellini, Pini Prato, & Tonetti, 1993a, 1993b).

Absorbable Membranes

Absorbable membranes appeared half a decade later. These membranes have various compositions. Absorbable membranes offer a distinct advantage over nonabsorbable barriers in that there is no need for a second surgery to retrieve the membrane. The barrier must remain in place a minimum of 3 to 4 weeks (Minabe, 1991) for proper wound healing. Several membranes are available commercially (Table 27–4■).

The general consensus seems to be that furcation closure in a horizontal dimension is better with absorbable membranes (Garrett, 1996). The clinician must choose the appropriate barrier for the appropriate defect. Although nonabsorbable barriers do not have breakdown products that can interfere with tissue healing, the need for a second procedure to remove the membrane is a distinct disadvantage to wound healing.

The membrane should be covered completely by the flap to prevent bacterial colonization on the outer part of the membrane. Membrane exposure may lead to early infection and poor results. Unfortunately, membrane exposure to the oral

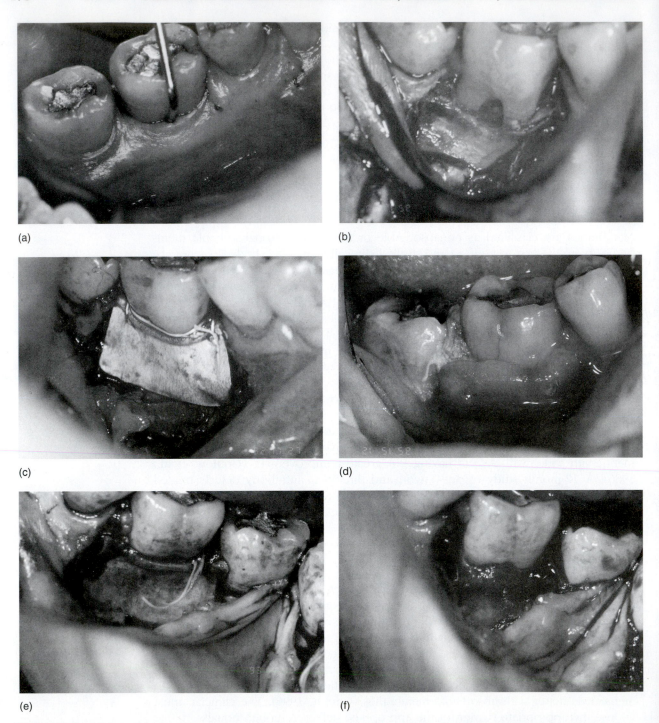

Figure 27–5   (a) A Grade II furcation defect on the buccal aspect of the mandibular first molar probed 10 mm. (b) Sulcular incisions were made, and a mucoperiosteal flap was reflected. (c) After the defect and root were thoroughly debrided, a barrier (Gore-Tex®) was adapted to the tooth and sutured. The flaps were sutured to cover the membrane. (d) Healing after 4 weeks. (e) Approximately 6 weeks later a flap was reflected to remove the membrane. (f) Early healing of site shows a closure of the furca.

Table 27–4	Absorbable Barrier Membranes	
Material	**Product**	**Manufacturer**
Polyglycolic acid, polylactic acid, and trimethylene carbonate	Gore OsseoQuest™ Gore Resolut® XT	W.L. Gore, Flagstaff, AZ; distributed by Nobel Biocare, Yorba Linda, CA
Polyglycolic acid and trimethylene carbonate	Gore Resolut® Adapt Gore Resolut® Adapt LT	W.L. Gore, Flagstaff, AZ; distributed by Nobel Biocare, Yorba Linda, CA
PLA (poly-DL-lactide)	Atrisorb® FreeFlow™ Atrisorb®-D FreeFlow™	CollaGenex, Newton, PA
Collagen (porcine)	BioMend™ BioMend Extend™ Bio-Gide®	Zimmer Dental, Carlsbad, CA Geistlich, Switzerland; distributed by Osteohealth Company, Shirley, NY

cavity occurs with both barrier types. Tissue management when membrane exposure occurs with nonabsorbable barriers may be a problem. Bacteria from the oral cavity may contaminate the exposed membrane by attaching to it. If complete flap closure is not possible, absorbable membranes may be the best choice.

Although GTR using nonabsorbable and absorbable membranes has revolutionized clinical practice, the technique is not as yet predictable for class II, class III, and horizontal bone defects. More research in regeneration of furcation and interproximal defects is needed.

Barrier membranes need to be secured around the tooth to hold it in place and prevent it from moving. Either sutures or bone tacks can be used to attach and immobilize the membrane. A mallet is used to secure the tacks in place. The bone tacks are either stainless steel or titanium. Most are nonresorbable, thus a second surgery is needed to remove the tacks. Osteo-Pin® (Osteohealth, Shirley, NY) is a bioabsorbable fixation pin that does not need to be removed. A periodontal surgical case using bone tacks to secure a barrier membrane is shown in Figure 27–6■.

Regenerative Surgery: Postoperative Care

The patient's oral home care is of utmost importance for a desirable outcome. The dental hygienist should give the patient thorough home care instructions. Guidelines for postoperative care are outlined in Table 27–5■ (Becker & Becker, 1993; Garret & Bogle, 1993; Yukna, 1993). An antimicrobial mouthrinse such as chlorhexidine gluconate may be prescribed. The patient may be prescribed an antibiotic before and after the surgery to prevent infection. The first postoperative visit is within 7 to 14 days.

Professional maintenance and plaque control have been repeatedly shown to correlate with successful clinical results of regenerative therapies including open flap debridement (Froum et al., 1982; Nyman, Lindhe, & Rosling, 1977; Rosling, Nyman, & Lindhe, 1976) bone grafting (Rosen, Reynolds, & Bowers, 2000), and guided tissue regeneration (Cortellini, Pini Prato, & Tonetti, 1994). The hygienist thus plays a key role in the short- and long-term success of regenerative therapy.

Complications can occur during the healing period after GTR surgery. Some complications (Becker & Becker, 1993) are outlined in Table 27–6■.

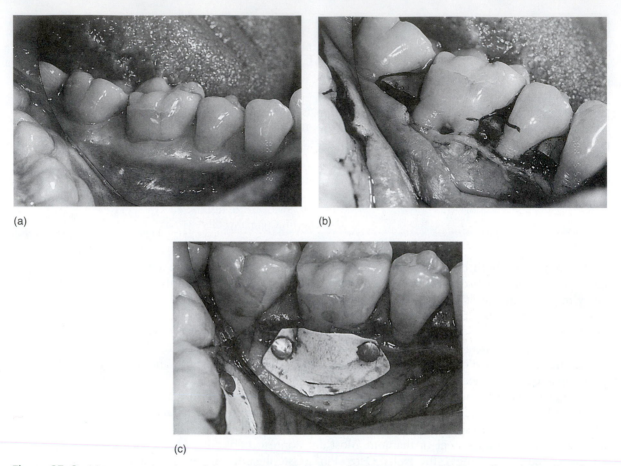

Figure 27–6   (a) Preoperative view of the mandibular first molar. (b) Surgical view with flap reflected showing a buccal Class II furcation involvement. (c) Bone grafting material was placed into the furcation defect and a Gore-Tex membrane placed over the defect and attached with non-resorbable bone tacks. (Courtesy of Dr. Yoon-Euy Hong, New York University Advanced Periodontics, New York, New York)

 Root Surface Treatment

Animal studies have shown that the root surface becomes contaminated by bacteria, bacterial by-products, and endotoxins that will prevent connective tissue attachment and regeneration (Garrett, 1977). The classic method of scaling and root planing, while effective in removing endotoxins from the root (Smart, Wilson, Davies, & Kieser, 1990) in most cases, will not result in new connective tissue attachment, but rather a long junctional epithelium. Use of an acid solution such as citric acid or tetracycline HCl has been studied to determine if a new connective tissue attachment results. The proposed purposes of using acidic solutions on contaminated root surfaces are to detoxify the root and expose collagen fibers for a connective tissue attachment. However, two recent reviews of periodontal regeneration studies with and without the use of citric acid root conditioning showed no clinical advantage to its use (Garrett, 1996; Mariotti, 2003).

Table 27–5	Periodontal Regenerative Surgery: Postoperative Care	
Surgical Procedure	**Postoperative Home Care**	**In-office Reevaluation Procedures**
Bone grafting	If a periodontal dressing is placed, instruct the patient not to brush the area. Instruct the patient to rinse with 0.12% chlorhexidine gluconate twice a day. Following suture removal the patient may start to brush (soft or ultrasoft brush) surgical site gently with a circular technique. Bleeding may occur but will gradually lessen, and the patient should continue to brush. If an antibiotic was prescribed, instruct the patient to continue until all medication is finished.	At the postoperative visit (7 to 14 days), carefully remove the dressing (cut sutures if embedded in dressing), and wipe off the white film (this consists of dead epithelial cells). Reapply dressing if needed (especially if sutures and dressing are removed before 10 days). Periodontal probing should not be done prior to 6 months after surgery. Final prosthetic restorations should not be completed until 6 months or more after surgery. Initial appointments for professional plaque removal should be every 2 to 3 weeks for the first month, then every month for 4 visits, followed by every 3 months (alternate with visits to the general dentist).
Guided tissue regeneration	A periodontal dressing is usually not placed. Instruct the patient not to floss or brush around the surgical area for 6 weeks after the surgery. However, a soft or ultrasoft toothbrush may be used for coronal brushing of the surgical area. Rinse with 0.12% chlorhexidine gluconate twice a day, and use cotton swabs saturated with chlorhexidine around the surgical area. Instruct the patient to continue to take the prescribed antibiotic until finished.	At the first postoperative visit (1 to 2 weeks), the surgical area is inspected. The patient should be seen every 2 to 3 weeks for supragingival scaling and tooth polishing with sterile water. Between 4 and 6 weeks, the membrane-attached sutures are removed. At 6 to 8 weeks, an incision is made to remove the nonabsorbable membrane. Periodontal probing should not be done prior to 6 months after surgery. Final prosthestic restorations should not be completed prior to 6 months after surgery.

Source: Yukna 1993; Becker and Becker 1993; Garrett and Bogle 1993.

Risk Factors for Regenerative Therapy

The same contraindications for any surgical periodontal therapy apply to regenerative therapies. These include any acute or chronic uncontrolled systemic diseases that put the patient at risk (e.g., diabetes mellitus), inadequate plaque control, and smoking (especially more than one pack per day). Smoking has been shown to have a negative influence on the results of regenerative therapy. Using GTR therapy, smokers had less than 50% gain in attachment levels compared to results in nonsmokers (Tonetti et al., 1996). Of the failures with GTR, the majority (80%) occurred in smokers (Rosenberg et al., 1984).

Summary

Today, the role of periodontics in dentistry focuses not only on stopping the progression of inflammatory periodontal diseases but also on the regeneration of periodontal structures (cementum, PDL, supporting alveolar bone) that were destroyed

Table 27–6	Complications after Periodontal Regenerative Surgery
Complication	**Procedures to Follow**
Membrane becomes uncovered	Instruct the patient to call the office. Most often the membrane will become exposed within a few weeks after surgery. If there is no infection, instruct patient to keep optimal oral hygiene. Place the patient on an antimicrobial mouth rinse such as chlorhexidine gluconate. Monitor the area. Instruct the patient not to disrupt the membrane.
Gingival recession at the surgical site	If recession occurs, it will usually happen within 1 to 3 weeks after surgery. Since increased plaque accumulation may result, optimal plaque control is stressed.
Pus	If an infection develops, it is most likely at the fourth and fifth postoperative visit. Remove the membrane and place the patient on an antibiotic. If the patient is already on an antibiotic, change to another antibiotic in a different classification.

by disease. Periodontal regenerative therapy uses bone replacement materials and guided tissue regeneration (GTR) techniques. The use of growth factors (e.g., bone morphogenic proteins, platelet derived growth factor, and tissue modifiers) holds great promise. These factors most likely will be the next addition to periodontal regenerative techniques.

Key Points

- Periodontal regeneration is defined as healing after periodontal surgery that results in the reproduction of cementum, PDL, and supporting alveolar bone that was lost or destroyed by periodontal diseases.
- Ideally, after periodontal surgery, healing by regeneration is preferred over repair.
- Periodontal regenerative techniques include the use of bone grafts, synthetic bone substitutes, guided tissue regeneration (GTR), and a combination of these.
- Bone-replacement materials may contribute to new bone formation or serve as a filler material for bone formation that starts from the adjacent bone and grows into the defect.
- GTR is used to delay apical migration of the junctional epithelium and exclude gingival connective tissue (inner flap) from the surgical site. The goal is to allow periodontal regenerative cells to repopulate the wound first.
- A barrier membrane is placed over the osseous defect and root to create a space for the migration of cells from the PDL and alveolar bone to repopulate the wound.

Web Sites

www.perio.org
www.goremedical.com

Self-Quiz

1. During periodontal surgery, bone is taken from a mandibular torus and placed into a three-wall periodontal osseous defect. Which one of the following types of bone graft is this? (pp. 469–470)

   a. allograft

   b. autograft

   c. alloplast

   d. xenograft

2. Which one of the following types of cells is required for successful periodontal regeneration? (p. 473)

   a. periodontal ligament

   b. odontoblasts

   c. gingival connective tissue

   d. gingival epithelial

3. Guided tissue regeneration (GTR) focuses on the isolation or exclusion of what type of tissue cells? (p. 473)

   a. junctional epithelial and gingival connective tissue

   b. alveolar bone and sulcular epithelium

   c. connective tissue and alveolar bone

   d. alveolar bone and junctional epithelial

4. Which one of the following types of material is nonabsorbable Gore-Tex® membrane? (p. 477)

   a. polytetrafluoroethylene (e-PTFE)

   b. poly-DL-lactide (PLA)

   c. polylactic acid/polyglycolate (PLA/PGA)

   d. bovine collagen

5. After surgical placement of a barrier membrane around an intraosseous defect, it is important to cover the membrane with the flap because (pp. 479–480)

   a. brushing the area is easier

   b. bacterial contamination can be prevented

   c. aesthetics are enhanced

   d. tooth mobility is reduced to pretreatment levels

6. Which one of the following defects heals best when treated with bone grafts/bone substitutes? (p. 469)

   a. one-wall

   b. two-wall

   c. three-wall

   d. Class III furcations

   e. horizontal bone loss

7. All the following are objectives of using bone-replacement materials in the treatment of infrabony defects except one. Which one is the exception? (p. 471)

   a. reduction in probing depth

   b. reduction of bleeding

   c. gain in clinical attachment

   d. fill of the defect

   e. regeneration of the attachment apparatus

8. Which one of the following materials is a type of allograft? (p. 470)

   a. bone from the patient's chin

   b. demineralized freezed-dried bone

   c. bone from the patient's hip

   d. enamel matrix protein derivatives

   e. bioactive glass particles

9. All the following complications may be seen after placement of barrier membranes except one. Which one is the least likely? (p. 481)

   a. suppuration

   b. gingival overgrowth

   c. soft tissue recession

   d. membrane exposure

10. All the following postoperative instructions apply to a patient after a regenerative procedure using a barrier membrane except one. Which one is the exception? (p. 480)

    a. Floss the surgical area.

    b. Rinse the area frequently with diluted salt water.

    c. Use an antimicrobial mouthrinse.

    d. Use antimicrobial impregnated swabs.

References

American Academy of Periodontology. 2001. *Glossary of periodontal terms,* 4th ed. Chicago: Author.

Becker, W., and B. E. Becker. 1993. Clinical applications of guided tissue regeneration: Surgical considerations. *Periodontology 2000* 1:46–53.

Brunsvold, M. A., and J. T. Mellonig. 1993. Bone grafts and periodontal regeneration. *Periodontology 2000* 1:80–91.

Camelo, M., M. L. Nevins, R. K. Schenk, M. Simion, G. Rasperini, et al. 1998. Clinical, radiographic, and histological evaluation of human periodontal defects treated with Bio-Oss and Bio-Guide. *Int J. Periodontics Restorative Dent.* 18:321–331.

Cortellini, P., G. Pini Prato, and M. S. Tonetti. 1993a. Periodontal regeneration in human intrabony defects: I. Clinical measures. *J. Periodontol.* 64:254–260.

Cortellini, P., G. Pini Prato, and M. S. Tonetti. 1993b. Periodontal regeneration in human intrabony defects: II. Reentry procedures and bone measurements. *J. Periodontol.* 64:261–268.

Cortellini P., G. Pini Prato, and M. Tonetti. 1994. Periodontal regeneration of human infrabony defects (V). Effect of oral hygiene on long-term stability. *J. Clin. Periodontol.* 21:606–610.

Fetner, A. E., M. S. Martigan, and S. B. Low. 1994. Periodontal repair using Perioglas® in nonhuman primates: Clinical and histologic observations. *Compend. Contin. Ed. Dent.* 15:932–939.

Fox, J. S. 1997. Bone grafting materials for dental applications: A practical guide. *Compend. Contin. Ed. Dent.* 18:1013–1038.

Froum S. J., M. Coran, B. Thaller, L. Kushner, I. W. Scopp, and S. S. Stahl. 1982. Periodontal healing following open flap debridement. *J. Periodontol.* 53:8–14.

Froum S. J., C. Gomez, and M. R. Breault. 2002. Current concepts of periodontal regeneration. *NYSDJ* 68(9):14–22.

Froum, S. J., M. A. Weinberg, J. Novak, J. Mailhot, J. Mellonig et al. A multicenter study evaluating the sensitization potential of enamel matrix derivative after treatment of two infrabony defects. *J. Periodontol.* 2004; 75:1001–1008.

Froum, S. J., M. A. Weinberg, E. Rosenberg, and D. Tarnow. 2001. A comparative study utilizing open flap debridement with and without enamel matrix derivative in the treatment of periodontal intrabony defects: a 12-month re-entry study. *J. Periodontol.* 72:25–34.

Froum, S. J., M. A. Weinberg, and D. Tarnow. 1998. Comparison of bioactive glass synthetic bone graft particles and open debridement in the treatment of human periodontal defects: A clinical study. *J. Periodontol.* 69:698–709.

Garrett, S. 1977. Root planing: A perspective. *J. Periodontol.* 48:553–557.

Garrett, S. 1996. Periodontal regeneration around natural teeth. *Ann Periodontol.* 1:621–666.

Garrett, S., and G. Bogle. 1993. Periodontal regeneration: A review of flap management. *Periodontology 2000* 1:100–108.

Giannobile W.V., and M. Somerman. 2003. Growth and amelogenin-like factors in periodontal wound healing. A systematic review. *Ann. Periodontol.* 8:193–204.

Gottlow, J., S. Nyman, T. Karring, and J. Wennström. 1986. New attachment formation in the human periodontium by guided tissue regeneration: Case reports. *J. Clin. Periodontol.* 13:604–616.

Hallmon, W. W., F. A. Carranza, Jr., C. L. Drisko, J. W. Rapley, and P. Robinson. 1996. Surgical therapy. In *Periodontal literature review,* 167–194. Chicago: American Academy of Periodontology.

Hench, L. L. 1988. Bioactive ceramics. *Ann. N.Y. Acad. Sci.* 523:54–71.

Hench, L. L., and J. K. West. 1996. Biological application of bioactive glasses. *Life Chem. Rep.* 13:187–241.

Laurell, L., J. Gottlow, M. Zybetz, and R. Persson. 1998. Treatment of intrabony defects by different surgical procedures: A literature review. *J. Periodontol.* 69:303–313.

Mariotti, A. 2003. Efficacy of chemical root surface modifiers in the treatment of periodontal disease. A systematic review. *Ann. Periodontol.* 8:205–226.

Marx, R. E., and E. R. Carlson. 1993. Tissue banking safety: Caveats and precaution for the oral and maxillofacial surgeon. *J. Oral Maxillofac. Surg.* 51:1372–1379.

Melcher, A. H. 1976. On the repair potential of the periodontal tissues. *J. Periodontol.* 47:256–260.

Melcher, A. H., C. A. G. McCulloch, T. Cheong, E. Nemeth, and A. Shiga. 1987. Cells from bone synthesize cementum-like and bone-like tissues in vitro and may migrate into periodontal ligament in vivo. *J. Periodontol. Res.* 22:246–247.

Mellonig, J. T. 1984. Decalcified freeze-dried bone allograft as an implant material in human periodontal defects. *Int. J. Periodont. Restor. Dent.* 4(6):41–55.

Mellonig, J. T., A. B. Preuett, and M. P. Moyer. 1992. HIV inactivation in a bone allograft. *J. Periodontol.* 63:979–983.

Minabe, M. 1991. A critical review of the biologic rationale for guided tissue regeneration. *J. Periodontol.* 62:171–179.

Nevins, M. L., M. Camelo, M. Nevins, C. J. King, R. J. Oringer, et al. 2000. Human histologic evaluation of bioactive ceramic in the treatment of periodontal osseous defects. *Int. J. Periodontics Restorative Dent.* 20:459–467.

Nyman, S., J. Gottlow, T. Karring, and J. Lindhe. 1982. The regenerative potential of the periodontal ligament: An experimental study in the monkey. *J. Clin. Periodontol.* 9:257–265.

Nyman, S., J., J. Lindhe, and B., Rosling. 1977. Periodontal surgery in plaque-infected dentitions. *J. Clin. Periodontol.* 4:240–249.

Reynolds, M. A., M. E. Aichelmann-Reidy, G. L. Branch-Mays, and J. C. Gunsolley. 2003. The efficacy of bone replacement grafts in the treatment of periodontal osseous defects. A systematic review. 8:227–265.

Rosen P. S., M. A. Reynolds, and G. M. Bowers. 2000. The treatment of intrabony defects with bone grafts. *Periodontology 2000* 22:88–103.

Rosenberg E. S., H. D. Dent, and S. H. Cutles. 1994. The effect of cigarette smoking on the long-term success of guided tissue regeneration: A preliminary study. *Ann. Royal Aust. Coll. Dent. Surg.* 112:89–93.

Rosling, B., S. Nyman, and J. Lindhe. 1976. The effect of systematic plaque control on bone regeneration in infrabony pockets. *J. Clin. Periodontol.* 3:38–53.

Schallhorn, R. G. 1977. Present status of osseous grafting procedures. *J. Periodontol.* 48:570–576.

Slavkin, H. C., and A. Boyde. 1975. Cementum: An epithelial secretory product? *J. Dent. Res.* 53:157 (Abstract 409).

Smart, G. J., M. Wilson, E. H. Davies, and J. B. Kieser. 1990. The assessment of ultrasonic root surface debridement by determination of residual endotoxin levels. *J. Clin. Periodontol.* 17:174–178.

Smith, D., W. Ammons, and G. van Belle. 1980. A longitudinal study of periodontal status comparing osseous recontouring with flap curettage: II. Results after 6 months. *J. Periodontol.* 51:367–375.

Tonetti M., G. Pini Prato, and P. Cortellini. 1993. Periodontal regeneration of human infrabony defects. IV. Determinants of the healing response. *J. Periodontol.* 64:934–940.

Tonetti M., G. Pini-Prato, and P. Cortellini 1996. Factors affecting the healing response of intrabony defects following guided tissue regeneration and access flap surgery. *J. Clin. Periodontol.* 23:548–556.

Wozney, J. M. 1995. The potential role of bone morphogenic proteins in periodontal reconstruction. *J. Periodontol.* 66:506–510.

Yukna, R. 1993. Synthetic bone grafts in periodontics. *Periodontology 2000* 1:93–99.

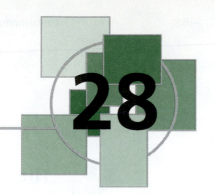

Implantology

Suzanne K. Farrar, R.D.H., B.S., M.S. HCM
Jeanne St. Germain, R.D.H., B.S
Raymond A. Yukna, D.M.D., M.S.

Outline

Goals

To provide an understanding of dental implants and the establishment of proper implant evaluation procedures and maintenance.

Educational Objectives

Upon completion of this chapter, the dental hygiene student should be able to:

Define the role of the dental hygienist in the management of patients with dental implants.

Explain the various types of dental implants currently in use.

Discuss the general sequence of implant placement, uncovering, and restoration.

Compare the tissues around natural teeth and dental implants.

Discuss the steps in evaluating tissue conditions around dental implants.

KEY WORDS

- dental implant
- osseointegration
- perimucosal seal
- peri-implant disease
- nonmetallic materials

We are indebted to Connie Holland Gandy and Marianne Gabb for assistance with the preparation of the original version of this chapter.

Describe proper instrument selection and therapeutic steps for in-office maintenance procedures.

Choose appropriate home-care techniques for patients with dental implants.

The Role of the Dental Hygienist

The dental hygienist plays a critical role in implant dentistry, providing valuable information on treatment and maintenance. The dental hygienist should know the types of implants used in his or her dental office. It is usually beneficial to have before and after pictures of patients who have undergone implant procedures in the office to show prospective patients potential end results.

A potential implant patient must be well educated about the entire procedure, especially the need for follow-up care. Although most implants now have a success rate of over 90%, they still require maintenance and routine care for long-term survival.

Age, Systemic, and Social Factors

The age of the patient has not shown to have an effect on the success or failure of implants (Dao, Anderson, & Zarb, 1993).

Implant therapy may not be an option for patients with certain systemic diseases or adverse risk factors. Systemic diseases such as reduced immune defense (HIV/AIDS) and uncontrolled diabetes mellitus can cause an increased susceptibility to infection and interfere with wound healing. Similarly, social risk factors such as smoking, excessive alcohol intake, drug abuse, and stress have been shown to be associated with an increased frequency of implant problems, including failure (Bain, 1996). Consultation with a patient's physician is required if a patient has disturbances of blood coagulation (including anticoagulation therapy), is on long-term steroids, or has a cancer that requires chemotherapy (Belser et al., 1996). An alternate method of replacing missing teeth should be pursued for such patients, such as fixed partial dentures, removable partial dentures, or complete dentures.

Types of Implants

Several types of implants have been used to replace teeth or support prostheses over the centuries. A few types have been developed that provide the predictable success rates that clinicians and patients expect (Albrektsson & Sennerby, 1991; Brånemark, Zarb, & Albrektson, 1985).

The components of a dental implant include the following (Fig. 28–1a■):

1. The implant body or fixture is the part that is surgically placed into the bone.
2. The abutment (or metal post) is the part that is attached to the implant body and will be fitted with a restoration that can be placed on top of it.

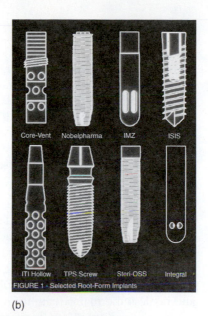

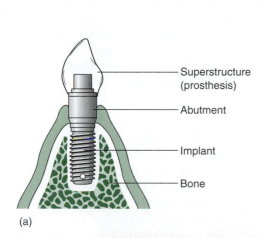

Superstructure
(prosthesis)

Abutment

Implant

Bone

(a)

(b)

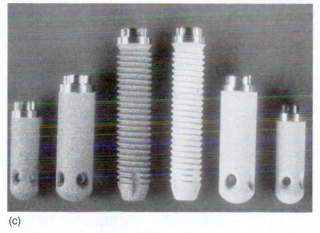

(c)

Figure 28–1   (a) Parts of a dental implant. Osseointegration occurs with direct anchorage of bone to the implant. Diagrammatic (b) and clinical (c) examples of different types of root-form dental implants showing different shapes, surfaces, and coatings.

3. The superstructure is the prosthetic replacement (e.g., crown or denture) that is either screwed or cemented to the abutment.

Implant success and survival rates are affected by the anatomic region of the jaw, the quality of bone, and the length and width of the implant (Cochran, 1996). Minimal criteria for success should include absence of clinical mobility, absence of persistent and/or irreversible signs and symptoms of pain or infections, no peri-implant radiolucency, no irreversible mechanical failures (e.g., implant fractures), support and/or retention of functional restoration(s), and lack of progressive bone loss beyond physiologic remodeling (0.2 mm per year after the first year of loading). There are four types of implants: endosseous, subperiosteal, transosteal, and endodontic.

Endosseous Implants

Endosseous means "within the bone." Endosseous implants have several different shapes, including blade, cylinder, and screw types, with each manufacturer having its own designs. These are the most commonly used implants, and they are placed in edentulous areas of the maxilla or mandible (endosseous). Blade-type implants were popular in the 1960s and 1970s and were associated with a fibrous type of attachment to bone (connective tissue found between the implant and bone). They have been replaced generally by root-form implants, which are associated with a direct bony attachment called osseointegration (see Fig. 28–1a).

Osseointegration

Osseointegration is a term introduced by Brånemark and coworkers in 1969 to describe the direct contact of a load carrying dental implant (inert metal) with bone without any intervening connective tissue. Thus the implant becomes an integral part of the bone and is, in effect, ankylosed, as seen at the light microscopic level (Brånemark et al., 1969). This phenomenon has revolutionized implant dentistry and made it the mainstream form of therapy it is today.

This description has been expanded by the same group of investigators to characterize the long-term success of an osseointegrated implant. Success rates have been reported to be greater than 90% in both fully edentulous and partially edentulous patients. Such success requires full occlusal function without pain and, most important, after an initial marginal bone height loss in the first year of 1 to 2 mm at the bone crest, a crestal bone height loss of no more than 0.1 to 0.2 mm per year. Inflammation of the gingiva around the implant neck is acceptable as long as it is contoured and does not affect the bone or jeopardize long-term implant success rates (Smith & Zarb, 1989).

The implant fixture that initially showed long-term success was made of machined pure titanium with a screw shape. The titanium surface oxidizes into a thin nonreactive titanium oxide layer to which bone adheres, at least at the light-microscopic level. This type of bone-implant interface is called osseointegration. While almost all dental implants today are titanium based (pure titanium or titanium alloy), some are coated, sprayed, or otherwise treated to create a rough surface, thus producing more surface area for the bone to contact or adhere to (see Fig. 28–1b, c). The coatings used are usually acid-etched and sprayed, a titanium plasma spray, titanium beads, grit blasted-acid etched, or calcium-phosphate ceramics (hydroxyapatite and others). Some research has shown that the initial bone bonding to hydroxyapatite may be greater and stronger than the bonding to titanium (Weinlander, 1991). Endosseous implants are the predominant type (>90%) used in current practice (Fig. 28–2a■).

Subperiosteal Implants

Subperiosteal means "on top of the bone." Subperiosteal implants are individually designed cast-metal frames that fit intimately over the bone and under the periosteum and gingiva. Resting on the bone for support, the frame may or may not be fixed by screws to the bone. Posts protrude through the gingiva as anchors for the replacement teeth (Fig. 28–2b). Currently, this type of implant is not used frequently except if there is insufficient bone mass for a root-type implant that cannot be corrected with surgery.

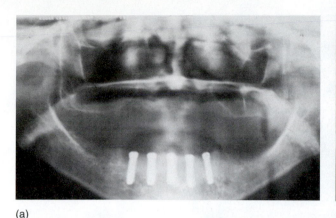
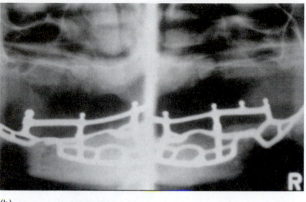

(a)   (b)

Figure 28–2   (a) Panoramic radiograph of root-form dental implants in mandible. (b) Panoramic radiograph of supraperiosteal dental implants on mandible.

Transosteal Implants

Transosteal means "through the bone." Transosteal implants are mandibular denture anchors placed all the way through the mandible from under the chin into the mouth. They are commonly called mandibular staple implants. A curved, flat plate fits under the anterior mandible and usually has five to seven pins. The pins are anchor screws to hold the plate, and the posts are drilled parallel through the mandibular alveolar ridge by means of a jaw-fixation jig with parallel drilling sleeves. This implant has a good success record and is used for very severely resorbed mandibles. However, complications may be more common and there is greater risk of tissue damage and infection.

Endodontic Implants

Endodontic implants are placed "in and through the tooth." They are also called endodontic stabilizers because they consist of a long, wide post inserted into the prepared root canal space that purposely extends at least a centimeter beyond the apex. The rationale is that this extension will stabilize the tooth and improve its usefulness as an abutment. However, this type of implant is not used commonly in the United States and has a poor prognosis because of the potential for root fracture, mechanical retention problems, and root resorption.

Surgical Procedure

Surgical protocol for implant placement varies from the two-stage surgery, to the single-stage surgery, and to the single-stage surgery with immediate or early loading.

Dental hygienists should be familiar with the basics of dental implant therapy, including the surgical procedures. While dental implant treatment may sound extensive, involved, and painful, most patients receive their dental implants in an outpatient setting and have few postoperative problems such as bleeding, infection, or pain. The general stages of dental implant treatment are outlined in Figure 28–3■.

Figure 28–3 Diagram of sequence of dental implant placement using two-stage technique. The body of the implant (fixture) is surgically placed in the bone under the gingiva, allowed to heal for several months, uncovered so that a healing post can be connected to the implant, and the restoration completed.

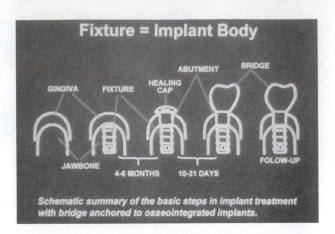

The patient should be aware that several preoperative steps usually are necessary before the actual implant surgery. The restorative dentist (and the surgeon) should do a full work-up on the patient. This includes mounted study casts, a wax-up of the planned restoration, fabrication of a radiographic and surgical guide stent, and appropriate pretreatment radiographs such as periapicals, panoramic, and computed or linear tomography for a three-dimensional view of the bone. These steps are needed to ensure accurate planning as to implant number, diameter, length, and location based on the restorative needs of the patient, bone quantity and quality, and anatomic structures.

Bone quantity and quality of the maxilla and mandible is also important for implant success. Bone quantity refers to the available bone at the future implant site. Bone quantity factors that must be evaluated are the bone width (distance between facial and lingual cortical plates of bone; a minimum of 5 mm is recommended), height (measured from the crest of the edentulous ridge to an anatomical structure such as the maxillary sinus or mandibular canal), and length (mesiodistal distance in an edentulous site or the distance between two adjacent implants (recommended distance between two implants is 3 mm). Determination of bone quality is based on bone density (Table 28–1■), which reflects the strength of the bone (Lekholm & Zarb, 1985). Types I, II, and III bone offer good strength, while type IV bone has poor strength because this type of bone has a thin cortical plate and low trabecular density.

Implant placement can be done as a two-stage or single-stage procedure in which the implant body is placed in the bone and following a healing period is surgically exposed to prepare the implant for a restoration. In the single-stage pro-

Table 28–1	Quality of bone for implant placement (Lekholm & Zarb, 1985)
Type of Bone	**Quality of Bone**
I	Homogenous cortical (compact) bone
II	Core of dense trabecular (cancellous) bone with a thick layer of compact bone surrounding it
III	Thin layer of cortical bone surrounding dense trabecular bone of favorable strength
IV	Thin layer of cortical bone surrounding a core of low-density trabeclar bone

Source: Lekholm & Zarb, 1985.

cedure the implant body is placed in bone with a portion of the implant body (collar) or abutment (post) left exposed until the time of restoration some time later.

Two-Stage Surgical Procedure

First-Stage Surgery

Once the patient is made comfortable and the areas of implant placement are anesthetized, the surgical guide stent is positioned and the specific implant locations marked. An incision is made through the crest of the gingiva, and flaps are reflected to expose the bone. A specific sequence of drills/burs is used to create a hole of specific diameter and depth for the implant(s) to be used. The drilling is done at relatively slow speed with copious irrigation to keep the bone cool and minimize trauma to the potential bone-healing cells. The root-form implant is then threaded or gently tapped into position so that its top is flush with the top of the bone. A cover screw is placed on top of the implant to seal the screwhole for cleanliness. The gingiva is then sutured to cover the implant(s) (Fig. 28–4■). The implant surgeon may prescribe analgesics and antibiotics as needed. Sutures are left in place for approximately 7 to 14 days. While most patients would like to have a temporary tooth replacement in the implant area immediately, pressure on top of the implant should be avoided. A fixed temporary restoration relieved over the implant sites often can be placed in the partially edentulous implant patient.

The implants are allowed to heal undisturbed for 3 to 6 months in order that osseointegration occurs before second-stage uncovering surgery is performed. The time period needed for osseointegration varies depending on the bone quality or density and therefore is shortest for the mandibular anterior area, which is composed of dense cortical bone (3 to 4 months), and longest for the maxillary posterior area, which is composed of more fragile cancellous bone (5 to 6 months). However, recent advances in implant surfaces have allowed manufactures to claim implants can be loaded as early as 2 months after placement.

Second-Stage Surgery

Second-stage or uncovering surgery is performed to expose the top of the implant to create a permanent opening and replace the cover screw with a temporary healing abutment or post that screws into the implant fixture and protrudes through the gingival tissue into the oral cavity. This surgery is usually performed using local anesthesia. After a small incision is made over the implants, the cover screw is removed, and the healing abutment is placed. The gingiva is then sutured tightly around the protruding abutment. After 2 to 3 weeks of soft tissue healing, the restoration process continues. Impressions of the implant(s) are taken and crowns are fabricated to cement or screw onto the implant abutments. A removable prosthesis can also be attached to the abutment, which allows the patient to remove and clean the tooth.

Single-Stage Surgical Procedure

Some implant systems avoid the second-stage surgery with one-stage implants. Single-stage implants are left exposed but not loaded at the time of surgery. This single-stage surgery still requires a 3- to 6-month healing time but rather than

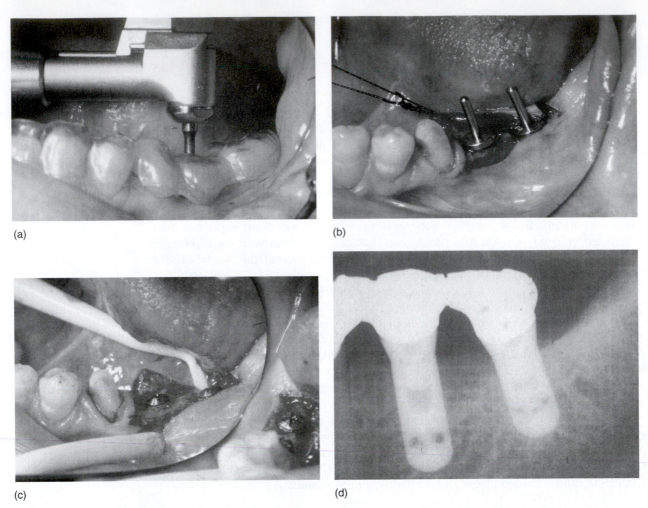

(a)

(b)

(c)

(d)

Figure 28–4   Clinical case illustrating implant placement. (a) Initial drill hole using surgical guide stent. (b) Test pins placed to verify position and angulation of the planned implants. (c) Two implants placed into properly drilled holes to be level with bone crest. (d) Five-year follow-up radiograph illustrating fixed-bridge design for good oral hygiene and maintenance of bone level.

performing a second surgery, the cover screw or healing abutment is removed and the final restoration (crown) is placed.

Single-Stage Surgical Procedure with Early/Immediate Loading

Implants placed with primary stability can be put into function immediately as long as the forces are controlled and below the critical movement threshold. If primary stability cannot be achieved then delayed (extended time for healing) loading is required. This procedure allows the attachment of a temporary prosthesis at the time of implant placement rather than waiting months until healing is complete. Early loading of implants with a dental prosthesis occurs at another visit after the surgery, whereas immediate loading of implants with dental prosthesis/tooth occurs at the same visit as the surgery.

Immediate Implant Placement in Extraction Sockets

Implants can also be placed at the same visit that a natural tooth is extracted. Immediately following extraction of a tooth, the implant is placed into the socket. Loading can be performed at a future time or in the same visit. There are a number of considerations for success including adequate availability of bone, primary stability of the implant, and absence of infection. Drawbacks to this type of surgery include protracted healing time, excessive pain and swelling, and a large ridge defect if the implant fails and has to be removed.

Single Tooth Replacements

Single tooth replacement with dental implants is a treatment option for anterior or posterior teeth. Single missing anterior and posterior teeth are generally caused by trauma/injury, congenitally missing, extensive caries, or failed endodontic procedures. In the past, the primary concern with anterior single tooth placements in the anterior maxilla was with esthetics and having the single dental implant closely resemble adjacent natural teeth (Fig. 28–5■). Advancements in clinical application,

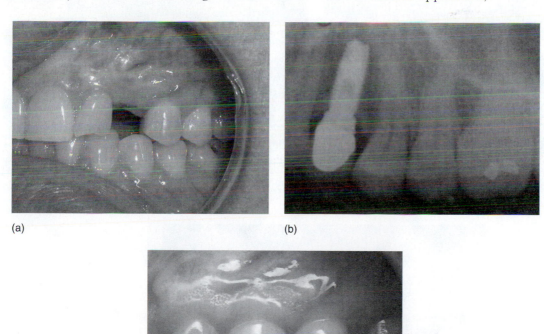

(a)   (b)

(c)

Figure 28–5   (a) Preoperative clinical view of a missing maxillary canine. (b) Radiograph of implant placement to replace maxillary canine. (c) Final clinical view of single tooth implant. (Courtesy of Dr. Stuart J. Froum, New York, New York)

concepts, and technology have developed into single tooth replacements with a high rate of success.

Special Considerations

While the surgical procedures outlined above are basic and apply to patients with good bone quantity, quality, and form, additional procedures often must be used to build up the bone or gingival tissues to allow proper implant placement and restoration. These extra procedures may include such therapy as bone-replacement grafts, guided bone regeneration, soft tissue grafts, sinus bone grafts (sinus lifts), distraction osteogenesis, or combinations of these. These additional procedures may extend the total treatment time until the final restoration can be delivered.

Sinus grafts are needed to increase the height of the posterior alveolus (Fig. 28–6■). Surgery is performed to expose and elevate the maxillary sinus membrane

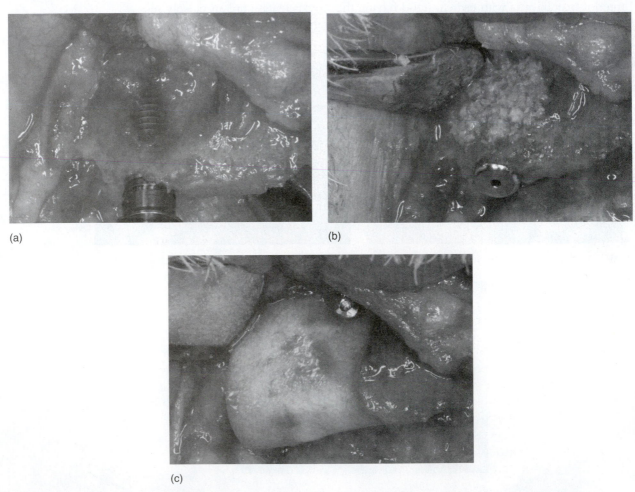

(a)   (b)

(c)

Figure 28–6   (a) Surgical exposure of an implant. Bone resorption has occurred on the buccal aspect. Note the dehiscence with exposure of the threads of the implant. (b) Placement of Bio-Oss® bone graft in the bony defect and (c) a barrier membrane attached to the bone with bone tacks. (Courtesy of Dr. Stuart J. Froum, New York, New York)

from the floor of the sinus and bone graft material is placed into this area. Onlay bone block grafts are required to augment thin ridges (buccal/lingual dimension).

Distraction osteogenesis is a surgical procedure used to increase the bone height of the alveolar ridges by cutting the bone into two pieces, which are gradually separated by 1 mm a day to form new bone in between the cut pieces of bone. This allows for the displacement of bone into the deficient site. This procedure does not require placement of bone grafts. Figure 28–7■ reviews a case involving distraction osteogenesis.

Implant patients and dental office personnel must realize the stages and timeline involved in dental implant therapy. Generally, it takes 9 to 12 months to arrive at the point of delivery of the desired restoration. Longer times are necessary if implant sites require bone grafts or guided tissue (bone) regeneration procedures prior to implant placement. After the final restoration is placed, patients must commit to long-term professional maintenance and optimal oral hygiene self-care.

Prostheses

The original Brånemark implant system in the 1980s was initially recommended for edentulous (no teeth) patients and used "hybrid" prostheses supported by implants in the anterior area of the maxilla or mandible with the abutments visible when the lips are retracted. The function was good but the appearance of these hybrid prostheses was not highly acceptable and alternative, more esthetic restorations were needed. Completely edentulous mouths may be treated with fixed prosthesis or overdentures, while partially edentulous mouths may be treated with fixed partial prosthesis and single tooth replacement.

Conventional dentures (for completely edentulous patients) rest on the alveolar ridge, which does not give much support when chewing and the bone under the gingival continues to resorb. If the patient has trouble with speaking and eating and more retention and stability is required, an implant-supported overdenture should be recommended. Overdentures are attached to multiple implants usually with an over bar (a supportive bar) connecting the implants. This implant-supported overdenture provides more stability to the denture and may help stop alveolar ridge resorption. These patients usually have adequate vertical bone height.

If the patient is not totally edentulous, fixed dentures (bridges) attached to multiple implants may be a treatment option. Although some studies showed that splinting of implants to natural teeth resulted in intrusion of the natural tooth (Sheets, 1993), a recent long-term study showed no higher risk for implant or prosthetic failure for implants splinted to teeth compared to implants splinted only to implants.

For the maxilla, treatment options include a fixed prosthesis supported by implants (in a patient with >10 mm of bone height) or an implant supported by a fixed removable denture or removable overdenture (in a patient that has lost teeth and some of the alveolar bone).

Implants versus Teeth

There are obvious differences between implants and teeth in structure and components (Table 28–2■). Implants are not prone to caries, endodontic (pulpal) problems, or root sensitivity, as are teeth. However, implants depend on proper

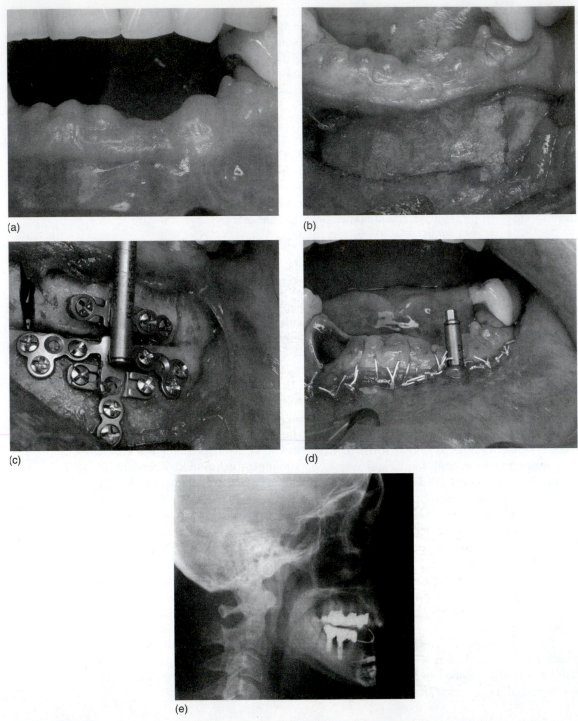

Figure 28–7 Distraction osteogenesis procedure. (a) Note the reduced alveolar ridge height of the mandible. The mandibular bone height must be lengthened to place dental implants. (b) Surgical procedure starts with raising a flap and exposure of the cortical bone. The area is outlined where the distraction device will be placed. This device is used to transmit controlled torque for elongation of the device thereby affecting distraction osteogenesis. (c) This device for lengthening bone by distraction osteogenesis (separating bone pieces) comprises a telescoping screw assemble. (d) The flap is repositioned to cover the device and sutured. The lead screw is exposed and is left in place until bone healing occurs. (e) Final case complete. (Courtesy of Dr. Stuart J. Froum, New York, New York)

Table 28–2	Biologic Environment
Natural Tooth	**Dental Implant**
Perpendicular connective tissue (PDL) attachment inserting into cementum	Parallel connective tissue attachment
Greater blood supply at neck	Less blood supply at neck (scar)
Plaque—less; more confined inflammation	Plaque—greater; more widespread inflammation
Transseptal/supracrestal fibers	No limiting fibers (circular)
Late, slow bone loss in suprabony or infrabony patterns	Earlier, faster bone loss—circumferential around the implant
Inflammation not found in bone marrow	Inflammation into bone marrow
May show slight mobility	Any mobility means implant failure

restoration and occlusion, good oral hygiene, and regular maintenance, just as teeth do. Having a healthy soft tissue barrier is very important. Superstructures should be designed to help facilitate this. It has been shown that plaque accumulation and excessive occlusal forces are primary causes for implant failures (Meffert, Langer, & Frutz, 1992).

Anatomy

Implant–Tissue Interface

Natural teeth are surrounded by the periodontium: alveolar and supporting bone, cementum, periodontal ligament, and gingiva. Dental implants are surrounded by peri-implant tissues, including osseointegrated bone surrounding the fixture. There is no periodontal ligament. The abutment, like the crown of a natural tooth, is surrounded by gingiva. After surgery, the gingiva heals around the abutment. During the healing process, a new free gingival margin forms, including a gingival sulcus.

On natural teeth, the junctional epithelium provides a seal at the base of the sulcus against the invasion of bacterial substances. If the seal is disrupted and/or the gingival fibers are destroyed, the junctional epithelium migrates in an apical direction onto the root surface and connective tissue fibers are destroyed, forming a periodontal pocket. The evidence supports the fact that a junctional epithelium adheres to implant component surfaces and has similar biologic features to the epithelial-tooth interface of a natural tooth. The junctional epithelium, which is referred to as a perimucosal seal, separates the inner tissues from the outside environment for both implants and teeth.

On the other hand, the implant–connective tissue interface shows marked differences when compared with teeth. There is a lack of cementum and no connective tissue fibers insert into the implant surface. Connective tissue fibers subjacent to the epithelium on implants have been shown to be either parallel or circular in orientation to the implant surface, but they do not insert directly into the implant surface. This is sometimes called a pursestring arrangement, and it helps to keep the soft tissues tightly adapted to the implant (Listgarten, Lang, Schroeder, & Schroeder, 1991).

Table 28–3	Pathogens Associated with Peri-Implantitis
Porphyromonas gingivalis	Fusobacterium nucleatum
Campylobacter recta	Eikenella corrodens
Bacteroides forsythus*	Eubacterium species
Prevotella intermedia	Selemonas species
Peptostreptococcus micros	Spirochetes
Actinobacillus actinomycetemcomitans	

*New name for *Bacteroides forsythus* is *Tannerella forsythensis*

Keratinized Gingiva

There are conflicting reports concerning the need for keratinized tissue around implants. However, multiple factors may influence the desirability for the presence of keratinized tissue (see Table 28–3■).

Blood Supply

Implants have less blood supply near their neck with more of a scar tissue appearance. Lack of a periodontal ligament limits the blood supply to the area to only the periosteal vessels and bone marrow spaces.

Inflammatory Lesion

Dental plaque has been shown to grow faster on titanium than on enamel (Quirynen, Van Steenberghe, Jacobs, Scotte, & Darius, 1986). When plaque accumulation occurs, it results in more widespread inflammation around implants than the confined nature of the inflammatory lesion seen around teeth (Ericsson, Berglond, Marinello, Liljenberg, & Lindhe, 1992; Lekholm, 1986). This is due primarily to a lack of limiting attached connective tissue fibers such as the transseptal and supracrestal fiber groups that are present on teeth. Similarly, natural teeth tend to exhibit slow bone loss, and the inflammation does not usually extend into the bone marrow to any great degree. Infected implants, however, tend to have earlier and more rapid bone loss that extends into the adjacent bone marrow, creating a low-grade osteomyelitis.

Bacteriology

Neither dental implants nor natural teeth are immune to plaque accumulation. Regular, effective plaque control is imperative for soft tissue health and a good long-term prognosis with both.

Several studies have investigated the amount, rate, and contents of plaque deposits on implants as compared with teeth. Virtually all these studies show that there are no differences in the amount of plaque or the type of bacteria that accumulate on teeth or various implant surfaces. The types of pathogens found on both teeth and implants are similar (Newman & Flemming, 1988; Table 28–4■). Peri-implantitis (inflammation of the soft tissues around the implant) and marginal bone

Table 28–4	Assessment of Dental Implants and Maintenance Procedures (In-Office)

1. Review medical history.
2. Head and neck examination, oral cancer screening.
3. Take radiographs every 3 months for first year after implant restoration is placed; then yearly to check for bone loss. Place radiographs in sequential mounts.
4. Remove superstructure if necessary and possible.
5. Clean superstructure.
6. Check tissues for surface inflammation.
7. Check for plaque, and review oral hygiene practices.
8. Record probing depths using a plastic or nylon periodontal probe.*
9. Record bleeding on probing.*
10. Clean implant abutments using special nonmetallic instruments.
11. Irrigate with antimicrobial solution if indicated.
12. Replace superstructure, if removed.
13. Have occlusion checked.
14. Review dental hygiene again with superstructure in place.
15. Reschedule for 3- or 4-month recall depending on evaluation of tissue and oral hygiene.

*Somewhat controversial.

loss have been associated with the presence of these pathogens in both partially and fully edentulous patients.

For both implants and teeth, smooth surfaces inhibit and roughened surfaces encourage plaque accumulation. Therefore, in-office maintenance procedures should not roughen the surface of implant components (or teeth). Care should be taken not to locally damage the implant surface with metal ultrasonic or manual instruments. Plastic instruments should be used instead.

In summation, the major difference between implants and teeth, therefore, is the mechanism by which they are attached to the jawbone. Teeth are connected to the bone by means of a connective tissue sling, the periodontal ligament, which is a dynamic, responsive, adjustable attachment mechanism. Implants, by design, become osseointegrated or ankylosed without the cushioning effect of a periodontal ligament. Teeth can move as a result of occlusal or orthodontic forces. Implants do not have any physiologic movement.

Implant Maintenance Program

Periodontal maintenance procedures (continuing care) provided by the dental hygienist for implant patients include assessment of the entire oral cavity as well as the implant sites. A thorough assessment of plaque and calculus accumulation, as well as evaluation of soft and hard tissues, should be a part of the protocol for each maintenance visit. Table 28–5■ reviews these assessment procedures.

The goal for maintenance therapy is to continually monitor the stable condition created by active treatment. Recall appointments should take place at 3-month intervals, and the frequency should be increased if that interval is not adequate to maintain health.

Some clinicians assumed that patients with a history of tooth loss caused by periodontal disease presented a potentially higher risk for implant failure. How-

Table 28–5	Periodontal Criteria for Success with Dental Implants

- No mobility
- Frequent inspection and debridement
- Shallow, stable pockets
- No bleeding on probing
- Effective oral hygiene
- Patient ability/accessibility
- Keratinized gingiva
- Accurate, secure fit of parts
- No trauma from occlusion
- Change in dental behavior pattern
- Maintenance of biocompatible interface

ever, several publications disproved this assumption demonstrating successful osseointegration in patients with different types of periodontal disease (Mengel, Stelzel, Hasse, & Flores-de-Jacoby, 1996; Ellegaard, Baelum, & Karring, 1997; Nevins & Langer, 1995). However, since the same periodontal microbiota colonizes teeth and implants placed in patients with periodontally compromised teeth, it is essential that optimum oral hygiene and plaque control be maintained prior to and following implant placement.

Clinical Parameters of Evaluation

Soft Tissue Evaluation

The clinical similarities between the natural dentition and dental implants have led to the use of similar parameters for evaluation of the periodontium and peri-implant tissues. This provides a means of monitoring and observing peri-implant health status and the effectiveness of treatment. Evaluation of the soft tissue surrounding dental implants is very similar to that of natural tooth structure. A basic assessment begins with the color, contour, and consistency (texture) of the surrounding soft tissue. The presence of erythema, edema, and suppuration, which are the traditional signs of inflammation, should be noted. Thorough documentation of the changes in the soft tissue is important because change may signify current disease activity.

Probing Depth Probing depth also can be used to assess the health of peri-implant tissues. However, the use of periodontal probes for evaluation of the peri-implant condition is highly controversial (Brägger, 1994). Some clinicians feel that probing depth is not an important clinical parameter in the success of an implant (Smith & Zarb, 1989). Concern has been expressed that probing for pockets around an implant may create a pathway for bacteria to attack the peri-implant seal. The probe may carry microorganisms from an infected site and seed a noninfected site. Also, different probing forces allow the probe to penetrate into the connective tissue/bone region easily because of the lack of a connective tissue attachment. No numerical value has been determined as a "healthy probing depth," as is the case with natural teeth (Rapley, 1995). These concepts have not been verified, and thus gentle probing is recommended around implants if the practitioner suspects pathology.

When probing is performed, four measurements around the circumference of the implant should be recorded. As with natural teeth, minimal probing depth (<4 mm) is preferable (Balshi, 1986; Orton, Steele, & Wolinsky, 1987). Changes in probing depth over a period of time around an implant may be more important as an indicator of disease activity than a single probe depth measurement (Balshi, 1986). The use of a plastic or nylon periodontal probe is recommended to prevent scratching of the titanium components. With some abutment and superstructure designs, accurate probing may be difficult because the probe is prevented from reaching the base of the sulcus; thus the probing depth may be underestimated. A more accurate measurement may be obtained by removing the superstructure, which would allow probe insertion parallel to the long axis of the implant. However, more important than the actual probing depth is detecting early changes in the depth of the pocket. Early detection provides an opportunity for therapeutic intervention before irreversible changes have occurred. Probing level has been demonstrated to correlate highly with the marginal bone level (Quirynen et al., 1991; Fig. 28–8■).

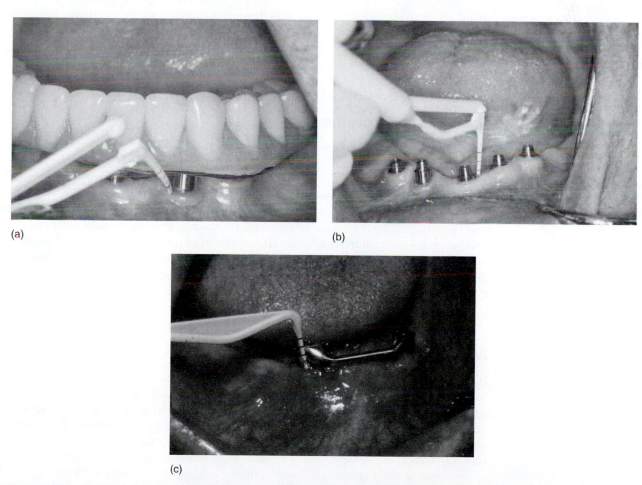

(a)

(b)

(c)

Figure 28–8 Periodontal probing around implants and tissue health. (a) Plastic probe with pressure-limiting mechanisms showing shallow probing depth. Note health of surface tissue. Also note relative lack of keratinized gingiva. (b) Probing access is easier with superstructure removed. Shallow probing depth and good zone of keratinized gingiva. (c) Inflamed tissue with deeper probing depth and bleeding on probing indicating an unhealthy implant site.

Bleeding on Probing   Controversy also can be found in the literature regarding the use of bleeding on probing as a clinical assessment parameter for implants. As with natural teeth, bleeding on probing can be a significant clinical finding. Despite the apparent healthy look of surface tissues and even shallow probing depths, bleeding on probing is an indication that there is underlying disease (Lekholm, 1986). Any bleeding site (especially if the same site bleeds from visit to visit) should be inspected closely for the presence of irritants, and appropriate therapy should be instituted. However, some researchers find that bleeding may be related to probing force and wounding of the tissue rather than actual inflammation (Esposito, Hirsch, Lekholm, & Thomsen, 1998; Rapley, 1995) and should not be used as an indicator of healthy or diseased peri-implant tissue.

Keratinized Gingiva

The presence of keratinized gingiva adjacent to implants is associated with improved tissue health. As with natural teeth, keratinization improves the strength and stability of the epithelium and promotes long-term implant success. An inadequate zone of keratinized gingiva may lead to increased recession, tissue soreness with toothbrushing or eating, and the ability of metallic components to be seen through mucosal tissues.

Hard Tissue Evaluation

Radiographic Procedures

Implant bone levels are best determined by regular accurate radiographic evaluations. Panoramic radiographs commonly are taken for baseline data following abutment placement; however, individual periapical or vertical bitewing radiographs should be taken using the paralleling technique with a gridded film (film with millimeter markings). Such radiographs are preferable for determining bone height and density. Marginal bone height should be measured both mesially and distally and recorded in relation to a landmark on the implant system. For dental implant success, 0.2 mm or less of bone loss annually along the implant surface is acceptable (Albrektsson, Zarb, Worthington, & Eriksson, 1986). For proper continued evaluation, radiographic examinations are recommended after prosthetic connection, at 6 and 12 months, and subsequently at 1- to 3-year intervals.

Mobility

It is recommended that the prosthesis be removed at least once a year to test for implant and abutment mobility. Since the truly osseointegrated implant has no periodontal ligament, there should be zero mobility around stable implants. Mobility of an implant after an appropriate healing period is a sign of implant failure, indicating lack of osseointegraton. Radiographic examinations together with implant mobility tests seem to be the most reliable parameters in the prognostic assessment of osseointegrated implants (Esposito, Hirsch, Lekholm, & Thomsen, 1998).

Mobility of the superstructure can be evaluated by wedging a curet between the prosthesis and the abutment head or by traditional mobility detection. If the abutment is loose, the screws may need to be examined and possibly tightened.

Identifying the Problem Implant

While endosseous root-form dental implants are quite successful, with most studies showing greater than 90% long-term success with a variety of systems, some do develop problems. Identification of these problems when they first begin is important for effective management.

Criteria for Success

The periodontal criteria for success are similar for dental implants and natural teeth. The basis of success is frequent inspection and debridement. As with natural teeth, shallow and stable probing depths are desirable at each visit. In addition, there should be no bleeding on probing at any evaluation site. An adequate zone of keratinized gingiva may be advantageous to protect the soft tissue interface (Brånemark, Zarb, & Albrektson, 1985). The main difference in success criteria involves mobility. While unchanging mobility within physiologic limits is acceptable with natural teeth, any implant mobility is unacceptable.

Restoratively, the prosthesis must fit accurately and securely. There should be no trauma from occlusion (excessive occlusal force on the implant), especially in lateral excursions. Moreover, there should be no mobility of the superstructure and especially of the implant itself. Radiographically, no radiolucency should be present around the implant, and less than 0.2 mm of bone loss per year should be present.

Perhaps the most important factor in success is to effect a change in the patient's dental behavior pattern. If this occurs, and the preceding technical aspects are achieved, then a biocompatible interface between the implant and the host tissues can be maintained for a long time. These criteria are summarized in Table 28–5 (Smith & Zarb, 1989).

Overloading of Implants

Mechanical failures of both the implant components and prosthetic superstructures have been associated with occlusal overload and ill-fitting restorative frameworks. Excessive occlusal force (overloading) generated either from improper placement/angular of implant, prosthesis design, and/or parafunctional activity may cause loosening and/or fracture of the screws through bending overload (Akca & Iplikcioglu, 2001). Marginal bone loss around implants also has been associated with implant overload.

Stages of Peri-Implant Disease

Plaque-induced inflammation occurs in a similar fashion around dental implants as around natural teeth. The pathogenesis is very similar for both entities, but there are several differences, as noted earlier in this chapter. Inflammation around implants generally is called peri-implantitis.

Peri-implantitis has many of the same clinical manifestations and stages as periodontitis. It can be graded from slight to severe, and its treatment parallels that of the stages of periodontitis (Fig. 28–9■). Slight problems are treated with improved oral hygiene and nonsurgical local therapy (controlled-release antibiotics, mouth rinses) (Ciancio, Lauciello, Shibly, Vitello, & Mather, 1995). Moderate

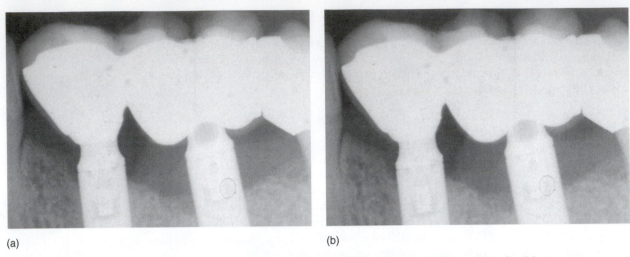

(a) (b)

Figure 28–9   (a, b) Radiographic evidence of bone loss around dental implants, indicating peri-implantitis.

problems usually require systemic antibiotics (Mombelli & Lang, 1992) or flap access surgery. Severe problems require flap surgery for access, with the likelihood of regenerative therapy, including bone-replacement grafts and guided tissue regeneration barriers. The latter has not been shown to be as effective with implants as with natural teeth. The best results in severe cases of peri-implantitis are obtained when the implant has the plaque removed and can be reburied to recapture the lost osseointegration. Sometimes, the problem is so advanced that the implant must be removed.

Instrumentation

Superstructure Removal

On some occasions, the prosthetic superstructure supported by an implant must be removed for better access for maintenance of the implant abutment posts. Some superstructures are removable prostheses anyway, and the patient is familiar with their removal and replacement. Others (increasingly common) are fixed prostheses (screw-retained or cemented) and must be removed by dental office personnel.

Since the hygienist may be asked to remove a superstructure, he or she must be familiar with the removal and replacement process (Table 28–6■).

Removing the superstructure generally entails unscrewing it from the abutments. This must be done in a systematic way. For example, a patient may have crowns and bridges from tooth 2 to tooth 15 with six implants under this superstructure. The hygienist should have six containers, small cups, or dappen dishes, with markings on them to correspond to the jaw location of the implants. When the screw from implant 2 is removed, it should be placed in the container marked 2. When the screw from implant 6 is removed, it should be placed in the container marked 6, and so on. The hygienist will want to back the screws off a little at a time, alternating among them, much in the way a tire is removed and replaced on a car. Unscrewing one side, for example, implant screws 2, 4, and 6 all the way, and not unscrewing implant screws 11, 13, and 15, may cause the integrity of the

Table 28–6	Removal and Replacement of Superstructure

1. Review radiographs and familiarize yourself with the implant location(s).
2. Note location of each implant under superstructure.
3. Have appropriately sized screws and instruments for removal and replacements available.
4. Remove any temporary filling material that may be in the screw hole area.
5. Have small containers, dappen dishes, or envelopes available. When removing the screws use a throat pack.
6. Once screws are removed, place in containers labeled as to location.
7. If removing extensive restorations, loosen screws a little at a time. Then return to each screw and loosen fully.
8. Remove superstructure and examine underside for debris.
9. Clean appropriately, keeping the integrity of the interface with the abutments and the screw holes free of debris.
10. Clean around implant abutments.
11. Replace superstructure.
12. Using correct screws, screw into place using same sequential technique as was used when removing superstructure.
13. Place temporary filling material over screws if indicated.
14. Check occlusion.

implants and superstructure to be compromised. When removing screws the hygienist should employ a throat pack (gauze) to block and prevent any loose screws or abutments from being accidentally swallowed by the patient. Once the superstructure is removed, better access is available to evaluate the soft tissue and gingiva and provide maintenance therapy to the individual implants. The superstructure itself should be thoroughly inspected and cleaned. The hygienist must be aware that the inside of the screw holes always must be kept free of debris or pumice, or the screws may not fit, and the superstructure may not seat properly.

When replacing the superstructure, begin with one implant, and slightly tighten the screw. Then move to the next implant, and so on, just like replacing a tire on a car. Once all the screws are in position and slightly tightened, the hygienist can begin to tighten them down fully. Since peri-implant bone loss may result from occlusal overload, always make sure the occlusion is checked once the superstructure is in place.

Appropriate Instruments for Implants

Deposits that accumulate on supra- and subgingival surfaces of dental implant components should be removed. Normally, calculus on these surfaces is not as tenacious as on natural teeth because the deposits do not penetrate or interlock with the implant component surfaces.

The nature of the surface of implant components must be considered when deciding which instruments to use during office procedures. Most implant components are titanium, a very tough but easily scratchable metal. Stainless steel and carbon steel instruments used directly on titanium can cause marring and scratching of the surface, resulting in roughness, which can increase plaque adherence. Curets made of nonmetallic materials, such as plastic, graphite, Teflon®, or nylon are recommended, and these are available from several manufacturers (Figs.

Figure 28–10   Several types of nonmetallic scalers and curets for use on dental implant components.

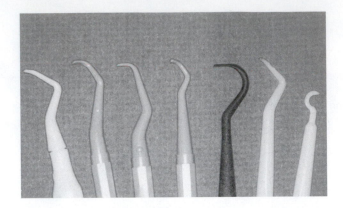

28–10■ and 28–11■). Cleaning around the tissue surface of the prosthesis and implant abutments also can be performed with gauze or tufted floss.

Air-powder abrasive units are effective, but they should not be used directly on implant components for any length of time. The use of ultrasonic- and sonic-powered scalers with metal tips is also contraindicated with implants. Specific plastic or nylon sleeves placed over the tip are available that allow cleaning of implants without scratching (Fig. 28–12■).

In-Office Irrigation

The purpose of in-office irrigation is to attempt to irrigate to the base of the pocket. Plastic rather than metal irrigation tips or needles should be used when irrigating around implants, and the hygienist should be careful not to become too aggressive in forcing the tip into the pocket. Using an irrigation device with an antimicrobial solution at every maintenance visit is considered to be of some benefit by certain practitioners. Irrigation can be used if pathologic changes are present (Meffert et al., 1992). However, this information is anecdotal, and there are not enough controlled clinical studies to support implant irrigation.

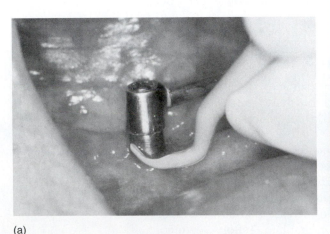

(a)

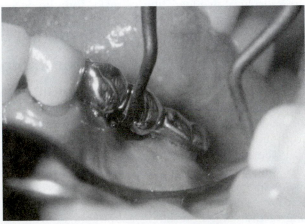

(b)

Figure 28–11   (a, b) Use of nonmetallic curets.

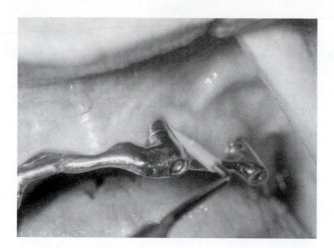

Figure 28–12 Nylon or plastic sleeve for ultrasonic or sonic instruments to prevent scratching of implant components.

Summary

Implant therapy is a rapidly growing part of dental care. With the growing number of implants being placed, the dental team will have an important role in helping attain and preserve the oral health of these patients. Patient education regarding the scope of implant procedures, recommendations for daily home-care regimens, periodic maintenance visits, and regular evaluations are all part of the role of the dental hygienist. The hygienist probably will spend the most time with the patient and can help contribute substantially to the success of dental implant treatment. The dental hygienist has a significant role not only in implant maintenance but also in patient motivation and education. It is important to keep in mind that implant therapy is not for everyone. For this reason, it is crucial that the dental hygienist be educated about implant types, the sequence of therapy, and the social and systemic factors that influence implant success.

Key Points

- Controversy exists regarding the use of periodontal probes around healthy implants.
- Progressive bone loss is a pathologic sign that can lead to implant failure.
- The implant should not be mobile; mobility indicates lack of osseointegration.
- Different prosthetic designs are used for final implant restorations.
- Implant placement can be done as a single-or second-stage procedure.
- Metal (e.g., stainless steel) instruments should never be used on dental implants; use only Teflon®, wood, nylon, graphite, rubber, or plastic instruments.

Web Sites

www.perio.org

www.aaid.-implant.org

www.osseo.org

Self-Quiz

1. All the following systemic conditions are contraindications to implant placement except one. Which one is the exception? (p. 488)
   a. uncontrolled diabetes mellitus
   b. controlled hypertension
   c. head and neck cancer
   d. AIDS

2. Which one of the following types of dental implants is used most commonly today to support prostheses? (p. 490)
   a. submucosal
   b. subperiosteal
   c. endosseous
   d. transosteal

3. Which one of the following similarities is common between dental implants and natural teeth? (p. 500)
   a. bone interface
   b. microbial flora
   c. connective tissue attachment
   d. probing depths topography

4. Routine periodontal probing around implants is controversial because probing may introduce bacteria into the perimucosal seal. (p. 503)
   a. Both the statement and the reason are correct and related.
   b. Both the statement and the reason are correct but not related.
   c. The statement is correct, but the reason is not.
   d. The statement is not correct, but the reason is correct.

5. Which one of the following terms is similar to the process of osseointegration? (p. 490)
   a. ankylosis
   b. cementosis
   c. gemination
   d. fusion

6. All the following types of instruments are used to clean implant abutments except one. Which one is the exception? (p. 508)
   a. Teflon®
   b. stainless steel
   c. nickel
   d. wood

7. Which one of the following is the major criterion for success of an implant? (p. 505)
   a. inflammation
   b. mobility
   c. bleeding
   d. bone level

8. Which one of the following parameters is most reliable in the assessment of the prognosis for osseointegrated implants? (pp. 503–506)
   a. color and contour of the gingiva
   b. bleeding on probing and mobility
   c. radiographic changes and mobility
   d. periodontal probing and color of the gingiva

9. Which one of the following signs indicates implant failure? (p. 505)
   a. deep probing depths
   b. edematous tissue
   c. bleeding
   d. mobility

10. Oral irrigation should be used routinely around dental implants because there is no periodontal ligament attachment to an implant, allowing for easy access of the irrigant to the implant surface. (p. 509)
    a. Both the statement and the reason are correct and related.
    b. Both the statement and the reason are correct but not related.
    c. The statement is correct, but the reason is not.
    d. The statement is not correct, but the reason is correct.
    e. Neither the statement nor the reason is correct.

References

Akca, K., and H. Iplikcioglu. 2001. Finite element stress analysis of the influence of staggered versus straight placement of dental implants. *Int. J. Ora Maxillofac. Implants* 16:722–730.

Albrektsson, T., and L. Sennerby. 1991. State of the art in oral implants. *J. Clin. Periodontal.* 16:474–481.

Albrektsson, T., G. Zarb, P. Worthington, and A. R. Eriksson. 1986. The long-term efficacy of currently used dental implants: A review and proposed criteria of success. *Int. J. Oral Maxillofac. Implants* 1:11–25.

Bain, C. A. 1996. Smoking and implant failure: Benefits of a smoking cessation protocol. *Int. J. Oral Maxillofac. Implants* 11:756–759.

Balshi, T. J. 1986. Hygiene maintenance procedures for patients treated with the tissue integrated prosthesis (osseointegration). *Quintessence Int.* 17:95–102.

Belser, U., R. Mericske-Stern, D. Buser, J. P. Bernard, D. Hess, and J. P. Martinet. 1996. Preoperative diagnosis and treatment planning. In eds. A. Schroeder, F. Sutter, D. Buser, and G. Krekeler, *Oral implantology,* pp. 231–255. New York: Thieme Medical.

Brägger, U. 1994. Maintenance, monitoring, therapy of implant failures. In eds. N. P. Lang and T. Karring, *Proceedings of the 1st European Workshop on Periodontology.* Chicago: Quintessence.

Brånemark, P. I., G. Zarb, and T. Albrektson. 1985. *Tissue-integrated prosthesis osseointegration in clinical dentistry.* Chicago: Quintessence.

Brånemark, P. I., U. Breine, R. Adell, O. Hansson, J. Lindström, and A. Ohlsson. 1969. Intraosseous anchorage of dental prosthesis. *Scand. J. Plast. Reconstr. Surg.* 3:81–100.

Ciancio, S. G., C. Lauciello, O. Shibly, M. Vitello, and M. Mather. 1995. The effect of an antiseptic mouthrinse on implant maintenance: Plaque and peri-implant gingival tissues. *J. Peridontol.* 66:962–965.

Cochran, D. 1996. Implant therapy I. *Ann. Periodontol.* 1:707–820.

Dao, T. T., J. D. Anderson, and G. A. Zarb. 1993. Is osteoporosis a risk factor or ossointegration of dental implants? *Int. J. Oral Maxillofac. Implants.* 8:137–144.

Ellegaard, B., V. Baelum and T. Karring. 1997. Implant therapy in periodontally compromised patients. *Clin. Oral Implants Res.* 8:180–188.

Ericsson, I., N. T. Berglund, C. Marinello, B. Liljenberg, and J. Lindhe. 1992. Long-standing plaque and gingivitis at implants and teeth in the dog. *Clin. Oral Implant Res.* 3:99–103.

Esposito, M., J.-M. Hirsch, U. Lekholm, and P. Thomsen. 1998. Biological factors contributing to failures of osseointegrated oral implants: I. Success criteria and epidemiology. *Eur. J. Oral Sci.* 106:527–551.

Lekholm, M. 1986. Marginal tissue reactions at osseointegrated titanium fixtures. *Int. J. Oral Maxillofac. Implants* 15:53–61.

Lekholm, M., and G.A. Zarb. 1985. Patient selection. In eds. P-I. Brånemark, G.A. Zarb, & T. Albrektsson. *Tissue integrated prosthesis. Osseointegration in clinical dentistry,* 199–209. Chicago: Quintessence.

Listgarten, M. A., N. P. Lang, H. E. Schroeder, and A. Schroeder. 1991. Periodontal tissues and their counterparts around endosseous implants. *Clin. Oral Implant Res.* 2:1–19.

Meffert, R., B. Langer, and M. Frutz. 1992. Dental implants: A review. *J. Periodontol.* 63:859–870.

Mombelli, A., and N. P. Lang. 1992. Antimicrobial treatment of peri-implant infections. *Clin. Oral Implants Res.* 3:162–168.

Newman, M., and T. Flemming. 1988. Periodontal considerations of implants and implant associated microbiota. *J. Dent. Ed.* 52:737–744.

Nevins, M., and B. Langer. 1995. The successful use of osseointegrated implants for the treatment of the recalcitrant periodontal patient. *J. Periodontol.* 66:150–157.

Mengel, R., Stelzel, M. Hasse, C. and Flores-de-Jacoby, L. 1996. Osseointegrated implants in patients treated for generalized severe adult periodontitis. An interim report. *J. Periodontol.* 67:782–787.

Orton, G. S., D. L. Steele, and L. E. Wolinsky. 1987. The dental professional's role in monitoring and maintenance of tissue-integrated prosthesis. *Int. J. Oral Maxillofac. Implants* 4:305–310.

Quirynen, M., D. van Steenberghe, R. Jacobs, A. Schotte, and P. Darius. 1991. The reliability of pocket probing around screw-type implants. *Clin. Oral Implant Res.* 2:186–192.

Rapley, J. 1995. Dental implants: Maintenance. In eds. P. F. Fedi, Jr. and A. R. Vernino, *The periodontic syllabus,* 3rd ed. pp. 183–186. Baltimore: Williams & Wilkins.

Sheets, C.G., and J. C. Earthman. 1993. Natural tooth intrusion and reversal in implant-assisted prostheses for the occurrence. *J. Prost. Dent.* 70:513–520.

Smith, D., and G. Zarb. 1989. Criteria for success of osseointegrated endosseous implants. *J. Prosthet. Dent.* 62:567–572.

Weinlander, M. 1991. Bone growth around dental implants. *Dent. Clin. North Am.* 35:585–601.

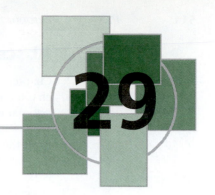

Periodontal Emergencies

Mea A. Weinberg, D.M.D., M.S.D., R.Ph.

Outline

Abscesses of the
    Periodontium
Necrotizing Ulcerative
    Gingivitis
Primary Herpetic
    Gingivostomatitis

Summary
Key Points
Web Site
Self-Quiz
Reference

Goal

*To provide an understanding of the etiology, identifying
features, and therapy of different emergency infections.*

Educational Objectives

*Upon completion of this chapter, the dental hygiene stu-
dent should be able to:*

Define the role of the dental hygienist in the treatment of
    abscesses.
Define the role of the dental hygienist in the treatment of
    necrotizing ulcerative gingivititis.
Define the role of the dental hygienist in the treatment of primary
    herpetic gingivostomatitis.
Define the role of the dental hygienist in the treatment of
    pericoronitis.

KEY WORDS

- pain
- gingival abscess
- periodontal
  abscess
- pericoronal
  abscess
- necrotizing
  ulcerative
  diseases
- primary herpetic
  gingivostomatitis

Abscesses of the Periodontium

Chapter 13 reviewed the different types of abscesses of the periodontium. This chapter reviews the treatment of these abscesses as well as other common periodontal emergencies that may be encountered in the dental office.

As mentioned in Chapter 13, an abscess is defined as an infection originating from the tooth or periodontium. Pain and swelling from an abscess usually brings the patient into the dental office as an emergency visit. Classification of abscesses is based upon the location of the infection. For example, a gingival abscess is an infection located in the gingival tissue, usually the free (marginal) gingiva; a periodontal abscess is an infection located within the tissues adjacent to the periodontal pocket; and a pericoronal abscess is an infection located within the tissue around the crown of a partially erupted tooth, usually the last tooth in the arch. Treatment of an abscess is based upon the origin of the abscess.

Gingival Abscess

A gingival abscess is an acute infection characterized by a localized, painful edema at the free gingival margin. Foreign objects such as popcorn kernels, fish bones, or seeds that become lodged in the gingival crevice are responsible for many gingival abscesses. Since the abscess develops fairly rapidly (within 24 to 48 hours), the patient often knows the cause. Calculus is usually *not* the etiologic factor. Often, there are no signs of periodontitis in the patient's mouth.

The differential diagnosis of a gingival abscess is a periodontal abscess or endodontic abscess. The gingival abscess is usually located more coronally than the periodontal or endodontic abscess. The gingival abscess is usually found just within the gingival sulcus, whereas the periodontal abscess is usually found at the lateral side (corresponding to a deep pocket) and the endodontic abscess is usually found at the apical area of the root. Treatment requires removal of the etiologic agent by periodontal debridement (Table 29–1■). Since the gingiva may be friable, careful tissue manipulation is advised. It is best to place the finger of the nondominant hand on the tissue to support it. Local anesthesia may be helpful but the injection should never be directly into the infection as the infection may spread. Scaling establishes drainage through the gingival crevice. The patient can be placed on a warm saline rinse (1/4 teaspoonful of salt to 8 oz of warm water; rinse every 1 to 2 hours for several days). The patient should be instructed to use a soft-bristled toothbrush. If treated adequately, the condition will resolve within a matter of days. Systemic antibiotics are not recommended, as there is no systemic infection.

Table 29–1	Treatment Steps for Gingival and Periodontal Abscesses	
Gingival	**Periodontal**
First probe the site: shallow	First probe the site: deep
Location is submarginal	Location is base of pocket
Incision and drainage: debride and irrigate area	Incision and drainage: debridement and irrigation/ periodontal surgery
	Systemic antibiotics if lymphadenopathy is present

Periodontal Abscess

A periodontal abscess, also called a lateral abscess, is a localized purulent nidus of acute inflammation within the periodontal tissues. A periodontal abscess develops as a result of a bacterial infection that eventually leads to the formation of pus (suppuration). Gram-negative anaerobic rods are the most common bacteria isolated in the exudate of periodontal abscesses (Meng, 1999). Thus, a periodontal abscess contains bacteria, bacterial by-products, inflammatory cells, tissue breakdown products, and serum et al., 2003). In the gingival connective tissues an inflammatory reaction occurs due to the bacteria and bacterial by-products resulting in the connective tissue becoming infiltrated with inflammatory cells (e.g., neutrophils, machrophages). As a result of the inflammatory infiltrate, there is destruction or breakdown of the gingival connective tissues (e.g., collagen). The bacterial mass becomes encapsulated with the resultant pus formation.

Periodontal abscess formation is often seen in deep periodontal pockets (Fig. 29–1■) and in furcation sites. Such patients usually have a number of sites with chronic periodontitis. Many patients with diabetes mellitus are more susceptible to periodontal abscess formation. Periodontal abscesses may also develop a few days after scaling and root planing, especially at sites with deeper probing pocket depths.

Periodontal abscesses can occur as a result of inadvertent embedding of a foreign body subgingivally (calculus fragment, popcorn husk, seeds, shellfish fragments, etc.) that obstructs the normal sulcular drainage of gingival crevicular fluid and inflammatory by-products of chronic periodontitis. To reestablish drainage, a fistula may form that drains pus through the otherwise intact surface of the gingiva or mucosa.

The periodontal abscess presents as a shiny, swollen, discolored mass on the gingiva or mucosa. Finger pressure may produce purulent drainage. The involved tooth is often tender to percussion, mobile, and may feel high to the patient. Patients usually complain of pain. Occasionally, patients may demonstrate localized lymphadenopathy and fever.

It is important to rule out a pulpal etiology prior to addressing the periodontal condition. To help confirm the diagnosis, an endodontic gutta percha point is placed into the fistula and positioned until resistance is felt. A radiograph is taken with the gutta percha point in place. The end of the point will end at the origin of

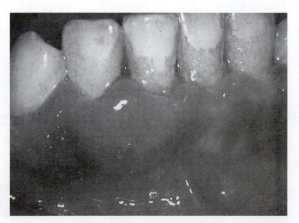

Figure 29–1
Periodontal abscess involving the mandibular central incisor. Note the heavy accumulation of plaque and calculus. Treatment involved is scaling and root planing. (Courtesy of Dr. Robert S. Schoor, NYU College of Dentistry)

the abscess. This will help to distinguish between a periodontal and endodontic abscess.

Treatment of a periodontal abscess consists of two phases. The first phase involves management of the acute signs and symptoms. Different therapies have been suggested for the acute lesion including incision and drainage, scaling and root planing, administration of systemic antibiotics, periodontal surgery, or tooth extraction (see Table 29–1). Some clinicians prefer to wait until the acute lesion has simmered down with the use of systemic antibiotics followed by scaling and root planing or periodontal surgery. Others prefer to initially establish drainage of the infection (pus) and remove any foreign causative agent (if applicable). Usually treatment consists of establishing drainage and removing any foreign causative agent (if applicable). Block anesthesia is likely necessary. When giving infiltration anesthesia the abscess should never be directly injected into. Generally, vigorous subgingival debridement reestablishes drainage and removes any foreign body. A soft diet, rest, analgesics, and warm salt water rinses are prescribed. Antibiotics may be prescribed if systemic involvement (e.g., fever and/or lymphadenopathy) is suspected. The successfully treated patient will notice improvement within 24 hours of treatment. If symptoms fail to improve promptly, emergency surgical access to the affected root surface may be necessary.

The second phase involves treatment of the underlying periodontal lesion. Once acute symptoms resolve, the second phase is done to treat the underlying original or residual periodontal lesion. This may consist of periodontal surgery to eliminate the deep periodontal pocket.

Pericoronal Abscess

The gingival flap (or operculum) overlying the erupting tooth (third molar) usually disappears once the tooth fully erupts, but many of these teeth remain partially erupted (Fig. 29–2■).

Treatment initially is toward controlling the infection. Food debris is often found under the operculum so irrigation with saline, iodine solution, or water is common therapy to flush out the debris. This area is very sensitive so care must be taken when manipulating the tissues. If the infection is severe or systemic involvement is suspected, systemic antibiotics such as penicillin VK are indicated. Ultimately, extraction of the erupting tooth may be necessary but is better performed when the patient no longer has acute local infection or trismus.

Figure 29–2
Pericoronitis. The third molar is partially covered by a "gingival flap." (Courtesy of Ann Goodwin, Formerly NYU College of Dentistry)

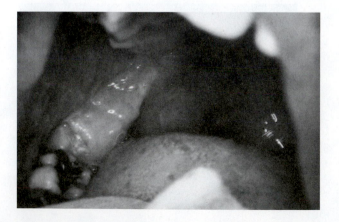

Necrotizing Ulcerative Diseases

It is important to distinguish between NUG and primary herpetic gingivostomatitis. The latter is highly contagious, and both are seen most commonly in young adult populations. Both are painful and can occur simultaneously. Patients with primary herpetic gingivostomatitis usually have a fever and show small ulcerations on the hard palate and attached gingiva remote from the gingival margins. NUG patients are often afebrile and show oral ulcerations extending from the marginal and papillary gingiva.

NUG is treated by addressing its causes. Since NUG is an infectious disease, treatment involves systemic antibiotics and mechanical debridement (Table 29–2■). The signs and symptoms of NUG are reduced when the microbial concentration is reduced. Systemic analgesics may also be used in the initial treatment due to the pain. If left untreated, extensive gingival tissue and bone destruction can occur. Even with treatment, recurrent lesions may occur.

Treatment on the first day the patient shows up in the dental office consists of data collection (e.g., medical/dental history, chief complaint, etc.) and making the correct diagnosis. Since the patient may be in too much pain to have mechanical debridement, the first step is to place the patient on a systemic antibiotic to eliminate the infection. Metronidazole is considered the drug of choice for spirochetes in NUG. Other antibiotics that may be used include tetracycline and penicillin. Additionally, an analgesic (e.g., ibuprofen) should be prescribed. Although symptoms diminish within 24 hours, the antibiotic should still be taken for the prescribed time. Patients are instructed to rinse with a mixture of 1 tablespoon of 3% hydrogen peroxide in 1/2 glass of warm water and to gently brush with a soft or extrasoft toothbrush twice daily. Placement on a multivitamin may also be helpful. The NUG patient is advised to avoid alcohol and tobacco, eat a balanced diet, and rest. In 1 to 2 days the patient should see much improvement with alleviation of pain and the infection under control. Instruct the patient to use chemical plaque control (saline, diluted hydrogen peroxide, or chlorhexidine gluconate) in place of toothbrushing. In 1–2 days the patient should return to the office for plaque control

Table 29–2	Treatment Steps for Necrotizing Ulcerative Gingivitis
1st appointment	Give systemic antibiotics and an analgesic. Rinse with warm water and salt, diluted hydrogen peroxide (1:4) or Gly-Oxide.
2nd appointment (Day 1–2)	When patient is out of pain, mechanical debridement (power-driven scalers and hand instrumentation) is started. Oral hygiene instructions given (ultrasoft toothbrush gently). Control of other risk factors (e.g., smoking cessation).
3rd appointment (same week and the following week)	Continued mechanical debridement under topical/local anesthesia
4th appointment	Collection of more data; gingival examination to see the gingival architecture
5th appointment	Definitive treatment planning
6th appointment	2-month periodontal maintenance
7th appointment	2-month periodontal maintenance. At this time evaluate the gingival architecture to determine the presence of residual gingival craters and the need for gingival surgery to recontour the interdental papillae to eliminate the craters.

instructions and education of the patient on elimination of other risk factors such as smoking cessation. At this time ultrasonic or sonic scalers and hand instrumentation (anesthesia is given) with irrigation are used. Complete debridement may not be accomplished at one visit and may return at least once a week. When debridement is finished, the patient will return in a few days so that a gingival examination can be done to evaluate the gingival architecture. The patient is placed on a 2-month maintenance schedule. After a few maintenance appointments, a definitive treatment plan is made. If gingival craters are present, surgical intervention may be needed to eliminate craters, which are plaque traps.

In NUP patients, treatment is aimed at periodontal debridement, improved oral hygiene self-care, and frequent use of an antiplaque rinse or irrigant such as chlorhexidine gluconate. Oral fungal infections are sometimes seen, and these may require antifungal medication. Referral to a periodontist is recommended.

AIDS-related oral lesions may not fully respond to therapy. Periodontal debridement may expose necrotic bone that should be removed. Local anesthesia, pain medication, and antibiotics may be necessary. Frequent periodontal maintenance visits are recommended. Oral care should be provided in collaboration with the patient's physician. Referral to a periodontist should be considered.

Primary Herpetic Gingivostomatitis

Primary herpetic gingivostomatitis is a condition of the oral mucosa characterized by a *previous* infection with herpes virus (HSV 1), which is mainly a disease of infants and children and only clinically detectable in about 90% of patients. After a brief prodromal period (1–2 days before development of blisters) of fever, headache, nausea, vomiting, and malaise, many small blisters (vesicles) form in the gingiva as well as other parts of the mouth including the hard palate and buccal and labial mucosa. These blisters quickly break and form painful, yellowish-gray ulcers, which form in groups surrounded by a red halo (inflammation). Rarely are the vesicles present at the time of the office visit because they quickly rupture (Fig. 29–3■). One of the most important distinguishing features, which is diagnostic for

Figure 29–3
Primary herpetic gingivostomatitis. Note lesions on the cheek and gingiva. (Courtesy of A. Ross Kerr, DDS, NYU College of Dentistry, Department of Oral Medicine)

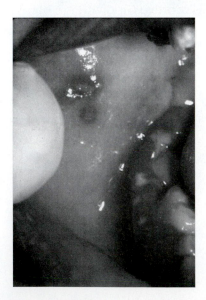

primary herpetic gingivostomatitis, is the presence of a generalized acute gingivitis. The gingiva is red (erythematous), and swollen (edematous). Submandibular lymphadenopathy is present. These patients do not have a past history of recurrent herpes labialis. When this disease is present in adults it may be more difficult to diagnose because the typical signs and symptoms may not be present. Most patients develop the infection through direct contact with another person with active recurrent lesions (e.g., through kissing). Symptoms usually last for 1 to 2 weeks. Patients with NUG have necrotic, punched out interdental papillae, while in primary herpetic gingivostomatitis the papillae are intact. However, a differential diagnosis would be aphthous stomatitis (canker sores). Aphthous stomatitis occurs only on unattached mucosa and there is a history of recurrence and usually there is no associated fever, whereas the ulcers in primary herpetic gingivostomatitis occur on both unattached and attached mucosa.

Treatment of primary herpetic gingivostomatitis in both children and adults is primarily palliative. The intense oral pain makes eating and drinking difficult. Dehydration must be prevented with frequent drinking of liquids. Rinsing with viscous xylocaine 2% before eating and drinking may be helpful to anesthesize the area. Antipyretics such as acetaminophen is recommended to reduce the fever and pain. Antiviral drugs such as acyclovir (Zovirax®; 400 mg four times daily for 1 to 2 weeks is recommended) is used to reduce the duration of the infection.

Summary

An abscess is an infection originating from the tooth or periodontium. It is important to determine the point of origin so that proper treatment is given. Treatment involves removal of the irritant, if possible, and establishing drainage. Once the acute infection is managed, further treatment of the underlying lesion may be necessary.

Treatment of necrotizing ulcerative gingivitis involves elimination of the bacterial infection with systemic antibiotics. Since the condition is very painful, once the patient is out of pain then mechanical debridement can be started.

A differential diagnosis of NUG is primary herpetic gingivostomatitis. Primary herpetic gingivostomatitis is treated with antiviral drugs, fluids, and acetaminophen.

Key Points

- Abscesses are bacterial infections.
- It is important to determine the origin of the abscess.
- Establish incision and drainage of the infection.
- Systemic antibiotics are only needed if there is systemic involvement.
- Necrotizng ulcerative gingivitis is confined to gingival tissues.
- Five to ten percent of patients initially infected with the herpes simplex virus develop primary herpetic gingivostomatitis.

Web Site

www.perio.org

Self-Quiz

1. Which of the following is usually the first treatment in the management of the acute periodontal abscess? (p. 516)
   a. site-specific antibiotics
   b. periodontal surgery
   c. incision and drainage
   d. leave alone until it becomes chronic

2. Which of the following diseases is a differential diagnosis of necrotizing ulcerative gingivitis? (p. 517)
   a. chronic periodontitis
   b. necrotizing ulcerative periodondititis
   c. primary herpetic gingivostomatitis
   d. aphthous ulcers

3. Which of the following is the first step in treating NUG? (p. 517)
   a. scaling and root planing
   b. systemic antibiotics
   c. irrigation and ultrasonics
   d. observation

4. Which of the following treatments is used for a patient with a gingival abscess? (p. 514)
   a. incision and drainage
   b. systemic antibiotics
   c. systemic analgesic
   d. controlled-drug delivery

5. Which of the following is not usually present in a patient with NUG? (p. 517)
   a. pain
   b. fetid odor
   c. fever
   d. bleeding
   e. ulceration of papillae

Reference

Meng, H.X. 1999. Periodontal abscess. *Ann. Periodontol.* 4:79–82.

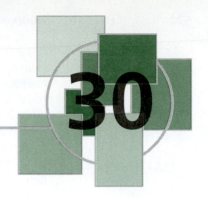

Periodontal Management of Medically Compromised Patients

Mea A. Weinberg, D.M.D., M.S.D., R.Ph.

Outline

- Cardiovascular Disorders
- Endocrine Disorders
- Pregnancy
- Kidney Diseases
- Systemic Corticosteroid Therapy
- Chemotherapy/ Radiotherapy
- Organ Transplants
- Seizure Disorders
- Liver Diseases
- Human Immunodeficiency Virus Infection
- Tuberculosis
- Infective Endocarditis
- Summary
- Key Points
- Web Sites
- Self-Quiz
- References

Goal

To provide an understanding of the identification and periodontal management of medically compromised patients.

Educational Objectives

Upon completion of this chapter, the dental hygiene student should be able to:

List the different categories of medically compromised patients.

Identify medically compromised patients.

Describe various dental care considerations for medically compromised patients.

Discuss the management of a patient requiring prophylactic antibiotics.

<table>
<tr><th colspan="2">KEY WORDS</th></tr>
<tr><td>•</td><td>medical risk</td></tr>
<tr><td>•</td><td>medically compromised</td></tr>
<tr><td>•</td><td>special care</td></tr>
<tr><td>•</td><td>universal precautions</td></tr>
</table>

Since more people are living longer today than ever before, there is an increased chance of encountering patients with medical conditions that may alter their dental treatment plan and care. Identification of these patients is necessary before treatment commences in order to avoid untoward medical emergencies. Recognition of these patients comes initially from reviewing their health/medical histories. It is the responsibility of every practitioner to identify any patient who may be at a potential medical risk and modify his or her care and/or consult with his or her physician. Since it is now recognized that medical conditions can develop as a result of a patient's preexisting periodontal disease, it is prudent to identify such conditions and make sure that they are well controlled. Different categories of medically compromised patients or patients with medical conditions that may require special care or alterations of the treatment plan will be discussed in this chapter: patients with cardiovascular disorders, endocrine conditions, hormonal conditions, kidney diseases, corticosteroid therapy, chemotherapy/radiotherapy, organ transplant, epilepsy, hepatitis, human immunodeficiency virus (HIV) infection, and tuberculosis.

Cardiovascular Disorders

Cardiovascular or heart disease is one of the more common medical conditions in the United States. Often cardiovascular disease may go undiagnosed. If it is not revealed in the patient's health/medical history, a dental hygienist can recognize certain signs and symptoms to help in the potential identification of patients with the disease.

Hypertension

Hypertension is defined as an elevation of arterial pressure. It is estimated that there are more than 50 million hypertensive people in the United States (Berkow, Fletcher, & Beers, 1992). Vital signs, including blood pressure and pulse, should be taken on the initial dental appointment and every subsequent office visit. Blood pressure increases with increasing age from under 110/75 mmHg in children less than 6 years of age to 140/90 mmHg in adults. When taking a blood pressure reading, position the patient's arm at chest level. If the blood pressure is elevated, the patient should be referred to a physician; it is not the responsibility of the dentist or dental hygienist to make a diagnosis of hypertension. Symptoms the patient may experience include headache, weakness, nosebleeds, and dizziness.

The Joint National Committee on Prevention, Detection, Evaluation, and Treatment of High Blood Pressure released its seventh report (JNC VII) in 2003. There is a new category entitled "prehypertension," which indicates patients that are at an increased risk of developing hypertension. Additionally, there is new emphasis on elevated systolic pressure (SBP) being an important risk factor for cardiovascular disease (CVD) rather than on elevated diastolic blood pressure (which has been for many years) (Chobanian et al., 2003). For patients older than 50 years, SBP > 140 mm Hg is considered a risk for future CVD. Additionally, the JNC recognized that most patients require at least two drugs for controlling their hypertension.

The newest classification of blood pressure is in Table 30–1■. Students can go directly to the websites: www.nhlbi.nih.gov/guidelines/hypertension/phycard.pdf

Table 30–1	Blood Pressure Classification (2003)		
Classification	**Systolic (mm Hg)**		**Diastolic BP (mm Hg)**
Normal	<120	AND	<80
Prehypertension	120–139	OR	80–89
Hypertension: Stage 1	140–159	OR	90–99
Hypertension: Stage 2	≥160	OR	≥100

Adapted from Chobanian AV, Bakris GL, Black HR, Cushman WC, Green LA, Izzo JL, et al. 2003. Seventh report of the Joint National Committee on Prevention, Dectection, Evaluation, and Treatment of High Blood Pressure. *JAMA* 289; 2560–2571.

and www.nhlbi.nih.gov/guidelines/hypertension/express.pdf for more information. This information should be printed out and kept in the office for handy reference.

The JNC recommends more invasive testing if the patient's hypertension is difficult to control, if blood pressure responds poorly to drug therapy, or if the hypertension developed suddenly (Chobanian et al., 2003). For most patients the treatment goal is having a BP of < 140/90 mm Hg; for patients with diabetes, the goal BP is < 130/80.

Periodontal Management of a Patient with Hypertension

Patients with Stage I hypertension (systolic 140–159 mm Hg or diastolic 90–99) may precede with periodontal treatment. However, risk assessment is necessary for all patients, especially those needing periodontal surgery (Herman et al., 2004). Risk factors for hypertension must be evaluated. The JNC VII recommends limiting the use of epinephrine in hypertensive patients because many older patients may have other CVDs. It is recommended that 2 to 3 carpules of lidocaine with 1:100,000 epinephrine is considered safe for most of these patients, except in cases of severe CVD (Herman et al., 2003).

Patients with Stage 2 hypertension (systolic ≥ 160 mm Hg or diastolic ≥ 100) should have their BP taken again. Proper referral to the patient's physician is recommended. Any patient with BP higher than 210/120 mm Hg should be referred immediately for medical treatment (Herman et al., 2004). If BP is elevated > 20 mm Hg over the goal BP of <140/90, referral to the patient's physician is necessary.

Hypertension can be treated with diet and/or antihypertensive medications. Nonpharmacologic methods for lowering blood pressure include weight reduction, elimination of smoking, change in dietary habits, and stress reduction (Kaplan, 1998).

The dental hygienist should ask the patient if he or she is taking the medication as directed, usually in the morning or at night. Sometimes patients forget to take the medication, or they feel that it is not necessary because they feel "good" today. Some medications can cause orthostatic hypotension. Orthostatic hypotension occurs when blood pressure falls quickly upon assuming an upright position. Dizziness and/or syncope (fainting) can result when the patient suddenly sits up after prolonged lying down. To avoid orthostatic hypotension, change the chair position slowly, have the patient sit upright in the dental chair for a few minutes, and then assist the patient in getting out of the chair. Another adverse side effect of antihypertensive drugs is xerostomia. Although not a medical emergency, this is an annoying problem for the patient. It may be necessary to discuss a change in the medication with the patient's physician. Numerous types of over-the-counter synthetic saliva replacements are available.

Anesthesia/Anesthetics

Periodontal patient care to prevent medical complications involves a stress-free and anxiety-free environment, short appointments, caution in chair positioning, proper medication use, and limited use of vasoconstrictors (e.g., epinephrine) in the local anesthetic. Epinephrine binds to receptors on the heart, causing vasoconstriction, which can increase the force and rate of heart contraction and result in elevated blood pressure. Epinephrine is not contraindicated but must be used with caution. In cardiac patients, the use of 0.036 mg of epinephrine is suggested; this corresponds to two carpules (1.8 ml) of 2% lidocaine with 1:100,000 epinephrine. Levonordefrin, a less potent vasoconstrictor found in the local anesthetic mepivacaine, also should be limited to two carpules. If a vasoconstrictor such as epinephrine is not used during painful dental procedures, the stress experienced by the patient most likely would cause more elevation in blood pressure and anxiety than use of a limited amount of epinephrine.

Caution should be employed in the use of nitrous oxide to avoid hypoxia, which also can elevate blood pressure. If the patient appears to be stressed or fearful of the procedure, treatment should be postponed to a later time.

Angina Pectoris

Angina pectoris is defined as pain or pressure in the chest due to a decrease in oxygen to the heart. Pain can radiate to the left shoulder, left arm, fingers, jaws, and teeth. Angina is usually experienced after exercise, excitement, stress, digestion of a heavy meal, or exposure to cold temperatures. Angina pectoris is classified as stable or unstable. Stable angina occurs when chest pain lasts between 3 and 5 minutes. These attacks typically are relieved by rest or nitroglycerin and are provoked by exercise and stress. Usually the patient can predict an attack. Nitroglycerin is a drug that causes vasodilation (dilates blood vessels to reduce the load to the heart). As part of the medical history, the patient should be asked when the last attack occurred. With unstable angina, chest pain occurs at rest or after exertion. Such attacks do not respond well to nitroglycerin and usually are very distressing and disabling. These patients should not have dental treatment and should be referred to a physician immediately.

Patients with stable angina may need to be premedicated with antianxiety drugs and/or nitrous oxide. Epinephrine is not contraindicated but should be used with caution. It is better to have profound analgesia than to have the patient release endogenous epinephrine as a result of uncontrolled pain. Cardiac patients generally are given 0.036 mg of epinephrine, which corresponds to two carpules (1.8 ml) of 2% lidocaine with 1:100,000 epinephrine.

Patients with angina always should keep their nitroglycerin tablets on the bracket table during dental treatment. If a patient has an angina attack in the dental chair, the dentist should be notified and the following steps should be taken (Rose, Steinberg, & Atlas, 1995):

- Stop the procedure.
- Place the patient in a supine position in the dental chair.

- Administer 100% oxygen.
- Administer sublingual nitroglycerin.
- Monitor vital signs.

If after three doses of nitroglycerin, given every 5 minutes, the patient does not respond and pain continues, lasting more than 15 to 20 minutes and accompanied by nausea, vomiting, or syncope, a more serious condition may be occurring. Emergency medical services should be called immediately. Cardiopulmonary resuscitation (CPR) may have to be implemented if cardiopulmonary arrest occurs.

Myocardial Infarction

Myocardial infarction (MI) occurs when heart cells are deprived of blood and oxygen, which causes them to lose the ability to contract and soon die. The result is known as a "heart attack." Most heart attack victims have atherosclerosis with occlusion of a coronary vessel due to an atherosclerotic plaque. Symptoms the patient may experience during an MI include deep chest pain radiating to the back, jaw, or left arm. The pain is similar in character to that of angina pectoris but is usually more severe and longer lasting and is relieved little or only temporarily by rest or nitroglycerin (Berkow et al., 1992).

Since patients who have had an MI within the last 6 months are more likely to have another MI, it is advised that minimal dental treatment be done within 6 months of an MI and only after a consultation with the patient's physician (Rose et al., 1995). The same management of patients with other cardiovascular conditions as described earlier should be followed with patients who have had an MI.

Cerebrovascular Accident

Cerebrovascular accident, or stroke, most commonly occurs when the oxygen flow to the brain is disturbed, resulting in neurologic changes. Risk factors for a stroke include smoking, hypertension, diabetes mellitus, advanced age, prior history of stroke, and atherosclerosis. Since recurrences are frequent, no dental treatment should be done (except emergency situations) within 6 months.

Most stroke victims will have some type of memory or speech impairment, paralysis with limited mobility (patient may be in a wheelchair), and impaired emotional status. The patient's appointments should be short, and vital signs should be monitored. The amount of vasoconstrictor (e.g., epinephrine) in the local anesthetic should be minimal; no more than five carpules of 1:1,000,000 epinephrine. Oral hygiene self-care may have to be modified, for example, through the use of powered toothbrushes and floss aids. Oral irrigation can be recommended. An antimicrobial mouthrinse such as chlorhexidine gluconate may help in dental plaque control.

Anticoagulation/Antiplatelet Medications

Patients with prosthetic valves or blood flow disturbances such as stroke are often required to take anticoagulation drugs. Most such patients take warfarin sodium (Coumadin®, DuPont Pharmaceuticals, Wilmington, DE); one tablet taken orally inhibits vitamin K, a natural coagulant (clotting) in the blood. This causes the blood to become "thin," with a resulting increase in flow. Since there is an increased risk of bleeding in these patients, any dental procedures that are likely to cause bleeding, such as an extraction or periodontal surgery, must be discussed with the patient's physician. The physician may decide to discontinue the warfarin for a few days before the surgical procedure but to reinstate it immediately after the procedure. The traditional method for determining the efficacy of anticoagulant therapy is the prothrombin time (PT). After a blood sample is taken from the patient, tests are done and the time until a fibrin clot forms, measured in seconds, is reported as the PT.

Because different methods and sources are used to determine the PT, it was necessary to standardize the technique. Thus, to resolve the problem of highly variable PTs, the use of the international normalized ratio (INR) or prothrombin time ratio (PTR) has been recommended for monitoring patients' oral anticoagulant therapy. The INR is the ratio of the patient's clotting time to the lab's mean reference value. This recommendation is supported by the American College of Chest Physicians, the National Heart, Lung and Blood Institute, and the British Society for Hematology (Nichols & Bowie, 1993).

Thus, INR is a good indicator of bleeding values. The higher the value, the greater are the anticoagulant effects. Nonsurgical or surgical dental procedures can be performed without discontinuation of warfarin if the patient's anticoagulation level (INR) is within the currently recommended therapeutic range and does not exceed 4 (Wahl, 2000) and the PTR does not exceed 2.2 (Wahl, 2000). If the patient's anticoagulation level exceeds the therapeutic range, the physician may decide to either discontinue the warfarin or reduce the dosage until the level returns to the therapeutic range.

Patients also may be taking aspirin prophylactically, either self-medicated or as prescribed by their physician, to reduce the risk of stroke or a heart attack. Many physicians recommend that aspirin be given prophylactically to patients with cardiovascular conditions at a dose of 81 to 325 mg per day. Platelets (disks found in the blood that are involved in blood clotting) tend to adhere to atherosclerotic plaques in coronary (heart) or cerebral (brain) arteries, increasing the risk of an MI or a stroke. During the medical history, the dental hygienist should ask patients if they are taking aspirin. Aspirin (acetylsalicylic acid), an antiplatelet drug, binds to and inhibits the action of cyclooxygenase, which is an enzyme in platelets that is involved in the formation of thromboxane A_2. Inhibiting the formation of thromboxane A_2 results in inhibition of platelet aggregation, which increases blood flow.

Endocrine Disorders

Diabetes Mellitus

Diabetes mellitus (DM) is a syndrome characterized by an absolute or relative lack of insulin. Insulin, a hormone produced by cells in the pancreas, allows sugar (glucose) in the bloodstream to enter all cells of the body and be used as energy. In diabetes, the glucose builds up in the blood instead of moving into the cells. This is termed hyperglycemia. Some, but not all, of the excess sugar is carried out of the body (in the urine), and the energy is wasted. Approximately 16 million Americans have diabetes, but only one-third to one-half have been diagnosed. Most of the deaths associated with diabetes are related to its chronic complications. Diabetes is currently the fourth leading cause of death by disease in the United States.

The American Diabetes Association (ADA) has established new guidelines and terms for diabetes mellitus. Formerly called insulin-dependent diabetes mellitus (IDDM), juvenile-onset diabetes, or type I diabetes, this form of DM is now called type 1 diabetes. Formerly called non-insulin-dependent diabetes mellitus (NIIDM), adult-onset diabetes, or type II diabetes, this form of DM is now called type 2 diabetes (American Diabetes Association, 1997).

In type 1 diabetes, the beta cells of the pancreas produce no insulin. Thus insulin must be reintroduced into the blood by injections of insulin. In type 2 diabetes, the pancreas produces insulin, but the tissues become insulin-insensitive and do not respond to the insulin. This is termed insulin resistance and is partly due to obesity and physical inactivity. These patients do not need injections of insulin but require oral medication and changes in diet and exercise levels. Classic signs and symptoms of diabetes include polyuria (excessive urination), polydipsia (excessive thirst), polyphagia (excessive desire for food), and weight loss, which is seen more commonly in type 1 diabetes but may be seen in type 2 diabetes. Plasma glucose levels are 200 mg/dl or greater.

When interviewing a diabetic patient, it must be determined if the patient's diabetes is controlled or uncontrolled. Discuss use of medications and self-testing at home (blood and urine glucose levels). Also inquire about a past history of periodontal disease, including periodontal abscesses. Evidence suggests that DM has an influence on the development of periodontal diseases (Cohen & Rose, 1998) not based on microbiologic etiology but rather on host immune responses. Diabetes per se does not cause periodontal disease. It is the altered metabolism of the tissues that lowers resistance to infection and local irritants. Elevated glucose levels decrease leukocyte chemotaxis and phagocytosis. Altered collagen metabolism and microvascular (small blood vessels) changes also may contribute to periodontal disease. The diabetic patient may present with numerous symptoms (Table 30–2■).

The level of metabolic control, duration of disease, types of medications used, and existence and severity of diabetes-related complications influence periodontal treatment care (Mealey, 1996). The patient's resistance to infection, wound-healing abilities, and cardiovascular and renal function should be assessed as components of the patient's medical and dental management (Little et al., 1997). Improved wound healing and decreased rates of postoperative infection are associated with good glycemic control.

Frequently, diabetic patients are not well controlled, and there is not enough insulin in their blood. Signs of hyperglycemia include decreased blood pressure and acetone breath. Unless treated in time, such patients may lapse into a state of unconsciousness (diabetic coma) that can terminate in death. Insulin must be injected, and CPR must be started. Immediate hospitalization is required.

Table 30–2 Oral Symptoms Presented in the Diabetic Patient

- Edematous and deep red color of the gingiva
- Multiple periodontal abscesses
- Lowered resistance to infection
- Poor tissue wound healing
- Dental and root caries
- Dry mouth (xerostomia)
- Burning mouth
- Candidiasis (yeast infection)

Hypoglycemia occurs when there are low levels of glucose and excessive amounts of insulin in the blood. Signs and symptoms of hypoglycemia, or insulin shock, include sweating, nervousness, fainting, and palpitations. Treatment includes the immediate ingestion of sugar (glucose or sucrose). Patients are advised to drink a glass of fruit juice or water with 3 tablespoonfuls of table sugar added or a soft drink and to carry candy or glucose tablets at all times. Hypoglycemia is the most common emergency likely to be encountered in a dental office during treatment of diabetic patients (Mealey, 1996). Hypoglycemia in diabetic patients is most likely caused by having taken too much insulin, missing or delaying meals, ingesting alcohol, and undergoing excessive stress (Mealey, 1996). If untreated, death can result. Referral to the patient's physician is necessary.

Periodontal Management of Diabetic Patients

The dental practitioner should evaluate the diabetic patient's level of glycemic control, including the ability to maintain optimal glycemic control during and following periodontal appointments. Glycated hemoglobin (HbA_{1c}) is a substance created as a result of the interaction between glucose and hemoglobin (blood). The level of glycated hemoglobin provides information on the average level of glucose in the body over a 3- to 4-month period of time. The glycated hemoglobin test should be performed two to four times a year to monitor blood glucose for long-term control. However, this test is not useful or necessary in the management of most patients with diabetes. The fingerstick test is usually done by the patient before meals, before bed, 1 to 2 hours after meals, and at 2:00 or 3:00 AM at least once a week, if they have type 2 diabetes. Ask the patient if he/she took their blood levels and the results. The average blood glucose levels are approximately between 100 to 120 mg/dl. If necessary, refer the patient to their physician before any dental treatment is started.

The dental hygienist should discuss with the patient the importance of blood glucose control. Meticulous home oral self-care is an important point to stress with patients. Well-controlled diabetics with good oral hygiene are at lower risk for periodontal diseases and respond better to periodontal therapy. Under good metabolic control, the diabetic patient shows no greater tendency to post-periodontal surgical complications than does the nondiabetic patient (Rose et al., 1995). However, stress reduction is also important in the diabetic patient because stress may increase epinephrine release, which raises glucose levels (Rose et al., 1995).

Treatment modifications include shorter periodontal maintenance visits, control of the environment to minimize stress, prevention of insulin shock or diabetic coma, meticulous plaque control, and dietary advice. It is important to make sure that patients have taken their insulin or oral medication as directed, and appointments should be scheduled approximately 1 1/2 hours following insulin administration and breakfast. Shorter, early-morning appointments are advisable. Epinephrine counteracts the hypoglycemic effects of insulin by elevating blood glucose levels; it causes the formation of glucose. Thus it is recommended to use the amount suggested for cardiac patients.

Pregnancy

Positioning of pregnant patients in the dental chair is critical. Avoiding a supine position (especially during the third trimester) allows better breathing and avoids hypotension (lowering blood pressure) and syncope (fainting) as a result of less uterine pressure on the inferior vena cava. A wedge may be placed under the patient's right side to take the pressure off the inferior vena cava.

Meticulous home oral self-care should be stressed. Appointments should be short, and the patient should be allowed to change position frequently. Periodontal maintenance visits can be scheduled throughout the entire pregnancy, but the second trimester is the safest. Lidocaine can be used safely during pregnancy. Use of radiographs during pregnancy has been controversial. Women should inform their dentists if they are pregnant, might be pregnant, or plan to become pregnant (American Dental Association, 2004). The American Dental Association (1989) states that radiographic specifications do not need to be changed because of pregnancy (see also Mealey, 1996). The decision to take radiographs must be based on need, which is determined by a health history and clinical examination. If dental X-rays are required during pregnancy, the American Dental Association recommends that a protective thyroid collar and apron be used (American Dental Association, 2004). The ADA further believes that the benefits of radiographs in diagnosing and managing oral conditions are very high and, when used prudently, can prevent the extension of many dental problems, such as infections, that may adversely affect the fetus. The American Dental Association recommends that elective dental radiographs should be postponed until after delivery. A study from the University of Washington in April 2004 reported that dental radiography during pregnancy is associated with low birth weight, specifically with preterm low birth weight (Hujoel, Bollen, Noonen, & del Aguila, 2004). The ADA (2004) responded to this article by stating that "studies have shown that pregnant women with severe periodontal disease may be at increased risk for preterm delivery and that professional oral health care administered during pregnancy to this at-risk group actually improved pregnancy outcomes."

If antibiotics are necessary, penicillins, clindamycin, cephalosporins, and erythromycins (except the estolate form and clarithromycin) are considered safe; however, consultation with the patient's physician is recommended before any drug is prescribed. All forms of tetracyclines are contraindicated. For pain control, acetaminophen, naproxen, and naproxen sodium are considered safe. Narcotics such as codeine should not be prescribed for a pregnant or nursing patient without consultation with the patient's physician.

Kidney Diseases

The most important function of the kidneys is the production of urine, which is the medium whereby the body eliminates excess water, waste products, salts, and so on. In renal failure, the kidneys do not function properly, and the excretion products accumulate in the body. Dialysis is necessary when a patient's kidneys have partly or completely stopped functioning. There are two common methods of dialysis: peritoneal dialysis (no machine is used; the solution is injected into the patient's abdomen) and hemodialysis (a machine acts as an artificial kidney). During this "purification" process, blood containing waste products for removal is passed through tubes consisting of thin synthetic membranes immersed in a dialyzing solution. In this way the waste products are removed from the bloodstream. Only patients undergoing hemodialysis need special precautions during dental treatment. On the day of the dialysis, an anticoagulant (a drug that prevents blood clotting) is administered to keep the blood flowing. Thus periodontal treatment should not begin until at least the day after dialysis (24 hours after) to allow for the effects of the anticoagulant to be removed. Of note, hemodialysis patients have a higher incidence of hepatitis (inflammation of the liver).

Bleeding during periodontal treatment is best managed by prevention (Mealey, 1996). Coagulation tests (e.g., bleeding time [BT], prothrombin time [PT], and partial prothrombin time [PPT]) should be ordered through the patient's physician. This will help determine the patient's susceptibility to bleeding (hemorrhage). Bleeding time is the time it takes for an incision to stop bleeding (this tells about platelet function). Partial prothrombin time is the time it takes for blood to clot (this tests for defects in the coagulation pathway).

All dialysis patients should receive initial comprehensive oral examinations with frequent follow-up care. Comprehensive oral hygiene instruction is essential in the overall oral health of such patients (Naugle, Darby, Bauman, Lineberger, & Powers, 1998).

The kidneys are a major route of excretion of many drugs. To avoid drug toxicity (elevated blood levels of a drug), only drugs (e.g., antibiotics or analgesics) that are not eliminated through the kidneys should be used. For example, doxycycline hyclate, minocycline HCl, penicillin V, amoxicillin trihydrate, clindamycin HCl, acetaminophen, and codeine (except if there is liver disease) are safe in patients with kidney disorders. Tetracycline HCl and aspirin should be avoided. Since hypertension is a cause of renal failure, blood pressure should be monitored closely.

Systemic Corticosteroid Therapy

Corticosteroids are hormones produced in the body by the adrenal cortex. The principal hormones produced by the adrenal cortex are cortisol (hydrocortisone) and aldosterone. Corticosteroids function primarily to maintain the chemical stability of the body despite changes in the environment; for example, they enable the body to withstand various stresses due to such causes as injury, disease, severe exertion, and mental strain. Steroids also have anti-inflammatory actions (reduce tissue inflammation).

Indications for systemic administration of steroids include asthma, rheumatoid arthritis, inflammatory bowel disease (e.g., ulcerative colitis), and connective tissue/skin disorders (pemphigus, systemic lupus erythematosus). Examples of systemic corticosteroids include prednisone, prednisolone, methyprednisolone, and dexamethasone.

Once systemic corticosteroids are administered, endogenous (within the body) production and secretion are shut down. Thus, when an individual is stressed or excited (e.g., undergoing dental treatment), not enough endogenous corticosteroids are present to allow the body to respond to the stress without leading to adrenal insufficiency. It is necessary to contact the patient's physician (always get approval from the patient to call his or her physician) to discuss this situation. Generally, however, most routine periodontal procedures, including periodontal debridement, do not require supplemental steroids (Little et al., 1997). Extractions and surgical procedures may need dosage adjustments (usually increase dosage).

Chemotherapy/Radiotherapy

Radiotherapy, or radiation treatment, uses the fact that rapidly growing young tissues, in particular cancerous tissues, are more sensitive to radiation than mature tissues. The treatment of cancer often requires high radiation doses, which are to some extent also harmful to normal healthy tissue.

Chemotherapy is the application of chemical agents that are not harmful to the patient but which have a specific suppressive or destructive effect on cancer cells. The problem is similar to that of radiotherapy in that cancer cells are degenerated cells of the human body itself that differ little in character from normal cells. The drawback of cancer treatment with such drugs is that they cannot distinguish cancer cells from healthy cells. Thus they also attack normal healthy tissue in the process of rapid growth, such as the bone narrow, oral mucosa, and intestinal cells.

Such treatments may result in the development of a wide range of oral conditions. There may be a reduction in the volume and character of saliva, resulting in xerostomia. There may be a disruption in the balance of the oral flora, resulting in a greater incidence of infections (Mealey, 1996). Patients may develop mucositis (inflammation of the mucous membranes), which is treated on a palliative basis by reducing or eliminating pain and discomfort until the radiation and chemotherapy treatment is completed. Oral candidiasis is the most common fungal infection in these patients. This may be treated with chlorhexidine gluconate rinses. Meticulous oral hygiene self-care is emphasized, as are frequent periodontal maintenance treatment visits. Gentle hand instrumentation is recommended; ultrasonic and sonic devices are not recommended. Saliva substitutes and viscous lidocaine are advised for oral discomfort. Consultation with the patient's physician is advisable before periodontal treatment is started.

Organ Transplants

After an organ transplant, patients are given a drug that will help prevent rejection of the new organ. The most commonly prescribed drug is cyclosporine. Patients also may be taking corticosteroids or azathioprine. Cyclosporine is an antibiotic that suppresses the immune system. Frequent adverse effects include renal impairment, hypertension, xerostomia, and gingival enlargement. Cyclosporine has been used in combination with corticosteroids and calcium channel blockers (for hypertension), which also may cause gingival overgrowth. Consult with the patient's physician regarding the use of steroids if periodontal surgery is to be performed; otherwise, no dosage adjustments are required for periodontal debridement.

Meticulous home self-care using a soft-bristled toothbrush and an antimicrobial mouthrinse such as chlorhexidine gluconate is important; however, removal of dental plaque alone does not prevent gingival overgrowth (Seymour & Smith, 1991).

Besides organ rejection, infection is another complication after transplant surgery. Therefore, in preparation for such surgery, all questionable and hopeless teeth should be extracted. Routine dental treatment should be avoided during the first three months after the transplant surgery until the physician gives clearance (Mealey, 1996; Rhodus & Little, 1993).

Seizure Disorders

Epilepsy is convulsions (seizures) due to disturbances in electrical activity of the brain. Patients presenting with a seizure disorder should have their condition and level of disease control reviewed. Asking the patient when his or her last seizure occurred may help determine this. Vital signs, including respiratory status, must be taken at every dental appointment. There are numerous types of seizures: grand mal, petit mal (absence), status epilepticus, and myoclonic syndrome. Different drugs are used for specific seizure types. A common adverse side effect of phenytoin and valproate is gingival enlargement. Phenytoin adversely interacts with many other drugs, including acetaminophen, alcohol, antidepressants, antacids, aspirin, barbiturates, benzodiazepines, corticosteroids, doxycycline, and metronidazole. A side effect of valproic acid is excessive bleeding and decreased platelet aggregation. Aspirin and nonsteroidal anti-inflammatory drugs (NSAIDs) such as ibuprofen should not be taken with valproic acid.

Blood tests should be performed before dental treatment. Morning appointments are preferred. Meticulous oral hygiene is stressed. If in the event of a seizure, remove objects around the patient, open the airway, and do not restrict patient movement.

Liver Diseases

Viral Hepatitis

Hepatitis is inflammation of the liver, usually as a result of a viral infection, but it also can be due to alcohol and drugs. There are at least five forms of infectious or viral hepatitis: hepatitis A, hepatitis B, hepatitis C, hepatitis D, hepatitis E, and hepatitis G. When the liver infection does not resolve after 3 to 6 months, the acute disease becomes chronic active hepatitis.

Hepatitis A is transmitted from person to person by direct contact or through contaminated food or water. Hepatitis A is caused by the hepatitis A virus (HAV), an RNA virus. There is no known chronic carrier state, and HAV plays no role in the production of chronic active hepatitis or liver cirrhosis. There is no evidence that HAV poses an occupational risk to dental personnel as a result of injury or puncture of the skin (Gilllcrist, 1999). In 1995, a vaccine became available for immunity against HAV.

Hepatitis B is transmitted from person to person by direct contact of contaminated blood or other body secretions such as saliva. Individuals at risk for hepatitis B include intravenous drug users; persons undergoing tattooing, acupuncture, or body piercing; health care workers; homosexual and bisexual men; patients receiving blood transfusions; and hemodialysis patients. Hepatitis B is caused by the hepatitis B virus (HBV), a DNA virus. Hepatitis B can lead to acute or chronic hepatitis, which causes many of the deaths from chronic liver disease. The presence of HBsAg (hepatitis B surface antigen) in the blood is indicative of ongoing HBV infection. The hepatitis B vaccine is available for prevention.

Hepatitis C is an RNA virus that is transmitted from person to person by direct contact of contaminated blood. Individuals at risk for HCV infection include intravenous drug users, hemodialysis patients, patients undergoing blood transfusions, persons who are sexually active, and health care workers (e.g., undergoing injuries from contaminated sharps) (Little et al., 1997). Onset is usually insidious, with anorexia, vague abdominal discomfort, and nausea and vomiting, progressing to jaundice less frequently than hepatitis B. Hepatitis C may be the most serious of the viral hepatitis infections because of its ability to produce chronic infection. Up to 85% of patients become chronically infected, resulting in liver failure, carcinoma, and cirrhosis (Gillcrist, 1999). Immunization against infections with hepatitis C virus is not available.

Routes of transmission of hepatitis D are similar to those of hepatitis B. Hepatitis D is caused by an RNA virus that is found in patients who are carriers of hepatitis B virus. In the United States, infections with HDV most commonly affect persons at high risk of hepatitis B, particularly intravenous drug abusers and persons with hemophilia. Immunization with the hepatitis B vaccine also confers protection against coinfections with HDV-HBV (Gillcrist, 1999).

At present, the modes of transmission for hepatitis E virus (HEV) are similar to those for HAV. Hepatitis E is seen more commonly in undeveloped countries with inadequate environmental sanitation and unsafe drinking water, such as India and certain countries in Africa and Asia. Both diseases usually resolve without complications. As with HAV, there is no concern about occupational exposure in health care workers. A vaccine for HEV is not yet available.

Hepatitis G virus (HGV), an RNA virus, was discovered in 1995 (DiBisceglie, 1996). The true modes of transmission are not clearly defined, but it is definitely a blood-borne virus. There is no evidence to show that HGV is transmissible by injury or breaking through the skin. Further studies are needed before the cause, clinical features, prevention, and treatment can be established (Gillcrist, 1999).

General Recommendations

Dental hygienists and dentists should keep up with the latest information regarding viral hepatitis (Gillcrist, 1999). All health care workers are advised to have the hepatitis B vaccine, which gives immunity to the virus. Consultation with the patient's physician is needed to determine the status of the patient's hepatitis. It is extremely important to determine whether the patient is a carrier of hepatitis B, C, or D because he or she could be infectious. These carriers of the virus show no symptoms, so the presence of the virus in their blood remains unsuspected. Many times an individual is unaware that he or she has or has had hepatitis. A blood test is needed to determine if the patient is a carrier. If a positive history of hepatitis is reported on the health/medical history, the dental hygienist should further question the patient as to the age of onset of the disease and the possible cause (e.g., food and blood transfusion). If the clinician finds that the information is incomplete, a medical consultation is required. There is no evidence that hepatitis A virus poses an occupational risk to dental personnel as a result of a skin puncture injury (Gillcrist, 1999).

If the hepatitis is chronic, active, and ongoing, as determined by the patient's physician, elective periodontal treatment should be postponed. Chronic active liver disease indicates that the virus is actively replicating in the liver. Such patients usually are ill and very weak.

Universal precautions should be used on all patients because many patients and clinicians are unaware of the presence of the disease. Universal precautions is the Occupational Safety and Health Administration's (OSHA) accepted method of control to protect employees from exposure to all human blood and other potentially infectious materials. The purpose in following specific guidelines is to prevent transmission of the infection. Precautions should be taken in using aerosol-producing instruments, including ultrasonic/sonic scalers, air polishers, and the air-water syringe.

In patients with significant liver damage, there is a possibility for abnormal bleeding (elevated prothrombin time). A medical consultation is necessary to find out the status of the liver function. The liver metabolizes several antibiotics and analgesics to prepare them for final elimination from the body. If these drugs are given to patients with severely impaired liver function, elevated blood levels could occur and could result in drug toxicity. These drugs either should not be given or should be administered in a limited amount (Table 30–3■).

Human Immunodeficiency Virus Infection

Acquired immune deficiency syndrome (AIDS) is the end stage of infection with the human immunodeficiency virus (HIV). AIDS is a complex illness that interferes with the body's immune system in a number of ways, particularly that portion responsible for cell-mediated immunity and tumor suppression. Thus the disease attacks the body's immune system, leaving a person vulnerable to otherwise rare life-threatening infections, cancers, and other conditions. The definition of AIDS has changed several times since monitoring began in the early 1980s. Many systems and tissues in the body are affected. HIV can be transmitted from person to person through blood and other bodily secretions. Three basic modes of HIV transmission are (1) sexual contact, (2) blood-to-blood contact, and (3) from mother to child.

HIV is a transmissible retrovirus containing an enzyme called reverse transcriptase that converts viral RNA into a proviral DNA copy that becomes integrated into

Table 30–3	Drugs Used in Dentistry That Are Primarily Metabolized by the Liver

Amide local anesthetics
  Lidocaine
  Mepivacaine
  Prilocaine
  Bupivacaine
Nonnarcotic analgesics
  Acetaminophen
  Nonsteroidal anti-inflammatory drugs (NSAIDs), including ibuprofen and naproxen
Narcotic analgesics
  Codeine
Antibiotics
  Tetracycline HCl (doxycycline hyclate and minocycline HCl are eliminated by the
    kidneys)
  Penicillin V
  Amoxicillin
  Amoxicillin and clavulanic acid
  Metronidazole
  Azithromycin
  Clindaymycin

the host cell DNA. HIV preferentially attacks T-lymphocytes, specifically T-helper cells (or CD4+ cells). A person is considered to have AIDS if the CD4 count is less than 200/mm³. T cells are important to an effective immune response. Because the T-helper cell count in the blood is currently the best indicator of the clinical manifestations of HIV infection, the progress of the chronic infection is now tracked by following the slow decline of patients' CD4+ cells over several years.

HIV infection can range from asymptomatic to full-blown AIDS. HIV affects almost every organ in the body, including the oral cavity. Symptoms associated with HIV infection include fever, fatigue, night sweats, weight loss, dry cough, swollen glands, and diarrhea. These symptoms explain a lot of other medical conditions. The only difference is that in HIV-infected persons, these symptoms are ongoing and do not go away.

The best way to reduce occupational risk of infection with HIV, as well as any other transmissible infectious disease, is to follow universal precautions. Consultation with the patient's physician is necessary before treatment to determine the patient's CD4 count. Many oral infections are seen in HIV-positive patients. These conditions include hairy leukoplakia (on the lateral border of the tongue), linear gingival erythema (distinctive marginal gingival redness), necrotizing ulcerative periodontitis, candidiasis (fungal infection), and Kaposi's sarcoma. Treatment of oral conditions is palliative. Consultation with the patient's physician should be done before prescribing antibiotics, antifungal agents, or pain medications. Meticulous oral hygiene should be stressed. Chlorhexidine gluconate oral rinse can be prescribed to help reduce supragingival plaque accumulation. Lidocaine 2% viscous solution can be prescribed as an analgesic rinse. There seems not to be any contraindications to routine dental treatment for most HIV-positive patients (Mealey, 1996). The incidence of postoperative complications following scaling and root planing or tooth extractions is low (Glick, Abel, Muzyka, & Delorenzo, 1994), although excessive bleeding, delayed healing, and infections can occur.

Tuberculosis

Tuberculosis (TB) is a chronic, recurring infection most common in the lungs. TB is caused primarily by *Mycobacterium tuberculosis,* which enters the body by inhalation. The presence of HIV infection accelerates the course of TB. Many medications to treat TB are not as effective today as they were in the past. Thus resistance to antituberculosis drugs is a problem with treatment. Also, many individuals infected with TB are not undergoing treatment.

It must be determined if a patient has active TB or if he or she was exposed previously and currently is not active. Often patients with TB remain asymptomatic. A cough is the most common symptom. The cough also may be due to smoking or a cold, but the cough in TB is usually productive (of yellow or green sputum).

If TB is suspected, the patient should be referred to a physician. The tuberculin skin test can be used to help determine if the patient has TB. The skin test is performed by injecting slightly under the skin an extract of the mycobacterium called purified protein derivative (PPD). A positive test occurs if the area becomes indurated or hard by two days after the inoculation. While this test is not very definitive, it is still a good way to screen individuals for TB. If a patient was exposed previously but did not develop signs and symptoms of TB, the test will be positive.

On the other hand, a patient with TB may not have a positive test. If a chest x-ray reveals a scar or cavity in the lung, then the patient is TB-positive.

If the patient has active TB, periodontal treatment should be postponed. If the patient reports a positive PPD test on the health/medical history but no chest x-ray was taken, referral to a physician is necessary. If the patient reports a positive PPD test and a positive x-ray and has not had medical treatment, referral to a physician also is necessary. If the patient reports a positive PPD test and a negative chest x-ray, proceed with periodontal treatment, but follow universal precautions.

Treatment

Isoniazid (INH) is used in adults whose tuberculin skin test converted from negative to positive within the previous two years. This is a form of prophylactic (preventive) treatment. Other antimicrobial drugs used in the treatment of TB include rifampin, ethambutol, pyrazinamide, and streptomycin.

Since the disease is transmitted through the air, precautions are necessary in the use of aerosol-producing instruments, including ultrasonic/sonic scalers, air polishers, and the air-water syringe.

Infective Endocarditis

Although its incidence is rare, infective endocarditis (IE) is a critical and potentially lethal condition. The older term, subacute bacterial endocarditis (SBE), is no longer used because IE can be caused by microorganisms other than bacteria. The risk of IE associated with dental procedures makes it an important condition for the dental hygienist to be aware of. Equally important is the need for the hygienist to be thoroughly familiar with its causes and prevention. With proper knowledge of what conditions to recognize, which procedures present a risk, and how to pretreat patients at risk, the chances of a dental procedure resulting in IE may be drastically reduced.

Endocarditis most often is the result of an infection of the valves of the heart. The heart valves are made of avascular tissue. In a healthy heart, the cusps of each valve are washed as blood passes over them with each heartbeat. In certain conditions, however, when one of the valves is functioning abnormally, the individual may be susceptible to infection. The avascular nature of the valve tissue enables foreign microorganisms to colonize and literally hide from the immune system. Once bacteria have colonized the valve(s), they continue to proliferate unbeknown to the immune system, and in time, they begin to affect the function of the valve(s). The valve affected most often by infection, be it congenital or acquired, is the mitral valve or bicuspid valve on the left side of the heart. Some medical conditions create a higher risk of IE than others. The conditions and associated risks of IE listed in Table 30–4■ are based on the potential of an infection resulting in endocarditis. High-risk patients are those patients considered to have the greatest risk of developing severe endocardial infections, often associated with morbidity and mortality. Moderate-risk patients are at a significantly lower risk for endocardial infections yet still must be monitored closely preoperatively for signs of infection. Patients should receive antibiotic coverage if the procedure to be done may cause

Table 30–4	Cardiac Conditions and Associated Risk of Endocarditis	
High-Risk Category	**Moderate-Risk Category**	**Negligible Risk**
Prosthetic cardiac valves	Other cardiac malformations (other than those in the right column)	Isolated secundum atrial septal defect
Previous bacterial endocarditis	Acquired valvar dysfunction (e.g., rheumatic heart disease)	Surgical repair of atrial septal defect
Complex cyanotic congenital heart disease	Hypertrophic cardiac myopathy	Previous coronary artery bypass surgery
Surgically constructed systemic pulmonary shunts	Mitral valve prolapse with valvular regurgitation and/or thickened leaflets	Mitral valve prolapse without valvular regurgitation Innocent (functional) heart murmurs Previous Kawasaki's disease without valve dysfunction Previous rheumatic fever without valve dysfunction Cardiac pacemakers and implanted defibrillators

Source: Adapted from Dajani et al. (1997).

bleeding. Antibiotic prophylaxis for certain dental procedures is recommended for patients in the high- and moderate-risk categories. The negligible-risk category has been designated to include conditions that do not predispose patients to endocardial infections.

Bacteremia may be caused by many different dental procedures, but it is important to take into account all conditions that may give rise to bacteria in the bloodstream. In addition to toothbrushing, chewing, or flossing, bacteremia has been associated with poor oral hygiene and periodontal or periapical infections. The incidence and magnitude of bacteremia are directly proportional to the degree of oral inflammation and infection. It is therefore essential for patients at risk for endocarditis to establish and maintain the best possible oral health in order to reduce the risk of bacteremia. The best oral health is maintained through regular professional care, as well as routine home care. Table 30–5■ represents the dental procedures for which prophylaxis is recommended and those for which it is not recommended.

The recommendations listed in Table 30–5 are guidelines and not a substitute for clinical judgment. If it is suspected that a patient will bleed during any dental procedures, it is advisable to premedicate the patient. Patients who have not been premedicated and those who are currently taking antibiotics for other reasons will be discussed later in more detail. It is important to note that it is not acceptable to premedicate every patient, since prolonged use or misuse of antibiotics can lead to drug resistance. Furthermore, although it can significantly reduce the risk, antibiotic prophylaxis does not eliminate the risk of endocarditis. Clinical judgment is always necessary to evaluate each patient's risk, and close attention should be paid to the patient when risk is suspected.

Table 30–6■ indicates recommended prophylactic antibiotic regimens for oral and dental procedures. The regimens are most effective when given around the

Table 30–5	Antibiotic Prophylaxis Recommendations for Dental Procedures	
Higher Incidence		**Lower Incidence**
Dental extractions		Restorative dentistry (operative and prosthodontic)
Periodontal procedures: surgery, scaling and root planing, probing and recall maintenance		Local anesthetic injections (all except intraligamentary)
Implant placement and reimplantation of avulsed teeth		Placement of rubber dams
Root canal instrumentation when beyond apex (endodontics)		Postoperative suture removal
Subgingival placement of antibiotic fibers or strips		Placement of removable prosthodontic/ orthodontic appliances
Placement of orthodontic bands (not brackets)		Taking oral impressions or radiographs
Intraligamentary local anesthesia injection		Fluoride treatment
Prophylactic cleaning of teeth and implants		

time of dental treatment in doses that allow for adequate levels of the drug in the serum before, during, and after the procedure. In order to reduce the development of antibiotic resistance and maintain minimum serum levels for prophylaxis, the regimens are designed to give the patient adequate serum levels of the drug no longer than necessary.

The bacteria most commonly associated with endocarditis following dental and oral procedures is *Streptococcus viridans* (a-hemolytic streptococci). Amoxicillin

Table 30–6	Prophylactic Antibiotic Regimens for Oral and Dental Procedures	
Situation	**Drug**	**Regimen**
Standard general prophylaxis	Amoxicillin	Adults: 2.0 g orally 1 h before dental procedure Children: 50 mg/kg orally 1 h before procedure
Unable to take oral medication	Ampicillin	Adults: 2.0 g intramusculory (IM) or intravenously (IV) Children: 50 mg/kg IM or IV within 30 min before procedure
Allergic to penicillin	Clindamycin *or* Azithromycin or clarithromycin *or* Cephalexin or cefadroxil*	Adults: 600 mg; children: 20 mg/kg orally 1 h before procedure Adults: 500 mg; children: 15 mg/kg orally 1 h before procedure Adults: 2.0 g; Children: 50 mg/kg orally 1 h before procedure
Allergic to penicillin and unable to take oral medications	Clindamycin *or* Cefazolin*	Adults: 600 mg; children: 20 mg/kg IV within 30 min before procedure Adults: 1.0 g; children: 25 mg/kg IM or IV within 30 min before procedure

*Cephalosporins should not be used in patients with immediate-type hypersensitivity reaction (urticaria, angioedema, or anaphylaxis) to penicillins.

remains the most recommended antibiotic for endocarditis prophylaxis. Agents such as ampicillin and penicillin V have an equal antimicrobial effect against these a-hemolytic streptococci, but amoxicillin is better absorbed in the gastrointestinal tract and provides higher, more sustained serum levels than the other penicillins.

Until 1994, the recommended pretreatment dose of amoxicillin for antibiotic prophylaxis was 3.0 g. However, a recent study has indicated that 2.0 g is sufficient to reach adequate serum levels for several hours (Dajani et al., 1997). Previously, it was recommended that a second dose be given postoperatively. Currently, it has been demonstrated that not only will the initial dose of amoxicillin remain above the minimal serum level for long enough following the procedure, but also the inhibitory effect of the drug is sufficient to eliminate the need for a postoperative dose.

Erythromycin, which was approved originally as an effective prophylactic agent for endocarditis in cases of penicillin allergy, is no longer among the recommended agents. Erythromycin can cause severe gastrointestinal upset, and certain formulations (e.g., erythromycin ethylsuccinate) have complicated pharmacokinetics. Instead, second-generation erythromycins, azithromycin, or clarithromycin can be used because they have better absorption and produce much less gastrointestinal upset.

Periodically, patients will present to the dental office for a routine visit during a course of antibiotic therapy with a drug used for endocarditis prophylaxis. Patients receiving antibiotics for other reasons at the time of a routine dental visit who are considered at risk for endocarditis have specific recommendations. Rather than increasing the dose of the drug currently being used, it is advisable to select an agent from a different class of antibiotic. Remember, if you have to choose another antibiotic, it must have the same bactericidal or bacteriostatic activity as the antibiotic taken for prophylaxis. For instance, if the patient is taking tetracycline (a bacteriostatic drug), he or she cannot take amoxicillin (a bactericidal antibiotic) but can take clindamycin, azithromycin, or clarithromycin, which are all bacteriostatic. If possible, the dental procedure is best postponed until at least nine (Leviner, Tzukert, Benoliel, Baram, & Sela, 1987) to 14 days (Simmons et al., 1986) after completion of the antibiotic. This will allow the normal oral flora to reestablish (Dajani et al., 1997).

Since repeated use of antibiotics can lead to the emergence of antibiotic-resistant microorganisms in the oral cavity, it is recommended that there be an interval of at least seven days between dental appointments.

Generally, patients with mitral valve prolapse do not require antibiotic coverage unless they have a heart murmur or regurgitation associated with the mitral valve prolapse. If at the time of the dental appointment the presence or absence of regurgitation has not been determined, it is best to premedicate the patient with antibiotics and then refer the patient to a physician (Ciancio, 1997).

Specific cardiac surgical procedures have varied implications in terms of risk for endocarditis (Steckelberg & Wilson, 1993). As the volume and frequency of successful coronary artery bypass graft surgery increase, so does the likelihood of seeing more of these patients in the dental office. There is no evidence to suggest that this type of surgery introduces risk for bypass surgery (see Table 30–4). In the case of prosthetic valve placement, the risk of postoperative endocarditis increases. There is no evidence to suggest that heart transplant patients are at an increased level of risk for endocarditis, but such patients are subject to an increased likelihood of valve dysfunction and are often treated as moderate-risk patients. Whenever possible, patients who plan to have any cardiac surgery should have a carefully executed dental treatment plan in order to complete any dental work necessary before the cardiac procedure. This may decrease the chance of late postoperative endocarditis.

According to the Council on Scientific Affairs, there is no need to premedicate patients with prosthetic joints except for high-risk patients. High-risk or medically compromised patients with prosthetic joints include immunocompromised/immunosuppressed patients (those with rheumatoid arthritis or systemic lupus erythematosus) or patients with disease-, drug-, or radiation-induced immunosuppression. Other high-risk patients include those with insulin-dependent (type 1) diabetes mellitus, patients during the first 2 years following joint placement, patients with previous prosthetic joint interfaces, and patients with evidence of malnourishment or hemophilia. Table 30–7■ lists recommendations for antibiotic prophylaxis in these patients.

Summary

A comprehensive health history is required on every patient. Numerous individuals with acquired diseases present for routine periodontal care and an understanding of these medically compromised states is fundamental for dental practitioners. The student and dental practitioner must be able to recognize these compromised states and prevent complications during periodontal treatment. Additionally, it is important to recognize when to use consultations and referrals to physicians.

Key Points

- Never treat a stranger; review the health/medical history and interview the patient thoroughly to determine if a medical condition requires physician referral or either special precautions or postponement of periodontal treatment.
- Prevention of disease transmission requires an understanding of infection control and modes of disease transmission in the dental office (e.g., power-driven scalers, air-water syringe, and air polisher).

Table 30–7	Suggested Antibiotic Prophylaxis Regimens in Patients at Potential Increased Risk of Hematogenous Total Joint Infection	
Situation	**Drug**	**Regimen**
Standard general prophylaxis	Cephalexin or amoxicillin	2 g orally 1 h before dental procedure
Patients unable to take oral medications	Cefazolin or Ampicillin	1 g IM or IV 1 h before procedure / 2 g IM or IV 1 h before procedure
Allergic to penicillin	Clindamycin	600 mg orally 1 h before procedure
Allergic to penicillin and unable to take oral medications	Clindamycin	600 mg IV 1 h before procedure

Web Sites

www.perio.org

www.aafp.org

www.hsc.stonybrook.edu/dental

Self-Quiz

1. Which one of the following procedures should be followed if a 50-year-old patient did not take his medication the morning of the periodontal appointment and has a blood pressure of 180/100 mmHg in the office? (p. 523)

   a. Call the physician immediately.

   b. Give the patient his medication and let him wait in the office.

   c. Notify the emergency medical service (EMS).

   d. Position the patient in a supine position in the dental chair.

   e. Retake blood pressure and/or refer to a physician.

2. A patient is taking an antihypertensive drug called prazosin. After periodontal treatment is completed at an office visit and the patient is ready to be dismissed, which one of the following procedures should be followed? (p. 523)

   a. Have the patient drink orange juice slowly.

   b. Have the patient sit in the dental chair awhile.

   c. Administer more epinephrine.

   d. Administer oxygen.

3. Which one of the following statements is true about use of epinephrine in a cardiac patient? (p. 524)

   a. Use similar amounts as in a noncardiac patient.

   b. Use higher concentrations than in a noncardiac patient.

   c. It is contraindicated.

   d. Use cautiously.

4. Which one of the following time periods should the patient wait after having a heart attack or heart surgery before having periodontal treatment? (p. 525)

   a. 1 month

   b. 3 months

   c. 6 months

   d. 1 year

   e. 2 years

5. Which one of the following medications may be taken prophylactically to prevent a stroke or heart attack? (p. 525)

   a. acetylsalicylic acid

   b. vitamin K

   c. isoniazid

   d. prednisone

6. Which one of the following guidelines have to be followed in a controlled diabetic? (pp. 526–527)

   a. Schedule short, quick appointments.

   b. Antibiotic prophylaxis is required.

   c. Treatment is the same as in a nondiabetic.

   d. Corticosteroid is required before invasive procedures.

7. A patient calls for a periodontal appointment. She has just had hemodialysis at 12:00 P.M. today. When should you make the appointment? (pp. 529–530)

   a. 8:00 A.M. the next morning

   b. 12:00 P.M. the next day

   c. 6:00 P.M. the next day

   d. 2:00 P.M. the same day

8. A patient has been taking prednisone for arthritis for the last year. Which one of the following precautions needs to be followed for periodontal debridement regarding the drug? (p. 530)

   a. Keep the same dose.

   b. Decrease the dose.

   c. Increase the dose.

   d. Change to a different drug.

9. How soon after a kidney transplant can a patient be seen by a dental hygienist for periodontal debridement? (p. 529)
   a. 2 weeks
   b. 3 weeks
   c. 1 month
   d. 2 months
   e. 3 months

10. Which one of the following medications is used in the prophylaxis of tuberculosis? (pp. 534–535)
    a. rifampin
    b. isoniazid
    c. prednisone
    d. phenytoin
    e. acetaminophen

References

American Dental Association. 2004. X-rays in spotlight. *American Dental Association News* 35(9):1, 12.

American Dental Association Council on Dental Materials, Instruments, and Equipment. 1989. Recommendations in radiographic practices: An update. *J. Am. Dent. Assoc.* 118:115–117.

American Diabetes Association. 1997. Guidelines: Report of the expert committee on the diagnosis and classification of diabetes mellitus. *Diabetes Care* 20(7): 1183–1197.

Berkow, R., A. J. Fletcher, and M. H. Beers. 1992. *The Merck manual,* 16th ed. Rahway, NJ: Merck Research Laboratories, Merck & Co.

Ciancio, S. 1997. Bacterial endocarditis prophylaxis guideline changed. *Biol. Ther. Dent.* 13(2):9–10.

Cohen, D. W., and L. F. Rose. 1998. The periodontal-medical risk relationship. *Compendium* 19(1):11–24.

Dajani, A. S., K. A. Taubert, W. Wilson, A. F. Bolger, A. Bayer, et al. 1997. Prevention of bacterial endocarditis: Recommendations by the American Heart Association. *JAMA* 277:1794–1801.

DiBisceglie, A. M. 1996. Hepatitis G virus infection: A work in progress. *Ann. Intern. Med.* 125:772–773.

Gillcrist, J. A. 1999. Hepatitis viruses A, B, C, D, E and G: Implications for dental personnel. *J. Am. Dent. Assoc.* 130:509–520.

Glick, M., S. N. Abel, B. C. Muzyka, and M. Delorenzo. 1994. Dental complications after treating patients with AIDS. *J. Am. Dent. Assoc.* 125:296–301.

Hujoel P.P., A. Bollen, C. J. Noonan, M.A. del Aguila. 2004. Antepartum dental radiograph and infant low birth weight. *JAMA.* 291:1987–1993.

Kaplan, N. M. 1998. Treatment of hypertension: Insights from the JNC-VI report. *Am. Fam. Physician* 58:1323–1330.

Leviner, E., A. A. Tzukert, R. Benoliel, O. Baram, and M. V. Sela. 1987. Development of resistant oral *Viridans streptococci* after administration of prophylactic antibiotics: Time management in the dental treatment of patients susceptible to infective endocarditis. *Oral Surg. Oral Med. Oral Pathol.* 64:417–420.

Mealey, B. L. 1996. Periodontal implications: Medically compromised patients. *Ann. Periodontol.* 1:256–321.

Naugle, K., M. L. Darby, D. B. Bauman, L. T. Lineberger, and R. Powers. 1998. The oral health status of individuals on renal dialysis. *Ann. Periodontol.* 3:197–205.

Nichols, W. L., and E. J. W. Bowie. 1993. Standardization of the prothrombin time for monitoring orally administered anticoagulant therapy with use of the international normalized ration system. *Mayo Clinical Procedure* 68:897–898.

Perusse, R., J. P. Goulet, and J. Y. Turcotte. 1992. Contraindications to vasoconstrictors in dentistry, part I. *Oral Surg. Oral Med. Oral Pathol.* 74:679–686.

Rhodus, N. L., and J. W. Little. 1993. Dental management of the renal transplant patient. *Compend. Contin. Educ. Dent.* 14:518–532.

Rose, L. F., B. J. Steinberg, and S. L. Atlas. 1995. Periodontal management of the medically compromised patient. *Periodontology 2000* 9:165–175.

Seymour, R. A., and D. G. Smith. 1991. The effect of a plaque control program on the incidence and severity of cyclosporin-induced gingival changes. *J. Clin. Periodontol.* 18:107–110.

Simmons, N. A., R. A. Cawson, C. A. Clark, S.J. Eykyn, A.M. Geddes, et al. 1986. Prophylaxis of infective endocarditis (letter). *Lancet* 1:1267.

Steckelberg, J. M., and W. R. Wilson. 1993. Risk factors for infective endocarditis. *Infect. Dis. Clin. North Am.* 7:9–19.

Wahl, M. J. 2000. Myths of dental surgery in patients receiving anticoagulant therapy. *J. Am. Dent. Assoc.* 131:77–81.

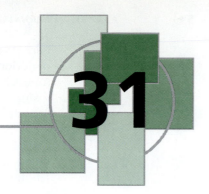

Periodontal Maintenance Therapy

Mea A. Weinberg, D.M.D., M.S.D., R.Ph.

Outline

Refractory Periodontal Diseases/Recurrent Periodontal Diseases

Objectives of Periodontal Maintenance

Components of the Periodontal Maintenance Visit

Periodontal Conditions and Smoking

Treatment: Recurrent Periodontal Disease versus a Well-Maintained Periodontium

Chemotherapeutics

Frequency of Intervals

General Dentist–Periodontist Relationship

Patient Compliance

Summary

Key Points

Web Sites

Self-Quiz

References

Goal

To provide an overview of the role periodontal maintenance has in the long-term management of inflammatory periodontal diseases.

Educational Objectives

Upon completion of this chapter, the dental hygiene student should be able to:

List the objectives of periodontal maintenance.

Describe the components of periodontal maintenance.

Describe the role of the dental hygienist in periodontal maintenance visits.

Define the role of the dental hygienist in smoking cessation.

Identify when retreatment is necessary.

Explain the factors involved in patient compliance.

KEY WORDS

- periodontal maintenance
- recurrence
- primary prevention
- secondary prevention
- smoking cessation
- retreatment
- patient compliance

543

Periodontal maintenance also has been referred to as periodontal recall, supportive periodontal care, and continuing care. All these terms are appropriate, but the American Academy of Periodontology (AAP) has adopted the term "periodontal maintenance," which may be a more up-to-date and inclusive term because it is a branch of periodontal therapy.

It is known generally that after periodontal treatment is completed, patients will exhibit a decrease in plaque control and a recurrence of gingivitis or periodontitis unless they are enrolled in a regular periodontal maintenance program (Axelsson & Lindhe, 1981). Patients must be informed of the need for periodic periodontal maintenance visits throughout their life. Since it cannot be predicted when and if gingivitis will progress into periodontitis, the disease must be monitored, and regular professional removal of dental plaque and calculus must be accomplished.

Refractory Periodontal Diseases/ Recurrent Periodontal Diseases

Refractory periodontal disease occurs in treated periodontal patients who fail to respond to periodontal treatment including maintenance therapy and who demonstrate meticulous oral hygiene. Patients may be refractory because of inadequate treatment, presence of systemic disease (e.g., diabetes mellitus), deficient immune response, or persistence of periodontal pathogens. On the other hand, *recurrent periodontal disease* occurs in patients who previously responded well to periodontal therapy but later showed signs of disease reactivation. In this situation, there was a recurrence of the disease. Recurrent disease sites also occur in patients demonstrating meticulous plaque control and on a regular maintenance program.

Treatment for refractory periodontitis may include adjunctive use of antibiotics. Treatment for recurrent disease sites is based on conventional periodontal therapy (e.g., scaling/root planing, surgery, good plaque control and maintenance).

Objectives of Periodontal Maintenance

The primary objectives of periodontal maintenance are (American Academy of Periodontology, 2003b) (1) to prevent or minimize the recurrence of periodontal diseases in patients by controlling risk factors known to contribute to the disease process (e.g., dental plaque, calculus); (2) to prevent or reduce the incidence of tooth or implant loss by monitoring the dentition and prosthetic replacements of the natural teeth; (3) to increase the probability of locating and treating other conditions or diseases found in the mouth; and (4) to preserve the health, comfort, and function of the teeth. Periodontal maintenance is also important for monitoring the overall dental health of the patient and to recognize, identify, and manage other diseases or conditions found within or related to the oral cavity (Wilson, 1996b).

Indications for Periodontal Maintenance

Periodontal maintenance is indicated for three types of patients: (1) peridontally healthy patients who have never had periodontal disease as a preventive procedure (this type of care is termed *primary prevention* and applies to a large section of the population), (2) patients after active periodontal therapy to prevent or minimize the recurrence and progression of periodontal disease and tooth loss (this type of care is termed *secondary prevention*), and (3) medically compromised patients or patients who maintain poor oral hygiene and are not considered candidates for periodontal surgery.

Components of the Periodontal Maintenance Visit

Patient needs at the periodontal maintenance visit vary widely and are modified on an individual basis. Regardless, standard periodontal maintenance procedures include the following steps (American Academy of Peridontology, 2003b):

1. an update of medical and dental histories;
2. extraoral and intraoral examinations;
3. dental examination and gingival and periodontal assessment;
4. radiographic review;
5. oral hygiene evaluation (amount of plaque, calculus, and stains);
6. review of the patient's plaque-control efficacy; and
7. removal of dental plaque from the supragingival and subgingival areas, root debridement where indicated, teeth polishing, and adjunctive chemotherapy if necessary.

The patient's chart should be reviewed for previous periodontal treatments, including periodontal maintenance care before any current treatment is initiated. Any medications needed before periodontal maintenance, such as antibiotic prophylaxis, can be determined before the patient is seen and acknowledged when the patient arrives at the dental office.

Two aspects emphasized and provided during periodontal maintenance are monitoring and therapy. The preceding examination steps should be performed on every patient at each periodontal maintenance visit but are subject to the judgment of the dentist and the dental hygienist. The clinical findings obtained at the periodontal maintenance visit should be compared with baseline findings. Baseline values are first established at the initial examination and again following active therapy.

Periodontal maintenance is designed to eliminate or reduce primary and secondary risk factors. The primary risk factor for inflammatory periodontal diseases is dental plaque. Secondary factors include plaque-retentive areas such as calculus and restorations with overhangs or defective margins. The patient removes supragingival dental plaque by toothbrushing and flossing, and the dental hygienist or dentist removes both supragingival and subgingival plaque and calculus by mechanical debridement. The dentist should replace or restore defective or failed restorations. Table 31–1■ provides a step-by-step review of the components of a periodontal maintenance visit.

Medical and Dental Update

The patient should be asked if there have been any medication or health changes, including hospitalizations, since the last appointment. Review current medications (prescription and over-the-counter) with the patient. Note any changes in dosage or instructions for use. A medical consultation with the patient's physician may be warranted if new illnesses are recognized or if a previous condition has changed significantly. A chief complaint should be noted, and this should be accompanied by a notation of the degree of comfort or discomfort. The patient and the dentist should sign the amended form.

Counseling of the patient on risk factors that contribute to periodontal diseases, such as cigarette smoking, stress, nutrition, medications (e.g., calcium channel blockers, phyentoin, cyclosporine, oral contraceptives), and systemic diseases (e.g., diabetes mellitus, AIDS), also should be done during the periodontal maintenance visit (Kerry, 1995). The patient should be informed about the availability of programs for smoking cessation in and outside the office.

Since many patients are on an alternating periodontal maintenance program, seeing both a general dentist and a periodontist, any communication from the last treating office should be reviewed. Any new restorative treatment should be indicated on the chart and evaluated clinically.

Extraoral/Intraoral Examination

An updated examination is performed in the head and neck area and intraoral tissues for the detection of any abnormalities, including enlarged lymph nodes or salivary glands and red, white, or pigmented lesions. If any suspicious lesions are found, the dentist should be informed for further examination or treatment.

Dental Examination

The dental examination at the periodontal maintenance visit includes caries assessment as well as documentation of the status of restorations. Restorations should be charted, noting any defective restorations or failures such as fractures or open margins of amalgams, composites, and crowns. The stability of bridges and removable partial dentures also should be noted. Documentation of tooth loss since the last charting should be recorded, including the cause. A good rule to follow is to always count the number of teeth present.

Gingival and Periodontal Assessment

Gingival Assessment

Initially, a visual examination of the gingival tissues is done to determine the condition of the gingiva. The color, contour, consistency, and surface texture of the gingiva are recorded. Any mucogingival involvement should be noted. If compromised teeth are to receive crowns, augmentation of the attached gingiva may be necessary. If gingival inflammation is found, the location and severity should be noted, as well as etiologic factors (e.g., dental plaque accumulation due to poor oral hygiene self-care, medication-induced, or resulting from a hormonal imbalance).

Periodontal Assessment

Next, a periodontal evaluation is performed. This includes recording of probing depths, gingival recession, clinical attachment level, furcation involvement, suppuration (pus), and tooth mobility. The Periodontal Screening and Recording™

Table 31–1 Components of a Periodontal Maintenance Visit

Examination	Remarks
Review and update medical and dental history, take blood pressure, pulse, respiration.	To determine if additional risk factors are responsible for recurrent or progressive periodontal breakdown.

Clinical examination, including
  Extra-intraoral examination
  Plaque evaluation/disclosing
  Evaluating the patient's oral hygiene technique
  Dental charting of caries, restorative care
  Periodontal charting of probing depths, gingival recession, furcation defects, bleeding on probing, exudation, tooth mobility, fremitus
  Implant evaluation: peri-implant tissues, probing depths, bleeding on probing, stability of dental implant (mobility), examination of abutment teeth, occlusal examination
	Changes that should be of concern during a periodontal maintenance visit include sites that have changed from nonbleeding to bleeding, sites that have increased 2 to 3 mm or more in attachment loss or probing depth, and any sites with pus or suppuration.

Radiographic review	Since radiographs only show past activity (e.g., bone loss occurred approximately 6 months ago, not yesterday or today), it is important to correlate the radiographic findings with clinical probing depths and clinical attachment levels.

Treatment options
  Removal of supragingival and subgingival plaque and calculus
  Selective polishing
  Oral hygiene reinstruction
	These treatment guidelines depend on the type of periodontal patient. Treatment should not be started unless the data collected are appropriately recorded.

Adjunctive therapy
  Antimicrobial therapy
  Occlusal treatment
  Counseling on control of contributing factors such as smoking cessation, stress reduction, and nutrition
  Restorative and prosthetic care	

Reevaluation 2 to 3 weeks after debridement	
Scheduling of next periodontal maintenance appointment	

(PSR™) system may be used for screening for patients with no history of periodontal disease susceptibility.

Gingival Recession   The position of the gingival tissues on the tooth is defined as the location of the gingival margin in relation to the cementoenamel junction (CEJ). Gingival recession that has progressed since the last appointment must be addressed and treatment options given to the patient. If the recession has remained unchanged, then monitoring is all that is needed. In order to treat gingival recession, the cause must be determined. Etiologic factors include inappropriate toothbrushing technique, attachment loss (disease process), and shrinkage of tissues after initial therapy. Treatment may include educating the patient on proper brushing technique or mucogingival surgery. Common patient complaints concerning gingival recession include poor aesthetics and tooth pain or hypersensitivity with air or cold application. Any dentinal hypersensitivity can be managed in most patients with desensitizing agents (e.g., potassium nitrate, sodium fluoride, or stannous fluoride).

Disease Stability: Probing Depth and Clinical Attachment Level   Monitoring of probing depths and clinical attachment levels (CALs) currently is the most reliable way to determine periodontal disease stability. It may be time-consuming to determine the CAL, but it is an extremely important measurement. Probing depth recordings should be taken at six sites per tooth. If a patient's periodontal condition has deteriorated rapidly since the last periodontal maintenance visit, systemic disease such as diabetes mellitus, smoking, stress, or use of alcohol must be considered as risk factors.

Measurement of the CAL is made from the CEJ to the apical extent of the tip of the probe. Such measurements are compared with measurements obtained at the last periodontal maintenance visit. A 2- to 3-mm increase in CAL loss indicates disease progression (Haffajee, Socransky, & Goodson, 1983; Kornman, 1987), and more aggressive treatment or retreatment may be justified. A patient with a 3-mm probing depth associated with 6 mm of gingival recession, for example, has a 9-mm CAL loss. In such patients, periodontal maintenance must be discontinued and active periodontal therapy started. However, a patient with a 3-mm probing depth without recession has a 3-mm CAL with no attachment loss, and this is not of great concern.

Bleeding on Probing   Probing depths should be interpreted on a patient-by-patient, site-by-site basis. For example, a 5-mm probing depth that does not bleed on probing is viewed differently from a 5-mm probing depth with bleeding on probing and suppuration. Bleeding on probing in deep pockets indicates inflammation within the connective tissue (Armitage, 1996), whereas bleeding while stroking the lateral wall of the gingival crevice indicates early gingival inflammation (Van der Weijden, Timmerman, Nijbor, Reijerse, & Van der Velden, 1994). Thus disease stability can be monitored during periodontal maintenance on the basis of bleeding on probing (Lang, Joss, & Tonetti, 1996). Bleeding sites in deep pockets seem to have an increased risk for progression of periodontitis (progressive attachment loss) in patients on periodontal maintenance care (Claffey, Nylund, Kiger, Gorrett, & Egelberg, 1990). The absence of bleeding on probing is a better indicator of gingival health than its presence is of periodontal disease (Lang et al., 1996). One should chart the sites that bleed on probing (e.g., use a red dot over the site). Thus sites that bleed warrant more attention during the periodontal maintenance visit and may have to be reinstrumented, whereas nonbleeding sites should be left without repeated subgingival instrumentation (Lang et al., 1996). Bleeding on probing generally is apparent 10 seconds after probing (Lang et al., 1996).

It should be emphasized that the force used while probing (probing force) varies considerably during probing depth measurements, even from tooth to tooth. Therefore, a tooth with healthy periodontium may bleed because "too much" force was used and not because of inflammation. Ideally, a probing force of 0.25 N (25 g) should be used, which clinically represents a "light probing force" (Joss, Adler, & Lang, 1994; Lang et al., 1996), or probe until slight resistance is felt. A nonmetallic probe should be used to probe around implants.

Furcation Involvement   Furcation involvement for each tooth is noted on the chart. Tooth mobility also should be measured and recorded on the chart as Grade I, II, III, or IV (Carranza & Takei, 1996). If there is increasing mobility since the last visit, the cause should be determined and appropriate treatment rendered. The presence of fremitus also should be recorded.

Radiographic Review

Radiographs show past periodontal tissue destruction. It is important to monitor the patient's periodontal status with clinical probing and standardized radiographs taken at appropriate intervals so as to compare with previously taken radiographs. In a periodontal patient with a history of bone loss and periodontal surgery, a full-mouth radiographic series should be taken every few years. Sites that have had bone (osseous) grafting or guided tissue regeneration should be evaluated with radiographs at least 6 months after surgery. In patients without a history of periodontal diseases, a longer interval for radiographs is acceptable. The need for bitewing and periapical radiographs depends on the stage and severity of the disease, risk for caries, and presence of implants. Vertical bitewing views are ideal for periodontal patients because they show more of the alveolar bone than do horizontal bitewings.

Oral Hygiene Evaluation and Patient's Plaque-Control Regimen

The next step is to evaluate gross plaque accumulation, determine the quality of oral hygiene self-care procedures, and conduct patient education. A disclosing agent is used for patient education and as a basis for recording a plaque index. Scoring of plaque at a periodontal maintenance appointment may be misleading because patients frequently brush very well just before coming to such an appointment. However, inflammation, if present, will be evident. In any event, monitoring of the plaque level can be used to evaluate the patient's compliance with oral hygiene self-care. The patient's oral hygiene practices are reviewed by asking the patient to brush and use interdental devices while the hygienist watches. The level of patient motivation to perform daily plaque removal must be determined. A patient may understand and show correct technique in the office but may not comply with instructions at home because of lack of interest or time constraints. It is important to recognize such patients and to spend more time explaining to them the importance of performing these tasks.

Dental Implants

Evaluation of a patient with dental implants is essentially the same as that of a patient with natural teeth. However, rather than teeth, the implants and peri-implant tissues are evaluated. If inflammation or disease is detected around an implant, the probing depth should be measured and bleeding and suppuration noted. The stability of the abutment teeth and prosthesis also should be noted by recording mobility. An abutment is a tooth or implant used for support and retention of a crown or removable partial denture. The prosthesis is checked for occlusal wear. Any loosened screws should be recorded.

Because there is a correlation between implant failure and bone characteristics, it is essential to take radiographs periodically. Generally, periapical films are indicated at 6-month to 1-year intervals to determine the height of bone around an implant. The accepted standard for a stable endosseous implant one year after placement is vertical bone loss less than 0.2 mm per year (Albrektsson, Zarb, Worthington, & Eriksson, 1986; American Academy of Periodontology, 1989). Radiographically, an ailing, failing, or failed implant will show varying amounts of alveolar bone loss (Meffert, 1992). Mobility will occur with the failed implant.

Periodontal Conditions and Smoking

The literature supports the conclusion that smokers, especially cigarette smokers, have increased calculus, greater bone loss, and increased pocket depths but have the same levels of plaque accumulation and the same or less gingival inflammation (American Academy of Periodontology, 1996; Haber et al., 1993). It also has been shown that surgical periodontal procedures are less effective for smokers (Bergström, Eliasson, & Preber, 1994). The amount and frequency of tobacco use are essential information when evaluating the risk factors associated with smoking (American Academy of Periodontology, 1996). Since smoking cessation may decrease the progression of periodontal diseases, it is important that the dental hygienist urge periodontal patients who smoke to stop and perhaps recommend an effective smoking-cessation program. The dental hygienist should perform periodic soft tissue evaluations and recognize any deleterious changes in the periodontium. The dental hygienist can provide assistance in guiding patients to stop smoking, yet he or she needs to realistically assess the effects of this habit on the gingival health and the resulting compromised healing. Education and continued support are beneficial factors influencing the patient's decision to stop smoking.

Practical Steps to Smoking Cessation

Smoking-cessation programs can be made available in the dental office. The dental office is a logical place to counsel patients on the effects of smoking on the periodontium and the importance of stopping smoking for improved long-term periodontal health and better results after periodontal treatment. Furthermore, it is important to stress to the patient that smoking cessation also can reduce the risk for other medical diseases such as cancer (Christen, McDonald, & Christen, 1991), heart disease, and respiratory disease (e.g., bronchitis). A smoking-cessation program should be a part of comprehensive preventive periodontal care. This includes behavior modification and, if necessary, medications.

The first step in establishing a smoking-cessation program is to get the office organized by selecting a director or coordinator such as the dental hygienist. The role of the director is to become familiar with the National Cancer Institute (NCI) manual and parts of the program, organize records and procedures, assist patients by reviewing self-help material with them, and involve the entire dental office team (Stone & Mattana, 1996).

Patients should be reassured that the entire office is going to help them. If a patient shows interest in quitting, then a program can be initiated. If a patient is not interested in quitting, do not force him or her, but rather counsel the patient and give him or her literature to take home. At the next visit ask the patient about smoking cessation again. Once the patient is enrolled in a program (yours or another one), continued maintenance or follow-up visits and communication through phone calls are important.

The role of the dental hygienist includes patient education and counseling in tobacco prevention and cessation. The patient should be informed that smoking influences periodontal conditions such as implant failure (Bain, 1996), oral cancer, and periodontal problems such as loss of clinical attachment (Grossi et al., 1994), impaired wound healing (Grossi et al., 1997; Jones & Triplett, 1992), halitosis, increased calculus formation, black-brown extrinsic staining, and bone loss (Bergström et al., 1991).

A set of guidelines is presented to the patient. Behavior modification should be part of a comprehensive smoking-cessation program. This includes talking to patients about their smoking habits and possibly incorporating hypnosis. Hypnosis has been used for many years in the treatment of habits. Hypnosis is a shift in awareness and not a state of concentration (Weinberg, 1986). Hypnosis allows patients to be more susceptible to accepting suggestions, such as quitting smoking. This allows the patient to be in full control of the situation, and responsibility is placed on the patient not to smoke (Weinberg, 1986). Patients are put into a situation where they see themselves not smoking anymore. The dentist can perform hypnosis on the patient in the office. The patient is never asleep during this procedure. The patient also can learn self-hypnosis, which can be used anytime and anywhere.

4A Smoking-Cessation Program

The Smoking, Tobacco, and Cancer Program of the National Cancer Institute (1996) recommends guidelines to help patients to stop using tobacco. The 4A Program consists of the following components that are reviewed with the patient during the initial examination and periodically:

Ask. Inquire whether your patient smokes and, if so, how long he or she has been smoking and how much.

Advise. Inform the patient of the benefits of quitting and the risks associated with continuing the tobacco habit; strongly suggest that your patient should work toward a goal of complete smoking cessation.

Assist. Give the patient behavioral self-monitoring techniques and, as appropriate, pharmacologic intervention such as nicotine gum, nicotine patches, or another agent. Encourage the patient to quit smoking. Let the patient set up a quitting date or discuss different therapies.

Arrange for follow-up. Set up follow-up visits. The patient should return to the office at regular intervals to observe his or her periodontium and to reinforce his or her quitting behavior.

Additionally, another "A" would be to assess for motivation to stop. The patient should be assessed for his/her reasons for quitting smoking and their thoughts for quitting.

Pharmacologic Agents

Acute physical withdrawal symptoms following smoking cessation are not usually long-lasting (seldom more than 1 to 2 weeks), but the success rates of smoking-cessation programs may be augmented by weaning smokers from nicotine gradually through the use of nicotine-replacement therapy. Table 31–2■ reviews various types of smoking-cessation methods.

Nicotine-replacement therapy by itself will not result in smoking cessation unless accompanied by counseling and behavior modification. Pharmacologic agents include nicotine gum, transdermal nicotine patches, nasal sprays, and a systemic dosage form. The nicotine-replacement drugs (gum or patches) work by replacing the nicotine that is absorbed in the body while smoking and act as a substitute for the cigarette. The manufacturers of these products claim that they help patients quit while lessening any concomitant nicotine cravings (Stone & Mattana, 1996). The efficacy of this method is questionable on a long-term basis. Patients must refrain from smoking while on the gum or patch because nicotine from these products is being introduced into the body. Nicotine therapy should not be used in a patient who continues to smoke. The importance of taking the gum as directed must be stressed to the patient. The gum should be chewed slowly between the cheek and gingiva for about 30 minutes and then thrown away. Currently, the gum is available over-the-counter without a prescription. Nicotine patches are available in different doses that are worn on the skin for variable amounts of time. Indications for use of these products is for the reduction of symptoms associated with smoking cessation, including nicotine craving.

Bupropion HCl (Zyban® Sustained-Release Tablets, Glaxo Wellcome, Research Triangle Park, NC) is an oral medication prescribed by dentists or physicians to help decrease the withdrawal symptoms and the urge to smoke that accompany smoking cessation. Advantages to this form of therapy are that it is nicotine-free and helps the patient to quit while still smoking. Bupropion is also used to treat depression. Adverse side effects include dry mouth (xerostomia) and insomnia (difficulty sleeping). Both nicotine gum and patches and bupropion should be used in conjunction with behavioral modification therapy.

Treatment: Recurrent Periodontal Disease versus a Well-Maintained Periodontium

Recurrent periodontal disease occurs when signs and symptoms of disease return after having subsided during active treatment. Clinical signs include bleeding on probing, increasing tooth mobility, continued soft tissue attachment loss (including deep pockets), suppuration from the pocket, and radiographic changes. Recurrent occlusal problems include increasing tooth mobility and fremitus. A good rule to follow may be that when bleeding on probing or the presence of suppuration is

Table 31–2   Smoking-Cessation Methods: Pharmacologic Therapy

Product	Directions for Use	Supplied
Nicotine Gum		
Nicorette® gum (2 mg; 4 mg) (GlaxoSmithKline)	One piece of gum every 1–2 hours for weeks 1–6, every 2–4 hours for weeks 7–9, and every 4–8 hours for weeks 10–12. Do not eat or drink for 15 minutes before chewing a piece of gum.	Over the counter; starter kit has 108 pieces, and refill kits have 48 pieces.
Nicotine Transdermal System		
Nicotrol® (Pharmacia Consumer Products)	Taper patches; up to 6 weeks.	Over the counter; 15-mg, 10-mg, and 5-mg nicotine patch.
Habitrol® (Novartis Consumer, East Hanover, NJ)	One patch daily; 21 mg/day for 6 weeks, then 14 mg/day for 2 weeks, then 7 mg/day for 2 weeks. Maximum therapy is 3 months.	Over the counter; patch containing 7 mg of nicotine, 14 mg, and 21 mg; 7-day supply.
Nicoderm® CQ (GlaxoSmithKline)	One patch daily; taper dosage as recommended by manufacturer (21 mg/day for 6 weeks, then 14 mg/day for 2 weeks, then 7 mg/day for 2 weeks). Maximum therapy is 3 months.	Over the counter; 7-mg patch, 14-mg patch, 21-mg patch; 7-day supply in 7-mg dose.
Prostep® (Lederle, Carolina; Puerto Rico)	One patch daily; 22 mg/day for 4–8 weeks, then 11 mg/day for 2–4 weeks. Maximum therapy is 3 months.	Over the counter; box contains 7 patches that deliver 22 or 11 mg/day.
Nicotine Nasal Spray		
Nicotrol® NS (McNeil Consumer Health Care, Fort Washington, PA)	Start with 2 sprays in each nostril every hour, which may be increased to 80 sprays per day (heavy smokers); maximum therapy is 6 months. Can cause nasal irritation.	Prescription; each spray delivers 0.5 mg nicotine; available in 10-ml bottles.
Nicotine Lozenge		
Commit® (GlaxoSmithKline)	Allow lozenge to dissolve slowly over 20–30 min, swallow as little as possible.	Over the counter; 2 mg and 4 mg lozenge
Nicotine Inhalation System		
Nicotrol® Inhaler (McNeil Consumer Health Care, Fort Washington, PA)	Reduces craving to smoke. Less nicotine per puff is released with the inhaler than with a cigarette. Best effect is achieved by frequent continuous puffing for about 20 minutes. The recommended treatment is up to 3 months and, if needed, a gradual reduction over the next 6–12 weeks. Total treatment should not exceed 6 months.	Prescription; the inhaler uses nicotine cartridges (10 mg/cartridge) that provide about 20 minutes of active puffing, or approximately 80 deep draws.
Oral Medications		
Bupropion HCl (Zyban®) Sustained-Release Tablets (Glaxo Wellcome, Research, Triangle Park, NC)	Start initial dose while the patient is still smoking to allow for higher blood levels; initial dose is 150 mg/day for 3 days. Maximum daily dose is 300 mg. Should stop smoking within 2 weeks of initiation of drug therapy. Continue drug therapy for 7–12 weeks after the patient stops smoking. Can be used with nicotine transdermal systems (nicotine patches).	Prescription; 150-mg sustained-release tablets.

seen 2 to 3 weeks following the periodontal maintenance appointment, then retreatment is plausible (Ramfjord, 1987). Another reason for retreatment includes a 2-mm or greater increase in probing depth or attachment loss. Depending on which of these the dental hygienist finds, or combinations thereof, the dentist should examine the patient to determine specific retreatment. This could include periodontal debridement (scaling and root planing), periodontal surgery, antimicrobial agents, occlusal adjustment, splinting, extractions, or a night guard. After the initial therapy is completed, reevaluation should be performed. If resolution does not occur after retreatment, then a systemic disease component must be considered.

In a well-maintained patient in whom inflammation is not present (no bleeding on probing) and for whom soft tissue attachment loss or bone loss is minimal, the following treatment is recommended at a periodontal maintenance visit:

1. Point out any areas in the mouth where the patient is having difficulty with plaque control, and correct the patient's technique, if necessary.
2. Deplaquing may be performed. In patients with little or no subgingival deposits (usually after active treatment), a deplaquing stroke can be used with a curet or ultrasonic or sonic scaler. The tip of the instrument is "floating" within the gingival sulcus, lightly touching the root surface.
3. Selective tooth polishing can be performed. Extrinsic stains may be derived from nicotine, tea, coffee, foods, and chlorhexidine oral rinse.
4. Determine the interval of the next periodontal maintenance visit.

Subgingival instrumentation, including root planing of shallow pockets, has been shown to increase soft tissue attachment loss (Lindhe, Socransky, Nyman, Haffajee, & Westfelt, 1982). Patients with dental implants should be questioned about any difficulty in oral hygiene self-care or discomfort or difficulty in chewing. Plastic periodontal probes, scalers, and curets should be used because stainless steel instruments can scratch the titanium surfaces of implants.

All patients must undergo oral hygiene reinstruction and counseling on control of contributing risk factors such as smoking. Patients should be kept informed of their current periodontal condition and treatment options. Consultation may be required with other dentists who will be providing restorative or prosthetic treatment or who will be involved in the periodontal maintenance program.

Chemotherapeutics

Chemotherapeutic agents may be beneficial in certain patients as an adjunct to standard oral hygiene procedures, but they do not replace brushing and flossing. Since chemotherapeutic agents help to prevent repopulation of potential gram-negative periodontal pathogens between periodontal maintenance appointments, medically compromised patients or those exhibiting poor oral hygiene may benefit from such agents. Since periodontitis is a subgingival malady, rinsing with an agent is ineffective. To target subgingival bacteria, oral irrigation may be helpful between periodontal maintenance visits to prevent repopulation of periodontal pathogens (Jolkovsky et al., 1990). Irrigation with water or a medicament detoxifies and removes unattached dental plaque. Systemic antibiotics are not recommended routinely during periodontal maintenance because of the potential development of bacterial resistance, although antibiotics occasionally may be of some benefit in recurrent and refractory periodontitis cases during periodontal maintenance. Controlled-release drugs such as Arestin™, PerioChip®, or Atridox® may be used in selected recurrent pockets of 5 mm or greater that bleed. Desensitizing agents may be applied at a periodontal maintenance visit to reduce or eliminate dentinal hypersensitivity in patients in whom gingival recession is present.

Frequency of Intervals

Periodontal maintenance intervals are determined on an individual basis according to periodontal disease severity, type of treatment performed, adequacy of oral hygiene self-care, presence of orthodontic and prosthetic appliances, systemic health, and patient compliance and cooperation (American Academy of Periodontology, 1998). The premise on which a time-interval frame for periodontal maintenance has been based is the repopulation time of periodontal pathogens after the last periodontal debridement. Data suggest that periodontal maintenance intervals of three months or less are indicated for continued suppression of potentially pathogenic microorganisms in susceptible patients (American Academy of Periodontology, 1998). A 12-month recall interval may be acceptable for patients with limited susceptibility to periodontitis (Rosén et al., 1999). Regardless, the periodontal maintenance interval is determined on a patient-by-patient basis, and the interval may be less or greater than 3 months. Figure 31–1■ is a schematic flowchart that reviews suggested time intervals for healthy and periodontal patients. Patients can return 2 to 3 weeks after periodontal debridement for further observations. Any time during a periodontal maintenance program, a patient may temporarily go back into active therapy.

The time required for the periodontal maintenance visit depends on the number of teeth; disease severity; amount of plaque, calculus, and stains; instrumentation access; presence of extensive prosthetic crowns and bridges; orthodontic appliances; depths of pockets; and patient cooperation. Although periodontal maintenance visits usually are scheduled for 45 to 60 minutes, the amount of time should be individualized (American Academy of Periodontology, 1998). A suggested schedule is as follows (Caffesse, Mota, & Morrison, 1996):

- 15 minutes for the oral/dental examination and oral hygiene evaluation;
- 30 minutes for scaling and selective root planing and fluoride application; and
- 15 minutes for the dentist to evaluate the procedures completed and future needs.

General Dentist–Periodontist Relationship

Periodontal patients should be monitored by both their general dentist and their periodontist, but they should be seen by the periodontist at least once a year for a thorough periodontal evaluation. Periodontal maintenance can be performed alternately by the general dentist and the periodontist.

Gingivitis or mild chronic periodontitis patients can receive total care, including chronic periodontal maintenance, by the general dentist. Moderate chronic periodontitis patients should alternate periodontal maintenance visits between the

At the completion of initial therapy (after reevaluation)

PERIODONTAL HEALTH (NO PREVIOUS HISTORY OF PERIODONTAL DISEASES)		GINGIVITIS
Compliant with oral hygiene self-care No extensive restorative or prosthetics No occlusal discrepancies No extensive restorative or prosthetics	No bleeding No periodontally comprised teeth Complaint with oral hygiene self-care hygiene	Generalized or localized bleeding No periodontally compromised teeth Noncomplier or irregular complier
6 months	6 months	3 months or less for the first periodontal maintenance visit; if patient responds to treatment with improvement in oral hygiene then increase interval between visits; if there is no improvement after a few periodontal maintenance visits enroll the patient into active treatment. Risk factors including smoking and systemic diseases (e.g., diabetes mellitus, medications, hormonal imbalance) must be considered.

SLIGHT TO MODERATE PERIODONTITIS (SURGICAL AND NONSURGICAL PATIENTS)	SEVERE PERIODONTITIS (SURGICAL AND NONSURGICAL PATIENTS)
No teeth with less than 50% bone remaining Localized or no bleeding on probing Localized shallow pockets remain A controlled systemic disease that contributes to periodontal destruction Compliers with oral hygiene self-care	If many of the following factors are present: Many periodontally compromised teeth (>50% bone loss) Generalized deep pockets Occlusal problems Systemic disease (uncontrolled or poorly controlled) that predisposes to periodontal destruction (e.g., diabetes mellitus) Extensive restorative and prosthetic appliances Periodontal surgery not performed for medical, psychological, or financial reasons Noncomplier or irregular complier with oral hygiene self-care
6 months to 1 year	3 months or less depending on the number of risk factors present.

Figure 31–1   Schematic illustration describing suggested time intervals for periodontal maintenance.

general dentist and the periodontist once active treatment is completed. Severe chronic periodontitis patients should be seen primarily by a periodontist, with annual appointments with the general dentist for general care. Refractory periodontitis and aggressive periodontitis patients should be seen exclusively by the periodontist for all active periodontal treatment.

Patient Compliance

An essential aspect of periodontal maintenance therapy is patient compliance. Most patients do not comply with long-term behavioral changes, especially for conditions that are not life-threatening. Wilson (1996a) identifies three types of compliers: full compliers, irregular compliers, and noncompliers. Periodontal maintenance appointments are essential and important for all groups, but noncompliers have less successful surgical outcomes over time. Better communication may contribute to more successful outcomes. Other methods of improving patient compliance include providing positive reinforcement and attempting to better accommodate patient needs (Wilson, 1996a). Furthermore, the severity of the periodontal problem should be stressed because the more threatening a patient perceives a disease, the higher is the compliance.

Wilson, Glover, Schoen, Baus, and Jacobs (1984) reported that of 100 treated patients who were given the opportunity for periodontal maintenance over an 8-year period in a private periodontal office, 34% never returned to the office for periodontal maintenance, and only 16% completed periodontal maintenance. Becker, Becker, and Berg (1984), in a study of 44 patients who refused to participate in periodontal maintenance, found that in the absence of periodontal maintenance, periodontal surgery was of questionable benefit in maintaining periodontal health.

Some common reasons for patient noncompliance with office visits include the expense, the belief by patients that they no longer require treatment because they no longer have any signs of disease, fear of dental treatment (Mendoza, Newcomb, & Nixon, 1991; Wilson, 1996a), or lifestyle changes (e.g., job change or move).

Most longitudinal studies have shown that patients who receive therapy maintain their teeth longer than those who do not. A study by Becker and colleagues (1984) looked at patients in three categories:

1. Patients with untreated moderate to advanced periodontal disease lost an average of 0.33 teeth per year.
2. Patients who had treatment but no periodontal maintenance lost an average of 0.22 teeth per year.
3. Patients who had treatment and periodontal maintenance lost an average of 0.11 teeth per year.

Providing patients with motivational strategies may help to improve compliance. Examples of such approaches include (1) giving patients printed self-care instructions at every periodontal maintenance visit, (2) noting the next periodontal maintenance appointment on the instructions, (3) counseling patients about their condition and the benefit-to-risk ratio of having periodontal maintenance, (4) seeking out patient concerns and responding to them, and (5) sending reminders or calling patients about their next periodontal maintenance visit.

Summary

Professional plaque control, oral hygiene self-care, and periodic periodontal maintenance are and will continue to be the foundation of periodontal therapy. Following periodontal and implant therapy, regular periodontal maintenance can encourage periodontal and peri-implant health. In the majority of patients, periodontal maintenance is started after completion of active periodontal therapy, but it can be used in other phases of treatment. Periodontal maintenance evolved from a dental prophylaxis and now emphasizes treatment of areas with previous attachment loss and areas where clinical signs of inflammation are found (Wilson, 1996a). Since the timing interval for periodontal maintenance appointments is not standardized, the decision is empirical, with no real scientific basis. An interval of three months between periodontal maintenance visits appears to be an effective schedule to follow, but this may vary according to the clinical judgment of the dentist, the periodontal disease severity of the patient, and clinical findings.

A number of risk factors must be identified and monitored during periodontal maintenance. Increases in bleeding, pockets, and tooth loss will occur in high-risk patients. Clinical decisions during maintenance therapy will be influenced by the presence of risk factors, and better knowledge of these risk factors may lead to improved and more efficient risk-management efforts during periodontal maintenance (Tonetti, Muller, Campanile, & Lang, 1998).

Dental hygienists play an important role not only in the mechanical aspects of periodontal maintenance but also in promoting preventive measures and explaining the importance of periodontal maintenance. Properly motivated patients will stay on a regularly scheduled periodontal maintenance regimen.

Key Points

- The desired outcome of periodontal maintenance in patients after active therapy is the maintenance of periodontal health.
- Noncompliance with regular periodontal maintenance visits may result in recurrence of progression of disease.
- Despite adequate periodontal maintenance and oral hygiene self-care, some patients may show recurrence or progression of disease, and thus active therapy should be reinstated.

Web Sites

www.perio.org
www.adrq.gov
www.nic.nih.gov

Self-Quiz

1. All the following are goals of periodontal maintenance except one. Which one is the exception? (p. 544)
   a. Maintain the patient's oral status and function.
   b. Minimize inflammation and bleeding.
   c. Prevent the recurrence of disease.
   d. Make professional referrals for consultation.

2. Which one of the following assessments best determines when periodontal disease activity or destruction is occurring? (p. 548)
   a. clinical attachment level measurement
   b. bleeding localized to certain teeth
   c. redness and edema of the gingival tissues
   d. suppuration

3. The absence of bleeding on probing is a better indicator of gingival health than its presence is of periodontal disease because bleeding only indicates inflammation. (p. 548)
   a. Both the statement and the reason are correct and related.
   b. Both the statement and the reason are correct but not related.
   c. The statement is correct, but the reason is not.
   d. The statement is not correct, but the reason is correct.
   e. Neither the statement nor the reason is correct.

4. Which one of the following procedures is appropriate if a nonbleeding site with a probing depth of 5 mm is found during a periodontal maintenance visit? (p. 548)

   a. Perform periodontal debridement.

   b. Immediately refer the patient to a specialist.

   c. Reevaluate the site at the next appointment.

   d. Prescribe systemic antibiotics.

5. All the following risk factors can be controlled during periodontal maintenance therapy except one. Which one is the exception? (p. 545)

   a. stress

   b. smoking

   c. interproximal plaque accumulation

   d. genetic susceptibility

6. Which one of the following protocols is most appropriate in a patient who shows generalized recurrence of disease at a periodontal maintenance visit? (pp. 552, 554)

   a. Perform periodontal surgery.

   b. Reinstate Phase I therapy.

   c. Insert tetracycline fibers into the sites.

   d. Prescribe a systemic antibiotic in conjunction with periodontal debridement.

7. All the following determine the most appropriate time interval for periodontal maintenance visits except one. Which one is the exception? (p. 555)

   a. medical condition

   b. level of plaque control

   c. severity of the disease

   d. number of medications taken

8. Which one of the following types of pockets is most appropriate for adjunctive controlled-release drug delivery? (p. 554)

   a. nonbleeding, >5 mm

   b. nonbleeding, <5 mm

   c. bleeding, ≥5 mm

   d. bleeding, ≤5 mm

9. All the following techniques the dental hygienist can use to improve patient compliance to periodontal therapy except one. Which one is the exception? (pp. 556–557)

   a. Print self-care instructions.

   b. Counsel patients about their condition.

   c. Call the patient every week.

   d. Seek out patient concerns and respond to them.

   e. Send patients reminders about their next visit.

10. All the following components of the 4A Program are introduced during smoking-cessation sessions except one. Which one is the exception? (pp. 551–552)

    a. ask

    b. advise

    c. agree

    d. assist

    e. arrange

References

Albrektsson, T., G. Zarb, P. Worthington, and A. R. Eriksson. 1986. The long-term efficacy of currently used dental implants: A review and proposed criteria of success. *Int. J. Oral Maxillofac. Implants* 1:11–25.

American Academy of Periodontology. 1989. *Proceedings of the World Workshop in Clinical Periodontics, Consensus report, Discussion section VIII: Implant therapy (VIII-11-18).* Chicago: Author.

American Academy of Periodontology. 1996. Tobacco use and the periodontal patient. *J. Periodontol.* 67:51–56.

American Academy of Periodontology. 1998. Periodontal maintenance (PM). *J. Periodontol.* 69:502–506.

American Academy of Periodontology. 2003a. *Current terminology for periodontics and insurance reporting manual,* 9th ed. Chicago: Author.

American Academy of Periodontology. 2003b. Periodontal maintenance. *J. Periodontol.* 74:1395–1401.

Armitage, G. C. 1996. Manual periodontal probing in supportive periodontal therapy. *Periodontology 2000* 12:33–39.

Axelsson, P., and J. Lindhe. 1981. The significance of maintenance care in the treatment of periodontal disease. *J. Clin. Periodontol.* 8:281–294.

Bain, C. A. 1996. Smoking and implant failure: Benefits of a smoking cessation protocol. *Int. J. Oral Maxillofac. Implants* 11:756–759.

Becker, W., B. E. Becker, and L. E. Berg. 1984. Periodontal treatment without maintenance. A retrospective study in 44 patients. *J. Periodontol.* 55:505–509.

Bergström, J., S. Eliasson, and H. Preber. 1991. Cigarette smoking and periodontal bone loss. *J. Periodontol.* 62:242–246.

Caffesse, R. G., L. F. Mota, and E. C. Morrison. 1996. The rationale for periodontal therapy. *Periodontology 2000* 9:7–13.

Carranza, F. A., and H. H. Takei. 1996. Treatment of furcation involvement and combined periodontal-endodontic therapy. In eds. F. A. Carranza and M. G. Newman, *Clinical periodontology,* 640. Philadelphia: W. B. Saunders.

Christen, A. G., J. L. McDonald, and J. A. Christen. 1991. *The impact of tobacco use and cessation on nonmalignant and precancerous oral and dental diseases and conditions.* Indianapolis: Indiana University School of Dentistry.

Claffey, N., K. Nylund, R. Kiger, S. Garrett, and J. Egelberg. 1990. Diagnostic predictability of scores of plaque, bleeding, suppuration and probing depth for probing attachment loss. 3 1/2 years of observation following initial periodontal therapy. *J. Clin. Periodontol.* 17:108–114.

Grossi, S. G., J. J. Zambon, A. W. Ho, G. Koch, R. G. Dunford, et al. 1994. Assessment of risk for periodontal disease: I. Risk indicators for attachment loss. *J. Periodontol.* 65:260–267.

Grossi, S. G., J. Zambon, E. E. Machtei, R. Shifferle, S. Andreana, et al. 1997. Effects of smoking and smoking cessation on healing after mechanical periodontal therapy. *J. Am. Dent. Assoc.* 128:599–607.

Haber, J., J. Wattles, M. Crowby, R. Mandell, K. Joshipura, and R. L. Kent. 1993. Evidence for cigarette smoking as a major risk factor for periodontitis. *J. Periodontol.* 64:16–23.

Haffajee, A. D., S. S. Socransky, and J. M. Goodson. 1983. Comparison of different data analyses for detecting changes in attachment level. *J. Clin. Periodontol.* 10:298–310.

Jolkovsky, D. L., M. Y. Waki, M. G. Newman, J. Otomo-Corgel, M. Madison, et al. 1990. Clinical and microbiological effects of subgingival and gingival marginal irrigation with chlorhexidine gluconate. *J. Periodontol.* 61:663–669.

Jones, J. K., and R. G. Triplett. 1992. The relationship of cigarette smoking to impaired intraoral wound healing: A review of evidence and implications for patient care. *J. Oral Maxillofac. Surg.* 50:237–239.

Joss, A., R. Adler, and N. P. Lang. 1994. Bleeding on probing. A parameter for monitoring periodontal conditions in clinical practice. *J. Clin. Periodontol.* 21:402–408.

Kerry, G. J. 1995. Supportive periodontal treatment. *Periodontology 2000* 11:176–184.

Kornman, K. S. 1987. Nature of periodontal diseases: Assessment and diagnosis. *J. Periodontol. Res.* 22:192–204.

Lang, N. P., A. Joss, and M. S. Tonetti. 1996. Monitoring disease during supportive periodontal treatment by bleeding on probing. *Periodontology 2000* 12:44–48.

Lindhe, J., S. S. Socransky, S. Nyman, A. Haffajee, and E. Westfelt. 1982. "Critical probing depths" in periodontal therapy. *J. Clin. Periodontol.* 9:323–336.

Medoza, A., G. Newcomb, and K. Nixon. 1991. Compliance with periodontal maintenance. *J. Periodontol.* 62:731–736.

Meffert, R. M. 1992. How to treat ailing and failing implants. *Implant Dent.* 1:25–33.

National Cancer Institute, U.S. Department of Health and Human Services. 1996. *Tobacco effects in the mouth,* eds. R. E. Mechlenburg, D. Greenspan, D. V. Kleinman, et al. Bethesda, MD: Author.

Ramfjord, S. P. 1987. Maintenance care for treated periodontitis patients. *J. Clin. Periodontol.* 14:433–437.

Rosén, B., G. Olavi, A. Baderstan, A. Rönström, G. Söderholm, and J. Egelberg. 1999. Effect of different frequencies of preventive maintenance treatment on periodontal conditions. *J. Clin. Periodontol.* 26:225–230.

Stone, C., and D. J. Mattana. 1996. The role of the dental team in helping patients stop using tobacco. *J. Mich. Dent. Assoc.* (Jan):58–66.

Tonetti, M., V. Muller-Campanile, and V. Lang. 1998. Changes in the prevalence of residual pockets and tooth loss in treated periodontal patients during a supportive maintenance care program. *J. Clin. Periodontol.* 25:1008–1016.

Van der Weijden, G. A., M. F. Timmerman, A. Nijbor, E. Reijerse, and U. Van der Velden. 1994. Comparison of different approaches to assess bleeding on probing as indicators of gingivitis. *J. Periodontol.* 21:589–594.

Weinberg, A. 1986. *Instructions in hypnosis,* unpublished findings.

Wilson, T. G., Jr., M. E. Glover, J. Schoen, C. Baus, and T. Jacobs. 1984. Compliance with maintenance therapy in a private periodontal practice. *J. Periodontol.* 55:468–473.

Wilson, T. G. 1996a. Compliance and its role in periodontal therapy. *Periodontology 2000* 12:16–23.

Wilson, T. G. 1996b. Supportive periodontal treatment introduction: Definition, extent of need, therapeutic objectives, frequency and efficacy. *Periodontology 2000* 12:11–15.

Appendices

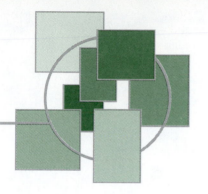

Periodontal Information Resources

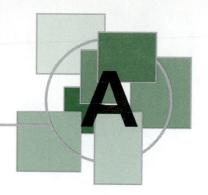

Mea A. Weinberg, D.M.D., M.S.D., R.Ph.

A great number of scientific and clinical resources on periodontology are available from organizations and various journals. This information should be used for continuing education so that the dental hygienist can keep up with current clinical studies and product availability. The Internet provides an excellent opportunity for dental professionals and patients to obtain information related to all aspects of dental hygiene.

Publications: American Academy of Periodontology

The American Academy of Periodontology (AAP) publishes patient education brochures, practice management resources, journals, and clinical publications. The Web site for the American Academy of Periodontology is www.perio.org.

The following materials are available:

1. Patient education brochures
2. 2003 Practice Profile Survey: Characteristics and Trends in Private Periodontal Practice
3. Practice management resources
   - "Designing Effective Practice Marketing Materials"
   - "Sample Periodontal Office Forms"
   - "Informed Consent for Surgical Periodontics"
4. Study club kits (binders containing slides, lecture script, consensus reports, article reprints, references)
   - "Periodontal Plastic Surgery"
   - "Implant Dentistry: A Team Approach to Optimal Patient Care" presentation kit
   - "Comprehensive Insurance Workshop: Reporting Periodontal Procedures to Third Parties" (CD-ROM)

- "Evidence-Based Periodontal Research: Set of Three Scientific Study Club Presentations"
- "Periodontal Medicine"
- "Introduction to Periodontal Surgery for Dental Hygienists" presentation kit
- "Classification, Epidemiology and Diagnosis of Periodontal Diseases"
- "The Role of Pharmacotherapeutics in Periodontal Diseases"
- "Periodic Reevaluation and Supportive Periodontal Therapy"

5. Clinical publications: *Journal of Periodontology* (monthly publication); also available on CD-ROM

6. *Annals of Periodontology*
   - *Annals of Periodontology* (1996 World Workshop in Periodontics), Vol. 1
   - *Annals of Periodontology* (1996 Joint Symposium on Clinical Trial Design and Analysis in Periodontics), Vol. 2
   - *Annals of Periodontology* (1997): New Directions in Periodontal Medicine, Vol. 3.
   - *Annals of Periodontology* (1999): 1999 International Workshop for a Classification of Periodontal Diseases and Conditions, Vol. 4.
   - *Annals of Periodontology* (2003): Proceedings of the Workshop on Contemporary Science in Clinical Periodontics, Vol. 8
   - *Periodontal-Systemic Links: An AAP Literature Compilation* (CD-ROM), 2003

7. *Periodontal Literature Reviews: A Summary of Current Knowledge* (1996)

8. *Periodontal Disease Management* (1993)
   - *2003 Current Procedural Terminology for Periodontics and Insurance Reporting Manual* (9th edition)
   - In-Service Exams (questions given to postgraduate students)

9. Audiotapes from past annual meetings (www.mobiltape.com or 1-800-369-5718).

10. Guidelines
    - Guidelines for Periodontal Therapy (1997)
    - Guidelines for In-Office Use of Conscious Sedation in Periodontics (2001)
    - Position Statement and Guidelines for Soft Tissue Management Programs (1996)

11. Parameters of care: Various papers on the parameters of care of periodontal diseases (2000)

12. Position papers (some position papers are listed below)
    - "Periodontal Diseases of Children and Adolescents" (2003)
    - "Diagnosis of Periodontal Diseases" (2003)
    - "Oral Features of Mucocutaneous Disorders" (2003)
    - "Modulation of the Host Response in Periodontal Therapy" (2002)
    - "Dental Implants and Periodontal Therapy" (2000)
    - "The Role of Controlled Drug Delivery for Periodontitis" (1999)
    - "Tobacco Use and the Periodontal Patient" (1999)
    - "The Pathogenesis of Periodontal Diseases" (1999)
    - "Periodontal Disease as a Potential Risk Factor for Systemic Diseases" (1998)
    - "Diabetes and Periodontal Diseases" (1999)

- "Treatment of Gingivitis and Periodontitis" (1997)
- "Epidemiology of Periodontal Diseases" (1996)

13. Product and procedure statements
    - "Tooth Extraction During Periodontal Therapy" (2003)
    - "The Use of Conscious Sedation by Periodontists" (2003)
    - "Gingival Curettage" (2002)
    - "Use of Dental Lasers for Excisional New Attachment Procedure (ENAP)"
    - "Periostat® Systemically Delivered Collagenase Inhibitor of Doxycycline Hyclate" (1998)

Other associations include:

- The American Dental Hygiene Association (ADHA). The Web site is www.adha.org.
- The American Dental Association (ADA). The Web site is www.ada.org.

Journals/Bulletins

1. *Journal of Periodontology* (American Academy of Periodontology, Chicago; Web site: www.perio.org).

2. *Journal of Dental Hygiene* (American Dental Hygiene Association, Chicago; Web site: www.adha.org).

3. *Practical Periodontics and Aesthetic Dentistry* (Montage Media Corp., Mahwah, NJ; 800-899-5350).

4. *Journal of Practical Hygiene* (Montage Media Corp., Mahwah, NJ; 800-899-5350).

5. *Periodontology 2000* (Musksgaard, Copenhagen; e-mail: fsub@mail.munksgaard.dk).

6. *Journal of Clinical Periodontology* (Munksgaard, Copenhagen; e-mail: fsub@mail.munksgaard.dk).

7. *Journal of Periodontal Research* (Munksgaard, Copenhagen; e-mail: fsub@mail.munksgaard.dk).

8. *Perio Reports* (www.PerioReports.com)—research articles are reviewed (Compendium of Current Research).

9. *International Journal of Oral and Maxillofacial Implants* (Quintessence Publishers, Carol Stream, IL; e-mail: quintpub@aol.com; Web site: www.quintpub.com).

10. *Clinical Oral Implants Research* (Munksgaard International Publishers, ltd., Malden, MA. e-mail: fsub@mail.munksgaard.dk; Web site: www.munksgaard.dk).

Other Web Sites

1. www.dentalcare.com (Procter & Gamble)

2. www.colgate.com (Colgate Oral Pharmaceutical)

3. http://jeffline.tju.edu/DHNet (National Center for Dental Hygiene Research)
4. www.oralhealth.org (Oral Health Letter)

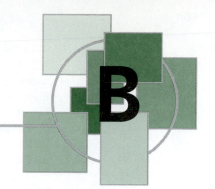

Reading the Literature

Trisha E. O'Hehir, R.D.H., B.S.

Article Classification

- Clinical trial (in vivo)
- Laboratory study (in vitro)
- Combination studies—part clinical, part laboratory
- Case studies—reports of individual patients and their outcomes
- Epidemiology—incidence and/or prevalence of disease in a population
- Informational
- Review

Research articles include several distinct sections. Each section provides valuable information. These sections do not have to be read in the order they are printed. It depends on what information is being requested. The following is a brief summary of each section.

Abstract

- Brief overview of the entire article
- Hypothesis being tested
- Number of subjects involved
- Methods used
- Results

The last sentence of an abstract often provides the essence of the project. The last sentence is where reading of a research article should begin.

Introduction

- Lays the groundwork for the project
- Historical information on the subject area
- Past research studies are sited in this area
- Author or authors have to make a case for their project
- Controversies in the area based on previously published work
- Statement of the hypothesis

Most often, a null hypothesis is stated, which says that if the researchers do what they propose, no changes will be seen. The goal of the researchers is to then disprove the null hypothesis. Approaching the hypothesis from the other direction requires stating that the drug, tool, or therapy to be tested will have a specific effect on the test subject, which necessitates quantifying the expected result. Guessing at the outcome before the study begins can be quite difficult. Therefore, disproving a null hypothesis allows for a positive result without the need to estimate the outcome at the start.

Some researchers state their purpose rather than formulating a hypothesis. The following is an example of stating a purpose:

> Thus, this study compares the amount of aerosol produced by a traditional ultrasonic scaler insert and that produced by a new focused style insert. In addition, the effect of using an aerosol reduction device with both types of inserts is evaluated. [Rivera–Hidalgo, F., Barnes, J., and Harrel, S. 1999. Aerosol and splatter production by focused spray and standard ultrasonic inserts. *J. Periodontol.,* 70:473–477]

Here is the same statement of purpose restated as a hypothesis:

> The hypothesis to be tested is that no difference in aerosol spray is expected comparing traditional and focused-style ultrasonic inserts, used either alone or with an aerosol reduction device.

The goal of the researchers remains the same—to determine if there is a difference, thus disproving the null hypothesis.

Methods and Materials

This section is often divided into subsections, providing some of the following information:

- *Study population.* Collection of people, items, or observations to be studied
- *People*
  - *Number of subjects.* Setting a desired outcome in statistical terms allows the statistician to calculate exactly how many subjects are needed.
  - *Random sample.* All subjects of a given population have an equal chance of being selected (e.g., picking names out of a hat or using a table of random numbers to select subjects).
  - *Convenience population.* Sample does not represent the population at large (e.g., dental or dental hygiene students).
  - *Volunteers or paid participants*
  - *Subject solicitation.* Clinic patients, newspaper ads, etc.
  - *Demographics.* Age, gender, general health, oral health, dental history
- *Location of the study.* University, clinical practice, community, etc.
- *Study design*
  - Timeline of events, including length of the study
  - Indices used and any modifications
  - Description of drugs, tools, or techniques to be tested
  - Who the examiners were and their preparation for the study
  - Characteristics of the clinical study design

(a) *Case control*. Subjects with a certain condition are selected and compared with controls (e.g., subjects without the condition). For example, a group of subjects with oral cancer is compared with a control group without oral cancer for smoking habits over the previous 5 years.

(b) *Crossover*. Each subject receives two or more treatments at different times, and end points are observed after each treatment.

(c) *Cross-sectional*. End points are observed at one given point in time.

(d) *Longitudinal*. End points are observed more than once over a period of time.

(e) *Observational*. Subjects or objects of interest (e.g., teeth) are observed in their natural state with no intervention by researchers.

(f) *Prospective*. Study subjects selected based on a certain treatment or exposure and observed for a specific outcome over a period of time (e.g., subjects selected based on smoking habits and observed for cancer development over a 5-year period).

(g) *Retrospective*. Study subjects are selected based on a certain outcome, and then data are gathered on previous exposure (e.g., subjects selected based on the presence of oral cancer and studied as to smoking habits during the previous 5 years).

(h) *Parallel group*. Experimental groups do not experience the same treatment or products (e.g., a control group and a test group).

(i) *Randomized*. Subjects or objects of interest (e.g., teeth) are assigned to different treatments or interventions randomly.

(j) *Split-mouth*. Each subject receives two or more treatments at different sites within the mouth, and outcomes are observed at a given point in time.

- *Details of laboratory tests*
  - How specimens are collected
  - How they are stored
  - How the tests are run
  - What equipment is used
  - Who does the testing
- *Statistical analysis*. Selection of mathematical techniques used to assist in the understanding and interpretation of data for the purpose of decision making.
- *Descriptive statistics*. Methods to simply describe data in a numerical way, such as frequency of a given parameter.
- *Inferential statistics*. Methods used to infer something about a population from a sample of observations from that population.

Results

- Factual presentation of the study data
- Statistics

Opinions or conclusion are left for the next section.

Discussion

- Limitations of the study
- Confirmation of earlier findings
- Integration of study findings with previously published data
- Unanswered questions
- New questions raised by the findings
- Interesting side findings that do not relate to this hypothesis
- Subjective opinions of the patients who participated
- Suggestions for future studies
- Conclusions that can be drawn from this study
- Significance of these findings, both statistical and clinical

Statistical significance might be better stated as "statistical difference," since the difference actually may not be clinically significant.

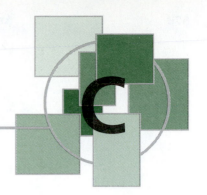

Health Insurance Portability and Accountability Act (HIPAA)

Mea A. Weinberg, D.M.D., M.S.D., R.Ph.

This section deals with the latest information concerning the **Health Insurance Portability and Accountability Act (HIPAA)** of 1996. The information in this chapter will be presented in a question-and-answer format.

1. What does HIPAA stand for?

   HIPAA is an abbreviation for The Health Insurance Portability and Accountability Act of 1996.

2. What is the primary objective of instituting HIPAA?

   HIPAA was developed to protect the privacy of patients' health (medical) information and records provided to health plans, doctors, hospitals, and other health care providers. This includes financial and administrative transactions such as electronic billing to insurance companies. Essentially, HIPAA maintains the confidentiality of patients' records, documents, agreements that are spoken, written, or electronic. Information and records of patients are to be used only for the purpose of caring for the patient. All paper and electronic records are not to be used for unauthorized purposes nor should there be disclosure of confidential information in casual conversation or in a public place. Additionally, patient information or other confidential information should not be shared in a place where the public or those not having a need to know can view it. Patients' records must be secured so that it is not readily available to those who do not need them.

   HIPAA also gives patients the right to find out how their information is being used, and gives patients the right to examine and obtain a copy of their own medical records and request corrections.

3. Who developed HIPAA?

   The Department of Health and Human Services (HHS) developed HIPAA.

4. When did compliance with HIPAA begin?

   The compliance date for the HIPAA regulations was April 14, 2003.

5. Who has to comply with HIPAA?

   Most health insurers, pharmacies, doctors, health care clearinghouses, and other health care providers must comply with these standards.

6. What are the standards of HIPAA?

   HIPAA calls for (1) standardization of electronic patient health, administrative, and financial data; (2) unique health identifiers for individuals, employers, health plans, and health care providers; (3) security standards protecting the confidentiality and integrity of "individually identifiable health information," past, present, or future; and (4) privacy and confidentiality standards.

7. What are some Web sites on the computer that further discuss HIPAA?

   http://www.hhs.gov/ocr/hipaa
   http://www.hipaadvisory.com/regs/HIPAAprimer1
   http://answers.hhs.gov/cgi-bin/hhs.cfg/php/enduser/prnt

8. What is PHI?

   PHI stands for protected health information. PHI is health information that relates to the health condition of patients. Use and disclosure of PHI is only allowed for purposes of treatment, payment, and health care operations, and when the patients gives written authorization.

9. Does the patient have to be notified of their privacy rights?

   Yes. Patients must be given written information about their rights as a patient and how this information can be used.

10. Can the PHI of patients in a teaching institution be used for the purposes of training students?

    Yes. But students must be taught on the appropriate uses of PHI. Disclosure of PHI outside the teaching institution or beyond the scope of their training activities is not permitted.

11. Can a PHI be shared between doctors?

    Yes, for the purposes of treating patients, doctors' payment, health care operations, and for limited health care operations outside of the health institution when related to patient treatment or payment.

12. Is the treating doctor permitted to discuss a patient's care with the patient's family and friends?

    Yes, if there is written HIPAA authorization by the patient, if the patient designates the family member or friend as a "personal representative," or if the patient brings a family member or friend with them and expresses by their conduct that this other person is involved in the patient's health care.

13. Can a health care provider leave a message at the patients' home or mail reminders to their home?

    Yes. The HIPAA Privacy Rule permits communication with the patient regarding their health care. This communication can be through the mail or the phone, including leaving messages for patients on their answering machine. It is up to the health care provider to limit the amount of confidential information left on an answering machine.

14. Can a doctor's office fax patient medical information to another doctor's office?

    Yes, for treatment purposes, but there must be appropriate administrative, technical, and physical safeguards to protect the privacy of protected health information.

15. Does HIPAA require health care providers document all oral communications?

    No. HIPAA does not require health care providers to document any oral information that is used or disclosed for treatment, payment, or health care operations. However, a record must be maintained of any disclosure made orally, by phone, or in writing.

16. Are patients required to pay for copies of their medical records?

    According to the HIPAA, the health care provider may charge reasonable, cost-based fees. This fee may include only the cost of copying (including supplies and labor) and postage.

17. Does HIPAA change the consent to treatment laws?

    No, HIPAA does not affect informed consent for treatment. This is governed by state law.

18. May health care providers have confidential conversations with other health care providers or patients considering that the conversation may be overheard?

    Yes. Oral conversations are permitted but reasonable safeguards must be implemented such as talking in a lower voice. HIPAA recognizes that some communications may be overheard and are unavoidable. Thus, HIPAA provides for these incidental disclosures.

19. Does a new, upgraded computer system need to be installed?

    No. However, every effort must be made to limit access to protect medical/health information to that in the office/workplace.

20. What does "privacy" mean in the context of HIPAA?

    Privacy pertains to who will have access to patients' health records.

21. What does "confidentiality" mean in the context of HIPAA?

    Confidentiality establishes how the patients' records or the systems that hold the records should be protected from inappropriate access.

22. What does "security" mean in the context of HIPAA?

    Security establishes the means by which the health care providers secure privacy and confidentiality.

23. What security standards are set forth in HIPAA?

    New security standards have been developed to protect the transfer of electronic health information (between health care provider [office/clinic] and health plans, insurance companies) from inappropriate access or alteration and to protect against loss of records.

24. Who is responsible to comply with these new standards for electronic transactions?

    All health care providers who choose to transmit health information electronically. Also, all health plans and health care clearinghouses that are involved in electronic transactions of health records of patients.

25. What information is covered by the Security Standards?

    Any health/medical information that identifies an individual through electronic exchange. A patient may sign a disclosure that permits individual authorization of health information. The authorization must specify the information to be disclosed, who will receive the information, and when the authorization expires.

26. Are there situations when individuals are exempted from signing authorization to transmit health information?

    Yes. Health care providers may use and disclose protected health information without individual authorization in the following circumstances:
    - Research
    - Law enforcement
    - Government health data systems
    - To provide information to the next-of-kin
    - For hospital directories
    - To financial institutions

27. Under HIPAA, may health care providers use either sign-in sheets or call out names in the waiting rooms of an office or clinic?

    Yes. Sign-in sheets and calling out a patient's name is permitted as long as the information disclosed is appropriately limited and reasonable safeguards are used, such as not disclosing the patient's medical diagnosis.

28. What is the latest, as of the time of publication of this textbook, HIPAA regulation established?

    As of October 16, 2003, all physicians, dentists, insurance providers, and claims clearinghouses must use new standard electronic formats for exchanging information. Medicare will only accept claims submitted electronically. This means that clinical practices need to have computer software that is able to meet HIPAA standards.

Selected References

United States Department of Health & Human Services. OCR Privacy Brief. Summary of the HIPAA. HIPAA Compliance Assistance. 2003. www.hhs.gov/ocr/hipaa/bkgrnd.html

United States Department of Health & Human Services. Fact Sheet. Protecting the Privacy of Patients' Health Information. 2003. www.hhs.gov/news/facts/privacy/html.

http://answers.hhs.gov/cgi-bin/hhs.cfg/php/enduser/prnt

http://www.wedi.org/snip/public/articles/details

http://www.hipaa.org/pmsdirectory

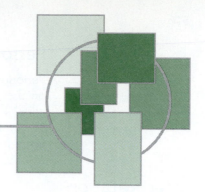

Case Study I

Medical History

The patient is a 65-year-old male who states he is in perfect health and goes to his physician once a year for a check-up. His blood pressure is 135/84 and he has a pulse of 72. He is 5 feet 9 inches tall and weighs 195 lb (88.6 kg). He denies taking any medications, including over-the-counter products. Occasionally he takes one aspirin when he has a headache.

Chief Complaint

"My gums look red and they bleed when I brush hard."

Dental History

The patient has not seen a dentist in the last 3 years because he states he is too busy with work and he thinks the condition of his gingiva is due to brushing too hard. He brushes twice a day but does not floss.

Social History

The patient is married with two grown-up children. He is the head of an investment company and travels frequently. The patient has smoked 1 pack of cigarettes a day for 30 years (30 pack/years) and drinks one or two cocktails every night at dinner as well as beer on the weekends.

Oral Hygiene Status

The patient has poor oral hygiene. An examination revealed generalized supra/subgingival plaque and calculus.

Dental Exam

The patient is missing all third molars.

Gingival Exam

The gingiva is red and edematous. There is generalized gingival recession.

Periodontal Exam

Periodontal probing depths range from 3 to 8 mm, with the deepest depths being on the maxillary molars. Radiographic survey reveals generalized bone loss with vertical bony defects on the mesial surface of the mandibular left first and second molar. There is red swelling at the mesial aspect of the right maxillary first molar upon probing the area, pus is evident.

Interpretation

Patient Problem	Basis For Discussion	Questions (Q)/Answers (A)	Chapter Location
Gingiva is red and bleeds	Inflammation is present	Q) What causes the erythema and bleeding? A) Erythema is caused by vascular proliferation. Sites that bleed have a greater area of inflamed gingival connective tissue	8, 9
Smokes	Patient needs to stop smoking. Talk to patient about a smoking cessation program.	Q) Does smoking affect the periodontium? A) Smoking is an important risk factor for inflammatory periodontal diseases. Smokers have greater probing depths, clinical attachment loss, and bone loss. Smoking can also impair the chemotaxis and phagocytosis of neutrophils.	6
Drinks	Patient needs to stop or reduce alcohol consumption.	Q) Does alcohol affect the periodontium? A) Chronic alcohol intake presents an increased risk for periodontitis because of increased bleeding tendencies, poor oral hygiene due to overall neglect, and a tendency to malnutrition.	6
Patient has poor oral hygiene	Generalized plaque accumulation	Q) What type of assessment procedure will best help the patient understand and improve his oral hygiene status? A) A plaque index. The O'Leary, Drake and Naylor Plaque Control Record shows the distribution rather than the amount of plaque. This will help to motivate the patient by showing him where most of plaque accumulates.	3
Generalized periodontal pockets and bone loss	Patient has generalized mild gingivitis and generalized moderate with localized areas of severe chronic periodontitis.	Q) What is the etiology of the periodontal pockets and the bone loss? A) The primary risk factor for periodontal diseases is dental plaque or biofilms. Bacteria and host cells synthesize toxins, by-products, and enzymes that cause bone destruction and pocket formation. Periodontal pockets form when the apical part of the junctional epithelium migrates apically along the root surface. This happens when the gingival fibers (gingival connective tissue attachment) is destroyed. This is referred to as attachment loss.	4, 8, 10

1. All of the following are contributing factors for this patient's periodontal condition EXCEPT one. Which one is the exception? (p. 64)
   a. pathogenic bacteria
   b. dental calculus
   c. smoking
   d. alcohol
   e. aspirin

2. Which one of the following types of pockets is found on the mesial surface of the mandibular left first molar? (p. 155)
   a. gingival
   b. pseudo
   c. suprabony
   d. infrabony

3. Which one of the following cells predominate in the area immediately below the junctional epithelium in this patient? (p. 128)
   a. mast
   b. melanocytes
   c. T lymphocytes
   d. B lymphocytes

4. Which one of the following parts of the periodontium is responsible for keeping the patient's mandibular left second molar in the tooth socket? (p. 20)
   a. gingival fibers
   b. periodontal ligament fibers
   c. alveolar bone proper
   d. junctional epithelium

5. Which one of the following findings is most consistent with gingival inflammation in this patient? (p. 238)
   a. bleeding on probing
   b. redness of the gingiva
   c. deep probing depths
   d. vertical bone loss

6. Which one of the following classification of periodontal diseases (American Academy of Periodontology) is characteristic of this patient? (pp. 31–38)
   a. plaque-induced gingivitis
   b. localized aggressive periodontitis
   c. generalized aggressive periodontitis
   d. chronic periodontitis
   e. necrotizing ulcerative periodontitis

7. High numbers of which of the following bacteria are most likely evident in this patient? (pp. 66–67)
   a. *Candida albicans*
   b. *Streptococcus sanguis*
   c. *Fusobacterium nucleatum*
   d. *Porphyromonas gingivalis*

8. All of the following features characterize this patient's periodontal condition except one. Which one is the exception? (pp. 149–160)
   a. apical migration of the junctional epithelium
   b. increased width of the attached gingiva
   c. supporting and alveolar bone loss
   d. loss of gingival connective tissue attachment

9. Which one of the following features in this patient is possibly responsible for a decrease in function of neutrophils? (p. 99–100)
   a. increased age
   b. cigarette smoking
   c. alcohol drinking
   d. high blood pressure
   e. aspirin tablets

10. Which one of the following substances is most likely the direct cause of the bone loss that has occurred in this patient? (pp. 74–75)
    a. lipooligosaccharides and enzymes
    b. bacterial waste products and enzymes
    c. cigarette smoke and dental calculus
    d. dental calculus and alcohol

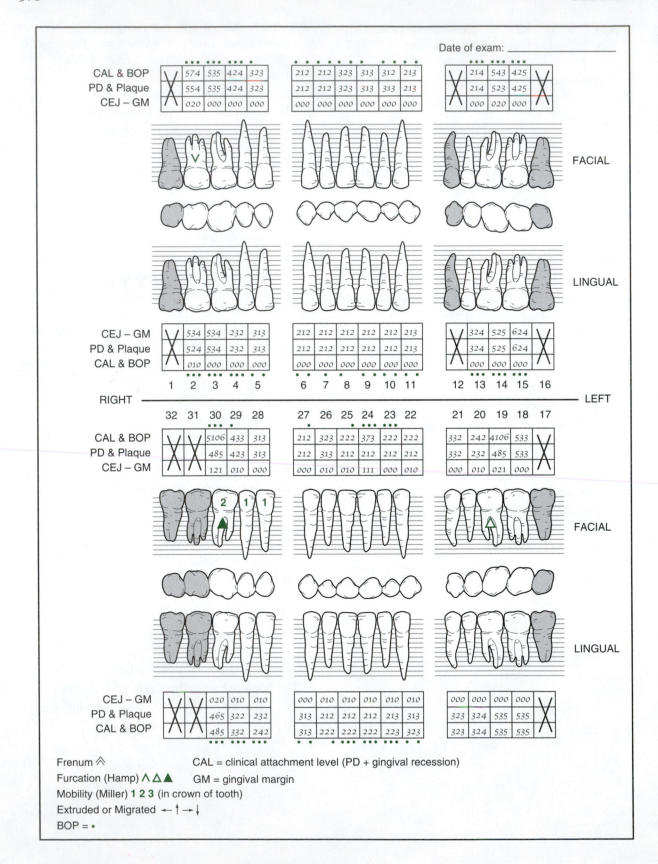

Date of exam: _____

		CAL & BOP																

Top section (Maxillary, Facial)

CAL & BOP | X | 574 | 535 | 424 | 323 | | 212 | 212 | 323 | 313 | 312 | 213 | | 214 | 543 | 425 | X
PD & Plaque | X | 554 | 535 | 424 | 323 | | 212 | 212 | 323 | 313 | 313 | 213 | | 214 | 523 | 425 | X
CEJ – GM | X | 020 | 000 | 000 | 000 | | 000 | 000 | 000 | 000 | 000 | 000 | | 000 | 020 | 000 | X

FACIAL

LINGUAL

CEJ – GM | X | 534 | 534 | 232 | 313 | | 212 | 212 | 212 | 212 | 212 | 213 | | X | 324 | 525 | 624 | X
PD & Plaque | X | 524 | 534 | 232 | 313 | | 212 | 212 | 212 | 212 | 212 | 213 | | X | 324 | 525 | 624 | X
CAL & BOP | X | 010 | 000 | 000 | 000 | | 000 | 000 | 000 | 000 | 000 | 000 | | X | 000 | 000 | 000 | X

 1   2   3   4   5   6   7   8   9   10   11   12   13   14   15   16

RIGHT ————————————————————————————————— LEFT

32   31   30   29   28   27   26   25   24   23   22   21   20   19   18   17

CAL & BOP | X | X | 5106 | 433 | 313 | | 212 | 323 | 222 | 373 | 222 | 222 | | 332 | 242 | 4106 | 533 | X
PD & Plaque | X | X | 485 | 423 | 313 | | 212 | 313 | 212 | 212 | 212 | 212 | | 332 | 232 | 485 | 533 | X
CEJ – GM | X | X | 121 | 010 | 000 | | 000 | 010 | 010 | 111 | 000 | 010 | | 000 | 010 | 021 | 000 | X

FACIAL

LINGUAL

CEJ – GM | X | X | 020 | 010 | 010 | | 000 | 010 | 010 | 010 | 010 | 010 | | 000 | 000 | 000 | 000 | X
PD & Plaque | X | X | 465 | 322 | 232 | | 313 | 212 | 212 | 212 | 213 | 313 | | 323 | 324 | 535 | 535 | X
CAL & BOP | X | X | 485 | 332 | 242 | | 313 | 222 | 222 | 222 | 223 | 323 | | 323 | 324 | 535 | 535 | X

Frenum ⋀   CAL = clinical attachment level (PD + gingival recession)
Furcation (Hamp) ∧ △ ▲   GM = gingival margin
Mobility (Miller) **1 2 3** (in crown of tooth)
Extruded or Migrated ← ↑ → ↓
BOP = •

Case Study II

Cheryl Westphal, R.D.H., M.S.

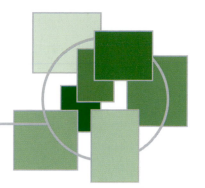

Medical History

This 25-year-old male patient denies allergies. The patient has a history of aphthous ulcers, otherwise there is a noncontributory health history. The patient uses Orabase®–HCA (hydrocortisone acetate).

Dental History

The patient has not had previous periodontal treatment. He says he brushes once a day and does not floss. Periodically, for the past 2 months he has experienced spontaneous bleeding.

Social History

The patient does not have a full time job. He is a 10 pack/years smoker and does not want to stop.

Chief Complaint

"My gums bleed and I have spaces between my teeth."

1. All of the following are etiologic or risk factors associated with this patient's periodontal condition EXCEPT one. Which one is the exception?

   a. smoking

   b. genetics

   c. aphthous ulcer

   d. pathogenic bacteria

2. Which one of the following classifications of periodontal diseases does this patient belong?

   a. plaque-induced gingivitis

   b. drug-influenced gingivitis

   c. chronic periodontitis

   d. aggressive periodontitis

   e. necrotizing periodontal diseases

3. Bleeding is evident after probing the maxillary anterior teeth. Which one of the following best explains the presence of the bleeding in this patient?

   a. laceration of the gingival tissue

   b. accumulation of calculus in the periodontal pockets

   c. increased production of gingival collagen in the connective tissue

   d. engorgement of connective tissue capillaries with ulceration of the sulcular epithelium

4. Which one of the following Angle's classifications is evident in this patient?

   a. right: I; left: I

   b. right: II; left II

   c. right: II; left: III

   d. right: III; left: II

   e. right: III; left III

5. Which one of the following instruments is best used to inspect and measure the amount of interradibular bone loss on the mandibular right first molar?

   a. William's probe

   b. Nabers probe

   c. CH3 explorer

   d. 11/12 explorer

   e. Columbia 13/14 curet

6. Which one of the following radiolucent areas is evident on the mandibular right second molar?

   a. amalgam restoration

   b. composite restoration

   c. dental caries

   d. root caries

   e. gold onlay

7. Which one of the following radiolucent findings is evident around the mesial root of the maxillary right second molar?

   a. subgingival calculus

   b. maxillary sinus

   c. dental caries

   d. bone loss

8. All of the following treatment procedures in this patient should be planned *except* one. Which one is the exception?

   a. prevention of future decay

   b. assessment of pockets for possible surgery

   c. assessment for prosthetic bridges

   d. exposure to panoramic radiograph

   e. possible antibiotics and periodontal debridement

9. Considering the probing depths, which one of the following plans would be most appropriate?

   a. Premedicate and perform supragingival debridement.

   b. Advise use of sanguinarine rinse and perform full mouth periodontal debridement.

   c. Advise use of chlorhexidine rinse and perform quadrant debridement.

   d. Prescribe tetracycline and reevaluate gingival tissues in 2 weeks.

10. Which one of the following tactics should the dental hygienist take when debriding the mandibular right lateral and central incisors?

   a. Do not debride because the teeth may exfoliate.

   b. Splint the teeth first before debridement procedures are started.

   c. Debride carefully to avoid pain.

   d. Perform supragingival debridement and wait 2 weeks.

PERIODONTAL EXAMINATION

PATIENT'S NAME:_____   DATE:_____

Facial (R → L, teeth 1–16)

| PD | 859 | 759 | X | 224 | 535 | 336 | 555 | 533 | 324 | 655 | 787 | 757 | 735 | 759 | 757 | X |

Lingual

| PD | 757 | 738 | X | 355 | 788 | 857 | 758 | 535 | 533 | 535 | 558 | 876 | 555 | 535 | 735 | X |

Lingual (teeth 32–17)

| PD | 555 | 335 | 555 | 757 | 737 | 557 | 753 | 323 | 232 | 337 | 737 | 775 | 533 | X | 555 | 523 |

Facial

| PD | 737 | 727 | 757 | 725 | 527 | 537 | 757 | 737 | 757 | 757 | 558 | 737 | 715 | X | 524 | 333 |

KEY TO CHARTING

Missing Tooth	Draw horizontal line through crown of missing teeth
AL, Attachment Level	CEJ to bottom of pocket
PD, Pocket Depth	Gingival margin to bottom of pocket
Plaque	+ or -
SUP	Suppuration or exudate, + or -
Overhang	˥ or L for mandible; ˥ or Γ for maxilla

Deficient Contacts	Draw 2 vertical lines and record space in mm
Endodontics	Draw vertical line through root if treated; draw circle at apex if lesion; indicate vitality response at apex V for max.; Λ for mand.
Muscle Attachment	+ or -
Calculus	+ or -
Micro	Site for microbiologic sampling

BOP	Bleeding on probing, + or -
Migration	Drifting, tipping or extruding - indicate an arrow in direction of movement
Mobility	Record I, II, or III on facial aspect of crown
Furcation	Place I in furca if incipient; II if partial; III if complete

Oral Examination

Poor oral hygiene

1. Generalized bleeding on probing
2. Generalized supra/subgingival plaque and calculus
3. Tooth mobility

Class I mobility: teeth #'s 2,4,6,7,8,9, 11,13,14,15,17,18,20,21,23,26,28,29,30,31

Class II mobility: teeth #'s 1,5,10,12,24, 25

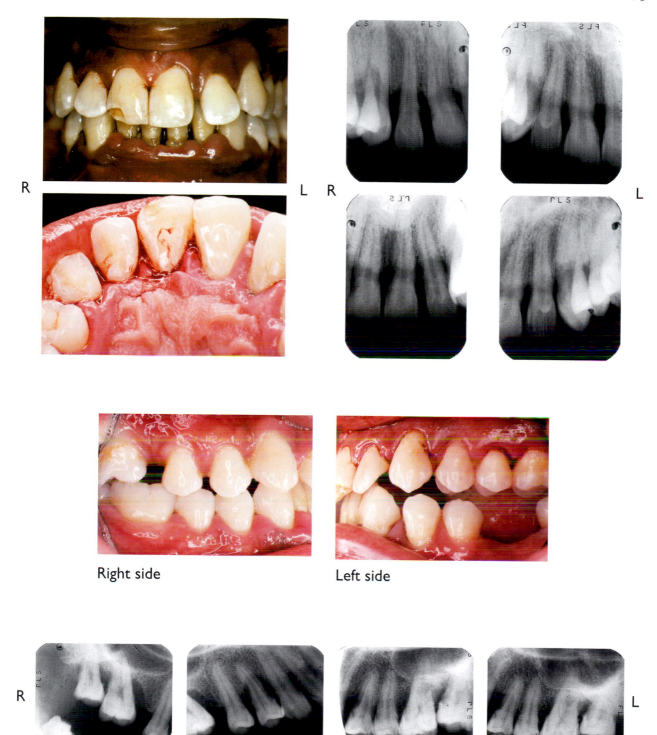

Right side

Left side

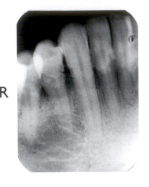
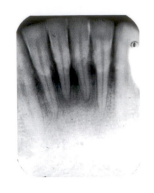
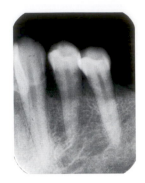

R L

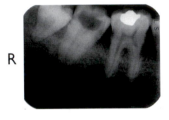
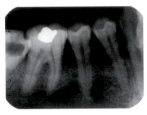
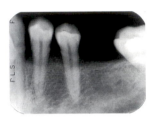
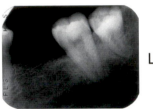

R L

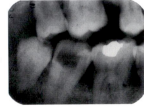
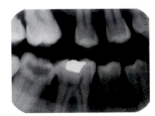
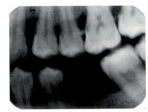
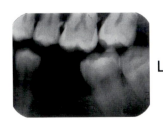

R L

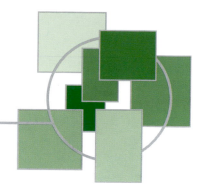

Case Study III

Medical History

This 55-year-old female patient was diagnosed with osteoarthritis 1 year ago and hypertension last month. Both conditions are controlled with medication. She is taking Prednisone 10mg/day and atenolol (Tenormin®) 50mg/day. She also has a functional heart murmur.

Dental History

The patient brushes twice a day with a soft bristle toothbrush and flosses occasionally.

Social History

The patient is married with two adult children. She has accepted her medical conditions, but at times feels stressed and depressed. She does not smoke.

Chief Complaint

"My upper right front tooth is loose and my mouth is dry."

1. Which one of the following pretreatment procedures should be followed in this patient?

   a. Medicate with 2g amoxicillin 1 hour before treatment.

   b. Medicate with 1g clindamycin 1 hour before treatment.

   c. Increase dosage of prednisone 2 hours before treatment.

   d. Decrease dosage of prednisone to 1/2 the original dosage.

   e. Increase dosage of atenolol to 100 mg/day.

2. Which one of the following should be avoided in this patient?

   a. use of epinephrine containing local anesthetic

   b. salivary substitutes for xerostomia

   c. stressful situations

   d. systemic antibiotics

3. Which one of the following factors is responsible for the patient's chief complaint?

   a. congenitally long clinical crown

   b. subgingival calculus

   c. primary occlusal trauma

   d. secondary occlusal trauma

4. To which of the following classifications of periodontal diseases does this patient belong?

   a. chronic periodontitis

   b. drug-induced gingivitis

   c. aggressive periodontitis

   d. periodontitis associated with systemic disease

5. Which one of the following is the most likely cause of the radiolucency at the junction of the mesial and distal root of the maxillary right second molar?

   a. periapical abscess

   b. periodontal abscess

   c. root caries

   d. furcation involvement

   e. maxillary sinus

6. Which one of the following teeth exhibits a mucogingival involvement or deformity?

   a. maxillary left central incisor

   b. maxillary left second premolar

   c. mandibular right central incisor

   d. mandibular right canine

7. Which one of the following oral hygiene aids is best for the proximal surface between the mandibular right central and lateral incisors?

   a. interdental brush

   b. tufted floss

   c. extra soft toothbrush

   d. toothpick-in-holder

8. Which one of the following factors is most likely the cause of the bone loss seen on the maxillary right first molar?

   a. occlusal trauma and subgingival bacteria

   b. bacteria and host response

   c. subgingival calculus

   d. periodontal abscess formation

9. Which one of the following instruments best accomplishes plaque and calculus removal on the mesial aspect of the mandibular left second molar?

   a. Gracey 1/2 curet

   b. Gracey 15/16 curet

   c. Gracey 13/14 curet

   d. Columbia 2R/2L curet

   e. Columbia 13/14 curet

10. Which of the following risk factors is associated with this patient's periodontal disease?

    a. osteoarthritis

    b. dental plaque

    c. heart murmur

    d. hypertension

PERIODONTAL EXAMINATION

PATIENT'S NAME:_____   DATE:_____

KEY TO CHARTING

Missing Tooth · Draw horizontal line through crown of missing teeth
AL, Attachment Level · CEJ to bottom of pocket
PD, Pocket Depth · Gingival margin to bottom of pocket
Plaque · + or -
SUP · Suppuration or exudate; + or -
Overhang · ⌐ or L for mandible; ⌐ or Γ for maxilla

Deficient Contacts · Draw 2 vertical lines and record space in mm
Endodontics · Draw vertical line through root if treated; draw circle at apex if lesion; indicate vitality response at apex
Muscle Attachment · V for maxil., Λ for mand.
Calculus · + or -
Micro · Site for microbiologic sampling

BOP · Bleeding on probing. + or -
Migration · Drifting, tipping or extruding · indicate an arrow in direction of movement
Mobility · Record I, II, or III on facial aspect of crown
Furcation · Place I in furca if incipient; II if partial; III if complete

PD (Facial, R–L, teeth 1–16):

| | 853 | 437 | 635 | 536 | 636 | 534 | 728 | 323 | 525 | 424 | 424 | 226 | X | 535 | X |

PD (Lingual, teeth 1–16):

| X | 825 | 646 | 436 | 533 | 333 | 333 | 727 | 423 | 333 | 332 | 233 | 216 | X | 535 | X |

PD (Lingual, teeth 32–17):

| X | 645 | 347 | 556 | 633 | 434 | 534 | 344 | 333 | 334 | 335 | 556 | 645 | 546 | 867 | X |

PD (Facial, teeth 32–17):

| X | 644 | 434 | 434 | 334 | 444 | 535 | 536 | 624 | 434 | 335 | 536 | 536 | 646 | 635 | X |

Oral Examination

Fair oral hygiene

1. Moderate supra/subgingival plaque
2. Localized bleeding on probing
3. Class I mobility #'s 4, 5, 25
   Class II mobility #'s 2, 3, 8

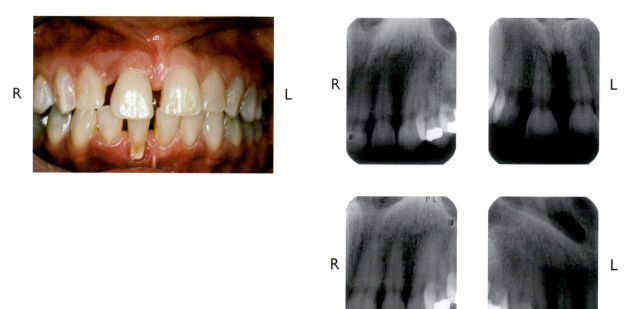

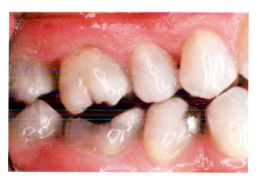

Right side

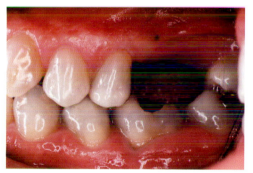

Left side

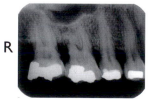

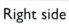

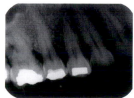

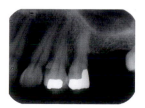

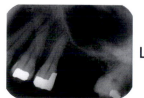

R 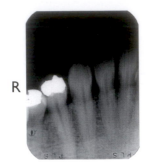 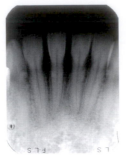 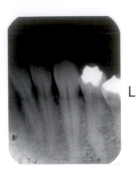 L

R 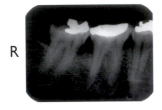 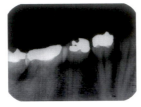 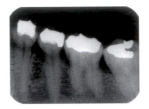 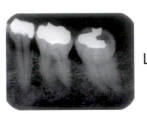 L

R 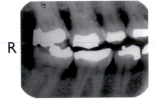 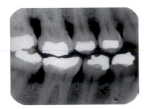 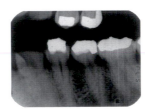 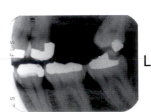 L

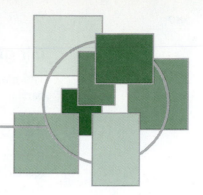

Case Study IV

Cheryl Westphal, R.D.H., M.S.

Medical History

The patient is a 39-year-old woman. Blood pressure is 130/82 mmHg, pulse rate is 64, and respiration rate is 16. The patient weighs 145 lb (65.9 kg). She is not under the care of a physician and has not had any illnesses requiring hospitalization within the last 5 years.

Current Medications

The patient is taking an oral contraceptive containing estrogen/progestin (Lo/Ovral®).

Dental History

The patient states that she brushes with a hard-bristled toothbrush twice a day and flosses only occasionally because she was never taught the proper technique. A previous dentist prescribed chlorhexidine oral rinse, which she is using twice a day. She has not used the rinse continuously and still has a few bottles left. She has not seen a dentist in about 9 months.

Social History

The patient is married with two young children. She denies drinking. The patient has a secure job, and she says she is under a lot of stress at home and work. The patient smokes low-tar cigarettes (10 pack/years) and has not attempted to stop.

Chief Complaint

The patient states that "my teeth are sensitive to cold, and I don't like the stains on my teeth. I want a cleaning."

Dental Exam

The patient has generalized gingival recession and localized tooth abrasion. The maxillary right first molar has an overhanging MOD amalgam.

Oral Hygiene Status

Fair. Generalized supra/subgingival plaque and calculus. Generalized staining.

579

Gingival Exam

The gingiva is red, edematous, enlarged, and shiny and smooth. The contour of the papillae is bulbous, and the margins are rolled. Generalized bleeding on probing.

Periodontal Exam

Probing depths range from 1 to 8 mm. The mandibular first molars have 8 mm on the direct facial surface and 2mm of gingival recession. There is no tooth mobility. Radiographs show bone loss around the mandibular first molars and the maxillary right first molar.

Interpretation

Patient Problem	Basis for Discussion	Questions (Q)/Answers (A)	Chapter Location
Wants teeth cleaned	Patient wants her teeth cleaned due to buildup of plaque, calculus, and stains—it has been 9 months since she last saw a dentist.	Q) Does accumulation of plaque and calculus affect the oral health of the patient? A) Dental plaque is the primary risk factor for periodontal diseases, and calculus is a secondary factor.	4, 5
Teeth are stained	Patient needs to stop smoking.	Q) Does cigarette smoking affect the periodontium and periodontal treatment? A) Greater probing depths, clinical attachment loss, gingival tissue changes, and bone loss have been reported in smokers; thus periodontal therapy may be less effective.	17, 18
	Patient needs teeth cleaned due to retention of stains.	Q) Do tooth stains from smoking and chlorhexidine adversely affect the teeth? A) Stains will not directly affect teeth, but the significance of stains is related to the rough surface they may create and the resulting plaque retention sites. Also, it may be unaesthetic to the patient and others.	5
Medication: Lo/Ovral®	Patient does not want to use an alternative birth control method.	Q) Do oral contraceptives affect the periodontium? A) Elevated hormonal levels (progesterone) aggravate the gingival response to local irritants—gingival inflammation. Good plaque control is important.	6, 17
Gingival recession and tooth abrasion	Patient should change the type of toothbrush and method used.	Q) What is the etiology of the gingival recession in this patient? A) Faulty toothbrushing	18
		Q) What is the etiology of the tooth abrasion? A) Over zealous toothbrushing technique with a hard-bristled toothbrush	16
Overhanging restoration on the maxillary right first molar	Patient experiences difficulty in flossing.	Q) Is an overhang of periodontal concern? A) Overhangs are plaque traps—could result in bone loss.	5 5, 16
Generalized bleeding and edematous tissue	Patient has generalized moderate gingivitis and localized (severe) chronic periodontitis.	Q) What is the etiology of the gingivitis? A) Dental plaque—hormones exaggerate the tissue response to plaque. Q) What is the etiology of the bleeding? A) Bleeding indicates inflammation in the lamina propria.	17 17
Localized bone loss		Q) What is the etiology of the bone loss in the furca? A) Same etiology as progressive periodontal disease—	10, 18

Localized furcation involvement

dental plaque. More difficult to control plaque in furcas.

Q) Are the periodontitis sites active or inactive (e.g., losing attachment)? 18, 20

A) Difficult to determine by conventional assessment tools. Currently, between 2 and 3 mm change in clinical attachment level must occur before a site can be labeled disease-active.

It is difficult to see the alveolar crest on the periapicals and bitewings molar films

Q) What technique can be used to allow visualization of the maxillary and manibular alveolar crest. 19

A) Use vertical bitewings.

1. Which one of the following statements is considered objective data in this patient's history? (p. 204–207)

   a. Cold hurts my teeth.
   b. My teeth have a lot of stains on them.
   c. The gingiva is erythematous and edematous.
   d. A hard-bristled toothbrush seems to work best.
   e. I occasionally use the mouthrinse that was prescribed.

2. Which one of the following assessment tests is most appropriate for this patient? (p. 297)

   a. genetic susceptibility testing
   b. gingival and periodontal
   c. culture and sensitivity
   d. DNA probe

3. The amount of clinical attachment loss on the facial surface of the mandibular right first molar is _____ mm. (p. 254)

   a. 2   d. 10
   b. 6   e. 12
   c. 8

4. Which one of the following treatment goals is most important to discuss with this patient? (pp. 201–207)

   a. Work out a financially acceptable plan that is affordable.
   b. Refer to a physician for smoking cessation.
   c. Stress the importance of keeping all appointments.
   d. Reduce plaque levels and stop the progression of periodontal disease.

5. The medications this patient is taking mimic which of the following medical conditions? (p. 237)

   a. diabetes mellitus   c. pregnancy
   b. hyperthyroidism   d. cirrhosis

6. Which one of the following types of radiographs would best show the overhang on the restoration on the maxillary right first molar? (p. 278)

   a. panoramic
   b. computed tomography
   c. horizontal bitewing
   d. digital subtraction radiology

7. Which one of the following Glickman's classification of furcation involvement is evident on the mandibular first molars? (p. 260)

   a. I   c. III
   b. II   d. IV

8. Which one of the following types of stains are present in this patient? (p. 221)

   a. extrinsic, endogenous
   b. extrinsic, exogenous
   c. intrinsic, endogenous
   d. intrinsic, exogenous

9. Which one of the following conditions is a consequence of the exposed root surfaces in the furca area of the mandibular first molars? (p. 217)

   a. caries
   b. fracture
   c. hypoplasia
   d. hypocalcification

10. Which one of the following histologic features explains the consistency of the interdental papillae in this patient? (p. 232)

    a. ulceration of the epithelium
    b. destruction of the gingival fibers
    c. accumulation of fluid in the tissue
    d. engorgement of blood in the tissue

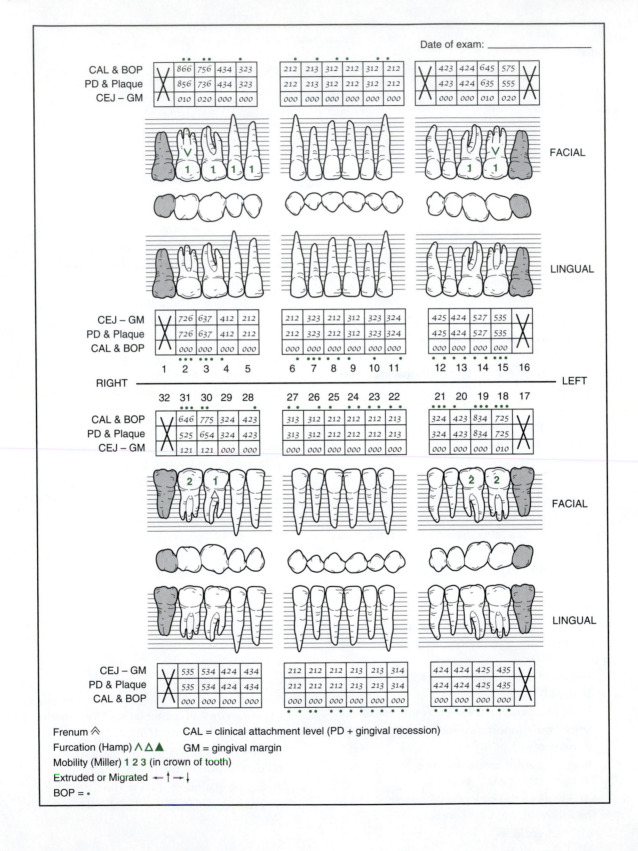

Date of exam: _____

Upper arch (teeth 1–16)

		1	2	3	4	5		6	7	8	9	10	11		12	13	14	15	16
CAL & BOP	X	866	756	434	323		212	213	312	212	312	212		423	424	645	575	X
PD & Plaque		856	736	434	323		212	213	312	212	312	212		423	424	635	555	
CEJ – GM		010	020	000	000		000	000	000	000	000	000		000	000	010	020	

FACIAL

LINGUAL

		1	2	3	4	5		6	7	8	9	10	11		12	13	14	15	16
CEJ – GM	X	726	637	412	212		212	323	212	312	323	324		425	424	527	535	X
PD & Plaque		726	637	412	212		212	323	212	312	323	324		425	424	527	535	
CAL & BOP		000	000	000	000		000	000	000	000	000	000		000	000	000	000	

RIGHT ———————————————————————————————— LEFT

		32	31	30	29	28		27	26	25	24	23	22		21	20	19	18	17
CAL & BOP	X	646	775	324	423		313	312	212	212	212	213		324	423	834	725	X
PD & Plaque		525	654	324	423		313	312	212	212	212	213		324	423	834	725	
CEJ – GM		121	121	000	000		000	000	000	000	000	000		000	000	000	010	

FACIAL

LINGUAL

		32	31	30	29	28		27	26	25	24	23	22		21	20	19	18	17
CEJ – GM	X	535	534	424	434		212	212	212	213	213	314		424	424	425	435	X
PD & Plaque		535	534	424	434		212	212	212	213	213	314		424	424	425	435	
CAL & BOP		000	000	000	000		000	000	000	000	000	000		000	000	000	000	

Frenum ⩓

Furcation (Hamp) ⋀ △ ▲

Mobility (Miller) **1 2 3** (in crown of tooth)

Extruded or Migrated ← ↑ → ↓

BOP = •

CAL = clinical attachment level (PD + gingival recession)

GM = gingival margin

Glossary

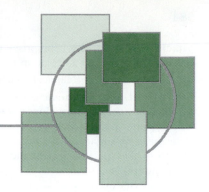

A

Abrasion Wearing away of a structure, such as a gingiva or the teeth, through an abnormal mechanical process. Examples would be gingiva or tooth abrasions due to incorrect brushing.

Abscess, periodontal (also called lateral periodontal abscess) Localized accumulation of pus in periodontal tissues formed by the disintegration of tissue.

Abutment (tooth) A tooth or implant used for support and retention of a crown or removable partial denture.

Abutment screw A screw that secures (holds) the abutment to the implant.

Accretions Accumulation of foreign materials on the teeth, such as dental plaque, materia alba, and calculus.

Acellular Without cells.

Acellular cementum Cementum that does not contain cementocytes.

Aerobic Utilizing and dependent on oxygen.

Air polishing A controlled stream of sodium bicarbonate used to remove extrinsic tooth stains and dental plaque.

Allograft See Graft, osseous.

Alloplastic See Graft, osseous.

Alveolar bone See Bone, alveolar.

Alveolar crest The most coronal part of the interproximal bone.

Alveolar mucosa See Mucosa, alveolar.

Alveolar process Compact and cancellous bone that surrounds and supports the roots of the teeth.

Anaerobic Non-oxygen utilizing. Oxygen is toxic to these organisms.

Angle's classification of malocclusion A classification of different types of malocclusion based on the relationship of the anteroposterior relationship of the dental arches.

Class I (neutroocclusion): The mesiobuccal cusp of the maxillary first permanent molar occludes in the buccal groove of the mandibular first molar. Crowding has to be present.

Class II (distoocclusion): The mesiobuccal cusp of the maxillary first permanent molar is mesial to the mandibular first molar; the mandibular dental arch is posterior to the maxillary arch.

Class II, division 1: Labioversion of the maxillary incisors.

Class II, division 2: Linguoversion of the maxillary central incisors.

Class III (mesioocclusion): The mesiobuccal cusp of the maxillary first permanent molar is distal to the mandibular first molar; the mandibular dental arch is anterior to the maxillary arch.

Ankylosis Fusion of the tooth with the alveolar bone without an intervening periodontal ligament.

Antibiotic A soluble substance produced by microorganisms that has the capacity to inhibit the growth of or to kill other organisms.

Antibiotic prophylaxis See Prophylaxis.

Antibodies Serum proteins synthesized and released by plasma cells. Antibodies bind to and neutralize bacterial toxins.

Antigen A foreign substance (e.g., bacteria, bacterial toxins, and by-products) that elicits the formation of antibodies.

Antimicrobials Chemical agents that inhibit the growth of or kill a microorganism. The terms antimicrobial and anti-infective are used interchangeably.

Antiseptic An antimicrobial applied to the skin surface or oral mucosa that inhibits the growth and development of microorganisms.

Apical Refers to the apical or anatomic end of the root of a tooth.

Attachment apparatus Comprises the cementum, periodontal ligament, and alveolar and supporting bone.

Attachment level See Clinical attachment level (CAL).

Attachment loss, connective tissue (also referred to as clinical attachment loss) A pathologic process whereby the gingival collagen fibers become detached from the root surfaces with the concomitant apical migration of the apical aspect of the junctional epithelium along the root surface.

Attrition The wearing-away of tooth structure by tooth-to-tooth normal or abnormal function.

Autograft See Graft, osseous.

Autoimmune disease Disease caused by the immunologic response against components of the body's own tissues.

Avascular Lacking in blood supply (e.g., tooth enamel, gingival epithelium, cementum).

B

Bacteremia Presence of bacteria in the bloodstream.

Bactericidal The ability of a drug or agent to kill bacteria.

Bacteriostatic Inhibiting the growth of bacteria.

Barrier membrane (occlusive membrane) Material placed over a bone graft (in a periodontal defect) that keeps the bone graft at the site and prevents the growth of epithelial cells into the site

Bifurcation The anatomic area where roots of a two-rooted tooth separate.

Biodegradable Resorbable.

Biofilm, plaque, dental Matrix-enclosed bacterial populations adherent to each other and/or to surfaces or interfaces.

Biologic width The combined height of the gingival connective tissue (1.07 mm) and the junctional epithelium (0.97 mm) present around natural teeth and implants.

Biota, oral The bacteria and other microorganisms that normally inhabit a bodily organ or part (also called oral flora)

Bone A hard type of connective tissue that contains collagen fibers, calcium phosphate, and hydroxyapatite.

Alveolar bone (also called alveolar bone proper): Compact bone that lines the tooth socket (alveolus).

Bundle bone: Alveolar bone with insertion of Sharpey's (principal) fibers.

Cancellous bone (spongy bone): Bone with trabeculae, located between the cortical plates and alveolar bone proper. It makes up the majority of a bone.

Compact bone: Bone that is hard and dense.

Cortical (plate) bone: Compact bone found on the facial and lingual aspects of the alveolar process.

Supporting bone: Surrounds and supports the alveolar bone proper. Is composed of the compact cortical plates of bone and cancellous trabecular bone.

Bone augmentation Correction of a bone defect or deficiency with the placement of a bone graft and/or bone replacement material.

Bone grafting A surgical procedure performed to re-establish bone volume. Placement of a bone graft or bone replacement material into an infrabony defect.

Bone loss

Horizontal bone loss: An equal amount of bone loss between two teeth.

Vertical bone loss (also called angular bone loss): Bone destruction that does not occur of the entire thickness of the alveolar process. Bone loss affects only a portion of bone surrounding the affected tooth. Examples include one-, two-, and three-wall bony defects. See Periodontal bony defect.

Bone resorption Bone loss.

Broad-spectrum (antibiotic) Antibiotic that affects a wide range of bacteria, including both gram-negative and gram-positive microorganisms.

Bruxism The involuntary and unconscious grinding or clenching of teeth. It is usually triggered by emotional stress, anxiety, or occlusal irregularities and usually results in abnormal wear patterns on the teeth.

Bundle bone See Bone, bundle.

C

Calculus Calcified microbial plaque. It is not viable (living bacteria) and thus is a local contributing risk factor for periodontal diseases. Bacteria embed into the porous surface.

Cancellous bone See Bone, cancellous.

Cementocytes Cementoblasts from the periodontal ligament that lie close to the root and become surrounded by forming cementum.

Cementoenamel junction The area at which the enamel and cementum are united at the cervical region of the tooth.

Cementum Thin, calcified layer of connective tissue that covers the root of teeth.

Centric occlusion See Occlusion, centric.

Centric relation The most posterior or retruded position of the mandible to the maxilla from which lateral movements of the jaw can be made.

Chemotaxis The process by which cells (PMNs, macrophages) are attracted toward an inflamed area, often by certain substances, including bacterial products, proteins, and interleukins.

Chemotherapeutics The prevention or treatment of a disease by chemical agents.

Cleft, gingival A vertical-shaped slit extending from and into the gingival margin, usually due to the start of pocket formation or improper flossing.

Clinical Pertaining to the signs, symptoms, and course of a condition or disease as observed by a clinician.

Clinical attachment level (CAL) Distance measured from the cementoenamel junction to the location of the tip of the periodontal probe at the most coronal level of the attached periodontal tissues (junctional epithelium). More reliable marker for disease progression than probing depth measurements.

Clinical attachment loss See Attachment loss, connective tissue.

Col A valleylike depression of the interdental gingiva that connects the facial and lingual papillae. It is just below the contact area of the tooth.

Collagen The most abundant protein of skin, bone, and other connective tissues. Synthesized by fibroblasts, osteoblasts, and odontoblasts.

Collagen fibers See Fibers, collagen.

Collagenase Belongs to a family of enzymes called matrix metalloproteinases, which are responsible for the normal turnover of connective tissue and destruction of host (body's) tissue (collagen). Produced and secreted by bacteria and host cells including PMNs and fibroblasts. Collagenase produced and secreted by PMNs is responsible for the host tissue destruction. Collagenase produced and secreted by fibroblasts is responsible for the normal remodeling and turnover of collagen.

Community periodontal index of treatment needs (CPITN) An index used in population studies of periodontal disease designed by the World Health Organization to assess periodontal treatment needs.

Compact bone See Bone, compact.

Complement A sequence of serum proteins that, when activated, attempt to destroy a foreign substance.

Compliance The patient's ability to adhere to the appointment schedule and oral home self-care instructions given by the dental hygienist or dentist.

Computed tomography (CT) Digitized tomography that results in an enhanced image that is much easier to read than a plane (conventional) tomogram. It measures the amount of energy transmission through an object. It produces a cross-sectional image of a slice of tissue (e.g., bone). Many slices are made of a given edentulous site.

Connective tissue attachment Mechanism of attachment of the connective tissue (gingival fibers) to the tooth or implant surface

Continuing care See Periodontal maintenance.

Contributing factor Does not initiate the disease process or act independently as an etiologic agent. Helps to allow a condition to become established and/or progress.

Coronal Toward the crown of a tooth.

Cortical bone See Bone, cortical.

Crater Interdental depressions in the gingiva or bone.

Crestal Of or pertaining to the crest or most coronal portion of the alveolar bone.

Curets

Area-specific curets (also called Gracey curets): Designed to be used on specific tooth surfaces of different teeth. Their design includes one cutting edge per end with a rounded back and toe.

Universal curets: Designed to be used on the mesial and distal surfaces of teeth without changing the instrument. Their design includes two cutting edges per end with a rounded back and toe.

Curettage, gingival Removal of the ulcerated soft tissue pocket wall.

Cytokines Proteins produced and secreted by host cells including macrophages and lymphocytes. These proteins signal and modify the behavior or actions of these cells and other cells. Examples are the interleukins, such as interleukin-1 (IL-1), which is responsible for bone destruction.

Cytoxic The ability to kill cells, including human cells.

D

Debridement The removal of inflamed, devitalized, or contaminated tissue or foreign material from or adjacent to a lesion.

Dehiscence Loss of radicular bone on a root or implant extending from the crest and proceeding apically.

Dental implant An artificial (usually titanium metal) post that substitutes for a tooth root and to which a prosthesis is attached.

Dental plaque Accumulations of bacteria and other microorganisms on tooth surfaces in the area of the sulcus or pocket. Referred to as plaque (dental) biofilm.

Dentifrice A powder, paste, or gel used in conjunction with a toothbrush to aid in the removal of plaque, materia alba, and stain from teeth.

Dentinal hypersensitivity The short, exaggerated, painful response elicited when exposed dentin is subjected to certain thermal, mechanical, or chemical stimuli.

Dentogingival junction (unit) Composed of two parts, the gingival connective tissue attachment and the junctional epithelium.

Deplaquing The removal of subgingival dental plaque after the completion of periodontal debridement. It is performed at the reevaluation/supportive periodontal therapy appointments.

Desensitization Reducing or eliminating dentin sensitivity.

Diagnosis

Dental diagnosis: Refers to the identification and naming of a disease.

Dental hygiene diagnosis: Identifies certain problems or the patient's response to the disease process that can be treated by a dental hygienist.

Diastema A space between two adjacent teeth in the same dental arch.

Digital imaging X-ray images that use a sensor to transmit the image directly to a computer via a cable link. X-ray image appears on a monitor and can be manipulated electronically to change contrast, orientation, resolution, and size of the image.

Disease A process characterized usually by at least two of these criteria: a recognized etiologic agent (or agents), an identifiable group of signs and symptoms, and consistent anatomic alterations.

Disease activity See Periodontal disease activity.

Disease severity See Periodontal disease severity.

Donor site Area in the mouth or body from which a graft (bone or soft tissue) is harvested.

Drifting Tooth migration as a result of loss of proximal contact of adjacent teeth in a healthy periodontium.

E

Edema An abnormal swelling caused by an accumulation of fluid in a tissue or part.

Edentulous Without teeth.

Embrasure The spaces that widen out from the proximal contact area. Each interdental space has four embrasures: facial embrasure, lingual embrasure, an occlusal or incisal embrasure, and a gingival embrasure. An open gingival embrasure is seen frequently in patients with periodontal disease.

Enamel matrix derivative (EMD) Protein obtained from amelogenin (enamel matrix precurser of enamel) of the developing tooth. Product called Emdogain.® Indicated for bone grafting.

Endosseous implant See Implant, endosseous.

Endotoxins Lipooligosaccharide (lipid) complexes formed by gram-negative bacteria. When the bacteria die and break apart (lysis), the endotoxin is released from the cell wall of the bacteria and is capable of having a toxic or harmful effect on the host tissue.

Enzyme A protein substance formed by living cells that acts to speed up metabolic processes or chemical reaction.

Epidemiology The study of the distribution and determinants of illnesses and their associated factors in the human population.

Epithelial ridges Ridgelike projections of epithelium into the underlying lamina propria.

Epithelium (oral) The tissue that lines the intraoral surfaces. It extends into the gingival crevice and adheres to the tooth at the base of the gingival crevice.

Erosion Chemical wearing-away of a structure, such as a tooth.

Erythema (erythematous) Redness of the mucous membranes due to inflammation.

Extent The number or percent of diseased teeth or sites in an individual.

Extrusion (extrude) Overruption of a tooth from its normal occlusal position in the dental arch.

Exudate A fluid substance formed within tissues as a result of inflammation. It consists of polymorphonuclear leukocytes, degenerated tissues, dead cells, bacteria, and tissue fluid.

F

Facial Pertaining to the face. The facial surfaces of the teeth are called buccal and labial.

Failed implant A dental implant that is mobile; lost failing implant osseointegration. A dental implant that is progressively losing bone around it.

Fenestration Root or implant surface is denuded (loss) of bone but the crestal bone is infact.

Fiber A filament or thread. In periodontics, the term usually refers to collagenous or connective tissue fibers.

Collagen fibers: White fibers composed of collagen. Found within connective tissue of the gingiva and periodontal ligament arranged in bundles or haphazardly distributed. Characterized by its hydroxyproline and hydroxylysine content.

Gingival fibers: (also called gingival connective tissue or supracrestal fiber apparatus) Fibers composed primarily of collagen that radiate from the cementum or bone into the lamina propria. Includes alveogingival, circular, dentogingival, dentoperiosteal, and transseptal.

Principle fibers: Collagen fibers of the periodontal ligament. Includes alveolar crest, apical, horizontal, interradicular, and oblique.

Fibroblast A cell found within connective tissue that synthesizes collagen and ground substance of connective tissue.

Fibrotic Tissue that is in a state of repair; tissue is hard and not resilient or spongy.

Filtration The use of absorbers for the selective reduction in intensity of radiation of certain wavelengths from a primary x-ray beam.

Flap A part of tissue (gingiva) separated from the underlying tissues except at its base.

Fluorosis, dental Enamel hypoplasia due to the ingestion of water containing excessive amounts of fluoride.

Food impaction The forceful wedging of food into the interproximal space by chewing pressure or tongue or cheek pressure.

Free gingival graft See Graft.

Fremitus Vibrational movement of the tooth under occlusal function.

Frenum A narrow band of alveolar mucosa radiates from a fixed part to a movable part and limits movement of that part. Example: Frenum runs from the gingiva to the lip, cheek, or under the tongue.

Frequency The number of times per second the insert tip moves back and forth during one cycle.

Furcation (also called furca) Anatomic area on multirooted teeth where the root base divides.

Furcation involvement (invasion) Pathologic loss of bone in the furcation of a multirooted tooth.

G

Genetic Inheritance or transmission of a disease or condition from a parent to a child.

Gingiva A part of the masticatory mucosa that is attached to the teeth and alveolar process.

  Attached gingiva: The portion of the gingiva that is firm, dense, and tightly bound down to the underlying periosteum, tooth, and bone.

  Free (marginal) gingiva: The portion of the gingiva that is unattached and forms the wall of the gingival crevice in health. It is continuous with the attached gingiva.

Gingival crevice A shallow opening between the free gingiva and the enamel or cementum. In gingival health it is called the gingival sulcus and in disease a pocket.

Gingival crevicular fluid Fluid originating in the gingival connective tissue that seeps through the sulcular and junctional epithelium. Flow increases in the presence of inflammation.

Gingival pocket (pseudopocket) See Pocket, gingival.

Gingival recession Apical migration of the marginal gingiva resulting in exposure of the root surface to the oral environment.

Gingival sulcus Space between the tooth and the marginal gingiva in gingival health. If bleeding is present, it is not a sulcus but a pocket.

Gingivitis Inflammation of the gingiva without involvement of the underlying bone or periodontal attachment. The following are gingival diseases listed in the new classification of periodontal diseases (American Academy of Periodontology, 1999):

  Drug-influenced gingivitis: Gingivitis or gingival enlargement caused by drugs (e.g., Ca channel blockers, phenytoin, cyclosporine, and oral contraceptives).

  Plaque-associated gingivitis: Gingivitis caused by dental plaque alone.

  Pregnancy-associated gingivitis: Hormonally influenced inflammation and enlargement of the gingiva during pregnancy.

  Puberty-associated gingivitis: Hormonally influenced inflammation of the gingiva during puberty.

Graft, osseous

  Allograft (allogenic graft): Bone taken from human beings (cadavers) other than the patient. Bone is bought from tissue banks. Three types: freeze-dried bone allograft (FDBA); demineralized freeze-dried bone allograft (DFDBA), and frozen.

  Alloplast (alloplastic graft): Synthetic or natural bone (inorganic) substitutes.

  Autograft: Tissue such as bone (osseous material; organic) taken from the patient's mouth or extraoral area such as the hip.

Graft, soft tissue

  Connective tissue graft: Connective tissue (donor) taken from underneath the epithelium and placed in a prepared recipient bed for the purposes of root coverage and increasing the amount of attached gingiva.

  Free gingival graft: Gingiva taken from an area in the patient's mouth, usually the palate (donor), and placed in a prepared recipient bed primarily to increase the amount of attached gingiva.

Grinding See Bruxism.

Guided bone regeneration (GBR) Bone regeneration (surgical) procedure using barrier membrane to regenerate bone.

Guided tissue regeneration Periodontal procedures performed in an attempt at regeneration. Barrier techniques are used with materials that exclude the junctional epithelium from the wound site in an attempt to allow periodontal ligament cells to populate the wound site.

H

Hemostasis Control of and stopping bleeding.

Histopathogenesis (histopathology) Pathologic (disease) changes within the periodontal structures at a microscopic level.

Host Referring to the body or self.

Host cells Cells normally present in the body (e.g., polymorphonuclear leukocytes [PMNs] macrophages, fibroblasts).

Host-derived enzymes Enzymes produced and secreted by cells in the human body such as neutrophils (PMNs) or fibroblasts.

Host response How the body responds to an implanted device or material.

Hypertropy Increase in bulk of a part or organ not due to tumor formation.

I

Iatrogenic Caused by dental or medical treatment; abnormal condition induced by a clinician.

Immune response Mechanisms used by the body as protection against environmental agents that are foreign to the body.

Immune system Components include the lymph nodes, thymus, spleen, and bone marrow.

Immunity The organism's (or body's) capacity for successfully resisting the actions of harmful foreign substances or pathogenic (disease-producing) microorganisms such as bacteria or viruses.

Immunodeficiency A deficiency in the immune system caused by an upset in the number of lymphocytes.

Implant, endosseous Dental implant placed within bone.

Incidence The rate of new occurrence of the disease in a population over a given period of time.

Index A screening tool designed to quantify and simplify the disease assessment in population surveys. Examples include plaque, debris, calculus, and periodontal destruction.

Infection Pathogenic invasion of the body and the body's response to these organisms.

Infective endocarditis Inflammation of the inner lining of the heart caused by a microbial infection.

Inflammation Protective response elicited by injury or destruction of tissues that attempts to destroy or wall off the injurious agent and tissue. It is also the cellular and vascular tissue reaction that occurs when tissue is injured.

Inflammatory cells Cells involved in the inflammatory response of tissues to injury or infection (e.g., PMNs, macrophages, mast cells).

Inflammatory periodontal diseases A group of inflammatory diseases of the periodontium including gingivitis and periodontitis.

Infrabony defect See Periodontal bony defects.

Interdental Between two adjacent teeth.

Interdental septum That part of the alveolar process extending between adjacent teeth.

Interproximal Pertaining to the area between two adjacent teeth. See Interdental.

Interradicular That part of the alveolar process between the roots of a multirooted tooth (e.g., molars, premolar).

K

Keratin A protein that is the main component of keratinized epithelium synthesized by keratinocytes.

Keratinocyte A cell found in the epithelium (a type of epithelial cell) that forms keratin.

L

Lamina dura A layer of compact bone forming the wall of a tooth alveolus (alveolar bone). In a radiograph, it appears as a thin radiopaque line separated from the tooth by the radiolucent image of the periodontal ligament space.

Lamina propria The gingival connective tissue layer under the epithelium.

Load External mechanical force applied to a tooth, implant, or prosthesis.

Lymphadenopathy Lymph nodes that are abnormal in size, consistency, or number.

Lymph nodes Small, round, or oval organs containing lymphocytes. Found in groups or chains in certain regions, often associated with large blood vessels.

Lymphocyte A type of white blood cell involved in the immune response. There are two types of lymphocytes: T cells and B cells.

M

Macrophage A large tissue cell responsible for removing damaged tissue, cells, and bacteria through phagocytosis. Increase in number in chronic inflammation.

Malocclusion Deviation from the acceptable relationship of opposing teeth. See Angle's classification of malocclusion.

Marginal Pertaining to the margin or edge.

Marginal ridge A ridge or elevation of enamel that is on the border of the occlusal surface of a tooth.

Mast cell A large tissue cell that releases inflammatory substances or mediators when damaged.

Masticatory (mastication) The process of chewing food.

Microbiota See Biota, oral.

Microflora Bacteria living in a part of the body (e.g., the mouth, intestines, nose). See also Biota, oral.

Migration, pathologic The movement of a tooth out of its natural position, usually as a result of advanced periodontal disease.

Mobility, tooth The degree of looseness of a tooth beyond physiologic movement. Tooth movement away from its normal position in a buccal/lingual or apical direction when slight pressure is applied.

Mucogingival involvement (defect) A discrepancy in the relationship between the gingival margin and the mucogingival junction. Usually there is minimal to no attached gingiva.

Mucogingival junction Demarcation between the attached gingiva and alveolar mucosa.

Mucosa A mucous membrane.

Alveolar mucosa: Mucosa covering part of the alveolar process and continuing into the vestibule and floor of the mouth. It is movable and loosely attached to the underlying periostium.

Masticatory mucosa: Mucosa of the gingiva and hard palate.

Murmur A sound produced within the heart at one of its orifices.

N

National Health and Nutrition Examination Survey (NHANES I) A national survey of adults from 1960 to 1962.

National Health and Nutrition Examination Survey (NHANES III) This is the seventh in a series, beginning in 1960, of national examination surveys of the U.S. population conducted by the National Center for Health Statistics in collaboration with the National Institute for Dental Research (NIDR). The survey was designed to collect data representative of the total U.S. civilian, noninstitutionalized population age 12 months and older.

National Institute of Dental Research (NIDR) Survey A national survey of employed adults between 18 and 64 years of age conducted by the National Institute of Dental Research. It was named the National Survey of Oral Health of U.S. Adults 1985–1986. More than 15,000 people were examined, representing over 100 million working adults in the United States.

Necrotizing periodontal diseases Formerly known as acute necrotizing ulcerative gingivitis (ANUG). Since acute is a clinical descriptive term, it should not be used as a diagnostic classification. Thus the correct term is necrotizing ulcerative gingivitis. In the new classification, NUG is a type of necrotizing periodontal disease. It is an inflammation of the gingiva characterized by necrosis of the gingival margin and interdental papillae. Included in this classification is necrotizing ulcerative periodontitis (NUP), which is characterized by necrosis of gingival tissues, periodontal ligament, and alveolar bone.

Neutrophil See Polymorphonuclear leukocyte.

O

Objective Based on facts; not affected by personal feelings.

Obligate Able to survive only in a specific environment (e.g., an obligate anaerobe is only able to live in a nonoxygen environment).

Occlusal adjustment (also called selective grinding or occlusal equilibration) Reshaping the occlusal or incisal surfaces of teeth by grinding to create harmonious contact relationships between the upper and lower teeth.

Occlusal trauma Injury to the attachment apparatus as a result of excessive occlusal forces.

Primary occlusal trauma: Excessive occlusal forces placed on a healthy periodontium that produces changes in the periodontal tissues. Examples include placement of a "high" restoration and orthodontic movement of teeth.

Secondary occlusal trauma: Normal forces of mastication on a periodontium with bone loss (periodontitis) that produce changes in the periodontal tissues.

Occlusion Contact of opposing teeth (maxillary and mandibular teeth); centric occlusion: maximum intercuspation of maxillary and mandibular teeth.

Open bite Anterior or posterior teeth do not occlude with the opposing teeth.

Oral hygiene self-care Removal of dental plaque with brushes, dental floss, and other oral aids.

Oral prophylaxis See Prophylaxis.

Osseointegration (osteointegration) The biologic phenomenon by which bone grows up to and contacts the surface of implants, thereby anchoring them to the jaw bone.

Osseous Referring to bone.

Ostectomy Surgical removal of supporting bone.

Osteoblast A cell that forms bone.

Osteoclast A cell that resorbs bone.

Osteoconduction Bone growth by laying down of form from the surrounding bone. Bone material acts as a scaffolding along which bone will be laid down.

Osteointegration New bone growth from osteoprogenitor cells.

Osteoplasty Surgical reshaping or removal of nonsupporting bone.

Overbite Vertical overlap of the upper incisor teeth over the lower incisor teeth.

Overdenture A removable partial or complete denture that is supported by implants or implant/tissue.

Overjet Horizontal projection of the upper teeth beyond the lower teeth.

P

Panoramic film A type of conventional radiograph showing the entire area of the mandible and maxilla.

Papillary Pertaining to the interdental papillae.

Parafunctional habit A habit characterized by abnormal (out of the normal range) function (e.g., bruxism, pencil chewing, nail biting).

Passive eruption Physiologic process with recession of the gingiva from the enamel apically toward the cementoenamel junction.

Pathogenic Disease-producing.

Pathologic mobility Horizontal or vertical displacement of a tooth beyond its physiologic movement.

Periapical film A type of conventional radiograph that shows the entire tooth, including the area around the root apex.

Periapical pathology Disease occurring around the apex of a tooth.

Pericoronitis (also termed pericoronal abscess) Inflammation of the operculum or tissue flap over a partially eurupted tooth, especially a third molar.

Peri-implant Around a dental implant.

Peri-implantitis Inflammation of the gingival tissues around an implant.

Periodontal Occurring around a tooth.

Periodontal bony defects A deviation from the normal form or contour of bone due to periodontal disease.

> Crater (interproximal crater): A two-wall infrabony defect (facial and lingual bony walls remain).
>
> Hemiseptum defect: The remaining interdental bone septum where the mesial or distal part has been destroyed, with one bony wall remaining (half of a septum).
>
> Infrabony defect: A general term to describe any periodontal bony defect associated with vertical (angular) bone loss. These defects are named according to the number of bony walls remaining in the interproximal area that surround the pocket (e.g., one-wall, two-wall, and three-wall).
>
> Intrabony defect: A type of three-wall defect with three bony walls remaining. The defect may or may not be totally lined by cortical bone and may have cancellous bone behind. Not all three-wall defects are intrabony.

Periodontal debridement The removal of a foreign material (e.g., plaque, calculus) or dead tissue from the crown, root surface, pocket space, pocket wall, and bone surface.

Periodontal disease activity (PDA) The ongoing loss of connective tissue attachment and bone at a particular point in time (e.g., at the clinical examination appointment). It is difficult to determine disease activity. A 2- to 3-mm change in clinical attachment level must occur before a site can be labeled disease-active.

Periodontal disease severity The total periodontal destruction and healing that occur prior to the clinical examination. Disease severity is determined after the periodontal assessment (visual, periodontal probing, radiographs) is completed. Severity can be classified as mild, moderate, or severe.

Periodontal ligament (fibers) See Principal fibers.

Periodontal maintenance Also referred to as recare, or continuing care. An extension of periodontal therapy. Procedures performed at selected intervals to assist the periodontal patient in maintaining oral health.

Periodontal pathogen Bacteria that cause periodontal disease.

Periodontal pocket See Pocket, periodontal.

Periodontal probing Measures the location where physical resistance of the probe is met by the junctional epithelial attachment to the tooth.

Periodontics The specialty of dentistry dealing with the prevention, diagnosis, and treatment of diseases of the tissues that surround the teeth.

Periodontist A dental practitioner who practices periodontics.

Periodontitis Inflammation of the supporting tissues of teeth where there is connective tissue attachment loss and alveolar and supporting bone loss. The following is a classification system developed by the American Academy of Periodontology (1999):

> Aggressive periodontitis: Formerly known as early-onset periodontitis (e.g., juvenile periodontitis, prepubertal periodontitis, and rapidly progressive periodontitis). Except for the presence of periodontitis, patients are otherwise clinically healthy. There is rapid attachment loss and bone destruction. Patients have defects in host defense. Includes prepubesent children who have periodontal destruction without any modifying systemic conditions. The following specific features are identified:
>
>> Generalized aggressive periodontitis: Formerly known as generalized juvenile periodontitis. Usually affects persons under 30 years of age, but patients may be older. Generalized interproximal attachment loss affecting at least three permanent teeth other than first molars and incisors.

Localized aggressive periodontitis: Formerly known as localized juvenile periodontitis (LJP). Circumpubertal onset. Primarily affects the first permanent incisors and first molars. Attachment loss may progress at a rate three to five times faster than chronic periodontitis. These patients are characterized by a lack of clinical signs of inflammation, harbor Actinobacillus actinomycetecomitans in their microflora, and display an altered immune response.

Chronic periodontitis: Formerly known as adult periodontitis. A form of periodontitis that usually is prevalent in adults but can occur in children and adolescents (formerly known as prepubertal periodontitis). The amount of periodontal destruction is consistent with the presence of local factors. Bone resorption usually progresses slowly.

Necrotizing periodontal diseases: Replaces necrotizing ulcerative gingivitis (NUG) and necrotizing ulcerative periodontitis (NUP). A form of periodontitis seen in the HIV/AIDS patient. (See necrotized periodontal diseases)

Refractory periodontitis: Patients who do not respond to conventional periodontal therapy treatment. It is not considered a single disease entity because it can occur in all forms of periodontitis.

Periodontium Comprises the periodontal tissues that support and surround the teeth, including the gingiva, cementum, periodontal ligament, and alveolar and supporting bone.

Periodontology The scientific study of the periodontal structures in health and disease.

Periosteum Connective tissue covering the outer surface of bone.

Phagocytosis The process of destroying bacteria by devouring and digesting them by phagocytic cells such as polymorphonuclear leukocytes and macrophages.

Pharmacokinetics What the body does to a drug (e.g., absorption, distribution, metabolism, and elimination).

Phase-contrast microscopy A method of using a microscope through which the shape, size, and mobility of bacteria can be viewed.

Phenytoin An anticonvulsant drug that can cause gingival enlargement.

Pocket

Gingival pocket: A deepening of the gingival crevice due to the coronal migration of the gingival margin without apical migration of the junctional epithelium (loss of attachment) and bone loss. Examples: drug-influenced gingival enlargement, inflammation of the gingiva. Also called a pseudopocket.

Periodontal pocket: A pathologic deepening of the gingival sulcus characterized by apical migration of the junctional epithelium and alveolar bone loss. Two types of periodontal pockets: infrabony and suprabony.

Infrabony pocket: A periodontal pocket that extends apical to the adjacent alveolar crest or into an infrabony defect (a defect with a vertical pattern of bone loss). There is apical migration of the junctional epithelium and bone loss; the base of the pocket is apical to the crest of alveolar bone.

Suprabony pocket: A periodontal pocket that extends coronal to the alveolar crest or into a suprabony defect with a horizontal pattern of bone loss. The base of the pocket is coronal to the crest of alveolar bone.

Polishing The removal of acquired pellicle, bacterial plaque, and stain from the external tooth surface through mechanical means and an abrasive agent.

Polymorponuclear leukocyte (PMN) The major mobile phagocytic white blood cell involved in engulfing, killing, and digesting microorganisms. The first cell to migrate to the acute inflammatory site. Impairment in their function is related to the pathogenesis of aggressive periodontitis.

Prevalence The proportion of individuals in a population having periodontal disease or the number of individuals expected to have periodontal disease in a specific time.

Primary occlusal trauma See Occlusal trauma, primary.

Principal fibers The connective tissue that surrounds the root surface of the tooth and attaches it to the alveolar bone.

Probing See Periodontal probing.

Probing depth The distance from the soft tissue (gingiva or alveolar mucosa) margin to the tip of the periodontal probe. The health of the attachment apparatus can affect the measurement.

Prognosis A prediction or forecast of the course and outcome of a disease.

Prophylaxis Prevention of disease.

Antibiotic prophylaxis: Antibiotic coverage necessary before invasive dental procedures that cause bleeding to prevent a bacteremia that ultimately could cause infective endocarditis or serious infections.

Oral prophylaxis: The removal of plaque, calculus, and stains from the exposed and unexposed surfaces of the teeth by scaling and polishing as a preventive measure for the control of local irritational factors.

Proximal Surface of a tooth next to another tooth.

Pseudocleft Slit or fissure of the gingiva associated with severe gingival inflammation or certain medications causing the papillae to enlarge and approach each other and not due to pocket formation.

Pseudopocket See Pocket, gingival or Pocket, pseudo.

Pus See Suppuration.

R

Radicular Pertaining to the root.

Recession See Gingival recession.

Recurrent When signs of disease return.

Regeneration, periodontal Formation of new alveolar and supporting bone, cementum, and periodontal ligament on a previously diseased root surface.

Resistance, antibiotic An antimicrobial agent no longer is effective in killing or inhibiting growth of microorganisms.

Rete pegs See Epithelial ridges.

Rheumatic heart disease A disease of the heart resulting from rheumatic fever, chiefly manifested by abnormalities of the valves.

Risk factors Characteristics that have been shown to directly cause periodontal disease (e.g., dental plaque, diabetes mellitus, tobacco smoking).

Risk indicators Behavioral and socioeconomic characteristics that are associated with periodontal diseases but are not considered to cause the disease (e.g., aging).

Root planing A treatment procedure designed to remove cementum or surface dentin that is rough, impregnated with calculus, or contaminated with toxins or microorganisms.

S

Scaler A periodontal instrument that is designed to scale primarily supragingival tooth surfaces.

Sonic: Produces mechanical vibrations by means of air pressure rather than electrical energy. The operating frequency is between 3,000 and 8,000 cycles per second.

Ultrasonic: Devices operating at frequencies between 18,000 and 50,000 cycles per second. They use electrical energy to produce mechanical vibrations that will remove calculus.

Magnetostrictive ultrasonic: Produces mechanical movement using a low-voltage magnetic signal. The operating frequency is between 18,000 and 45,000 cycles per second. The handpiece contains coils that activate the interchangeable inserts, causing them to vibrate. The working ends can be used on all sides, providing better adaptation to the tooth surfaces.

Piezoelectric ultrasonic: Produces mechanical movement using a high-voltage magnetic signal. The operating frequency is between 25,000 and 50,000 cycles per second. Only two sides of the working end are adapted to the tooth surface.

Scaling The removal of dental plaque, calculus, and stains from the crown and root surfaces.

Screening A single examination to separate periodontally healthy from diseased patients and to determine the patient's dental needs. It does not make a specific dental hygiene diagnosis or tell the type of treatment to be given. It simply requires probing depth measurements and conventional radiographs.

Secondary occlusal trauma See Occlusal trauma, secondary.

Selective grinding See Occlusal adjustment.

Severity Degree of disease involvement, quantifying the amount of attachment loss or probing depth. May be expressed as mild or slight, moderate, and severe.

Sign Any abnormality indicative of disease, discoverable by the clinician at the evaluation of a patient.

Single-stage implant An implant placed in a one-stage surgery.

Sonic See Scaler, sonic.

Stem cells Cells from which all the blood cells "stem" or come.

Stippling The "orange peel" appearance (depressions) on the attached gingiva. Stippling is not present on the free gingiva.

Subgingival (submarginal) Beneath the gingiva or gingival margin; into the crevice.

Subjective As described in an individual's words or opinions rather than facts.

Substantivity Ability of a substance to absorb or bind to a surface such as the tooth root, tissues, bacterial plaque, or enamel and slowly released over time in its active form.

Sulcus See Gingival sulcus.

Supporting bone See Bone, supporting.

Suppuration The formation of pus. An inflammatory or purulent exudate formed within the tissues. It consists of neutrophils, bacteria, degenerated and liquefied cells, and tissue fluids that form within the tissues in disease and escape through the ulcerated pocket epithelium into the oral cavity.

Supragingival Coronal (above) to the free gingival margin.

Surface texture The tactile quality of a material or tissue; the arrangement of parts of the tissue as it affects the appearance or feel of the surface.

Surgery The act and art of treating injuries or disease by manual operations.

Mucogingival surgery: Periodontal surgery involving the soft tissue (gingival) aspects such as root coverage or increasing the height and width of the alveolar ridge.

Osseous surgery: Periodontal surgery involving the addition or resection (removal) of bone.

Symptom A departure from the normal in function, appearance, or sensation experienced by a patient. A subjective sign.

Syndrome The aggregate of signs and symptoms associated with any morbid process and constituting together the picture of the disease.

Systemic Affecting or pertaining to the whole body.

T

Temporomandibular joint The connecting sliding hinge mechanism between the mandible (lower jaw) and the base of the skull (temporal bone).

Therapeutic levels (of a drug) Concentration of a drug in body fluids that causes a pharmacologic effect.

Toxin Substance that is harmful to the body (e.g., endotoxin).

Trifurcation Anatomic area where roots diverge in a three-rooted tooth.

U

Ultrasonic See Scaler, ultrasonic.

V

Vascular Refers to blood.

W

Wear facet A flattened, highly polished worn spot on the occlusal or incisal surface of a tooth (usually seen on the side of a cusp). It may be a clinical sign of attrition.

World Health Organization A specialized agency of the United Nations with primary responsibility for international health matters and public health.

X

Xerostomia Dryness of the mouth due to inadequate salivary secretion as a result of aging, salivary gland conditions, or medications.

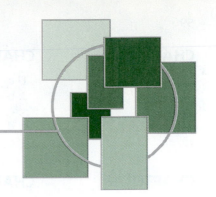

Answers to Self-Quiz Questions

CHAPTER 1

1. c	6. c
2. c	7. a
3. c	8. a
4. c	9. d
5. b	10. d

CHAPTER 2

1. a	
2. c	
3. a	
4. c	
5. c	

CHAPTER 3

1. b	6. a
2. b	7. c
3. c	8. a
4. b	9. b
5. c	10. a

CHAPTER 4

1. d	6. a
2. a	7. c
3. b	8. b
4. a	9. d
5. c	10. c

CHAPTER 5

1. b	
2. d	
3. a	
4. c	
5. c	

CHAPTER 6

1. b	6. e
2. c	7. b
3. c	8. d
4. a	9. c
5. b	10. a

CHAPTER 7

1. c	
2. c	
3. a	
4. a	
5. a	

CHAPTER 8

1. c	
2. c	
3. d	
4. c	
5. d	

CHAPTER 9

1. c	
2. c	
3. a	
4. b	
5. c	

CHAPTER 10

1. d	
2. a	
3. d	
4. d	
5. d	

CHAPTER 11

1. c	
2. a	
3. b	
4. a	
5. b	

CHAPTER 12

1. c	6. b
2. a	7. a
3. d	8. b
4. a	9. b
5. c	10. d

CHAPTER 13

1. a	
2. b	
3. b	
4. b	
5. c	

CHAPTER 14

1. b	
2. c	
3. a	
4. d	
5. b	

CHAPTER 15

1. a	
2. d	
3. c	
4. a	
5. d	

CHAPTER 16

1. b	
2. a	
3. b	
4. c	
5. e	

CHAPTER 17

1. d
2. a
3. a
4. c
5. e

CHAPTER 18

1. b
2. b
3. a
4. c
5. c

CHAPTER 19

1. a   6. b
2. c   7. a
3. d   8. c
4. c   9. a
5. c   10. c

CHAPTER 20

1. c   6. b
2. d   7. c
3. b   8. b
4. d   9. c
5. b   10. c

CHAPTER 21

1. a   6. c
2. c   7. a
3. b   8. b
4. e   9. a
5. a   10. a

CHAPTER 22

1. c   6. a
2. b   7. b
3. c   8. e
4. d   9. c
5. c   10. c

CHAPTER 23

1. d
2. d
3. c
4. c
5. a

CHAPTER 24

1. d   6. a
2. d   7. b
3. b   8. c
4. b   9. a
5. c   10. b

CHAPTER 25

1. c
2. d
3. c
4. d
5. a

CHAPTER 26

1. a   6. b
2. c   7. d
3. b   8. a
4. e   9. d
5. d   10. e

CHAPTER 27

1. b   6. c
2. a   7. b
3. a   8. b
4. a   9. b
5. b   10. a

CHAPTER 28

1. b   6. c
2. c   7. b
3. b   8. c
4. a   9. d
5. a   10. e

CHAPTER 29

1. c
2. c
3. b
4. a
5. c

CHAPTER 30

1. e   6. c
2. b   7. b
3. d   8. a
4. c   9. e
5. a   10. b

CHAPTER 31

1. d   6. b
2. a   7. d
3. a   8. c
4. c   9. c
5. d   10. c

CASE I

1. e   6. d
2. d   7. d
3. d   8. b
4. b   9. b
5. a   10. a

CASE II

1. c   6. c
2. d   7. d
3. d   8. d
4. b   9. c
5. b   10. c

CASE III

1. a   6. c
2. c   7. a
3. d   8. b
4. a   9. b
5. d   10. b

CASE IV

1. c   6. c
2. c   7. b
3. d   8. b
4. a   9. b
5. d   10. b

Index

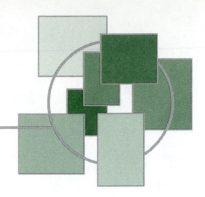

SINGLE PC LICENSE AGREEMENT AND LIMITED WARRANTY

READ THIS LICENSE CAREFULLY BEFORE OPENING THIS PACKAGE. BY OPENING THIS PACKAGE, YOU ARE AGREEING TO THE TERMS AND CONDITIONS OF THIS LICENSE. IF YOU DO NOT AGREE, DO NOT OPEN THE PACKAGE. PROMPTLY RETURN THE UNOPENED PACKAGE AND ALL ACCOMPANYING ITEMS TO THE PLACE YOU OBTAINED THEM. *THESE TERMS APPLY TO ALL LICENSED SOFTWARE ON THE DISK EXCEPT THAT THE TERMS FOR USE OF ANY SHAREWARE OR FREEWARE ON THE DISKETTES ARE AS SET FORTH IN THE ELECTRONIC LICENSE LOCATED ON THE DISK:*

1. GRANT OF LICENSE and OWNERSHIP: The enclosed computer programs and data ("Software") are licensed, not sold, to you by Pearson Education, Inc. ("We" or the "Company") and in consideration of your purchase or adoption of the accompanying Company textbooks and/or other materials, and your agreement to these terms. We reserve any rights not granted to you. You own only the disk(s) but we and/or our licensors own the Software itself. This license allows you to use and display your copy of the Software on a single computer (i.e., with a single CPU) at a single location for <u>academic</u> use only, so long as you comply with the terms of this Agreement. You may make one copy for back up, or transfer your copy to another CPU, provided that the Software is usable on only one computer

2. RESTRICTIONS: You may <u>not</u> transfer or distribute the Software or documentation to anyone else. Except for backup, you may <u>not</u> copy the documentation or the Software. You may <u>not</u> network the Software or otherwise use it on more than one computer or computer terminal at the same time. You may <u>not</u> reverse engineer, disassemble, decompile, modify, adapt, translate, or create derivative works based on the Software or the Documentation. You may be held legally responsible for any copying or copyright infringement which is caused by your failure to abide by the terms of these restrictions.

3. TERMINATION: This license is effective until terminated. This license will terminate automatically without notice from the Company if you fail to comply with any provisions or limitations of this license. Upon termination, you shall destroy the Documentation and all copies of the Software. All provisions of this Agreement as to limitation and disclaimer of warranties, limitation of liability, remedies or damages, and our ownership rights shall survive termination.

4. LIMITED WARRANTY AND DISCLAIMER OF WARRANTY: Company warrants that for a period of 60 days from the date you purchase this SOFTWARE (or purchase or adopt the accompanying textbook), the Software, when properly installed and used in accordance with the Documentation, will operate in substantial conformity with the description of the Software set forth in the Documentation, and that for a period of 30 days the disk(s) on which the Software is delivered shall be free from defects in materials and workmanship under normal use. The Company does not warrant that the Software will meet your requirements or that the operation of the Software will be uninterrupted or error-free. Your only remedy and the Company's only obligation under these limited warranties is, at the Company's option, return of the disk for a refund of any amounts paid for it by you or replacement of the disk. THIS LIMITED WARRANTY IS THE ONLY WARRANTY PROVIDED BY THE COMPANY AND ITS LICENSORS, AND THE COMPANY AND ITS LICENSORS DISCLAIM ALL OTHER WARRANTIES, EXPRESS OR IMPLIED, INCLUDING WITHOUT LIMITATION, THE IMPLIED WARRANTIES OF MERCHANTABILITY AND FITNESS FOR A PARTICULAR PURPOSE. THE COMPANY DOES NOT WARRANT, GUARANTEE OR MAKE ANY REPRESENTATION REGARDING THE ACCURACY, RELIABILITY, CURRENTNESS, USE, OR RESULTS OF USE, OF THE SOFTWARE.

5. LIMITATION OF REMEDIES AND DAMAGES: IN NO EVENT, SHALL THE COMPANY OR ITS EMPLOYEES, AGENTS, LICENSORS, OR CONTRACTORS BE LIABLE FOR ANY INCIDENTAL, INDIRECT, SPECIAL, OR CONSEQUENTIAL DAMAGES ARISING OUT OF OR IN CONNECTION WITH THIS LICENSE OR THE SOFTWARE, INCLUDING FOR LOSS OF USE, LOSS OF DATA, LOSS OF INCOME OR PROFIT, OR OTHER LOSSES, SUSTAINED AS A RESULT OF INJURY TO ANY PERSON, OR LOSS OF OR DAMAGE TO PROPERTY, OR CLAIMS OF THIRD PARTIES, EVEN IF THE COMPANY OR AN AUTHORIZED REPRESENTATIVE OF THE COMPANY HAS BEEN ADVISED OF THE POSSIBILITY OF SUCH DAMAGES. IN NO EVENT SHALL THE LIABILITY OF THE COMPANY FOR DAMAGES WITH RESPECT TO THE SOFTWARE EXCEED THE AMOUNTS ACTUALLY PAID BY YOU, IF ANY, FOR THE SOFTWARE OR THE ACCOMPANYING TEXTBOOK. BECAUSE SOME JURISDICTIONS DO NOT ALLOW THE LIMITATION OF LIABILITY IN CERTAIN CIRCUMSTANCES, THE ABOVE LIMITATIONS MAY NOT ALWAYS APPLY TO YOU.

6. GENERAL: THIS AGREEMENT SHALL BE CONSTRUED IN ACCORDANCE WITH THE LAWS OF THE UNITED STATES OF AMERICA AND THE STATE OF NEW YORK, APPLICABLE TO CONTRACTS MADE IN NEW YORK, AND SHALL BENEFIT THE COMPANY, ITS AFFILIATES AND ASSIGNEES. HIS AGREEMENT IS THE COMPLETE AND EXCLUSIVE STATEMENT OF THE AGREEMENT BETWEEN YOU AND THE COMPANY AND SUPERSEDES ALL PROPOSALS OR PRIOR AGREEMENTS, ORAL, OR WRITTEN, AND ANY OTHER COMMUNICATIONS BETWEEN YOU AND THE COMPANY OR ANY REPRESENTATIVE OF THE COMPANY RELATING TO THE SUBJECT MATTER OF THIS AGREEMENT. If you are a U.S. Government user, this Software is licensed with "restricted rights" as set forth in subparagraphs (a)-(d) of the Commercial Computer-Restricted Rights clause at FAR 52.227-19 or in subparagraphs (c)(1)(ii) of the Rights in Technical Data and Computer Software clause at DFARS 252.227-7013, and similar clauses, as applicable.

Should you have any questions concerning this agreement or if you wish to contact the Company for any reason, please contact in writing: Prentice-Hall, New Media Department, One Lake Street, Upper Saddle River, NJ 07458.